Physiother
Respiratory and
Cardiac Care

an evidence-based approach

Alexandra Hough

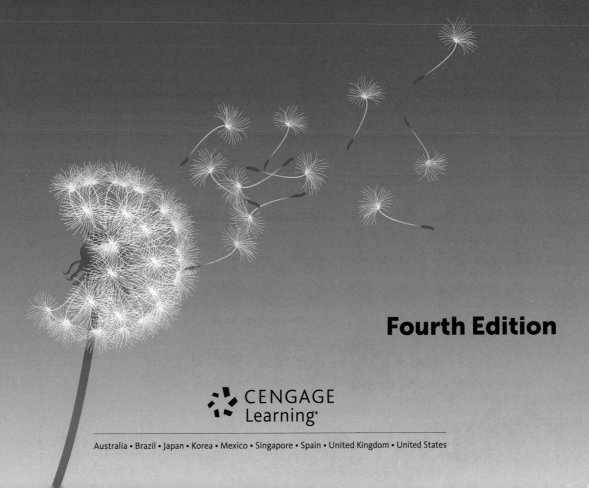

Fourth Edition

CENGAGE
Learning

Australia • Brazil • Japan • Korea • Mexico • Singapore • Spain • United Kingdom • United States

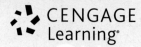
CENGAGE
Learning®

Physiotherapy in Respiratory and Cardiac Care, 4th edition

Alexandra Hough

Publisher: Andrew Ashwin

Commissioning Editor: Annabel Ainscow

Senior Production Editor: Alison Burt

Senior Manufacturing Buyer: Eyvett Davis

Typesetter: Cenveo Publisher Services

Cover design: Adam Renvoize

For product information and technology assistance, contact **emea.info@cengage.com**.

For permission to use material from this text or product, and for permission queries, email **emea.permissions@cengage.com**.

British Library Cataloguing-in-Publication Data
A catalogue record for this book is available from the British Library.

ISBN: 978-1-4080-7482-4

Cengage Learning EMEA
Cheriton House, North Way, Andover, Hampshire, SP10 5BE United Kingdom

Cengage Learning products are represented in Canada by Nelson Education Ltd.

For your lifelong learning solutions, visit **www.cengage.co.uk**

Purchase your next print book, e-book or e-chapter at **www.cengagebrain.com**

Printed in Singapore by Seng Lee Press
1 2 3 4 5 6 7 8 9 10 – 16 15 14

BRIEF CONTENTS

CONTENTS

PART I PHYSIOLOGY AND PATHOLOGY

1 Physiological basis of clinical practice

2 Assessment

3 Respiratory disorders

11   Physiotherapy for children

12   Physiotherapy for people with cardiovascular disorders

13   Physiotherapy for people with hyperventilation syndrome

14   Physiotherapy for elderly people with cardiorespiratory disease

15   Palliative respiratory physiotherapy

16   Physiotherapy for people undergoing surgery

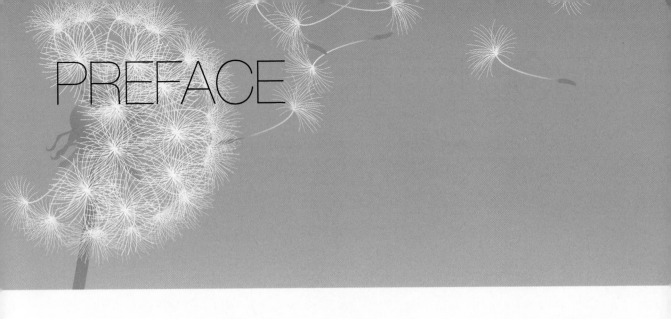

PREFACE

Good facts make good ethics.

Ashwal (2013)

Cardiorespiratory care is an immensely satisfying branch of physiotherapy. It challenges our intellect, exploits our handling skills and employs our humanity to the full.

The specialty is both art and science, but not an exact science. Effectiveness depends on problem-solving, which requires evidence-based information and a clear perspective of patients' needs. Clinicians, students and educationists expect integration of theory and practice, explanations that are referenced and physiologically sound, and exact detail of technique. This book is written for such readers and for those who question traditional assumptions.

Critical thinking is facilitated with clinical reasoning boxes in the text, and problem-solving is aided by case studies at the end of each chapter. Problems and diseases have comprehensive lists of validated outcome measures. Clarity is assisted by Glossary terms highlighted throughout.

The fourth edition includes online case studies, X-rays and patient handouts, which can be downloaded and personalized, Qs and As, extensive links for clinicians and patients, expanded tables to develop subjects such as medication, exercises and protocols, and extended Recommended Reading lists.

The book is suitable for physiotherapists from student level to accomplished practitioner because problem-solving requires thinking rather than experience. It would also suit domiciliary physiotherapists, for whom there is greater emphasis in this edition to reflect the trend in home management, and specialist respiratory nurses. The clinician will find here the opportunity to achieve clarity of thought and develop mastery in respiratory care.

ABOUT THE AUTHOR

Alexandra Hough is a clinician and lecturer. She has taught in the Bahamas, Canada, Chile, Denmark, Gibraltar, Greece, Ireland, Israel, Malta, Oman, Portugal, Singapore, South Africa and around the UK. When not teaching, she works clinically with respiratory patients in Eastbourne. She has also worked with torture survivors, who develop hyperventilation syndrome, and her royalties go to the charity Reprieve.

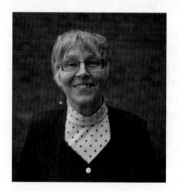

About the contributors

Alison Draper worked as a clinician in Birmingham and then Liverpool for ten years and became a lecturer in the School of Health Sciences, Liverpool University after completing her Masters degree.

Paul Ritson works at the Royal Liverpool Children's NHS Trust (Alder Hey), specialising in the respiratory speciality of Paediatric Intensive Care and lectures on the Mersey Region On Call Course for newly qualified Physiotherapists and delivers the Paediatric respiratory module at the University of Liverpool and the University of Salford.

Jo Sharp specialised in cardiorespiratory physiotherapy as a clinician and is a lecturer in the School of Health Sciences, Liverpool University.

ACKNOWLEDGEMENTS

Profound thanks to the patients who have taught me much over the years. I am also indebted to Paula Agostini for her clinical expertise, Veronica Bastow for her wisdom, Anne Canby for her invaluable neurological input, Charles Deakin for the depth of his critical care knowledge, Peter Dick for his helpful feedback on the imaging section, Kiran Katikaneni for his thoughtful understanding of the elderly population, Nikki Petty for her acumen, Jenny Taylor for her deep knowledge of palliative care, and Carol Usher my editor for her patience.

The publishers would like to thank Fiona Roberts, Janis Harvey, Una Jones, Caroline Belchamber, Elaine Dhouieb, Billie Hurst, Anna Murphy and Melanie Reardon, for their insightful review comments on the manuscript.

Dedicated to Marian.

DIGITAL SUPPORT RESOURCES

Dedicated Instructor Resources

To discover the dedicated instructor online
support resources accompanying this textbook,
instructors should register here for access:
http://login.cengage.com

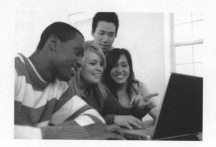

Resources include:

- Teaching Notes
- PowerPoint slides

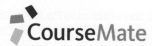

Instructor access

Instructors can access CourseMate by registering at
http://login.cengage.com or by speaking to their local
Cengage Learning EMEA representative.

Instructor resources

Instructors can use the integrated Engagement Tracker in CourseMate to track students'
preparation and engagement. The tracking tool can be used to monitor progress of the class as
a whole, or for individual students.

Student access

Log In & Learn In 4 Easy Steps

1. To register a product using the access code printed on the inside front-cover of the book
   please go to: **http://login.cengagebrain.com**
2. Register as a new user or log in as an existing user if you already have an account with
   Cengage Learning or CengageBrain.com
3. Follow the online prompts
4. If your instructor has provided you with a course key, you will be prompted to enter this after
   opening your digital purchase from your CengageBrain account homepage.

Student resources

CourseMate offers a range of interactive learning tools tailored to the fourth edition of
Physiotherapy in Respiratory and Cardiac Care, including:

- Self-test multiple choice questions
- Interactive eBook
- Critical Thinking Questions
- Appendices
- References
- Flashcards

COURSEMATE FEATURES BY CHAPTER

ONLINE FEATURE	CHAPTERS IT APPLIES TO
Multiple Choice Questions	Provided for all 20 chapters
Critical Thinking Questions	Provided for all 20 chapters
Ch 1	App C • Acid-base interpretation • Relation between P_aCO_2 and pH • Shunt fractions and biochemistry values
Ch 2	App C • Symptom scoring tools • Sputum induction
Ch 3	App B • What is COPD? • What is bronchiectasis? App C • Features of severity of acute asthma • Asthma drug guidelines • Prevention of aspiration during feeding
Ch 5	App B • How to manage your oxygen • How to use your inhaler • How to use your spacer
Ch 6	App B • How to use your incentive spirometer
Ch 7	App B • Breathlessness and exercise • Yoga breathing • How to relax • How to breathe efficiently • Keeping your legs strong

ONLINE FEATURE	CHAPTERS IT APPLIES TO
Ch 8	App B • Using your PEP tube, Acapella, Flutter, BreatheMAX • Controlling your cough • Pelvic floor exercises
Ch 9	App B • Exercise instructions and exercise diary • Inspiratory muscle training instructions and diary • Sex when you are breathless • Your future App C • Assessment for rehabilitation • Welcome booklet • Topics for education and discussion
Ch 12	App C • Stratification of risk for cardiac events • Exercise prescription for people with heart failure • Phase 1 cardiac exercise prescription • Exercise record
Ch 13	App B • What is hyperventilation syndrome? • How to control panic attacks
Ch 16	App B • Exercises after breast surgery App C • Preoperative education
Ch 17	
Ch 18	App B • ICU chart • Clinical decision making tool • On call criteria
Ch 20	App C • Cardiorespiratory standards, criteria and measurement • Competencies for cardiorespiratory physiotherapy • Referral criteria for nursing and medical staff • On call record • Cardiorespiratory team information
References	Relevant to all chapters
Recommended reading	Provided for all chapters
Glossary	Relevant to all chapters
Flashcards	Provided for all chapters
eBook	Provided for all chapters
Appendices	Appendix A – guidelines and links for health professionals Appendix B – handouts and links for patients Appendix C – extra tables Appendix D – links to radiology case studies Appendix E – patient experiences Appendix F – postural drainage positions Appendix G – conversions

PART I
PHYSIOLOGY
AND PATHOLOGY

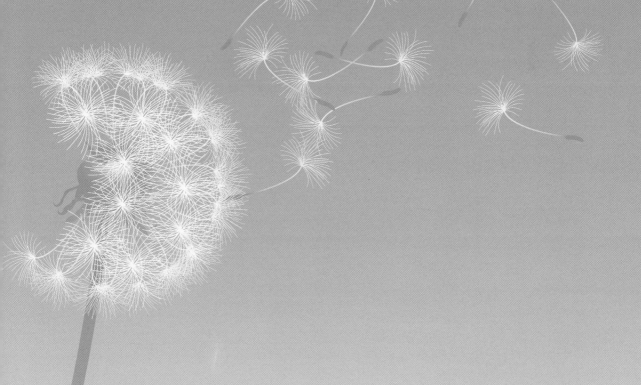

CHAPTER 1
Physiological basis of clinical practice

LEARNING OBJECTIVES

On completion of this chapter the reader should be able to:

- understand how the respiratory system defends the body against the elements

- recognize how the control of respiration adapts to different situations

- understand the mechanics of breathing and its relation to the work of breathing

- use clinical reasoning to relate ventilation and perfusion to clinical practice

- interpret arterial blood gases and apply them to a problem-based approach to treatment

- understand how the respiratory and cardiovascular systems contribute to oxygen delivery and its relationship to oxygen consumption

- recognize how the cardiorespiratory system responds to a variety of individual circumstances.

INTRODUCTION

Breathing is a forbidden fruit on the tree of knowledge.

Gilbert 1999a

Breathing is unique. Most of us give it little thought, yet it can be voluntary or automatic and is preserved in unconsciousness. It is associated with a respiratory system of remarkable ingenuity, being responsible for gas being pumped into the lungs, diffused into the circulation, transported around the body and passed into cells. It is also involved in speaking and laughing, balancing pH and controlling metabolism.

An understanding of how this system works creates the foundation for evidence-based practice. This chapter covers not just the textbook lungs of hefty young healthy males but also those of people who may smoke or be stressed or overweight.

Cardiovascular physiology is in Chapter 4, and the 'oxygen cascade' section in this chapter brings the workings of the respiratory and cardiovascular systems together.

DEFENCE

> *Imagine wearing your insides on the outside.*
> British Lung Foundation

The lung is an 'outdoor' organ that has to interact with the environment while facilitating ventilation, and is the body's primary route of infection (Waterer 2012). Every day, up to 480 million alveoli in the adult lungs (Nyengaard 2004) allow a surface area the size of a tennis court to be exposed to a volume of air and pollutants that could fill a swimming pool (Hanley & Tyler 1987). It is only by means of a sophisticated biological barrier that the body does not succumb to this onslaught.

Defence against the outside world is based on a network of filters, reflexes, secretions and specialized cells. Physiotherapists treat patients whose defences are breached when the nose is bypassed by mouth-breathing or an artificial airway, cilia are damaged by smoking or disease, and cough is inhibited by pain or weakness.

Nose

The nasal passages are the gatekeeper of the respiratory tract, providing the first line of defence by means of:

- sensing suspicious smells
- sneezing in response to irritating substances
- filtering large particles
- insulating against swings in temperature and humidity.

Mouth

The oral cavity, from the lips to the junction of the hard and soft palates, is home to over 700 species of microbe which contribute to the immune system (Gupta 2011). They are harmful only if they reach sites to which they do not normally have access: most hospital-acquired pneumonias are caused by endotracheal tubes or nebulizers (Guggenbichler *et al* 2011).

Pharynx

The pathways for air and food converge in the pharynx. When a person chews, breathing continues through the nose, but during swallowing the pharynx can only deal with food and the airway is closed off.

The **nasopharynx** exposes inspired and expired gas to a large surface area of highly vascular, moist mucous membrane (Fig 1.1). This nasal mucosa delivers warmth and humidity to the inspiratory breath and recovers a third of it on the expiratory breath (Richards *et al* 1996).

The **oropharynx** extends from the oral cavity to the tonsils. The tonsils are lymphoid tissue which defend against foreign pathogens. Surgical removal of tonsils and adenoids renders children more vulnerable to passive smoking (Chen *et al* 1998).

The **hypopharynx** is responsible for the tricky process of swallowing, in which 56 muscles are required to ensure airway protection while giving food the right of way (Higashijima 2010).

The epiglottis is a leaf-like lid which snaps shut over the larynx during swallowing to prevent aspiration into the trachea. The functions of the larynx are primarily to elevate during swallowing in order to protect the airway, secondarily to stabilize the transition between inhalation and exhalation (p. 8), and only as an afterthought to provide speech.

Cortical, subcortical and brainstem neural control centres help co-ordinate breathing and swallowing while ensuring that this is followed by exhalation, which further helps to prevent aspiration. This tight respiratory–swallowing coupling is compromised by hypercapnia (Nishino 2012) and neurological impairment.

Airways

Inhaled irritant particles increase bronchoconstrictor tone in order to narrow the airways. This is protective in normal airways but becomes exaggerated in asthma, when it is called bronchospasm.

FIGURE 1.1 The humidifying effects of nose breathing on inspiration (left) and expiration.

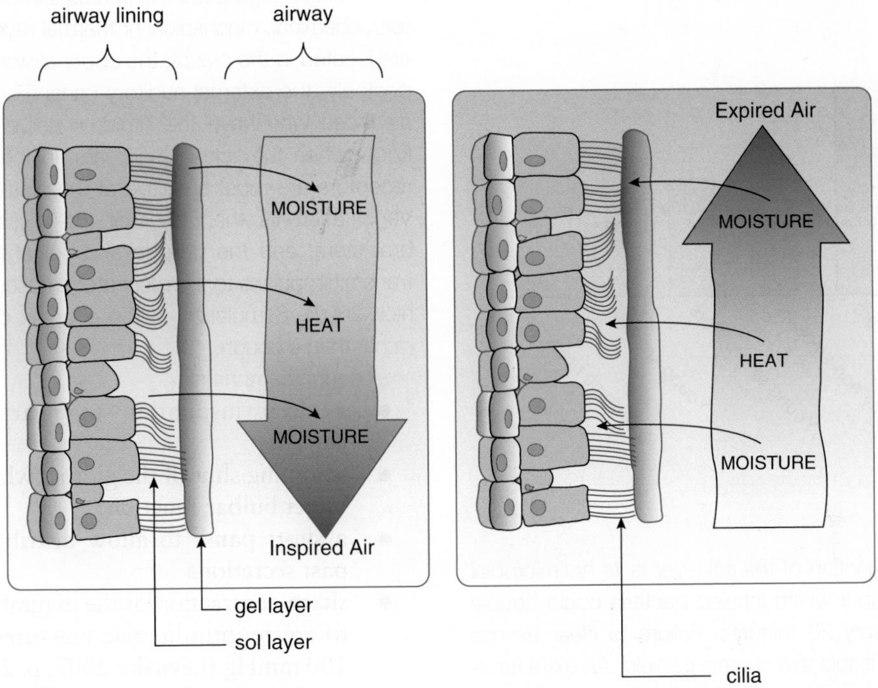

Other particles are trapped on a layer of sticky mucus lining the airways from the nasopharynx to the terminal bronchi. This mucous blanket is gripped from underneath by tiny hooks on the tips of hair-like cilia attached to the epithelium. These move the mucus up to the throat, from where it is swallowed or expectorated. This 'mucociliary escalator' can cleanse the lungs in 20 minutes, moving particles at an average 1–2 cm/min, most rapidly in the trachea and decreasing with each airway generation as the total cross section widens (Morris & Afifi 2010, p. 163).

The cilia beat in a 'sol' layer of watery fluid, reaching up to penetrate the 'gel' layer of mucus, hooking onto it with the onward stroke and diving beneath it into the sol layer on the recovery stroke at 20 beats a second (Fig 1.1). Balanced systemic hydration keeps the fluid in the sol layer the same height as the cilia. If the sol layer is too deep, or the cilia shortened by smoking (Leopold 2013), the hooks cannot reach the mucus. If it is too shallow, as in cystic fibrosis (CF), mucus clogs the delicate cilia. Systemic hydration is also relevant to the gel layer because water constitutes 95% of respiratory mucus and helps maintain mucociliary clearance (Nakagawa et al 2004).

Other protective functions of the mucus are insulation, antibacterial action and preventing the patient from drying out (Button & Boucher 2008). Moisture in inspired air maintains optimum ciliary beat frequency and acts as a buffer against extremes of temperature because water requires four times more energy to change temperature than air (Williams et al 1996).

This finely co-ordinated mechanism is compromised by smoking, disease, age (Fig 1.2), immobility, hypoxia, inflammation, dehydration and prolonged coughing which narrows the airways (Wanner et al 1996).

KEY POINT

Optimizing systemic hydration should be the first intervention for people with sputum retention.

FIGURE 1.2 Mucous velocity with different ages and conditions.

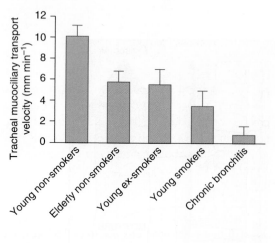

An extra function of the sol layer is its antimicrobial property, without which inhaled bacteria could double in number every 20 minutes. Failure to clear excess mucus may disable this chemical shield. An extra function of the gel layer is to engulf particles as well as carry them along on its surface (Knowles & Boucher 2002).

Airway epithelial cells contain pattern recognition receptors which warn downstream immune cells of approaching bacteria, and some interesting taste bud cells have relocated to the airway and respond to noxious particles by stimulating the cilia (Kinnamon 2011).

Cough

> *A cough is only as effective as the deep breath preceding it.*
>
> Sobush (2008)

The cough is the body's strongest physiological reflex and has been known to fracture brittle ribs, cause pneumothorax (Khajotia 2012) and in extremis rupture the diaphragm (Reper *et al* 2012). Its protective function is to expel secretions and debris when mucociliary clearance is damaged, as in bronchiectasis, or overwhelmed, as with some chest infections. Like swallowing and

belching, it is subject to higher cortical control, either as cough inhibition or voluntary cough.

A reflex cough occurs if irritants stimulate inflammatory, chemical, mechanical or thermal receptors. These are located in the pleura, the upper airways and, unexpectedly, the external auditory canal (Polverino 2012), as those who have the Arnold's nerve cough reflex know when they clean their ears. In the airways, the receptors are most sensitive at the glottis and carina. Vagal afferents then transmit the messages to the brainstem, and the phrenic and spinal motor nerves transmit impulses to the respiratory musculature (Homnick 2007). Stimulation of the pharynx causes a gag rather than a cough.

A cough comprises:
- a deep inspiration to near total lung capacity
- snapping shut of the glottis (which requires intact bulbar function)
- a short pause to allow distribution of air past secretions
- sharp contraction of the expiratory muscles to create intrathoracic pressures of at least 100 mmHg (Levitzky 2007, p. 219)
- sudden opening of the epiglottis, exploding the trapped gas outwards at up to 800 km/hr (Polverino 2012).

The resulting shear force overcomes viscous, frictional and gravitational resistance so that secretions are cleared from the upper airway and deeper secretions are squeezed from the lower airway (Pitts *et al* 2013).

Coughing is accompanied by violent swings in intrapleural pressure, which cause dynamic airway compression (p. 9). This is initiated in the trachea during the cough and extends peripherally as lung volume decreases, ensuring that the full length of the tracheobronchial tree is involved. The airways normally re-open with a subsequent deep breath, but for people unable to take a deep breath, they stay closed for lengthy periods. Coughing is inhibited by postoperative pain, and the mechanism is less efficient in some people with obstructive airways disease if they have poor expiratory flow or airways that collapse on expiration. It is weakened with neurological disease or if the glottis is bypassed by intubation or tracheostomy.

Complications of coughing include bronchospasm, exhaustion and stress incontinence. Despite high pressures, barotrauma is usually avoided by the support of the ribcage and by contraction of intercostal and abdominal muscles which buttress the chest wall and prevent overdistension of alveoli.

Other lung defences

Pollutants which manage to reach the alveolar secretions are met with scavenger macrophages and proteolytic enzymes which would be powerful enough to destroy the alveoli themselves except for the presence of an inhibitor secreted by the liver called alpha$_1$-antitrypsin (AAT), a deficiency of which causes AAT deficiency (Ch. 3) and predisposes to HIV (Ferreira 2014). Pathogens which survive this still have to resist a barrage of inflammation (Eisele & Anderson 2011). Asbestos particles circumvent all these defences because of their peculiar shape.

The function of the wafer-thin alveolar-capillary membrane is to allow efficient gas exchange, but this also allows carbon monoxide and chemical warfare to cause their mischief.

The entire blood volume passes through the lungs, which help detoxify foreign substances that have made it into the circulation. The pulmonary circulation also performs a range of metabolic functions and acts as a filter to help protect the systemic arterial system, particularly the coronary and cerebral circulations, from blood clots, fat cells, detached cancer cells, gas bubbles and other debris. Extracorporeal support systems such as cardiopulmonary bypass (Ch. 16) include a filter to perform some of these functions.

CONTROL

Breathing is the basic rhythm of life.
Hippocrates

Breathing is normally controlled with such exquisite sensitivity that pH in the blood is maintained within precise limits despite unpredictable metabolic demands. Carbon dioxide (CO_2) and oxygen are also controlled, but less tightly.

Clusters of neurons in the pons and medulla receive and integrate stimuli from the ribcage, lungs, chemoreceptors and cortex. They then discharge impulses to the respiratory muscles, triggering contraction.

The respiratory centres also perceive and respond to posture, coughing, hiccupping, defaecating, stepping into a cold shower and the lactic acid produced by intense exercise (de Souza 2010). Respiratory control occurs at a subconscious level but can be overridden by breathing exercises and modified by emotion, pain and some pathological states. Chronic obstructive pulmonary disease (COPD) for example, shows less precise control over breathing during sleep and exercise (Dempsey 2002), and some COPD patients have an altered chemoreceptor response, becoming dependent on low oxygen (hypoxic respiratory drive) rather than high CO_2 (hypercapnic respiratory drive) as a stimulus to breathe.

Yawning is controlled by the hypothalamus and is thought to relate to thermoregulation of the brain. The open mouth promotes pharyngeal cooling and the deep inspiration increases flow down the internal jugular vein. Boredom and the evening are associated with higher brain temperature. Contagious yawning appears to have evolved in order to coordinate arousal and vigilance in budgerigars and some mammals (Gallup & Eldakar 2012).

MECHANICS

When you can't breathe, nothing else matters.
Patient

The respiratory muscles

The lungs hang from whichever part of the chest wall is uppermost at the time and are attached to each other medially by their roots, but do not directly touch any muscle. The chest wall comprises the thoraco-abdominal wall and diaphragm, which are expandable. The diaphragm contracts downwards against the abdominal contents, which are themselves incompressible (but push out the abdominal wall), and the pelvic bowl which is rigid. The respiratory muscles extend from the mastoid process to the pubic symphysis and are the only skeletal muscles vital to life, providing the power for the respiratory pump and delivering oxygen to the distal airways while removing CO_2.

Inspiration

The diaphragm, the seat of the soul according to the ancient Greeks, is a dome-shaped sheet of muscle on which the upright lungs rest, separated by the pleura. It is innervated from C3–5 via the phrenic nerves and generates 70% of tidal volume. Attached to the bottom of the ribcage, it separates two compartments of markedly different densities, the thorax and abdomen (Mangera et al 2012).

At rest, or if paralyzed, the diaphragm extends upwards almost to nipple level (see Fig 19.8). Contraction flattens it, pressing down against the fulcrum of the abdominal contents, displacing the abdominal viscera by 5–7 cm, protruding the abdominal wall (unless prevented voluntarily or by tight clothing) and when the limit of abdominal wall compliance is reached, levering the lower ribcage upwards and outwards in a bucket handle action, causing expansion of the lower chest. This displacement downwards and outwards creates negative intrathoracic pressure, which sucks air into the lungs.

Muscles assisting this process are:

- the external intercostals which stabilize the chest wall so that diaphragmatic contraction can create these pressure changes
- the scalenes which stabilize the upper ribcage to prevent it being pulled downwards
- pharyngeal muscles which prevent collapse of the upper airway from the negative pressure.

These and other accessory muscles become major inspiratory muscles when there is increased work of breathing (WOB) such as with airflow obstruction or exercise.

During upper limb activity, intercostal and accessory muscles are obliged to stabilize the torso, forcing the diaphragm to take a greater load. People with COPD may find daily activities daunting because of the sustained arm movement required, especially in standing when the diaphragm also contributes to postural stability.

The diaphragm's role in core stability is controlling intra-abdominal pressure and reducing the stress on the spine through co-operative action with the abdominal and pelvic floor muscles (Noh et al 2014).

The postural functions of the respiratory muscles have led to links between increased WOB and impaired balance (David et al 2012) and between diaphragm fatigue and recurrent back pain (Janssens et al 2013).

Expiration

The transition between inhalation and exhalation is smoothed by a brake on expiratory flow caused by airflow resistance, especially at the larynx, and by continued low-grade diaphragmatic activity. When the larynx is bypassed by intubation, positive end-expiratory pressure (PEEP) is applied to the airway to support this function, thus avoiding fatigue of the diaphragm during exhalation. This function of the larynx is called 'physiological PEEP'.

Normal exhalation is largely passive, lung elastic recoil providing the driving force. This recoil is created first by surface tension acting throughout the vast gas/liquid interface lining the alveoli, and second by elasticity of the lung tissue which has been stretched during inspiration. Elastic recoil is reduced at low lung volumes, like a slack elastic band, and in emphysema because of damaged alveolar septa.

Active expiration becomes stronger with speech, exercise, coughing, sneezing, giving birth and obstructive airways disease. Abdominal, internal intercostal and pelvic floor muscles may then be recruited to augment passive recoil. Latissimus dorsi is enlisted during singing, and in COPD during forced exhalation, which may explain the benefit found by some patients on joining a choir (Watson et al 2012).

Speech is created when the expiratory column of air is interrupted by vibrating vocal cords, which break it into sound waves. The sound is then modified by the oropharynx, nasopharynx and oral cavity. A person with COPD may have a weak voice because of inability to generate sufficient expiratory pressure, and a person with neurological disease may have poor articulation because of weakness of the oropharyngeal musculature.

Respiratory muscle dysfunction can occur with COPD, thoracic deformity, critical illness or neurological disease (Gea 2012).

PRACTICE TIP

Drop your pen and then pick it up. Did you hold your breath? This illustrates the postural work of the diaphragm.

Pressures

Alveolar pressure: pressure inside the lung.
Pleural (intrapleural/intrathoracic) pressure: pressure in the pleural space.

Pressure equivalents
- $1 \text{ mmHg} = 1.36 \text{ cmH}_2\text{O}$
- $1 \text{ kPa} = 7.5 \text{ mmHg}$
- $1 \text{ torr} = 1 \text{ mmHg}$.

Alveolar pressure is negative on inspiration and slightly positive on expiration. Pleural pressure needs to be constantly negative to keep the lungs open. This negative pressure is achieved by inward pull from lung elastic recoil and outward pull from ribcage recoil, which attempts to spring outwards at all but the highest volumes (Dominelli & Sheel 2012). Outward recoil is assisted by the pumping out of pleural fluid by the lymphatics, leading to a total negative pleural pressure of about −6 cmH$_2$O, modulated by the breathing pattern (Negrini 2013). Inward and outward forces are in equilibrium at the end of a quiet exhalation, this resting lung volume being termed the functional residual capacity (FRC). Outward recoil of the chest wall assists inspiration, especially from low lung volumes.

These pressures are disturbed by:
- a large pneumothorax, which neutralizes pleural pressure so that the lung's inward pull is unopposed and it shrivels inwards
- emphysema, which reduces lung elastic recoil so that the outward pull of the chest wall is less opposed and the lung hyperinflates.

Increasing expiratory pressure by more forceful expiration can only generate extra flow in the early stages because, as airways narrow and frictional resistance increases, pleural pressure will exceed airway pressure, thus counteracting expiratory effort by compressing the airways. This 'dynamic airway compression' occurs at about 40 cmH$_2$O (De Beer 2013), presaging the effort-independent portion of the flow-volume relationship (see Fig 2.33) and can make forceful coughing counterproductive for people with obstructive airways disease.

Resistance

Resistance: force that must be overcome during breathing

$$= \frac{\text{pressure change}}{\text{flow change}}$$

Airflow resistance

Resistance to airflow is caused by friction, which is created in the airways when gas slides against the walls and over itself. Airflow resistance depends on the speed of airflow and calibre of the airway.

Peripheral airflow resistance is low because at the level of the terminal bronchioles the large number of small airways creates a wide total cross-sectional area of 180 cm^2, causing laminar flow. The cross section reduces to 2.5 cm^2 in the trachea, where there is higher total resistance, creating turbulent and disorganized airflow (Fig 1.3). Figure 1.4a shows increased resistance due to airflow obstruction. Frictional resistance must also be overcome in the chest and abdomen as organs are displaced by the moving lung.

Elastic resistance

Lung tissue, alveolar surface liquid and parts of the chest wall contribute to elastic resistance, which is increased by conditions such as pulmonary oedema, lung fibrosis (Fig.1.4b), ribcage deformity, obesity or a slumped posture.

FIGURE 1.3 Increase in total cross section of the airways as they divide, creating less frictional resistance as airflow becomes more laminar and streamlined.

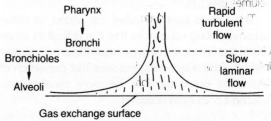

FIGURE 1.4a Both alveoli are normal, but the airway supplying alveolus B shows airflow obstruction, which is causing frictional resistance to airflow.

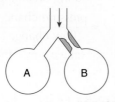

FIGURE 1.4b Both airways are normal, but alveolus B shows reduced compliance caused by a thickened alveolar-capillary membrane or raised surface tension, which increases elastic resistance.

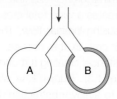

Compliance

$$\text{Compliance} = \frac{\text{volume change}}{\text{pressure change}}$$

Compliance describes the willingness of the lungs to distend, and elastance the willingness to return to their resting position. Compliance is represented by the relationship between volume and pressure, i.e. how much pressure (work of breathing) is required to expand the lung. This relationship is curved rather than linear due to a variation in the effort to breathe at different lung volumes (Fig 1.5).

The lung is least compliant, i.e. stiffest, at either extreme of lung volume, so that it is difficult to inflate alveoli that are closed or hyperinflate those that are fully inflated. Clinical reasoning indicates that prevention of atelectasis would therefore be more sensible than treating it once it has occurred.

FIGURE 1.5 Pressure-volume (compliance) curve indicating reduced compliance at either extreme of lung volume. The symbols represent alveolar size at different volumes. V: lung volume; P: pressure, i.e. work to expand the lung.

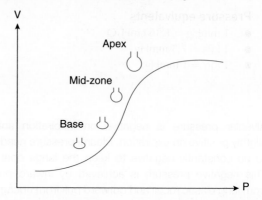

> ### PRACTICE TIP
>
> Blow up a balloon and feel your work of breathing at low, mid and high volumes.

Compliance is lower on inspiration, i.e. it is harder to breathe in than out, due mostly to alveolar fluid surface tension. This process is known as hysteresis and is demonstrated by the pressure-volume loop (Fig 1.6).

Alveoli are vulnerable to injury at excessively high or low volume, and mechanical ventilation (MV) aims to avoid either extreme, especially in patients with damaged lungs as with acute respiratory distress syndrome.

The contribution of airways to compliance relates to their calibre, resistance being increased and compliance decreased if airways are narrowed by bronchospasm, oedema, the collapsing airways of emphysema, and sometimes secretions in the large airways where there is greater overall resistance and less collateral ventilation.

The surface tension of alveolar fluid is partially counteracted by surfactant, a constituent in the fluid that acts like detergent, preventing the alveolar walls sticking together. Small alveoli are, therefore, less likely to collapse and empty their contents into large alveoli.

FIGURE 1.6 Pressure-volume loop showing how expiration requires less effort, i.e. less pressure for the same change in volume, than inspiration.

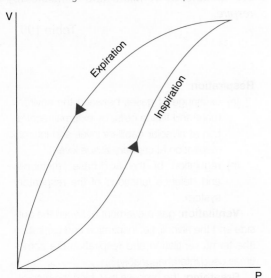

PRACTICE TIP

Pour some water into a plastic bag, empty the excess and then pull the bag open. The forces of surface tension are what makes this difficult. Repeat with a few drops of washing-up liquid.

The contribution of extra-pulmonary structures to compliance relates to the ease with which the chest wall can be pushed away on inspiration. Kyphoscoliosis or a distended abdomen reduce compliance.

Static compliance is measured during a breath-hold so that equilibrium is achieved between alveolar pressure and mouth pressure, alveoli being filled to a volume determined by their regional compliance. **Dynamic compliance** is measured during breathing. It normally approximates static compliance, but may be less in diseased lungs if regional variations in compliance and resistance mean that alveolar filling is not completed during inspiration.

Work of breathing (WOB)

Work is done during inspiration to overcome the resistive and elastic forces of airways, lungs and chest wall. This work can be defined in two ways:

- the pressure required to move a volume of gas, i.e.:
  transpulmonary pressure × tidal volume
- oxygen consumed by the respiratory muscles, i.e. the oxygen cost of breathing.

Elastic resistance contributes 80% of the WOB and airflow resistance the remaining 20% (Levitzky 2007 p. 32). Relative contributions to airflow resistance are:

- nasal passages: 50%
- larynx: 25%
- trachea to 8th generation: 20%
- peripheral airways: 5% (Eriksson 1996).

Normally, breathing is surprisingly efficient, helped by fluid coating the moving surfaces of the pleura, assuring a tight lung–chest wall coupling and allowing lung volume to faithfully follow changes in chest wall volume during the respiratory cycle (Negrini 2013). The pleural cavity, however, does not appear to be essential: people who have had a pleurectomy, and elephants (West 2001), have no functioning pleura but are able to breathe quite happily. However, it is handy for thoracic surgeons who would have difficulty if the lung was attached directly to the chest wall.

A change in alveolar pressure of only 1 cmH$_2$O is usually enough for airflow (Negrini 2013) and WOB uses just 2–5% of total oxygen consumption at rest, but this may be increased to 40% in people with obstructive airways disease (Cairo 2012, p. 194).

Deep breathing increases the work performed against elastic resistance, while rapid breathing increases the work against airways resistance. Most patients find the right balance, but some need breathing re-education to find the optimal breathing pattern to minimize their WOB.

Inspiratory muscle fatigue

Fatigue is loss of the capacity to develop force in response to a load. When acute, it is reversible by rest.

Fatigue is usually associated with a more abrupt decrease in respiratory muscle strength than weakness. It can be due to failure of any of the links in the chain of command from brain to muscle. Failure within the central nervous system is called central fatigue, and failure at the neuromuscular junction or in the muscle is called peripheral fatigue.

The diaphragm differs from other skeletal muscles in that it has to provide a lifetime of sustained action against elastic and resistive loads rather than irregular action against inertial loads. It is equipped for this by its comparative resistance to fatigue (Polla *et al* 2004) and the unusual way in which perfusion increases during contraction (Anzueto 1992).

Fatigue occurs if energy demand exceeds supply, as when WOB is increased by airflow obstruction, or when the ability of the respiratory muscles to contract efficiently is impaired by hyperinflation, scoliosis or a flail chest.

Fatigue serves a protective function to avoid depletion of enzymes. Procedures that force patients to overuse fatigued muscles can cause muscle damage (Kallet 2011), which is most likely to occur when weaning patients from MV.

Inspiratory muscle weakness

Weakness is failure to generate sufficient force in an otherwise fresh muscle. It is not reversible by rest, but is treated by addressing the cause and encouraging activity. Causes in the respiratory muscles include:

- neuromuscular disorder
- disuse atrophy
- malnutrition
- hypoxia, hypercapnia or acidosis
- low calcium, potassium or phosphate levels
- steroids
- inflammation, as occurs with COPD, sepsis or multisystem failure.

Weakness predisposes a muscle to fatigue. Fatigue differs from weakness in that a normal muscle can become fatigued if faced with excess WOB. Fatigue and weakness often coexist, especially in respiratory failure or during weaning from MV. The clinical features of fatigue and weakness are similar (Ch. 2). Both are experienced as breathlessness.

VENTILATION

We breathe to ventilate and ventilate to respire.

Tobin 1991

Respiration:

(a) exchange of gases between the environment and tissue cells, by external respiration at alveolar-capillary level, and internal respiration at capillary-tissue level

(b) regulation of the acid-base, metabolic and defence functions of the respiratory system.

Ventilation: gas movement between the outside and the alveoli, i.e. inspiration and expiration (the terms ventilation and respiration are sometimes used interchangeably).

Breathing: the process by which the respiratory pump creates ventilation.

Minute ventilation or minute volume ($\dot{V}_E$): amount of gas breathed per minute, i.e.:

Tidal volume × respiratory rate

Tidal volume (V_T): volume of air inhaled and exhaled at each breath.

Alveolar ventilation:

(tidal volume – physiologic dead space) × respiratory rate

A healthy spontaneously breathing adult maintains an approximate $\dot{V}_E$ of 5–9 litres, moving a V_T of 450–600 ml with a respiratory rate of 10–15 breaths per minute.

Gas that moves in and out of the lungs is made up of:

- alveolar ventilation, which is the fresh air that gets into alveoli and participates in gas exchange, defined above
- dead space ventilation (V_D), which does not contribute to gas exchange.

Most dead space is made up of **anatomical** V_D (Fig 1.7) which is air in the conducting passages that does not reach the alveoli, i.e. that which is last in and first out. It comprises one-third of V_T in a human, more in a giraffe. **Alveolar** V_D, representing air that reaches

FIGURE 1.7 Average volumes and flows of gas and blood in the lungs. *Frequency* = average breaths per minute

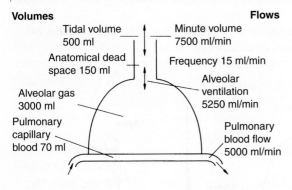

the alveoli but does not get into the blood, is minimal in normal lungs. The sum of anatomical and alveolar V_D is called **physiological** V_D. The presence of V_D is one reason why it is more efficient to increase $\dot{V}_E$ by breathing deeper than by breathing faster. Dead space is most usefully expressed in relation to tidal volume (V_D/V_T) and is normally 30% of V_T (Gott & Dolling 2013).

Ventilation is not distributed evenly within the lungs (Fig 1.8). In most healthy young adults, dependent regions are better ventilated for two reasons:

1   In the upright position, alveoli in upper regions are more inflated, but mostly with V_D gas. Gas travels more easily at first to the open spaces of these non-dependent regions, but they are rapidly filled and gas then travels to the dependent regions below. Alveoli in dependent regions are partially compressed by the weight of the lungs, heavy with blood above and around them. They therefore have more potential to expand, i.e. they are more compliant, allowing greater ventilation with fresh gas. This reasoning carries through to whatever position a young adult is in. If the alveoli are collapsed or heavily compressed, e.g. if the patient is slumped in a chair, elderly, or obese, they will be lower on the compliance curve (Fig 1.5) and less easy to inflate.

2   In the horizontal position, dependent fibres of the diaphragm contract from a

position of mechanical advantage because they are more stretched. Side-lying augments this because the shape of the chest creates a greater vertical distance. Although fresh gas in the lower lung provides a greater contribution to gas exchange, the upper lung is more expanded and therefore responds earlier to deep breathing exercises for increasing lung volume. For patients with atelectasis, therefore, and indeed for most clinical problems, patients are placed with the affected lung upwards (Ch. 6).

However, unlike the perfusion gradient, the ventilation gradient is only slight and responds to minor fluctuations, so that:

- it is reversed in elderly people (Lowe 2005), who have a higher closing volume (Fig 1.9), (and most patients are elderly)
- it is reversed in obese people (Pedoto 2012), those on some modes of MV, those who spend time in slumped positions without taking deep breaths, and sometimes in children
- in prone, pressure from the abdominal contents obliterates the gradient so that the lungs are uniformly inflated (Marcucci 2001).

PRACTICE TIP

Auscultate (Ch. 2) colleagues' lungs in standing, sitting, slumped sitting, supine, side-lying and prone.

If airways are obstructed, ventilation can continue through collateral channels. These are unimportant in normal lungs and ventilating through them is less efficient than using the main airways because airflow resistance is 50 times greater. This difference is eliminated in emphysema, when collateral ventilation promotes more homogeneous ventilation (Cetti *et al* 2006).

Normal breathing creates a V_T of one-tenth the vital capacity, but oscillations in V_T and involuntary sighs every 5–10 minutes help prevent alveolar collapse. Patients who are drowsy or sedated lose this mechanism.

FIGURE 1.8 Effect of gravity on the distribution of ventilation and perfusion (left), with position of alveoli on compliance curves (right).   V: lung volume, P: pressure required to expand lung.

(a) Upright lungs in a healthy young non-obese person, showing slight downward ventilation gradient and strong downward perfusion gradient.

(b) In supine, pressure from the abdominal contents stretches the dependent portion of the diaphragm, compressing dependent alveoli but facilitating more efficient diaphragm contraction.

(c) Side-lying shows greater volume change in the dependent lung due to pressure from the abdominal contents stretching this side of the diaphragm.

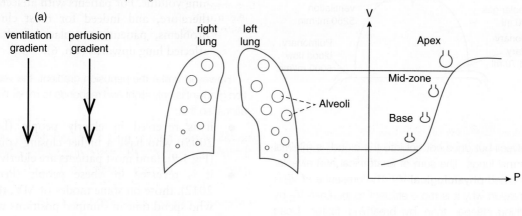

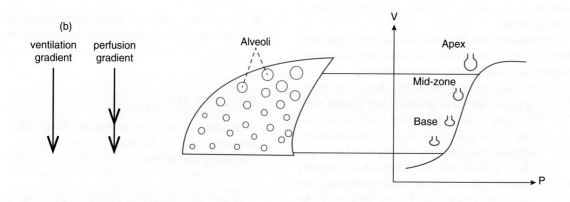

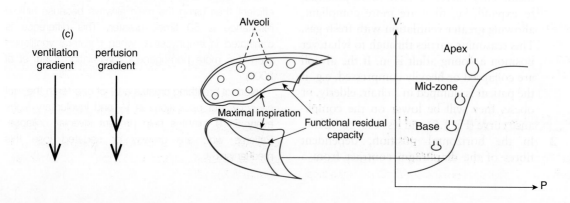

FIGURE 1.9 Factors that shift tidal breathing into the closing volume range, leading to airway closure in the lung bases during quiet breathing. V_T: tidal volume

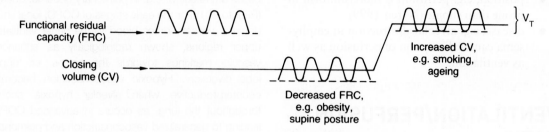

DIFFUSION

The wide total cross section of the peripheral airways means that airflow here essentially ceases, and gas movement from the respiratory bronchioles to alveoli continues by gaseous diffusion. In the alveoli, oxygen dissolves in alveolar fluid and is then driven across the alveolar-capillary membrane by the partial pressure difference, with CO_2 coming the other way.

The alveolar-capillary membrane is 50 times thinner than airmail paper (Weibel 2013), comprising two sheets of endothelium held together by wisps of connective tissue support. It is semipermeable, preventing plasma proteins and water leaking into alveoli but allowing gas exchange. Oxygen tension is equalized in one-third of the time that the blood takes to pass each alveolus, while CO_2 diffuses 20 times more quickly (Goodman 2001).

Defective diffusion across this membrane does not play a major role in gas exchange abnormalities except sometimes during exercise (Garvey *et al* 2012) or when sepsis causes high cardiac output and shortened transit times (Townsend & Webster 2000).

Gases such as ethanol, which are more soluble than oxygen or CO_2, are able to diffuse directly from the airways into the bronchial circulation, rendering, it is claimed, some alcohol breath tests inaccurate (Hlastala *et al* 2013).

PERFUSION

The lungs have a dual circulation. The high-pressure **bronchial** circulation, from the aorta, supplies the lung tissue itself but is not essential to survival, as shown after lung transplant when the bronchial vessels are tied. However, the lungs are awash with blood from the dominant low-pressure **pulmonary** circulation, which bathes the surfaces of the alveoli in order to exchange gases. The pulmonary vasculature consists of the equivalent of 7000 km of capillaries (Denison 1996) and can act as a blood reservoir in case of need such as haemorrhage.

The pulmonary circulation can respond to changes in flow with little change in pressure, reducing resistance by dilating, recruiting closed capillaries or shifting blood to the systemic circulation.

The effect of gravity on the low pressure pulmonary circulation is to create a perfusion gradient with more blood in dependent regions (Fig 1.8). This is steeper than the ventilation gradient because of the density of blood. The perfusion gradient is represented by Zones (West 2012 p. 45):

- Zone I is in the upper non-dependent lung, where alveolar pressure exceeds pulmonary arterial pressure so that capillaries are squashed and no blood flows.
- Zone II is in the middle, where pulmonary arterial pressure exceeds alveolar pressure, which in turn exceeds venous pressure.
- Zone III is in the dependent lung, where venous pressure exceeds alveolar pressure.

Zone I in health is small or non-existent. However, if hypovolaemic shock reduces arterial pressure, or MV increases alveolar pressure, Zone I becomes significant. MV also pushes blood downwards (Ch. 17) and the pressure of this blood may lead to airway closure in Zone III.

In addition, lung perfusion is affected by:

- lung volume, the vessels being stretched in the hyperinflated state
- position, e.g. perfusion is more uniform in prone than supine (Nyren 1999)
- disease, e.g. alveolar destruction in emphysema causes disruption of perfusion as well as ventilation.

VENTILATION/PERFUSION RATIO

It is no good having a well-ventilated alveolus if it is not supplied with blood, nor a well-perfused alveolus that is not ventilated. Fresh air and blood need to be in the same place at the same time for gas exchange to occur. The matching of these two is expressed as the ratio of alveolar ventilation to perfusion ($\dot{V}_A$/QT).

A degree of $\dot{V}_A/\dot{Q}$ mismatch is normal because of dissonance between ventilation and perfusion gradients, the lung bases receiving 18 times more blood and 3.5 times more gas than the apices in the upright lung (Thomas 1997).

Pathological $\dot{V}_A/\dot{Q}$ mismatch is due to a high or low $\dot{V}_A/\dot{Q}$ ratio. A high ratio occurs when the alveoli are ventilated but perfusion is impaired so there is nowhere for the oxygen to go, causing increased dead space. A low $\dot{V}_A/\dot{Q}$ ratio occurs where lung units are perfused but not adequately ventilated, which is the condition most frequently dealt with by physiotherapists. This creates a shunt, defined as the fraction of cardiac output that is not exposed to gas exchange in the lung. A shunt over 20% limits the utility of oxygen therapy because added oxygen cannot reach the shunted blood.

The shunt (App. C) is measured by comparing arterial and mixed venous blood, expressed as a percentage of cardiac output. A small shunt is normal because part of the bronchial circulation mingles with pulmonary venous drainage.

The mixing of shunted venous blood with oxygenated blood is known as venous admixture, which is normally 5% of cardiac output (Takala 2007).

Systemic hypoxia stimulates selective vasodilation to assist perfusion of vital tissues. Pulmonary hypoxia stimulates the opposite response: if a fall in alveolar oxygen tension is detected, an ingenious mechanism called hypoxic vasoconstriction helps maintain gas exchange by constricting capillaries adjacent to these alveoli, thus limiting wasted perfusion and improving $\dot{V}_A/\dot{Q}$ match (Ariyaratnam et al 2013). When the lung bases are affected, e.g. in pulmonary oedema, obesity (Pedoto 2012) or the early stages of COPD, local shutdown of vessels forces blood to the better ventilated upper regions, shown radiologically as enhanced vascular markings towards the apices, or 'upper lobe diversion'. Hypoxic vasoconstriction becomes counterproductive when alveolar hypoxia occurs throughout the lung, as occurs in advanced COPD, leading to generalized vasoconstriction and pulmonary hypertension.

ARTERIAL BLOOD GASES

PO_2: partial pressure or tension of oxygen (in kPa or mmHg)

P_aO_2: partial pressure of oxygen in arterial blood, i.e. oxygen dissolved in plasma (normal 11–14 kPa or 82.5–105 mmHg)

S_aO_2: extent to which haemoglobin in arterial blood is saturated with oxygen, i.e. capacity of blood to transport oxygen

S_pO_2: as above, but described in terms of measurement by pulse oximetry (the distinction is rarely important and normal values are the same)

Haemoglobin (Hb): molecule in erythrocytes that binds to and transports oxygen and some CO_2 around the body

P_aCO_2: partial pressure of CO_2 in arterial blood; basis of respiratory acid-base balance

F_iO_2: fraction of inspired oxygen.

Arterial blood gas (ABG) analysis identifies if breathing is effective by giving an indication of gas exchange, ventilation and acid-base status. Readings should be related to the level of inspired oxygen (F_iO_2) and previous values.

Arterial blood samples are taken either from an indwelling arterial catheter or by intermittent puncture of the radial artery using local anaesthesia. Local anaesthesia is stipulated in the UK Guidelines (BTS 2008), not just for humanity but also because the pain of a needle going through the arterial wall may lead to hyperventilation or apnoea, which can invalidate the results (Lee 2012). Table 1.1 relates the different measurements of arterial oxygenation.

P_aO_2 describes the 2% of oxygen that is dissolved in plasma, and reflects the pressure needed to push oxygen from blood into tissue cells. **S_aO_2** describes the 98% of oxygen that is bound to Hb for transport. These do not give a measure of oxygenation at tissue level, and resting levels do not reflect oxygenation during exercise, nor predict nocturnal gas exchange.

Gas exchange entails:

- oxygen dissolving in alveolar lining fluid
- diffusion of oxygen through the alveolar-capillary membrane into plasma
- oxygen binding to Hb for transport around the body
- at its destination, oxygen from Hb dissolving back into plasma
- diffusion of oxygen across the capillary wall and delivery to the tissues.

The reverse is happening to CO_2, but much is carried dissolved in blood and it slips back and forth with ease. The movement of CO_2 traditionally does not come under the term 'gas exchange'.

Oxygen dissociation curve

The relationship between S_aO_2 and P_aO_2 is not direct but expressed by the oxygen dissociation curve (Fig 1.10). Its S-shape illustrates the protective mechanisms that function in both health and disease.

TABLE 1.1 Relationship between oxygen saturation and tension in arterial blood under normal conditions

S_aO_2 %	P_aO_2 (kPa)	P_aO_2 (mmHg)
97	12.7–14.0	95–105
94	9.3–10.0	70–75
92	8.9–9.7	67–73
90	7.7–8.3	58–62
87	6.9–7.7	52–58
84	6.1–6.9	46–52

FIGURE 1.10 Oxygen dissociation curve relating oxygen saturation to oxygen tension. 2.3.DPG is an enzyme in red blood cells which increases in chronic hypoxaemia and allows easier unloading of O_2 to hypoxic tissues. P_{50} is the P_aO_2 at which Hb is 50% saturated and is the most sensitive indicator of a shift in the curve, a high value suggesting poor affinity of Hb for O_2. The shaded area represents critical tissue hypoxia.

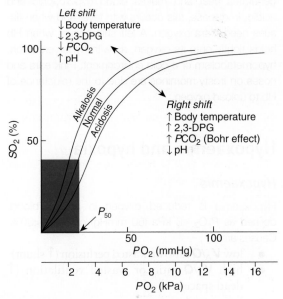

Upper flat portion of the curve

At the plateau of the curve, the combination of oxygen with Hb is favoured by a high PO_2, and its stability is not unduly disturbed by changes in P_aO_2. In health, this encourages loading of oxygen in the high PO_2 environment of the lung, and discourages unloading of oxygen before blood reaches the capillary bed. In disease, there can be a significant change in P_aO_2, e.g. a reduction to 10.7 kPa (80 mmHg), with little change in S_aO_2.

Steep portion of the curve

The dissociation of Hb becomes proportionately greater as PO_2 falls, so that small changes in P_aO_2 greatly affect S_aO_2. In health, this means that Hb can offload quantities of oxygen at cellular level while maintaining oxygen tension in the blood. In disease, large amounts of oxygen can be unloaded when tissues are hypoxic. A P_aO_2 of 7.3 kPa (55 mmHg) tips the patient into a slippery slope where further small drops in P_aO_2 result in tissue hypoxia.

Shift of the curve

Another singular way in which the body responds to need is to adjust the affinity of Hb for oxygen, as reflected by a shift of the curve. A right shift means that Hb unloads oxygen more easily at a given PO_2. In health, this occurs during exercise, when active muscle generates heat and makes blood hypercapnic and acidic. In disease, this occurs with fever and when tissues need extra oxygen. A left shift occurs when Hb holds tightly onto its oxygen, as with hyperventilation, hypometabolism or a cold environment. Pink ears and noses on frosty mornings are due to the reluctance of Hb to unload oxygen.

Hypoxaemia and hypoxia

Hypoxaemia

Hypoxaemia is reduced oxygen in arterial blood, defined as P_aO_2 <8 kPa (60 mmHg) or S_aO_2 <90%. Causes are:

- low $\dot{V}_A/\dot{Q}$ ratio or wasted perfusion (↑ shunt)
- high $\dot{V}_A/\dot{Q}$ ratio or wasted ventilation (↑ dead space)
- hypoventilation

- diffusion abnormality
- ↓ F_IO_2.

Low $\dot{V}_A/\dot{Q}$ occurs when blood is shunted through consolidated, collapsed or damaged lung without seeing any oxygen, somewhat attenuated by hypoxic vasoconstriction. **High $\dot{V}_A/\dot{Q}$** occurs, for example, when a pulmonary embolus blocks perfusion, thus increasing alveolar dead space and causing $\dot{V}_A/\dot{Q}$ mismatch at the other end of the spectrum (Fig 1.11).

Hypoventilation can be caused by respiratory depression (e.g. from over-sedation), respiratory muscle weakness (e.g. with neuromuscular disorder), or sometimes with COPD if patients chronically hypoventilate in order to rest the diaphragm (Ch. 3).

Diffusion abnormalities occur in disorders such as pulmonary oedema or fibrosing alveolitis, when a thickened alveolar-capillary membrane increases $P_AO_2–P_aO_2$.

↓ F_IO_2, is due to inadequate oxygen therapy, high altitude or fire entrapment.

Hypoxia

The term hypoxia is sometimes used interchangeably with hypoxaemia but it means oxygen deficit at tissue level, when demand exceeds supply, leading to anaerobic metabolism once P_aO_2 reaches 4.5 kPa (33.8 mmHg) (Townsend & Webster 2000). It is more relevant to body function than hypoxaemia but more difficult to measure.

FIGURE 1.11 Alveoli and surrounding capillary network, showing how impaired ventilation or perfusion upsets $\dot{V}_A/\dot{Q}$ matching.

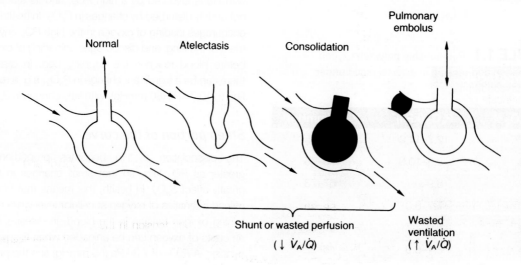

Hypoxaemic hypoxia occurs when hypoxia is caused by hypoxaemia. **Anaemic** hypoxia is when Hb levels are reduced or abnormal Hb cannot carry enough oxygen. **Ischaemic** hypoxia indicates impaired oxygen transport, e.g. haemorrhage, myocardial infarct or peripheral arterial disease. **Histotoxic** hypoxia occurs when cells cannot extract or utilize oxygen, e.g. following cyanide poisoning or in septic shock.

Effects of hypoxaemia and hypoxia

Acute hypoxaemia induces vasodilation of the peripheral vascular beds, increasing cardiac output and improving oxygen delivery. Chronic hypoxaemia thickens the blood and may strain the right heart (see Fig 3.4) and even transient hypoxaemia may shorten life (Criner 2013).

Hypoxia progressively causes the following:

$P_aO_2 < 7.3$ kPa (55 mmHg): memory defect, impaired judgment

< 5.3 kPa (40 mmHg) : tissue damage

< 4 kPa (30 mmHg) : unconsciousness

< 2.7 kPa (20 mmHg) : death, except in the bar-headed goose when it migrates over the Himalayas.

The brain is the first organ to be affected, followed by the gut lining. The kidney is also sensitive to hypoxia and manifests its distress more obviously, reducing urine output and increasing potassium, creatinine or urea levels. Cardiac arrhythmias may occur when S_aO_2 drops below 80%.

Hypercapnia

Hypercapnia is high P_aCO_2 and reflects hypoventilation, leading to respiratory acidosis or compensated metabolic alkalosis. An acutely rising P_aCO_2 is a danger sign if it presages exhaustion (see Fig 3.30), and with acidosis is an indication for mechanical ventilatory assistance. But chronic hypercapnia is neither dangerous nor damaging, sometimes accompanying advanced but stable lung disease.

CO_2 is also required to transmit nerve impulses, control blood flow to the brain and shift the oxygen dissociation curve when required.

The clinical signs of hypoxaemia and hypercapnia are insensitive and non-specific, but Table 1.2 indicates some similarities and differences.

Interpretation

Examples of ABG abnormalities are:

- $\downarrow P_aO_2$ with $\uparrow PaCO_2$: exacerbation of lung disease (causing $\downarrow$ oxygenation) in a patient who is becoming too exhausted to ventilate adequately (causing CO_2 retention)
- $\downarrow P_aO_2$ with $\downarrow P_aCO_2$: hypoxaemia in a patient who is breathless (which pushes

TABLE 1.2 Clinical features of hypoxaemia and hypercapnia

Hypoxaemia	Hypercapnia
Cyanosis	Flapping tremor of hands
↑ Respiratory rate	↑ Respiratory rate
↑ Heart rate	↑ Heart rate
Peripheral vasoconstriction	Peripheral vasodilation leading to warm hands and headache
Respiratory muscle weakness	Respiratory muscle weakness
Arrhythmias or bradycardia	Bradycardia
Restlessness → confusion → coma	Drowsiness → hallucinations → coma

down CO_2), e.g. pneumonia, fibrosing alveolitis, pulmonary oedema, pulmonary embolus

- normal P_aO_2 with ↓ P_aCO_2: emotion causing hyperventilation, e.g. painful arterial puncture or hyperventilation syndrome.

Hypercapnia is likely to be longstanding if pH is >7.35 (BTS 2008).

Reduced minute volume raises P_aCO_2 and lowers S_aO_2, but the reverse is not true. Increased minute volume blows off CO_2, but S_aO_2 does not rise above normal because Hb cannot be supersaturated. However mechanical ventilation with a high F_iO_2 can raise P_aO_2 above normal when the extra oxygen dissolves in the plasma.

Other indices of oxygenation

Gas exchange is best documented in relation to the inspired oxygen (Karbing et al 2007), described as the **P_aO_2:F_iO_2** ratio (see Glossary). Less easy to measure, but useful in identifying the cause of hypoxaemia, is the difference between alveolar and arterial oxygen, known as the alveolar-arterial oxygen gradient, the 'A-a gradient', or **P_AO_2–P_aO_2**. A raised gradient indicates greater difficulty in getting oxygen across the alveolar-capillary membrane, as occurs in diffusion impairment. Hypoventilation or reduced F_iO_2 do not affect the P_AO_2–P_aO_2.

Acid-base balance

Normal pH in the human body: 7.35–7.45

The degree of acidity or alkalinity is measured by pH, which measures hydrogen ions (H^+) in solution, but negatively, i.e.:

- low pH means more hydrogen ions and greater acidity
- high pH means fewer hydrogen ions and greater alkalinity.

Neutral is 6.8, but body functions occur on the alkaline side of neutral. **Acidosis** occurs when arterial pH falls below 7.35. The term means increased acidity in the body, while **acidaemia** means increased acidity of

blood plasma, but the former is normally used for both. Acidosis can lead to myocardial depression, arrhythmias and hypotension, while hypercapnic acidosis weakens the respiratory muscles and can increase inflammation (Bruno 2012). **Alkalosis** occurs at pH over 7.45. The pH responds to metabolic and respiratory change but cannot differentiate between them.

The following identify acid-base imbalances:

- **Respiratory acidosis** occurs when the drop in pH is caused by increased P_aCO_2. It is caused by hypoventilation, leading sometimes to ventilatory failure.
- **Respiratory alkalosis** occurs when a patient hyperventilates, thereby pushing down P_aCO_2 and raising pH. This always accompanies a raised minute volume and often accompanies breathlessness, though the rapid shallow breathing pattern of a breathless person is not necessarily efficient, nor synonymous with hyperventilation.
- **Metabolic acidosis** occurs when the body produces too much acid or the kidneys cannot remove enough acid. Metabolic acids include all the body acids except dissolved CO_2. They are not respirable and have to be neutralized, metabolized, or excreted by the kidney. Lactic acidosis is a distinct form of metabolic acidosis caused by the build-up of lactic acid if oxygen supply is inadequate.
- **Metabolic alkalosis** raises pH out of proportion to changes in P_aCO_2, a common occurrence in critically ill patients due to volume loss, diuretics or low potassium (Oh 2010).

Patients can have mixed acid-base disorders, e.g. a patient with acute hypercapnic COPD may have CO_2-induced respiratory acidosis, but comorbidities such as diabetes or the side effects of diuretics can induce a metabolic alkalosis, with the knock-on effects of a depressed respiratory drive and increased airway resistance (Terzano et al 2012).

Buffers

A buffer is a weak acid or base which mitigates a deranged pH by mopping up or squeezing out hydrogen ions like a chemical sponge. **Bicarbonate** (HCO_3^-)

is the most important buffer and its value provides an estimate of the metabolic component of acid-base balance, although it is affected by both metabolic and respiratory components. Values are:

- normal: 22–26 mmol/l
- metabolic acidosis: <22 mmol/l
- metabolic alkalosis: >26 mmol/l.

The effect of P_aCO_2 on pH is in App.C.

Standard bicarbonate (SBE) is the bicarbonate concentration under standard conditions, being adjusted as if P_aCO_2 were 5.3 kPa, i.e. it is similar to bicarbonate in a person with normal acid-base status.

Base excess (BE) is a calculated value from SBE, being positive in metabolic alkalosis and negative in metabolic acidosis. It represents the quantity of acid required to restore pH to normal if PCO_2 were adjusted to normal. Like HCO_3^-, it measures metabolic acid-base balance, but takes buffering by red blood cells into account and provides a more complete analysis of metabolic buffering than HCO_3^-. BE is calculated from pH, P_aCO_2 and haematocrit. Values are:

- normal: minus 2 to plus 2 mmol/l
- metabolic acidosis: < minus 3 mmol/l
- metabolic alkalosis: > plus 3 mmol/l.

Along with clinical assessment, arterial blood gas analysis helps identify the main causes of acidosis or alkalosis, although one may dominate and the other partially compensate (Fig 1.12). The prime mover is the one on which to focus and it is a mistake to treat a compensation.

A quick tip, as seen in Fig 1.12 is that if the primary acid-base disturbance is metabolic, pH and bicarbonate/BE change in the same direction, while if the primary problem is respiratory, pH and P_aCO_2 change in opposite directions.

Regulation

Acid-base balance is disturbed if removal of CO_2 from the lungs is abnormal (respiratory acidosis or alkalosis) or production of acid from the tissues or elimination elsewhere is abnormal (metabolic acidosis or alkalosis). Any deviation of pH from normal is fiercely resisted, at whatever cost, by three homeostatic mechanisms:

1 The buffer system neutralizes acids or bases by giving up or absorbing hydrogen ions, all within seconds. The following equation represents the dissociation of

FIGURE 1.12 Four examples of acid-base imbalance showing the process of compensation. Thick arrows in each box indicate which way a value has gone in order to create the acidosis or alkalosis. Thin arrows indicate which way the other value is going in order to compensate.

	Respiratory	Metabolic
Acidosis pH↓	$[HCO_3^-]$ ↑ PCO_2 ↑	$[HCO_3^-]$ ↓ PCO_2 ↓
Alkalosis pH↑	$[HCO_3^-]$ ↓ PCO_2 ↓	$[HCO_3^-]$ ↑ PCO_2 ↑

carbonic acid in solution, acting as a sink for hydrogen ions:

$$H_2O + CO_2 \leftrightarrow H_2CO_3 \leftrightarrow H^+ + HCO_3^-$$

An increase in P_aCO_2 shifts the equilibrium to the right, increasing H^+ and causing respiratory acidosis. A decrease in P_aCO_2 shifts it to the left.

2 If buffering is not adequate, the lungs then present an avenue for regulating CO_2. Hyper- or hypoventilation can stabilize acid-base balance in 1–15 minutes.

3 If this is still not adequate, the kidneys take over, but they need 3–5 days to do so (Ayers & Warrington 2008).

These mechanisms work to dispose of the acids that are continually produced by the body's metabolic processes, caused mostly by the hydration of CO_2 to create carbonic acid.

Interpretation

Step 1: look at the pH:

- ↓ pH means acidosis
- ↑ pH means alkalosis.

Step 2: look at the P_aCO_2: does it account for an abnormal pH? If breathing is the prime mover:

- ↑ P_aCO_2 means respiratory acidosis
- ↓ P_aCO_2 means respiratory alkalosis.

Step 3: look at the HCO_3^- or BE: does it account for an abnormal pH? If breathing is not the prime mover:

- ↓ HCO_3^- or BE means metabolic acidosis
- ↑ HCO_3^- or BE means metabolic alkalosis.

To help decide if a change in pH is respiratory or metabolic (if this is not obvious clinically), any change greater than the following is likely to be metabolic in origin (Williams 1998):

- for every increase in P_aCO_2 of 2.6 kPa (20 mmHg) above normal, pH falls by 0.1
- for every decrease in P_aCO_2 of 1.3 kPa (10 mmHg) below normal, pH rises by 0.1.

When pH is restored to normal, full compensation has occurred. The stages can be identified as follows:

- abnormal pH + change in P_aCO_2 or bicarbonate/BE = non compensation, i.e. an acute process

- abnormal pH + change in P_aCO_2 and bicarbonate/BE = partial compensation
- normal pH + change in P_aCO_2 and bicarbonate/BE = full compensation.

Table 1.3. clarifies the causes, effects and recognition of arterial blood gas imbalances. Examples are in App.C.

Table 1.4 shows how two respiratory disorders can affect arterial blood gas readings. P_aCO_2 values reflect breathlessness in acute asthma and hypoventilation in COPD. HCO_3^- and pH values reflect an acute non-compensated condition in acute asthma, and full compensation in COPD.

THE OXYGEN CASCADE

The *raison d'etre* of the cardiorespiratory system is to get oxygen to the tissues by means of oxygen cascading from the outside to the subcellular environment. Even when ventilation, diffusion and perfusion are in order, oxygen still has to reach and get into the tissues.

TABLE 1.3 Interpretation of arterial blood gas trends (N = normal)

Status	Causes	Effects	Recognition
Acute respiratory acidosis	Hypoventilation, e.g. exhaustion, weakness	P_aCO_2 ↑, pH ↓, HCO_3^- N (no renal compensation yet)	Shallow breathing, drowsiness, severe acute respiratory disease
Chronic (compensated) respiratory acidosis	Chronic hypoventilation	P_aCO_2 ↑, pH N, HCO_3^- ↑ (retention of HCO_3^- to restore pH, i.e. full compensation)	Severe chronic respiratory disease, e.g. COPD
Respiratory alkalosis	Acute hyperventilation, e.g. anxiety, pain, acute cardiorespiratory disease, fever, CNS injury	HCO_3^- ↓, P_aCO_2 ↓, pH ↑ (partial compensation)	Breathlessness
Metabolic acidosis	Shock, lactic acidosis, diabetic acidosis, severe diarrhoea or dehydration, kidney failure	HCO_3^- ↓, pH ↓, P_aCO_2 ↓, BE < −2 (partial compensation)	Hyperventilation (respiratory compensation to blow off PCO_2)
Metabolic alkalosis	Sepsis, heart failure, diuretics, severe vomiting, ↓ albumin	HCO_3^- ↑, pH ↑, P_aCO_2 ↑, BE > +2 (partial compensation)	Delirium

TABLE 1.4 Examples of arterial blood gas values in two disorders (numbers in brackets indicate mmHg).

	Normal	Acute asthma	COPD
P_aO_2	12.7 (95)	9.3 (70)	7.3 (55)
P_aCO_2	5.3 (40)	3.3 (25)	8 (60)
pH	7.4	7.5	7.4
HCO_3^-	24	24	29

Oxygen **transport** is the passage of oxygen to the tissues via the arteries and capillaries. The arterial circulation also acts as a cushion to soften the pulsations generated by the heart so that capillary blood flow is stable. The term 'oxygen transport' is often used synonymously with, and is virtually the same as, oxygen **delivery**, which is the oxygen presented to the tissues. Oxygen **consumption** or **uptake** by the tissues is usually equivalent to oxygen demand, determined by the metabolic needs of the tissues.

Oxygen availability to the tissues depends on:
- S_aO_2, P_aO_2 and Hb
- cardiac output (CO)
- distribution of CO and local perfusion
- oxygen extraction
- the oxygen dissociation curve.

Tissue oxygenation reflects the balance between supply (oxygen delivery or DO_2) and demand (oxygen consumption or $\dot{V}O_2$). The respiratory system, as with most other systems, has plenty of reserve capacity, and DO_2 is normally four times greater than $\dot{V}O_2$, creating an oxygen extraction ratio ($\dot{V}O_2/DO_2$) of 25% (Fawcett et al 2006).

$\dot{V}O_2$ varies with metabolic rate. An increase is usually met without difficulty by increased DO_2 (mostly through increased CO, partly through increased minute ventilation) and increased oxygen extraction by the tissues. Once maximum oxygen extraction is reached, consumption no longer drives delivery but becomes dependent on it. Further increase in demand, or reduced supply, leads to hypoxia.

Some organs are greedier than others, e.g.:
- The brain comprises 2.2% of body weight and receives 1.5% of CO.
- The myocardium comprises 0.5% body weight and receives 5% of CO.
- The kidneys comprise 0.5% body weight and receive 20% of CO.

- Skeletal muscle and skin comprise 50% body weight and receive 10% of CO (Epstein 1993).

Tolerance to hypoxia also varies:
- The brain suffers irreversible damage within three minutes.
- The kidneys and liver can tolerate 15–20 minutes of hypoxia.
- Skeletal muscle tolerates 60–90 minutes and vascular smooth muscle 24–72 hours.
- Hair and nails continue to grow for some days after death (Leach & Treacher 2002).

Septic patients may need 50–60% extra oxygen delivered to their tissues, while patients with multiple trauma, septic shock or burns may require 100% extra (Epstein 1993). At the same time, critically ill patients may be affected by:
- impaired DO_2 because of cardiorespiratory dysfunction
- cellular oxygen extraction hindered by toxins associated with sepsis, leading to mitochondrial dysfunction (Van Boxel et al 2012)
- loss of autoregulation, leading to disordered regional distribution of blood flow, both between and within organs
- hypoxic kidneys and liver unable to detoxify by-products of the shocked state.

If the body is not able to acquire, transport, extract and utilize sufficient oxygen, lactic acidosis occurs.

Compared to gas exchange in the lung, which is easily monitored in arterial blood, tissue oxygenation is usually estimated indirectly from the leftover oxygen in pulmonary artery blood, where it is at the end of its journey before being reoxygenated in the lungs (Ch. 17).

VARIATIONS

Effects of obesity

Obesity is the most common metabolic disease world-wide (Sood 2009), the commonest chronic disorder in the US (O'Donnell *et al* 2010), and Britain is catching up. The condition has more than doubled globally since 1980 and is now the fifth leading mortality risk (WHO 2012). Obesity places a significant load on the respiratory system, pushing up the diaphragm and restricting lung volumes so that FRC may approach residual volume (Fig 1.13) and overlap with closing volume (see Fig 1.9), leading to closure of dependent airways and $\dot{V}_A/\dot{Q}$ mismatch (Salome *et al* 2010). Breathing patterns tend to be rapid, shallow and apical, and breathlessness is common.

FIGURE 1.13 Effect of obesity on lung volumes, showing how FRC can approach RV. Compare with Fig 2.30a *TLC:* total lung capacity, *IC:* inspiratory capacity, *FRC:* functional residual capacity, *RV:* residual volume

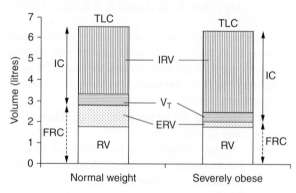

Obesity may also cause:

- a mixed obstructive/restrictive respiratory defect (Reynolds 2011) and ↑ risk of cardiovascular disease (Capodaglio 2013)
- ↓ chest wall compliance, which can triple elastic resistance and increase the work of breathing 10-fold (Sood 2009)
- attenuated response to hypoxic and hypercapnic ventilatory drives, ↑ work of breathing, ↓ work capacity, ↑ risk of falls

(Capodaglio 2013), exaggerated blood pressure (BP) response to exercise (Dipla *et al* 2012) and, with exercise, stress on the heart (Vella *et al* 2012)

- systemic inflammation which reduces muscle mass (King *et al* 2013), worsens airway inflammation, and reduces response to steroids and bronchodilators (Sismanopoulos 2013)
- urinary incontinence (Krause 2010), osteoporosis, sleep apnoea (Capodaglio 2013), some cancers (Kaaks 2013) and barotrauma during mechanical ventilation (Pedoto 2012)
- ↓ testosterone through the endocrine-modulating effect of adipose tissue (Woodard *et al* 2012)
- ↓ life expectancy (Jiang *et al* 2013)
- bias in the health care system (O'Brien *et al* 2012).

On the surgical wards, an obese patient should barely have emerged from anaesthesia before the physiotherapist becomes involved in pain control and positioning, closely followed by incentive spirometry (IS) and early mobilization (Reynolds 2011). Morbidly obese people show a greater propensity for thrombosis and wound infections, demonstrate a 30% likelihood of atelectasis or pneumonia after abdominal surgery (Licker *et al* 2007), and are three times more likely to die after lung transplant (Kanasky *et al* 2002).

On the medical wards, obesity is associated with asthma (Shore 2013) and COPD (O'Donnell *et al* 2010). For patients with lung disease, steroid medication can augment obesity, and obesity can disrupt pharmacokinetics (Cooper 2011).

On the intensive care unit, obesity increases the risk of sepsis and the complications of immobilization, the latter being moderated by early rehabilitation (Genc *et al* 2012).

Multidisciplinary rehabilitation is required if comorbidities are present (Capodaglio 2013) and oxygenation may actually increase during exercise because of the effect of deep breathing on expansion of collapsed lung units (Sood 2009).

Effects of smoking

> *Tobacco is the single most preventable cause of death in the world today … it kills up to half of those who use it.*
>
> WHO 2008

Smokers lose at least a decade of life (Jha *et al* 2013). Causes are the 4000 chemicals in tobacco smoke, including cyanide, carbon monoxide, arsenic and 43 known carcinogens (Aslani & Rafiei 2012). The smoke causes mucus obstruction (Randall *et al* 2006) and inflammation from oxidative tissue injury (Pignataro 2012). Carnage to the cardiorespiratory systems is well known (Ch. 3/4), but virtually every system is affected and the litany of destruction is outlined below.

Smoking is associated with back pain, other musculoskeletal pains (Pignataro 2012), including osteoarthritis (Amin *et al* 2007), muscle weakness, osteoporosis (Pignataro 2012) and exacerbation of other chronically painful conditions (Ditre 2012). It compromises immunity (Bauer *et al* 2013) and plays a major role in autoimmune diseases, e.g. rheumatoid arthritis, SLE (Ch. 3) (Pignataro 2012) and ankylosing spondylitis (Ward *et al* 2008). It impairs cognition, increases the risk of developing some neurological diseases and neuropathic pain (Pignataro 2012), wrinkles the skin (Patel 2006), disturbs sleep (Ezzie 2011), increases depression (Berk *et al* 2013), doubles the risk of dementia (Pignataro 2012) and shortens life by 11 minutes for each cigarette smoked (Warren 2001). It depletes vitamin C, which would otherwise repair some of the lung damage (Banerjee *et al* 2008). It leaches muscle mass (Van den Borst 2011) and damages the diaphragm and quadriceps (Ramirez-Sarmiento 2004). It ulcerates the gut (Bao *et al* 2010), rots teeth (Kubota *et al* 2011) and causes cataract (Glynn *et al* 2009) and ulnar neuropathy (Richardson 2009). It increases the risks of diabetes (Anon 2011) and many cancers (Blakely *et al* 2013). It quadruples the risk of postoperative complications (Bluman *et al* 1998), although smoking eases postoperative nausea and vomiting (Chimbira & Sweeney 2000) in patients who can escape the ward. Smoking doubles the risk of developing macular degeneration (Evans *et al* 2005) and increases the risk of subarachnoid haemorrhage 6-fold (Partridge 1992) and pneumothorax 13-fold (Light

1993). Smoking impairs wound healing and drug metabolism (Licker *et al* 2007), and the effects can even jump a generation, the grandchildren of smokers being more likely to develop asthma (Leslie 2013).

Smoking is neither virile nor sexy, and tobacco is toxic to both testes and ovaries. Smoking during pregnancy increases preterm birth (Cox *et al* 2013), and causes as much damage to the foetus as if it was smoking itself (Le Souëf 2000) including a future risk of obesity (Behl *et al* 2013). The BMA (2004) has found the following:

- Fertility is reduced in men and women, women smokers being twice as likely to be infertile as non-smokers, and both sexes showing reduced response to fertility treatment.
- For men, damage to blood vessels leads to male smokers being at least 50% more likely to be impotent, while those who succeed are more likely to produce damaged, malformed or mutated sperm.
- In women, smoking can cause dysmenorrhoea and a 25% increased risk of miscarriage.
- Smoking is the largest preventable cause of infant ill health and death, as well as risking birth defects. Damage persists into later life, and children whose mothers smoked during pregnancy are more likely to develop obesity, COPD and possibly cancer.
- The risk of cot death is trebled in infants whose mothers smoke, and increased 2.5 times if the father smokes. Babies of smokers cry more, and later have poorer performance at school.

> **KEY POINT**
>
> It is never too late to quit (Schroeder 2013).

Passive smokers increase their lung cancer risk by 30% (Pentz 2010) and suffer more postoperative complications than non-smokers (Licker 2007). Marriage to a smoker increases the risk of lung cancer by 26% (*BMJ* 1997). Children have more dental caries (Tanaka *et al* 2010), asthma and glue ear (Rouch *et al* 2010), some of these effects being attenuated by breast feeding (Woodward *et al* 1990). Passive smoking also increases the risk of stroke (Cao *et al* 2013), eye disease (Kahn 2006) and exercise limitation (Arjomandi *et al* 2012).

Nicotine is more addictive than heroin and seven times as addictive as alcohol (Haas & Haas 2000). Its one redeeming feature is that, according to patients, it aids relaxation and acts as a social crutch (*Lancet* 2013).

> *A custom loathsome to the eye, hateful to the nose, harmful to the brain and dangerous to the lungs.*
>
> King James I

Effects of stress

All ill people suffer stress, usually as a result of and sometimes as a predisposing factor to illness. The following effects of stress have been identified:

- ↑ respiratory rate, heart rate and BP (Schwartz *et al* 2011)
- ↑ sympathetic and platelet activation, which impairs vascular function, progresses heart disease (Staniute *et al* 2013) and predisposes to arrhythmias (Brame & Singer 2010)
- ↑ circulating catecholamines (Friedrich 2013)
- hyperglycaemia, immunosuppression, ↑ catabolism (Fawcett *et al* 2012)
- inflammation (Maslanik 2013), possibly explaining a link with asthma (Lehrer *et al* 2008) and Gulf War syndrome (Broderick *et al* 2013)
- in children, impaired immune function which can last into adult life (Slopen *et al* 2013)
- before birth, inflammatory changes that may permanently alter the function of the nervous and immune systems (Diz-Chaves *et al* 2013).

Effects of sleep

> *Sleep is something of a mystery.*
>
> Primhak & Kingshott, 2012

The effects of sleep on breathing include (Thompson 2001):

- ↓ respiratory drive and ↑ P_aCO_2, especially during rapid eye movement (REM) sleep (Fig 1.14), the reduced minute ventilation being out of proportion to the lower metabolic rate
- dips in S_aO_2 to 90% or less (BTS 2008) which may drive S_aO_2 down the steep part of the dissociation curve
- ↓ lung volume due to the horizontal position
- the above causing $\dot{V}_A/\dot{Q}$ mismatch and a doubling of airway resistance (Xie 2012)
- bronchoconstriction which is only of consequence with asthma (Kamdar *et al* 2012)
- ↓ mucociliary clearance.

Most people can accommodate all this quite happily, but those with little cardiorespiratory reserve can suffer dramatic nocturnal desaturation (Ch. 5) as well as nights that are disturbed by breathlessness or coughing.

FIGURE 1.14 Control of ventilation during sleep, showing reduced respiratory drive at deeper sleep stages. *REM:* rapid eye movement

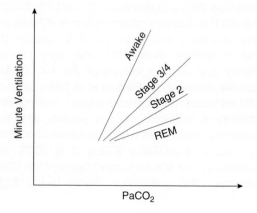

Sleep fragmentation brings further tribulation. A full 90 minute cycle is needed to gain the benefits of REM sleep, which comprises about a quarter of the sleep cycle and is associated with dreaming and perceptual learning. The brain is highly active during this restorative phase and consumes more oxygen than when awake at rest. It is the time when memories are processed (Cipolli *et al* 2013) and is particularly important for critically ill patients to prevent memory distortion.

Sleep deprivation contributes to toxin accumulation (Xie *et al* 2013) stress (Kerkhofs 2012), inflammation (Ingiosi 2013), stroke, multiple sclerosis, Alzheimer's disease, epilepsy, pain (Palma 2013), impaired cognition, inflammation, depression, diabetes, obesity and cardiovascular disease (Porkka-Heiskanen 2013). Cardiac complications can develop from too much or too little sleep (Ramos *et al* 2013).

> *Nurses and doctors frequently overestimate how much sleep patients are getting, and underestimate the importance of sleep.*
> Gelling 1999

Effects of immobility

> *Inactive people are contributing to a mortality burden as large as tobacco smoking.*
> Wen & Wu 2012

It is estimated that 60% of world's population is not physically active enough (Vrdoljak 2014). Immobility is now known to cause:

- cardiac atrophy, ↓ blood volume, orthostatic intolerance, ↓ $\dot{V}O_2max$ (Fig 1.15) and cardiovascular instability during position change (Vollman 2013)
- ↓ DO_2, accelerated ageing and hypertension (Bortz 1984)
- for critically ill patients: pneumonia, delayed weaning, pressure sores (Vollman 2013), myopathy, delirium (Pawlik 2012), loss of muscle mass (Parry *et al* 2012), ICU psychosis and urine infection (Olivier 1998)
- ↓ exercise tolerance (Kim & Thompson 2012)

FIGURE 1.15 The effect of immobility on maximum oxygen consumption

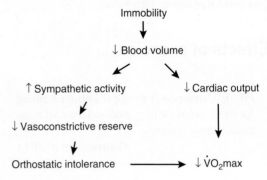

- ↓ cognitive function (Misak 2011) and depression (Hamer *et al* 2013)
- constipation and incontinence (Nurko & Scott 2011)
- cardiovascular deconditioning, thromboembolism, muscle mass by up to 1–5% per day (Mah 2013)
- survival and quality of life, healthcare utilization (BTS 2013)
- obesity, insulin resistance, high cholesterol, hypertension (Vrdoljak 2014)
- joint contractures (Brower 2010).

Contractures begin immediately, especially for joints held in extension (Trudel *et al* 1999), although this is unlikely to be significant for a patient who is immobile for a few days.

Loss of gravitational stimulus to the cardiovascular system causes a negative fluid balance within 24 hours, impairing vasoconstrictive ability and augmenting deconditioning. Deterioration occurs more rapidly in the cardiorespiratory system than the musculoskeletal systems, and deterioration is quicker than recovery (Dean & Ross 1992).

Turning, sitting and standing up

Regular position change as a preventive measure reduces haemodynamic instability on movement (Vollman 2013). Moving from supine to standing increases minute volume (Bahadur *et al* 2008) and redistributes blood from the thorax to the lower body, followed by compensatory vasoconstriction in most patients to restore BP (Fig 1.16).

Orthostatic intolerance occurs with inadequate haemodynamic compensation, e.g. with hypovolaemia or autonomic dysfunction, after prolonged bed rest or if the patient is elderly or dehydrated.

Effects of exercise

> *Physical exercise is the best known training for the cardiovascular, pulmonary and musculoskeletal systems.*
>
> Lainscak *et al* 2013

Exercise increases oxygen delivery, consumption and extraction by several mechanisms:

- The cardiovascular response can increase cardiac output (CO) 5-fold, accomplished by a near-doubling of stroke volume and an increase in heart rate (HR) to about 220 minus the person's age (MacIntyre 2000).

FIGURE 1.16 Typical circulatory response to postural change. *HR*: heart rate *MAP*: mean arterial pressure

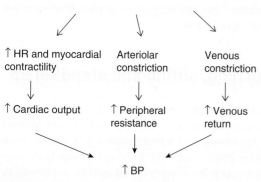

Moving from supine to standing
↓
500 ml blood migrates to pelvis and legs
↓
↓ Venous return, cardiac output and MAP
↓
↓ BP detected by aortic arch and carotid baroreceptors
↓
Information sent to brainstem
↓
↑ Sympathetic activity and ↓ parasympathetic activity

↑ HR and myocardial contractility → ↑ Cardiac output

Arteriolar constriction → ↑ Peripheral resistance

Venous constriction → ↑ Venous return

→ ↑ BP

- The respiratory response is represented by increased diffusion, more uniform lung perfusion, recruitment of dormant capillaries and, except with asthma, bronchodilation (Dominelli & Sheel 2012).
- Intense exercise can increase $\dot{V}O_2$ 20-fold (Owens 2013). Cerebral oxygenation rises during mild exercise and drops during intense exercise (Peltonen 2012). P_aO_2 remains steady throughout.
- Acid-base balance is usually maintained by increased ventilation, but metabolic acidosis may develop if buffering mechanisms are unable to cope with the extra CO_2 and lactic acid.

Exercise also enhances mucous transport (Houtmeyers 1999), aids sleep (Hargens *et al* 2013), induces a cascade of molecular and cellular processes that dampens chronic inflammation and pain in knee osteoarthritis (Gomes 2013) and other musculoskeletal conditions (Hagen 2012) and reduces the risk of developing chronic pain (Sluka *et al* 2013).

Cardiovascular performance imposes the primary limit to exercise (Trinity 2012), but with lung disease, dyspnoea may be the limiting factor (Stickland *et al* 2012). Exercise above a certain level for each individual is accompanied by inefficient anaerobic metabolism (Garvey *et al* 2012). Exhaustive training can impair immunity (Xiang *et al* 2013).

Exercise training or regular exercise is an accepted treatment for two of the main disorders that lead to an early death, cardiovascular disease and COPD (Woodard & Berry 2001). It also shows the following benefits:

- ↑ $\dot{V}O_2$max (Mendes 2013), i.e. ↑ fitness
- ↓ cardiovascular disease and quality of life (Vrdoljak 2014)
- ↓ respiratory disease (Williams 2014)
- oxidative stress and cellular ageing (Corbi *et al* 2012)
- ↑ immune function (Navarro *et al* 2013)
- ↑ bone mineral density to a greater degree than the drug alendronate (Macias *et al* 2012)
- ↓ inflammation related to COPD (Davidson 2012), heart failure (Vlist & Janssen 2010) and sepsis (Araújo *et al* 2012)
- ↓ cancer risk (p.119)

- ↓ risk of developing stress-related disease (Puterman *et al* 2012)
- healthier semen in men (Vaamonde *et al* 2012)
- ↑ cognition and longevity, ↓ risk of dementia (Joyner & Barnes 2013)
- ↓ falls (Yoo *et al* 2013).

Community-based exercise groups are particularly popular with elderly people (Reuter 2012).

Exercise is 'a miracle drug'.
Wen & Wu 2012

CASE STUDY : Ms LL

A 62 y.o. patient from Cape Town is admitted with an exacerbation of COPD.

Relevant medical history

- heart failure
- hypertension
- increased dyspnoea for two weeks.

Subjective assessment

- can't stop coughing
- occasionally brings up phlegm
- can't sleep
- daren't lie down
- exhausted.

Objective assessment

- apyrexial
- oxygen via nasal cannulae at 2 l/min
- rapid shallow breathing with prolonged expiration
- fluid chart and clinical assessment indicate dehydration
- no oxygen chart
- speaking sets off paroxyms of wheezy coughing, usually non-productive
- clutches between legs when coughs
- sits in chair day and night
- can mobilize slowly
- blood gases on air: P_aO_2 10.2 kPa (76.7 mmHg), P_aCO_2 6.4 kPa (48.1 mmHg), pH 7.4, HCO_3^- 28 mmol/l

Questions

1 Analysis?
2 Problems?
3 Goals?
4 Plan?

CLINICAL REASONING

Comment on the logic of the following conclusion to a research study.

> *'Our data suggest that the use of postural drainage and chest percussion in patients without sputum production is not indicated . . .'*
>
> Chest (1980), 78, 559–64

Response to Case Study

1   Analysis

- breathing pattern suggests ↑ work of breathing
- blood gases indicate hypoxaemia, hypercapnia and compensated respiratory acidosis
- oxygen therapy is uncontrolled
- coughing is largely ineffective and contributes to fatigue
- coughing, stress incontinence, immobility and fluid restriction are likely to be interrelated.

2   Problems

- inaccurate and unmonitored oxygen
- dyspnoea
- uncontrolled cough
- fatigue
- anxiety
- sputum retention
- stress incontinence
- ↓ mobility.

3   Goals

- short term: optimize oxygen, control cough, clear chest, balance rest and exercise
- long term: educate patient and family for home management.

4   Plan

- Liaise with the team about the need for a Venturi mask, oxygen prescription and monitoring (Ch. 5).
- Position for comfort, breathlessness and sputum clearance.
- Identify cause of poor sleep e.g. dyspnoea/cough/noise/anxiety, then remedy as possible with the team.
- Educate on cough suppression for use when cough is uncontrolled and non-productive.
- Educate on mucociliary clearance, including fluid intake. Patient chose manual techniques at first, then autogenic drainage.
- Educate on effective cough for when secretions are accessible.
- Explain connection between coughing and stress incontinence, teach preliminary pelvic floor exercises, refer to continence service.
- Show breathless management strategies.
- Mobilize to toilet.
- Provide written daily programme for self chest management and mobility.
- Liaise with ward staff regarding getting dressed and mobility.
- Rehabilitate to independence, including family.

Response to Clinical Reasoning

It is not indicated to do an unnecessary treatment.

RECOMMENDED READING

Ayers P, Warrington L (2008) Diagnosis and treatment of simple acid-base disorders. *Nutrition Clin Pract;* **23**(2): 122–7

Baillie K (2008) Simple, easily memorised "rules of thumb" for the rapid assessment of physiological compensation for respiratory acid-base disorders. *Thorax;* **63**: 289–90

Bain AR, Lesperance NC, Jay O (2012) Body heat storage during physical activity is lower with hot fluid ingestion under conditions that permit full evaporation. *Acta Physiologica;* **206**(2): 98–108

Bertuzzi R (2013) Energy system contributions during incremental exercise test. *J Sports Sci Med;* **12**(3): 454–60

Cetti EJ, Moore AJ, Geddes DM (2006) Collateral ventilation. *Thorax;* **61**(5): 371–37

Crimi E, Taccone FS, Infant T (2012) Effects of intracellular acidosis on endothelial function: An overview. *J Crit Care;* **27**(1): 108–118

Curley G, Laffey JG, Kavanagh BP (2010) Bench-to-bedside review: carbon dioxide. *Crit Care;* **14**(2): 220

Dominelli PB, Sheel AW (2012) Experimental approaches to the study of the mechanics of breathing during exercise. *Resp Physiol Neurobiol;* **180**: 2–3

Dunham C, Harms C (2012) Effects of high-intensity interval training on pulmonary function. *Eur J Appl Physiol;* **112**(8): 3061–8

Edwards SL (2008) Pathophysiology of acid base balance. *Int Crit Care Nurs;* **24**(1): 28–40

Elstad M (2012) Respiratory variations in pulmonary and systemic blood flow in healthy humans. *Acta Physiologica;* **205**(3): 341–8

Fähling M, Persson PB (2012) Oxygen sensing, uptake, delivery, consumption and related disorders. *Acta Physiologica;* **205**(2): 191–3

Fronius M, Clauss WG, Althaus M (2012) Why do we have to move fluid to be able to breathe? *Frontiers Physiol;* **3**: 146

Glenny RW, Bauer C, Hofmanninger J et al (2013) Heterogeneity and matching of ventilation and perfusion within anatomical lung units in rats. *Resp Physiol Neurobiol;* **189**(3): 594–606

Harris RS (2005) Pressure-volume curves of the respiratory system. *Respir Care;* **50**(1): 78–99

Lamberg E, Hagins M (2012) The effects of low back pain on natural breath control during a lowering task. *Eur J Appl Physiol;* **112**(10): 3519–24

Massery M, Hagins M, Stafford R et al (2013) Effect of airway control by glottal structures on postural stability. *J Appl Physiol;* **115**(4): 483–90

Matsuo K, Palmer JB (2010) Coordination of mastication, swallowing and breathing. *Jpn Dent Sci Rev;* **45**(1): 31–40

McCool FD, Tzelepis GE (2012) Dysfunction of the diaphragm. *N Engl J Med;* **366**: 932–94

Pitts T, Rose MJ, Mortensen AN et al (2013) Coordination of cough and swallow. *Resp Physiol Neurobiol;* **189**(3): 543–551

Smith MT (2013) Sleep, respiration and pain. *Anesthesiology;* **119**(5): 1011–13

Sundelin T (2013) Sleep loss and subjective health. *Brain Behavior Immunity;* **32**: e22

Taylor CE, Willie CK, Atkinson G et al (2013), Postural influences on the mechanical and neural components of the cardiovagal baroreflex. *Acta Physiologica;* **208**: 66–73

Waterier GW (2012) Airway defense mechanisms. *Clin Chest Med;* **33**(2): 199–209

Weibel ER (2013) It takes more than cells to make a good lung. *Am J Respir Crit Care Med;* **187**(4): 342–6

Weier AT, Pearce AJ, Kidgell DJ (2012) Strength training reduces intracortical inhibition. *Acta Physiologica;* **206**(2): 109–11

Yu Y-B, Liao Y-W, Su K-H et al (2012) Prior exercise training alleviates the lung inflammation induced by subsequent exposure to environmental cigarette smoke. *Acta Physiologica;* **205**(4): 532–54

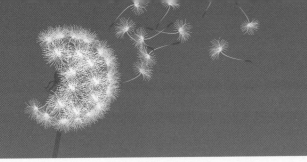

CHAPTER 2
Assessment

LEARNING OBJECTIVES

On completion of this chapter the reader should be able to:

- interpret medical notes and nursing charts

- analyze a patient's subjective report in order to develop, with the patient, problem-based goals and plans

- develop the skills of observation, palpation and auscultation

- analyze radiology findings

- interpret respiratory function tests

- use clinical reasoning to identify cardiorespiratory problems.

INTRODUCTION

It is more important to know what sort of a patient has a disease than what sort of disease a patient has.

William Osler

Accurate assessment is the linchpin of physiotherapy and forms the basis of clinical reasoning. A problem-based assessment leads to thinking such as:

- This patient cannot cough up her sputum by herself. Why?

- Because it is thick. Why?
- Because she is dehydrated. Why?
- Because she feels too ill to drink.

Illogical assessment leads to reasoning such as: 'This is COPD therefore I will turn the patient side-to-side and shake her chest'.

A thoughtful assessment encourages both efficiency and effectiveness. Efficiency saves time by avoiding unnecessary treatment. Effectiveness is assisted by incorporating the domains of the International Classification of Functioning, Disability and Health (ICF), which includes environmental and social factors, removes the negative concept of disability and provides a standardized language on what matters to the patient, i.e.:

- body function and structure
- activity limitation
- participation (Vidmar 2013).

The last two concepts relate in particular to the multidisciplinary team within which the physiotherapist works. Patient participation is embedded in shared decision-making, but individual preferences should be sought (Schoeb & Bürge 2012), particularly for patients who have difficulty communicating due to dyspnoea, learning disabilities or mechanical ventilation.

Relevant parts of the patient assessment should be repeated after treatment to assess outcome. Specific assessment and outcomes for rehabilitation, paediatrics and critical care are in Chapters 9, 10, 11 and 18.

BACKGROUND INFORMATION

> *Not everything that counts can be measured. Not everything that can be measured counts.*
>
> Albert Einstein

Handover

It is the physiotherapist's job to clarify the indications for physiotherapy to other staff, and to explain which changes in a patient's condition should be reported. No patient is 'too ill' or 'too well' for physiotherapy.

The ward report or handover also provides the opportunity to ask three of the most important, and oft-neglected, questions:

1 Is the patient drinking?
2 Is he eating?
3 Is he sleeping?

Apart from a daily report from the nurse in charge, any other opportunity to communicate should be taken, such as ward rounds and meetings. For physiotherapists working in the community, much communication will be on the phone, but visits to other teams usually benefit all concerned, including the patient.

If physiotherapy notes are kept separate from the medical notes, verbal communication can be reinforced by writing physiotherapy information in the medical notes, e.g. a résumé of treatment or request for a minitracheostomy.

Patient's notes

Relevant details from the medical notes include:

1 Past and present medical history, including other disorders needing physiotherapy and conditions requiring precautions in relation to certain treatments, e.g. light-headedness, bleeding disorder, history of falls, swallowing difficulty.
2 Relevant investigations, medical treatment and response.
3 Social history and home environment.
4 Recent cardiopulmonary resuscitation (requiring x-ray inspection for aspiration or fracture).
5 Possibility of bony metastases.
6 Long-standing steroid therapy, leading to a risk of osteoporosis.
7 History of radiotherapy over the chest.

The last four findings are a warning to avoid percussion or vibrations over the ribs until sufficient information is available to ensure that there is no risk of rib fracture.

Patient charts

The charts record:

- the vital signs of temperature, blood pressure (BP), heart rate (HR), respiratory rate (RR) and arterial oxygen saturation (S_pO_2)
- prescription for oxygen and drugs
- fluid balance.

Core temperature is one of the most tightly guarded of physiological parameters and is usually maintained at 37.7°C. For acute patients, the chart should be checked at every visit because fever is the main harbinger of infection.

Fever may be accompanied by increased RR and HR because excess heat raises oxygen consumption and metabolic rate. Clinical examination helps distinguish respiratory from other infection. Pyrexia can also have a non-infectious origin, e.g. atelectasis, dehydration, thromboembolism, blood transfusion or drug reaction (Cunha 2013). The mechanism of fever is thought to be phagocytosis.

KEY POINT

A pyrexial patient may be referred for physiotherapy with a 'chest infection'. Sputum retention can accompany a chest infection but does not itself cause pyrexia. The treatment for a bacterial chest infection is antibiotics while the treatment for sputum retention is physiotherapy. Clearing secretions may help the chest infection, but the physiotherapist works on the problem rather than on the diagnosis.

Blood pressure indicates the force that the blood exerts on the walls of the vessels. Normal at rest is 120/80. Hypotension in adults is indicated by systolic BP below 90 mmHg. These patients should be mobilized only with close observation for light-headedness, and with a chair close behind. A systolic pressure >140 or a diastolic pressure >90 indicates hypertension. The relevance of BP to exercise training, heart surgery and manual hyperinflation is discussed in Chapters 9, 12, 16 and 18.

Normal **heart rate** at rest is 60–100 beats per minute. More than 100 bpm (breaths per minute) indicates tachycardia, which increases myocardial oxygen demand and may reflect sympathetic activity, hypoxaemia, hypotension, hypoglycaemia, dehydration, anxiety, pain or fever. Less than 60 bpm indicates bradycardia, which may indicate profound hypoxaemia, arrhythmias, heart block or vagal stimulation due to suctioning. Moderate bradycardia is normal during sleep and in the physically fit. Both tachycardia and bradycardia impair cardiac output.

Oximetry gives instant feedback on S_pO_2. The different absorption of light by saturated and unsaturated haemoglobin (Hb) is detected by a pulse oximeter, which displays the percentage of Hb saturated with oxygen. The sensor is attached close to a pulsating arteriolar bed on the ear, finger or toe. Adequate arterial oxygenation is indicated by 94% saturation (BTS 2008), and is interpreted in relation to the F_IO_2.

The relationship between S_pO_2 and arterial blood gases (ABGs) is in Fig 1.10 and Table 1.1. Oximetry becomes less accurate if Hb desaturates below 83% (NGC 2001). Other factors are: too much noise (motion or ambient light), too little signal (cold peripheries, anaemia, vasoconstriction, peripheral arterial disease, hypotension, hypovolaemia., hypothermia, nail polish or, for an ear probe, pierced ears). The delay between application and an accurate reading may be 30 seconds for a finger probe, and most probes have a light to indicate maximum pulsation. Gentle rubbing may be needed to encourage vasodilation.

ABGs may be required in the following situations:

- unreliable oximetry readings
- critically ill patients (Perkins 2003)
- if there is an unexplained drop in S_pO_2
- clinical signs of hypercapnia (p.19)
- breathless patients at risk of metabolic conditions such as diabetic ketoacidosis or renal failure.

In smokers, a fall in S_pO_2 during a 20-second breath-hold at end-exhalation may identify lung damage before symptoms become apparent (Inoue 2009).

The vital signs can be correlated (Table 2.1) by a 'track-and-trigger' system (Hammond et al 2013) or an electronic automated system (Bellomo 2012) to identify patients at risk.

Prescribed **drugs** and **oxygen** are documented on the prescription chart and their effects documented on the observation chart, e.g. peak flow or S_pO_2.

The **fluid** chart documents input and output. It should show a positive daily balance of about 500–1000 ml due to insensible loss from the skin and respiratory tract. There are many reasons for a wide variation in fluid balance, including ambient temperature and major fluid shifts after surgery.

Fluid overload might be accompanied by pulmonary oedema. Dehydration is accompanied by reduced urine output and may be caused by diuretics, laxatives, lack of thirst in old age, dementia, inability of a patient to reach or manage their drink or conscious fluid restriction due to anxiety about reaching the toilet. A urine colour chart can be used to assess patients at home or in residential care (Mentes et al 2006), but is only reliable for early morning specimens and if the colour has not been affected by medication

TABLE 2.1 Examples of a MEWS (Modified Early Warning Score) system for calling the outreach team

Vital sign	Patient at risk
Airway	Threatened airway, excessive secretions or stridor.
Breathing	RR < 8 or > 25 breaths/min.
Circulation	HR < 50 or > 150 beats/min. Systolic BP < 90 mmHg, > 200 mmHg, or drop of > 40 mmHg. BP below patient's normal values.
Consciousness	Sustained fall in Glasgow coma scale of > 2 in past hour.
Oxygen	S_pO_2 < 90% on > 50 F_iO_2.
Urine output	< 30 ml/hr for > 2 hours (unless normal for the patient).
General	Clinically causing concern. Not responding to treatment.

(Heneghan *et al* 2012). Table 2.2 shows the fluid balance of a healthy adult.

Dehydration predisposes to:

- sputum retention
- pressure sores
- constipation
- confusion, short-term memory loss and impaired cognition
- kidney dysfunction
- headache
- muscle cramps
- fatigue
- impaired motor control (Holdsworth 2012)
- exercise intolerance (Barr 1999).

Fluid loss from the vascular to the interstitial space is caused by altered hydrostatic or oncotic pressures, or increased capillary membrane permeability, leading to effective hypovolaemia.

Biochemistry

Urea and electrolytes

'U&Es' are the most frequent biochemistry tests. Below are those relevant to physiotherapy.

Sodium is the commonest electrolyte in the blood and is regulated by the kidney. Low levels (hyponatraemia) are due to fluid retention or inappropriate antidiuretic hormone (ADH) secretion, while high levels (hypernatraemia) indicate dehydration.

Potassium is the principal intracellular electrolyte. High or low values can weaken muscles including the diaphragm. Low levels (hypokalaemia) predispose to cardiac arrhythmias, and can be caused by respiratory alkalosis, loss from diarrhoea, vomiting or inappropriate steroids (Blann 2006 p. 62). High levels (hyperkalaemia) suggest acidosis or kidney failure and are the commonest electrolyte emergency, requiring insulin and glucose to force potassium back into cells.

TABLE 2.2 Sources of normal fluid gain and loss over 24 hours in a 70 kg male

Intake and innate production		Output	
Water via fluids	1500 ml	Urine	1500 ml
Water via food	500 ml	Evaporation from skin and lungs	800 ml
Water via metabolism	400 ml	Faeces	100 ml
Total	2400 ml	Total	2400 ml

Urea is formed from protein breakdown and is excreted by the kidneys. High levels are caused by renal failure due to kidney disease or impaired kidney perfusion from heart failure or shock. **Creatinine** is formed from muscle breakdown and is also renally excreted. Levels rise with kidney failure and drop with malnutrition. Both urea and creatinine rise with dehydration.

Albumin

This antioxidant is the main protein in plasma and the interstitium, providing 15% of the buffering capacity and 80% of the osmotic pressure of blood (Vincent 2001). Reduced levels, due to hypermetabolism, malnutrition, blood loss, liver or kidney problems, burns, ascites, chronic inflammation or critical illness, cause metabolic alkalosis and reduce osmotic pull from the vascular space so that fluid escapes, causing systemic and pulmonary oedema.

Microbiology

Micro-organisms are identified by culturing specimens, e.g. blood, sputum or pleural fluid, on various media which promote their growth. Most bacteria grow in 24–48 hours, but the tubercle bacillus may require six weeks. Sensitivity tests identify which antibiotics can then tackle the bacteria.

Haematology

A full blood count (FBC) analyzes the components of blood to assess blood cells and coagulation.

Red blood cells (erythrocytes) contain no nucleus so they can penetrate the smallest capillaries and are the most abundant cell in blood:

- Reduced haemoglobin indicates anaemia, which causes fatigue and is poorly tolerated in people with lung or heart disease. Mobilizing a patient with low Hb requires close attention to a patient's colour and the same precautions as for hypotension. A high concentration, known as polycythaemia, is the body's response to chronic hypoxaemia due to disease or living at high altitude.
- Haematocrit (packed cell volume) is the proportion of total blood volume that is composed of red cells. Red blood cell count provides the same information.
- Erythrocyte sedimentation rate (ESR) is raised following myocardial infarction or if there is inflammation, TB, cancer or anaemia.

White blood cells (leucocytes) are part of the immune system, working to ingest unwelcome microorganisms by phagocytosis. A raised white cell count (WCC) indicates infection or other condition such as cancer, rheumatoid arthritis or the postoperative state. Neutrophils are the commonest white cells and are raised with bacterial infection or inflammation. They become over-enthusiastic in sepsis and start to destroy healthy tissue as well as pathogens. Cytotoxic drugs reduce WCC (leukopaenia) e.g. with cancer or following transplant, indicating that the patient is immunocompromised and extra infection control precautions are required.

Clotting studies which indicate that a patient might bleed easily include low platelet count (thrombocytopaenia), prolonged prothrombin time or raised INR. Patients on heparin are at risk.

Cytology and histology

Cytology is the study of fluids to identify abnormal or cancerous cells, e.g. in sputum or blood. Histology does the same with tissues such as biopsied lung tissue.

Arterial blood gases

Arterial blood is usually taken from the radial artery by a doctor, as opposed to other blood tests in which blood is taken from a vein by the phlebotomist. Patients should be undisturbed and stay in the same position for 20 minutes beforehand. Interpretation is in Chapter 1.

SUBJECTIVE ASSESSMENT

Osler supposedly said, 'Listen to the patient. He is telling you the diagnosis', to which I would add 'And she just might be telling you the best management too'.
Pitkin 1998

The subjective assessment is what matters to the patient. Problems such as breathlessness are more closely related to quality of life than physiological measurements, and subjective wellbeing is associated with longevity (Xu & Roberts 2010).

When possible, patients are assessed in a well-lit area that is quiet, private, warm and well ventilated. Respect for privacy includes awareness of those within hearing.

> ## KEY POINT
>
> If a patient's curtain is drawn, it is equivalent to their front door and you need to knock.
>
> Beaven (2012)

The patient requires an explanation because the public perception of physiotherapy is often limited to football and backache.

The inequality of the relationship can be minimized by:

- positioning ourselves at eye level if possible
- addressing adults by their surname (Wilkins *et al* 2010, p. 12), unless they ask otherwise
- asking permission before assessment.

Permission not only encourages patients' self-respect, it is a legal necessity in most countries. It is also good practice to ask before moving a patient's personal items or opening their locker.

Patients are asked to define their problems and how these influence their life. Active listening from the physiotherapist requires 'sustained, vivid, stable, effortful and non-judgmental attention' (Halifax 2011). Empathy is facilitated by using the patient's words and phrases rather than our own. Acknowledging a patient's experience and respecting their opinion are also potent motivating factors.

Patient history

> *I know what my body is telling me.*
> Patient quoted by Morgan 2012

The history from the notes needs to be supplemented with questions about how the patient's condition is affecting their lifestyle, from which goals can be developed. Unreliability of recall may be caused by anxiety, according to Barsky (2002), who advises on the use of historical anchor points as memorable milestones, and

suggests that patients recall the most recent events first. History-taking is assisted by listening to patients' stories attentively, empathically and mindfully (Mohrmann 2012). If the patient is unable to give a history, relatives can be questioned, but there is usually some disparity between relatives' and patients' perception of their quality of life (Carr 2001).

Cardiorespiratory symptoms

How long have symptoms been troublesome? What is their frequency and duration, their quality and severity? Are they getting better or worse? What are aggravating and relieving factors?

Breathlessness

Shortness of breath (SOB), or dyspnoea, is the most common symptom in advanced cardiopulmonary disease (Booth *et al* 2008), but it can also be metabolic, neurogenic or neuromuscular in origin. Respiratory causes reflect excess work of breathing, which is abnormal if inappropriate to the level of physical activity. Significant SOB is indicated by inability to complete a full sentence. Visual analogue scales (Fig 2.1) and numeric rating scales are validated for SOB (Johnson *et al* 2010), or a key question at each visit can be a comparative measurement, e.g. how much they can do at their best or worst, or what they are unable to do now because of their breathing.

If SOB increases in supine it is called **orthopnoea**. In lung disease, this is caused by pressure on the diaphragm from the abdominal viscera. In heart failure, a poorly-functioning left ventricle is unable to tolerate the increased volume of blood returning to the heart in supine. **Paroxysmal nocturnal dyspnoea** (PND) is

---

FIGURE 2.1 Visual analogue scale for shortness of breath

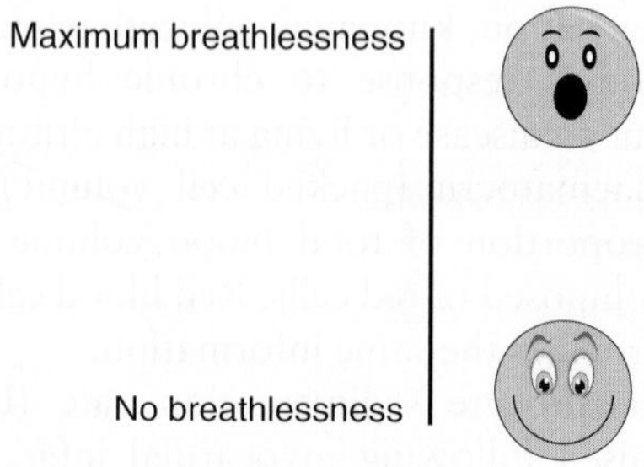

Maximum breathlessness

No breathlessness

caused by orthopnoeic patients sliding off their pillows during sleep, leading them to seek relief by sitting over the edge of the bed.

Distinguishing SOB due to lung or heart disorder is achieved by clinical reasoning using peak flow readings, auscultation, imaging, exercise testing and history. The quality of SOB can only be judged by the patient, typical descriptors being identified by Scano *et al* 2005, and specifically for heart failure by Parshall (2012). Patients may deny SOB if it has developed gradually, but they are likely to complain of its functional effects such as difficulty in getting upstairs, which underlines the relevance of the ICF approach. Detailed measurement of SOB is in Ch. 7. Table 2.3 indicates possible causes in relation to onset.

Cough

Coughing is abnormal if it is persistent, painful or productive of sputum. It may be underestimated by smokers and people who swallow their sputum. Acute cough is normally benign, self-limiting and commonly associated with upper respiratory tract infection. A post-viral dry cough is also benign but can continue for 3–8 weeks (Irwin *et al* 2006). Chronic cough (lasting more than eight weeks) is associated with disorders such as asthma, gastroesophageal reflux (GOR) (Fekri 2014), chronic obstructive pulmonary disease (COPD), bronchiectasis, interstitial lung disease, pleural effusion, heart failure, habit, Tourette's syndrome and some drugs.

> ## KEY POINT
>
> A cough should be reported if it is chronic and of unknown cause, or if it is accompanied by unexplained haemoptysis.

Serious conditions presenting as an isolated cough include cancer, TB or foreign body aspiration. A chronic cough is only considered idiopathic after assessment at a specialist cough clinic (Morice 2006).

Suggested questions relating to a cough are:

- What started it (e.g. infection)?
- What triggers it (e.g. smoking)?
- Is there sputum?
- Does the cough occur at night (GOR and/ or asthma)?
- Does it cause pain (see 'pleuritic pain', overleaf)?

Clinical reasoning can then be used, with the help of Table 2.4, to identify possible causes.

Chronic cough can cause musculoskeletal chest pains, sleep disturbance, a hoarse voice, vomiting, blackouts and sometimes social withdrawal or depression. It has been associated with urinary incontinence in 55% of women (Morice 2006).

A cough caused by asthma or GOR should disappear once the condition is controlled. A quarter of patients taking ACE inhibitor drugs develop a dry cough, which often disappears in 2–3 months (Li *et al* 2012). Other non-productive and habit coughs, such as those following viral infection, usually disappear over time, but dry coughs can perpetuate themselves by irritating the airways, in which case they can be controlled by the measures in Ch. 8.

The cough reflex can be over-sensitized by upper respiratory tract infection, mouth-breathing, GOR or irritants such as aerosols and cigarette smoke (Morice 2013).

Listening to the cough will help identify weakness and pick up sounds that may be missed on auscultation but stimulated by a cough. It is best to ask patients to show how they would cough to clear phlegm rather than to ask them to 'show me a cough'. Cough questionnaires include the Leicester Cough Questionnaires (Berkhof *et al* 2012) and those created by Murray *et al* (2009) and Polly (2008).

TABLE 2.3 Approximate time to the onset of dyspnoea

Immediate	Hours	Days or weeks	Months or years
Pneumothorax	Asthma	Pleural effusion	COPD
Pulmonary embolus	Pulmonary oedema	Lung cancer	Lung fibrosis
Foreign body aspiration	Chest infection		Heart failure
Myocardial infarct ⟶		Neuromuscular disorder ⟶	

TABLE 2.4 Characteristics of cough

Type of cough	Possible causes
Dry	Chronic asthma, ILD, pollutants, hyperventilation syndrome, airway irritation, ACE inhibitor drugs, viral infection
Productive	COPD, bronchiectasis, CF, PCD, acute asthma, chest infection
With position change	Asthma, bronchiectasis, CF, PCD, pulmonary oedema
With eating or drinking	Aspiration of stomach contents (e.g. with neurological disease or in elderly people)
With exertion	Asthma, COPD, ILD
Inadequate	Weakness, pain, poor understanding
Paroxysmal	Asthma, aspiration, upper airway obstruction, croup, whooping cough

ACE: angiotensin-converting enzyme, *CF:* cystic fibrosis, *ILD:* interstitial lung disease, *PCD:* primary ciliary dyskinesia

Secretions

Can the patient clear their secretions independently? If not, do they need advice or physical assistance? For acute patients, are secretions interfering with gas exchange? For patients with a chronic condition, are secretions impairing their lifestyle or contributing to a vicious circle that perpetuates hypersecretory disease (Ch. 8)? Has sputum changed in quality or quantity?

Wheeze

Airways narrowed by bronchospasm increase the work of breathing and may cause wheezing. The feeling should be explained to patients as tightness of the chest on breathing out, not just noisy, laboured or rattly breathing. If aggravated by exertion or allergic factors, asthma is a likely cause. Airways which are narrowed by factors other than bronchospasm may also cause a wheeze, but less consistently. Objectively, wheeze is confirmed by auscultation.

Other symptoms

Pain shares physiological mechanisms with SOB (Bentsen *et al* 2012). Chest pain may be musculoskeletal, cardiac, alimentary or respiratory in origin. Many patients associate chest pain with heart attacks, and anxiety may modify their perception and description of it. Lung parenchyma contains no pain fibres, but chest pains relevant to the physiotherapist are the following:

1 Pleuritic pain, which denotes the nature of the pain rather than the pathology. The pleura is replete with nerve endings, and pleuritic pain is sharp, stabbing and worse on deep breathing, coughing, hiccupping, talking and being moved. Causes include pleurisy, lobar pneumonia, pneumothorax, fractured ribs and pulmonary embolism.

2 Angina pectoris, a crushing chest pain due to myocardial ischaemia, which should be reported.

3 Musculoskeletal pain, e.g. costovertebral tenderness, which may be due to hyperinflation, when the muscles are obliged to work inefficiently, or chronic coughing, which may cause muscle strain.

4 Raw central chest pain, worse on coughing, caused by tracheitis and associated with upper respiratory tract infection or excessive coughing.

5 Bronchiectasis pain, which is a deep ache localized to areas of inflammation.

Musculoskeletal pain around the neck or shoulders may interfere with the accessory muscles of respiration. Postoperative pain is discussed in Ch. 16.

Fatigue is a common and often wretched symptom, closely associated with SOB and depression (Radbruch 2008). Patients may prefer to say that they are tired rather than admit to depression, which can be stigmatizing. The word 'fatigue' is not found in all languages, in which case the word 'weakness' can be used for the physical dimension and 'tiredness' for the cognitive dimension. Cognitive fatigue complicates activities such as reading, driving and other activities of daily living.

The sensation fits all domains of the ICF and is characteristic of many chronic conditions which may overlap, including COPD, heart failure, cancer and neurological conditions. Causes include inflammation, anaemia, infection, stress, dehydration, cachexia or sedatives (Radbruch 2008). Fatigue is severe if it cannot be relieved by rest or sleep.

Fatigue and weakness feel similar but may require opposite management strategies, e.g. exercise for weakness and rest for acute fatigue. However, many patients have both and require energy conservation, pacing and graded exercise.

If a patient is not able to describe the sensation, it is noteworthy that carers may overestimate and staff may underestimate its severity (Radbruch 2008). Visual analogue scales fail to assess the impact of fatigue on daily functioning, and valid measurements are in App. C or described by Butt *et al* (2013). Exhaustion is at the end of the fatigue continuum and if accompanied by ventilatory failure may indicate the need for non-invasive ventilation.

Sleep may be impaired by anxiety, SOB, a noisy environment, loss of day/night rhythm, pain or depression. **Appetite** may be impaired by depression, feeling ill, hospital food or the side effects of drugs.

Dizziness may be associated with postural hypotension, hyperventilation syndrome or a lesion of the 8th cranial nerve or brain stem. A history of **falls** may be caused by the factors in Ch. 14. **Fainting** (syncope) or near-fainting may be caused by hyperventilation syndrome, prolonged coughing or cardiovascular disorder.

KEY POINT

If the patient spends the day flopped in front of the TV, is this because of preference, exercise limitation or depression?

How does the patient feel about the disease? This question provides the opportunity for patients to describe their feelings but does not pressurize them. **Anxiety** affects the neural processing of respiratory sensations, which may underlie the increased perception of respiratory sensations in anxious individuals

(Leupoldt *et al* 2012), particularly if symptoms are unpredictable. Anxiety may reinforce other distressing factors such as frustration, embarrassment, restricted social function and loss of control.

It is useful to adopt the practice of asking patients what they think is the cause of their symptoms because their perceptions are often surprisingly accurate. People in some cultures may express emotions in terms of bodily sensations.

Activities of daily living (ADL)

Many patients express a desire for quality of life equal to or greater than their desire for quantity of life.

O'Neil *et al* 2013

Is it difficult to bathe, dress or shop? How much daily exercise does the patient take? Reduced mobility can lead to constipation, which is exacerbated by dehydration, and to urinary incontinence, which is exacerbated by coughing.

Limitation of activity is not an accurate indicator of cardiorespiratory disease because patients gradually reduce their ADL as they experience slowly-increasing breathlessness, fatigue or weakness, thus perpetuating a vicious cycle. But questions can be asked such as 'what have you stopped doing because of your breathing'?

How many stairs are there at work or home? Is the environment well-heated, smoky, dusty? Does the patient live alone, smoke, eat well? Is nutrition affected by dyspnoea or dysphagia? What support is available? Problems with personal care, employment, finance and housing loom large for people with cardiorespiratory disease.

The subjective assessment, particularly the functional element, is usually the basis of realistic goal-setting, which should be patient-led and regularly reviewed. Goals and family involvement help to ensure that the ICF approach is maintained. Measures of physical functioning are more related to quality of life than spirometry (Geijer *et al* 2007) and questionnaires are described in the relevant chapters.

OBSERVATION

Any part of the body not being observed should be kept covered throughout, with awareness of the needs of different cultures (Wilson *et al* 2012).

Breathing pattern

The breathing pattern should be observed while approaching the patient because it will change once they are aware of the physiotherapist's presence. Normal breathing is rhythmic, with active inspiration, passive expiration and an inspiratory to expiratory (I:E) ratio of about 1:2. There should be synchrony between chest and abdominal movement, but a relaxed person may show only abdominal movement. Individual variations achieve the same minute volume by different combinations of rate and depth or varied chest and abdominal movements.

Laboured breathing may be unavoidable, but increases the work of breathing (WOB), e.g.:

- forced exhalation with active contraction of the abdominal muscles to propel air out through narrowed airways
- obvious accessory muscle contraction (Fig 2.2)
- indrawing/recession/retraction of the soft tissues of the chest wall on inspiration (Fig 2.3), caused by excess negative pressure in the chest which sucks in supraclavicular, suprasternal and intercostal spaces, thus destabilizing the chest wall and further increasing the WOB.

Paradoxical breathing also increases WOB, e.g.:

- indrawing of soft tissues (as above)
- Hoover's sign, which occurs in a hyperinflated chest when the flattened diaphragm pulls in the lower ribs on inspiration, becoming in effect an expiratory muscle
- flail chest due to rib fractures (Ch. 19)
- abdominal paradox, in which a weak or fatigued diaphragm is sucked up into the chest by negative pressure generated during inspiration so that the abdomen is sucked in (Fig 2.4) instead of swelling outwards. Palpation distinguishes this from active abdominal muscle contraction. It is associated with poor exercise tolerance (Chien *et al* 2013) either because it indicates advanced disease or because energy is wasted on the inefficient breathing pattern.

The following may indicate inspiratory muscle fatigue, weakness and/or overload:

- abdominal paradox, as above
- ↑ RR

FIGURE 2.2 Soft tissues draped over the bones and prominent sternomastoid muscles, indicating malnutrition and muscle hypertrophy.

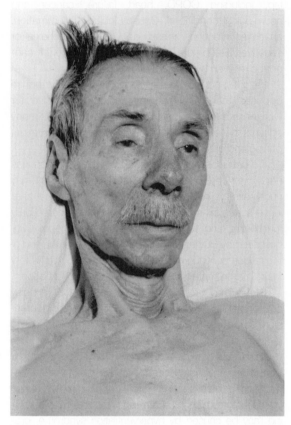

- ↓ P_aCO_2, ↑ pH (alkalosis)
- shallow breathing, which reduces elastic loading
- less commonly, alternation between abdominal and ribcage movement so that each muscle group can rest in turn, similar to shifting a heavy bag between arms.

Exhaustion, indicating that the patient requires mechanical assistance, is evident by:

- ↓ RR
- ↑ P_aCO_2, ↓ pH (acidosis).

Periods of apnoea interspersed with waxing and waning of the rate and depth of breathing are called Cheyne-Stokes breathing when regular or **Biot's** breathing when irregular. These indicate neurological damage, but Cheyne-Stokes breathing is also associated with heart

FIGURE 2.3 Indrawing of the soft tissues between the ribs due to extra work of breathing during inspiration.

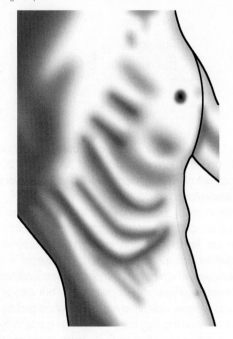

FIGURE 2.4 Paradoxical inward movement of the abdomen on inspiration due to weakness or fatigue of the diaphragm.

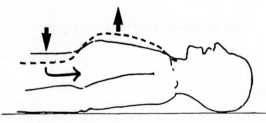

failure (Olson 2014), or it may be normal in some elderly people.

Irregular breathing indicates tension or may occur during normal rapid eye movement sleep. **Sighs** may indicate hyperventilation syndrome.

General appearance

Is the patient obese, thus compromising diaphragmatic function, or cachectic, indicating poor nutrition and weakness? If the patient is unkempt, does this reflect difficulty with self care or a measure of how disease has affected self esteem? Is the patient restless or incoherent, possibly due to hypoxia?

Does the posture suggest fatigue, pain, altered consciousness or respiratory distress? Breathless people characteristically brace their arms so that their shoulder girdle muscles can work unhindered as accessory muscles of respiration. For mobile patients, gait gives an indication of mood, balance, co-ordination and dyspnoea.

Confusion

Clinical reasoning helps to identify which of the following could be triggering confusion:

- hypoxia
- hypercapnia
- infection
- pain
- polypharmacy
- poor sleep
- fatigue
- constipation
- depressive illness
- sensory deficit
- disorientation, e.g. from 'relocation stress'
- dementia
- dehydration or electrolyte imbalance.

A notorious case occurred in the UK in 2009 when a young man became confused from dehydration, was sedated, and subsequently died from the dehydration.

Respiratory rate

Average RR is 12–16 breaths/minute (bpm) but there is a wide adult range of 10–20, and a full minute's count is required for accuracy.

A rate below 8 bpm increases P_aCO_2 and may lead to respiratory acidosis. Above 40 bpm (tachypnoea) blows off P_aCO_2, sometimes leading to respiratory alkalosis, and increasing WOB because of the extra turbulence. Rapid breathing is inefficient and if combined with shallow breathing increases dead space so that breathless patients can also be acidotic. Table 2.5 outlines abnormalities.

Chest shape

The chest and abdomen should be as visible for observation as the patient feels comfortable with. The chest

TABLE 2.5 Causes of abnormal respiratory rate

↑ RR	↓ RR
Lung or heart disease	Drug overdose
Inspiratory muscle fatigue or weakness	Exhaustion
Brain injury	Brain injury
Anaemia	Diabetic coma
Pain, nausea, anxiety or fever	
Pulmonary embolism or pneumothorax	

should be mobile and normally inflated (Fig 2.5). Obstructive lung disease can hyperinflate the chest by increasing its anteroposterior diameter (Fig 2.6). Hyperinflation may assist in keeping obstructed airways open, but at the cost of increased WOB.

Other abnormalities of the chest wall may increase WOB, e.g. a restrictive defect can be caused by kyphoscoliosis. Rarer conditions are pigeon chest (pectus carinatum) which protrudes the sternum, and funnel chest (pectus excavatum) (Binazzia 2012) which depresses the sternum; these rarely restrict lung function but occasionally require surgery (Schewitz 2013).

Colour

Pallor is associated with anaemia, reduced cardiac output or hypovolaemic shock. A **plethoric** appearance is a florid colour indicating polycythaemia. Haemoglobin is red when saturated with oxygen, but desaturation turns it blue, leading to a dusky blue colour of the skin known as **cyanosis**, best appreciated under fluorescent lighting (McMullen 2013). Causes are circulatory disorder for peripheral cyanosis and respiratory disorder for central cyanosis.

Peripheral cyanosis shows at the fingers, toes and ear lobes, and indicates stagnant blood which has given up its oxygen and is not being replenished. Causes include peripheral arterial disease or a cold environment which causes peripheral vasoconstriction.

Central cyanosis shows peripherally but also at the lips and tongue, indicating a gas exchange problem. It is a useful warning sign but an unreliable guide to hypoxaemia, being identified at S_pO_2 levels that vary from 72% to 95% (Martin 1990). Its detection depends not just on haemoglobin in the blood, but also on skin pigmentation and patency of vessels. It can be masked by anaemia or exaggerated by polycythaemia.

> *When the lips are blue the brain is too*
> Clapham 2005

FIGURE 2.5 (a) normal chest shape with (b) domed diaphragm and oblique ribs

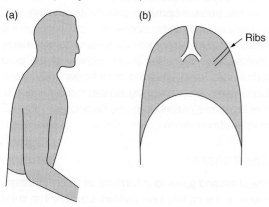

Hands

The hands are a rich source of information. Poor cardiac output causes cold hands. CO_2 retention is indicated by warm hands due to peripheral vasodilation, plus a coarse flapping tremor of the outstretched hands which disappears when the hands drop to the patient's side. A fine tremor may be a side effect of bronchodilator drugs, particularly in the elderly. For patients who are unable to give a smoking history, nicotine stains provide irrefutable evidence of the deadly habit.

Finger clubbing is a reduced angle between the nail and nail bed, developing into bulbous enlargement of the ends of the fingers, or in extreme cases a drumstick appearance (Fig 2.7), possibly related to endothelial

FIGURE 2.6 (a) hyperinflated, barrel-shaped and rigid chest with (b) flat diaphragm and horizontal ribs

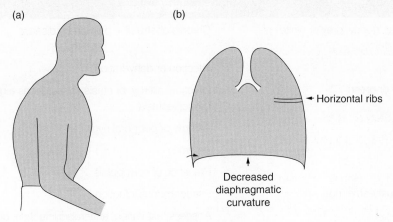

(a)   (b)

Horizontal ribs

Decreased
diaphragmatic
curvature

growth factor (Sarkar *et al* 2012). Causes are (Jefferies & Turley 1999 p. 117):

- pulmonary: 75%
- cardiac: 10%
- liver or gut: 10%
- other, e.g. thyroid disease or laxative abuse: 5%.

Pulmonary causes include fibrosing alveolitis and suppurative disorders such as bronchiectasis, cystic fibrosis, empyema or abscess. Clubbing is of supreme disinterest to the physiotherapist because it is not affected by physiotherapy, but it should be reported if it appears unexpectedly in a smoker because it may be the first sign of lung cancer (Rutherford 2013).

FIGURE 2.7 Clubbed fingers

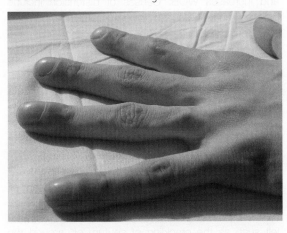

Oedema

Oedema is excess fluid in interstitial spaces. Peripheral oedema accumulates around the ankles or sacral area, depending on posture, and is usually caused by kidney, liver or cardiorespiratory disease such as COPD or heart failure.

Sputum

Sputum is mucus that has been expectorated. It is always abnormal because bronchial secretions are swallowed in healthy people. Characteristics are in Table 2.6.

Haemoptysis is expectoration of sputum containing blood, which can be an alarming experience for patients who see TV dramas in which coughing up blood is followed by instant death. Haemoptysis varies from slight streaking to frank bleeding. It is bright red if fresh, pink if mixed with sputum, or rusty brown if it is old blood. Causes are:

- bronchiectasis (intermittent, fresh)
- lung cancer (persistent)
- pulmonary tuberculosis (intermittent)
- lung abscess (copious)
- pneumococcal pneumonia (rusty red)
- pulmonary oedema (frothy, and pink or white)
- pulmonary embolus (bright red)
- blood clotting abnormality (fresh)
- trauma such as intubation, tracheostomy, lung contusion or frequent/rough tracheal suction (fresh).

Haematemesis occurs when blood is vomited, and it may be confused with haemoptysis. It is more likely to be

TABLE 2.6 Characteristics of sputum

Appearance	Possible causes
Mucoid, i.e. clear, gooey, grey or white (like raw egg white)	Chronic obstructive pulmonary disease
Thick	Infection or dehydration
Purulent, yellow or green	Infection, allergy, or stasis of secretions e.g. neglected bronchiectasis
Stringy	Asthma or poor oral hygiene
Plugs	Asthma
Green or yellow	Presence of eosinophils
Thick, green, musty-smelling	Pseudomonas infection
Smelly	Abscess, aspiration, anaerobic infection, bronchiectasis
Frothy (mixed with air) and sometimes pink (blood squeezed into alveoli)	Pulmonary oedema
Containing blood	see Haemoptysis, previous page

mixed with food than with mucus, and is distinguished by acidity and a dark brown colour which resembles coffee grounds. It may be associated with melaena (digested blood passed per rectum) or nausea. Careful questioning is needed to identify whether expectorated blood has been swallowed and vomited, or if vomited blood has been aspirated and expectorated.

Green or yellow samples were most likely to contain bacteria (Miravitlles *et al* 2012), but if secretions are not cream, white or clear (Johnson *et al* 2008), a sputum specimen may be sent for culture to identify the pathogen responsible for a likely chest infection so that an accurate antibiotic can be given. Eosinophils or neutrophils can also be identified, which indicate allergy or inflammation respectively, and occasionally some cancers may be identified (Yu *et al* 2010).

Most specimens have low sensitivity and specificity because of contamination with upper respiratory organisms (Kang & Kim 2012), but this can be minimized by patients blowing their nose, rinsing their mouth and spitting out saliva before expectorating. For patients who require suction, a sterile mucous trap is incorporated into the circuit. This should be kept upright during suction to prevent the specimen bypassing the trap.

Table 2.7 helps distinguish sputum and pulmonary oedema.

If a specimen cannot be produced by chest clearance and coughing or suction, or if specimens are required from the lower respiratory tract, for example to identify inflammation, sputum induction using hypertonic saline can be used to facilitate the production of a specimen (App. C)

PALPATION

Abdomen

The abdomen enjoys a close relationship with the diaphragm. After obtaining permission it should be palpated at every assessment. A distended abdomen inhibits diaphragmatic movement, restricts lung volume and increases WOB. Causes of distension include pain and guarding spasm, obesity, flatulence, paralytic ileus, enlarged liver, ascites, acute pancreatitis and constipation.

Chest expansion

Chest movement reflects lung expansion. The patient sits over the edge of the bed if possible and their chest observed or palpated from behind as they take a deep breath (Fig 2.8), unequal expansion suggesting loss of lung volume.

While palpating for expansion, other signs may be felt such as the crackling of sputum or, around the

TABLE 2.7 Comparative signs of excess bronchial secretions and pulmonary oedema secretions

	Bronchial secretions	Pulmonary oedema
History	Lung disease or chest infection	Heart disease (may be secondary to lung disease)
Temperature	May be raised	Normal
Fluid balance	Normal	Fluid retention usually
Crackles (heard at the mouth or by auscultation)	Patchy	Bilateral, late inspiratory, dependent
Cough	Caused by secretions, productive	Caused by irritation of lung receptors, usually dry
Secretions if present	Mucoid or purulent	Frothy, white or pink
Clearance of secretions	Cough or suction	Diuretics
Radiology	Normal, or related to lung disease	Bilateral hilar flare, often enlarged heart, sometimes pleural effusion
Albumin	Normal	May be reduced

neck and upper chest, the popping of subcutaneous emphysema which feels like Rice Krispies under the skin.

Percussion note

The percussion note (PN) is elicited by tapping the chest wall with a stiff curved finger from the dominant hand onto a finger from the other hand placed flat on the patient's chest (Fig 2.9). To avoid dampening the sound, the dominant finger should recoil sharply, like a woodpecker striking a tree. All the movement is in the wrist.

The PN evaluates the density of underlying tissue to a depth of 5–7cm (Wilkins *et al* 2010, p. 79). It is useful

FIGURE 2.9 Eliciting a percussion note. One finger is placed firmly along an intercostal space and this finger is struck by a finger of the opposite hand

FIGURE 2.8 Palpation for rib cage expansion. The fingers hold the sides of the chest and the thumbs rest lightly on each side of the spine. On inspiration, symmetrical separation of the thumb tips indicates equal chest expansion

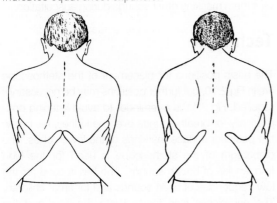

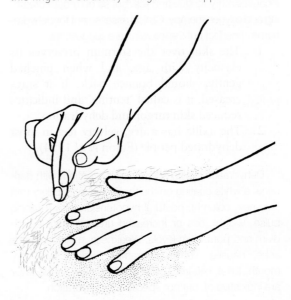

for confirming breath sounds, and is especially helpful if patients are unable to take a deep breath or if breath sounds are obscured by a noisy environment or loud wheezy crackles. Each side of the chest should be percussed alternately for comparison, remembering that the upper lobe predominates anteriorly and the lower lobe posteriorly (Fig 2.11).

The PN is **resonant** over normal lung tissue. **Hyperresonance** indicates excess air, as with hyperinflation or a large pneumothorax. A **stony dull** note is unmistakable and heard over a pleural effusion larger than 500 ml. However, both these conditions are detected radiologically unless the patient is supine. Most useful to the physiotherapist is the **dull** note of atelectasis or consolidation, in which the air that should be in the lung is replaced by solid (albeit squashy) tissue.

Hydration

The 1500 ml fluid intake that is normally required per day may not be achieved by people who are ill or in an unfamiliar environment. Patients at risk are:

- elderly people
- those who feel too sick to drink
- some who are not on intravenous fluids
- those who are constipated or pyrexial.

A patient who has heart failure and does not have swollen ankles should be closely examined for dehydration.

Dehydration causes inelastic skin, but so does ageing; it causes a dry tongue and lips, but so do mouth breathing and oxygen therapy. Clinical assessment for dehydration is imperfect but the following are suggestions:

1. The skin over the sternum preserves its elasticity with age, and when pinched gently, should bounce back. If it stays creased, it is called 'tenting' and indicates reduced skin turgor and dehydration.
2. The axilla has a dry, velvety feel in most dehydrated people (Eaton *et al* 1994).

Dehydration is also suspected in a patient with dark urine, a white coating on the tongue, slow capillary refill (see next column), postural hypotension with a racing pulse, weight loss or increased urea, creatinine, sodium and potassium levels. Weakness, malaise, headache, nausea, vomiting, cramps, weight loss, dry mouth, thirst, oliguria, tachycardia and low-grade fever are indicative of, but not specific to, dehydration.

Trachea

Tracheal deviation is detected by gentle palpation in the suprasternal notch. In the absence of thyroid enlargement, deviation is due to a shift of the mediastinum away from a large pleural effusion or tension pneumothorax, or a shift towards upper lobe atelectasis or fibrosis, which can be confirmed radiologically (see Fig 2.16). A hyperinflated chest causes a **tracheal tug**, which is descent of the trachea on inspiration.

Capillary refill time

With good circulation, pressing briefly on the nail or pulp of a finger to obstruct the circulation is followed by rapid return of normal colour. If this capillary refill is >2 seconds, reduced cardiac output or hypovolaemia is suspected.

Tactile vocal fremitus

A hand flat on the chest can feel the vibration of the voice, which is the palpatory equivalent of vocal resonance (p.52).

AUSCULTATION

Auscultation is used to verify observed and palpated findings before and after treatment. Prior to reaching for the stethoscope, it is worth listening for sounds at the mouth, which are just audible in a person with normal lungs. Noisy breathing indicates airflow turbulence due to obstructed upper airways. Crackles heard at the mouth should be cleared by coughing in order to prevent them masking other sounds during auscultation.

Technique

The basic positions for placement of the stethoscope are in Fig 2.10, but further positions may be necessary if required. Fig 2.11 is a reminder to avoid listening optimistically for breath sounds over the kidney, i.e. below the posterior surface markings of the lower lobes. The diaphragm of the stethoscope is used for the high frequencies of breath sounds. The bell is used for the low frequencies of heart sounds and for small children. The ear pieces face forward into the ears and the

FIGURE 2.10 Locations for stethoscope placement

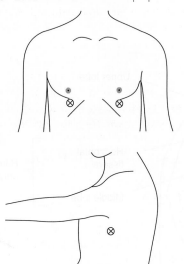

diaphragm is pressed firmly on the skin to reduce extraneous sounds including the rustle of chest hair. The patient is asked to breathe steadily in and out through the mouth. Each area of lung is compared on alternate sides, asymmetrical sounds usually indicating pathology.

The patient is best positioned sitting upright over the edge of the bed with arms forward to protract the scapulae and the physiotherapist standing behind. A compromise is with the patient in bed leaning forward from long-sitting, but this position compresses the lung bases so that breath sounds over this important area may be indecipherable. In patients who cannot sit up, side-lying may be used, with allowance for sounds from the underneath lung usually being quieter. The diaphragm of the stethoscope should be cleaned between patients.

Breath sounds

Breath sound intensity indicates regional ventilation or factors which affect the transmission of the sound. Breath sounds are generated by turbulent airflow in the large airways and then transmitted through air, liquid and solid to the chest wall, each medium attenuating the sound to a different degree. Sounds at the surface are filtered versions of those in the trachea and central airways. Sounds are not generated beyond lobar or segmental bronchi because the total cross-sectional area is too wide to create turbulence (see Fig 1.3).

The term 'breath sounds' is more accurate than 'air entry' because air may enter the lung but the transmission of sound can be affected by pathology. Breath sounds may be normal, abnormal or diminished.

Normal breath sounds are muffled because air in the alveoli is a poor conductor of sound. They are quieter in the base than the apex because the greater volume in the lung bases filters the sound further. Inspiration is louder than expiration because of turbulence created by airway bifurcations (Fig 2.12).

PRACTICE TIP

If the patient is unable to take a deep enough breath, the deep breathing following exertion can be utilized by listening immediately after the patient has talked, coughed, turned or been suctioned.

Bronchial breathing is an abnormal sound that is distinguished by a hollow blowing quality on expiration and a pause between inspiration and expiration. It indicates loss of functioning lung volume and is heard over the following:

- consolidation, which acts acoustically like a lump of meat in the lung, the solid medium transmitting sounds more clearly than an air-filled lung (Fig 2.13)
- small area of collapse, i.e. there is a patent airway to transmit the sound, but it then

FIGURE 2.11 Lateral and posterior views of the lobes and fissures of the lungs

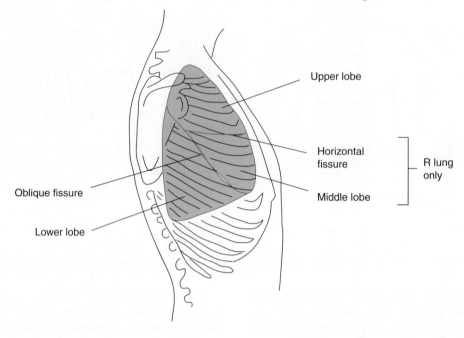

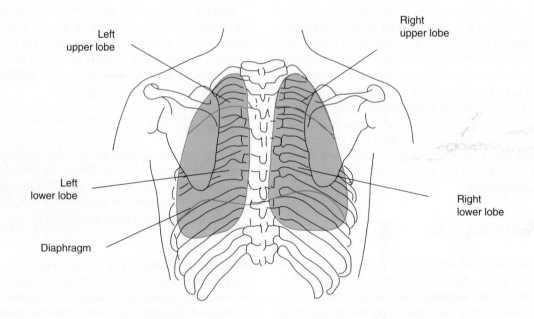

has to pass through collapsed lung tissue before reaching the surface

- above a pleural effusion because the compressed lung increases sound transmission (Sapira 1995).

Diminished breath sounds are heard if:

- the patient is obese, in a poor position or not breathing deeply
- there is no air entry to generate the sound, e.g. a larger area of collapse than that

FIGURE 2.12 Turbulence at airway bifurcation creating noisier sounds on inspiration than expiration

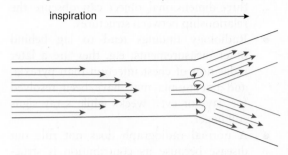

causing bronchial breathing, with an occluded airway
- there is air entry but transmission of the sound is blocked by an acoustic barrier such as the air/solid or air/liquid interface of a pneumothorax or pleural effusion (Fig 2.13)
- there is air entry but excess air in the lung filters the sound, e.g. hyperinflation as in emphysema or acute asthma.

Inaudible breath sounds over the chest of a person with acute asthma are a danger sign (Ch. 3).

Added sounds

Added sounds are superimposed on breath sounds. They are sometimes more obvious and can mask breath sounds. Non-respiratory sounds occur independent of

FIGURE 2.13 Mechanism of the creation of different breath sounds. *BS:* breath sounds

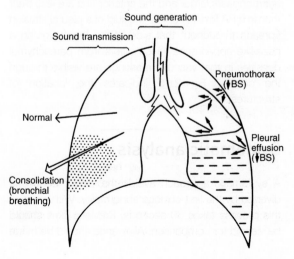

the breathing cycle and may be transmitted from the abdomen, the patient's voice, or the environment.

PRACTICE TIP

If added sounds are louder on one side, this may be due to increased added sounds on this side, or reduced breath sounds through which to hear the added sounds on the other side.

Crackles indicate secretions or parenchymal disorders such as pneumonia, fibrosis or pulmonary oedema (Vyshedskiy *et al* 2011). They are created when air is forced through airways which have been narrowed by excess secretions or pulmonary oedema fluid that has migrated up from the alveoli, or when collapsed airways snap open (Majumdar *et al* 2009). They are principally heard on inspiration, and their timing depends on the source. As a generalization:
- early-inspiratory crackles arise in the large airways, are sometimes heard at the mouth and are often heard with COPD
- early and mid-inspiratory crackles are characteristic of bronchiectasis or cystic fibrosis
- late-inspiratory crackles originate in alveoli and peripheral airways as they open at the end of inspiration; they are associated with pneumonia, fibrosis or pulmonary oedema.

The weight of the lung itself causes a degree of airway closure so that late-inspiratory crackles may be heard in dependent regions, especially in elderly obese people who have been recumbent for some time. Late-inspiratory crackles are sometimes called fine crackles, dry crackles, velcro crackles or crepitations. Crackles are heard predominantly on inspiration, but both inspiratory and expiratory crackles are heard in bronchiectasis (coarse) and fibrosing alveolitis (fine). Absence of coarse crackles does not always indicate absence of secretions (Jones & Jones 2000).

Wheezes are generated by the vibration of narrowed airways as air rushes through. Expiratory wheeze, combined with prolonged expiration, is usually caused by bronchospasm. Wheeze on inspiration and expiration can be caused by inflammation, pulmonary oedema, bronchial secretions, tumours or foreign bodies. These are termed polyphonic wheezes. A monophonic (single note) wheeze denotes upper airway obstruction from a foreign body or tumour. It is greater on inspiration and is also heard without a stethoscope.

Stridor is an inspiratory strangled sound that can also be heard without a stethoscope. It denotes laryngeal or tracheal narrowing to a diameter of just 5 mm (Thomas & Manara 1998) and a warning that nasopharyngeal suction should be avoided and the patient's head kept elevated to minimize oedema. Treatment of stridor is by steroids, Heliox (p.157) or stenting.

A **pleural rub** occurs in pleurisy, when the roughened inflamed pleural surfaces rub on each other and produce a sound similar to boots crunching on snow. It is localized to the affected area, but may be heard best over the lower lobes because excursion of the pleura is greater basally.

Voice sounds

The vibrations of speech can be felt by the hands (tactile vocal fremitus), or heard through the stethoscope (vocal resonance). The patient is asked to say '99' or engaged in conversation.

Voice sounds are normally an unintelligible mumble because vowels are filtered through air-filled lungs. **Increased voice sounds** create a clearer sound, heard when it is transmitted through a denser medium, e.g. consolidation, or atelectasis with a patent airway. This is usually associated with bronchial breathing and is sometimes known as bronchophony. Voice sounds transmitted above the liquid/air interface at the top of a pleural effusion have a characteristic nasal bleating quality, a slightly different form of increased vocal resonance called aegophony.

Reduced voice sounds are heard when there is a pneumothorax, pleural effusion or atelectasis with a blocked airway. Voice sounds tend to follow the breath sounds, i.e. they increase with bronchial breathing and decrease with quiet breath sounds.

Another confirmatory test is to ask the patient to whisper '99'. Over normal lung tissue, whispered words are barely audible, but through a solid medium such as consolidation, individual syllables are recognizable. This is known as **whispering pectoriloquy.**

IMAGING

AP: *anteroposterior*
PA: *posteroanterior*
L: *left,* **R:** *right,*
LL: *lower lobe,* **UL:** *upper lobe*

The chest radiograph provides a unique insight into the lungs and chest wall, but it has limitations:

- A two-dimensional representation of a three-dimensional object can obscure the relationship between structures.
- Radiology findings tend to lag behind other measurements, e.g. they are a later indication of chest infection than pyrexia, and pneumonia may have been resolved for days or even weeks while x-ray signs still linger.
- A normal radiograph does not rule out disease because its contribution is structural only, e.g. the physical damage of emphysema is more apparent than the hypersecretion of chronic bronchitis because secretions do not normally show on x-ray.

If possible, a PA view is taken, in which the beam is directed from the back, the patient standing up and taking a deep breath with shoulders abducted so that the scapulae do not obscure the lungs. The posterior ribs are clearly visible but become more obscure anteriorly (Fig 2.14). In the erect position a pneumothorax is easier to detect because gas passes upwards, and the fluid of a pleural effusion is visible as a fluid line.

An **AP** film is used when it is unsafe for patients to go to the radiology department due to immobility or impaired immunity. Patients sit up ('erect portable') or lie down, and a portable machine sends the rays from front to back. The patient may not be able to raise their arms or take a deep breath, leaving the lung fields partly obscured by the scapulae and diaphragm. The heart appears larger and the anterior ribs are less clear than in a PA film. In supine, the fluid of a pleural effusion spreads throughout that side of the thorax, giving a haze-like appearance which differs from parenchymal densities in that vascular markings are visible through the density. Fig 2.15 indicates the location of structures.

Systematic analysis

A systematic approach avoids the viewer becoming diverted by the first obvious abnormality. With practice this process takes 30 seconds. Previous films should be viewed for comparison. Allowance should be made

FIGURE 2.14 Normal PA film

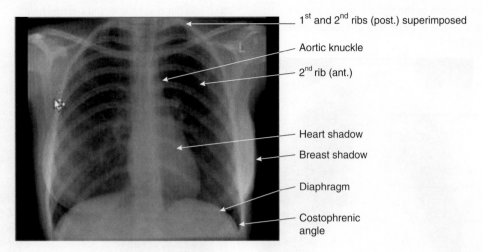

- 1st and 2nd ribs (post.) superimposed
- Aortic knuckle
- 2nd rib (ant.)
- Heart shadow
- Breast shadow
- Diaphragm
- Costophrenic angle

for normal variations between individuals such as different shaped diaphragms. Chest films show bilateral symmetry for many structures, enabling opposite sides to be compared.

Abnormalities can be classified into whether they are:

- too white
- too black
- too big
- in the wrong place (Corne & Pointon 2010).

Dense structures absorb rays and are opaque, with air having low density and appearing black.

FIGURE 2.15 Structures on PA film

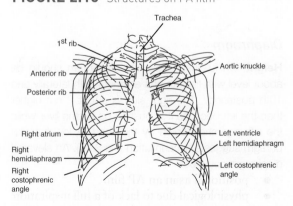

Trachea, 1st rib, Anterior rib, Posterior rib, Right atrium, Right hemidiaphragm, Right costophrenic angle, Aortic knuckle, Left ventricle, Left hemidiaphragm, Left costophrenic angle

Preliminary checks

The patient's **name** and the **date** should be noted. Then the **projection** is checked to see whether it is a PA or AP film. The **exposure** is then noted: an overexposed film appears too black and low density lesions can be missed, while an underexposed film appears falsely white. Correct exposure allows vertebral bodies to be visible through the upper but not the lower heart shadow.

Symmetry is correct if the spinous processes, which appear as tear-drop shapes down the spine, are midway between the medial ends of the clavicles. This check avoids misinterpretation about displacement of the heart, which is at the front of the chest so that if the patient is rotated to either side, the heart shadow appears shifted towards that side.

Trachea

The dark column of air overlying the upper vertebrae represents the trachea, which is in the midline down to the clavicles, then displaced slightly to the right by the aortic arch, before branching into the main bronchi. Abnormal deviation occurs if it is pushed, for example by a tumour, or pulled, for example by atelectasis or fibrosis (Fig 2.16).

Heart

The heart is sandwiched between the lungs and is the main occupant of the mediastinum. Points to note are:

FIGURE 2.16 Fibrosis in the R upper lobe pulling the trachea to the right. Fibrosis and an abscess are visible in the R mid and lower zones. The patient has TB

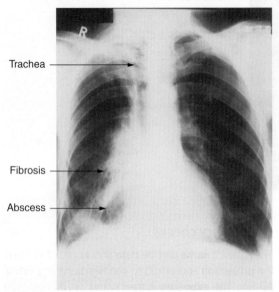

Trachea

Fibrosis

Abscess

FIGURE 2.17 Hyperinflated chest as indicated by a low flat diaphragm and narrow heart

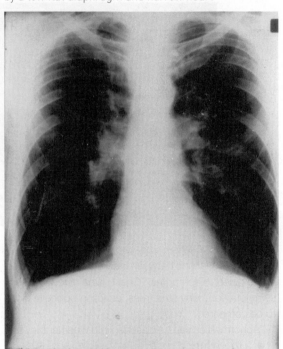

Size. The transverse diameter is normally less than half the internal diameter of the chest in a PA film. An apparently big heart could be due to ventricular enlargement, a PA film or poor inspiratory effort. A narrow heart is caused by hyperinflation, when the diaphragm pulls down the mediastinum (Fig 2.17), or it may be normal in tall thin people.

Shape. In right ventricular hypertrophy, the heart is enlarged and boot-shaped. A rounded heart might indicate pericardial effusion.

Position. The heart normally extends slightly left of midline. If displaced, it is pushed away from a large pleural effusion (Fig 2.18), empyema or tension pneumothorax (Ch. 18), and pulled towards a significant unilateral collapse (Fig 2.19), resection (see Fig 16.13) or fibrosis (Fig 2.16).

Borders. These are obscured (silhouette sign) if there is a lesion abutting the heart, e.g. middle lobe consolidation or collapse. Apposition of dense lung tissue with a contiguous structure such as the diaphragm or heart obliterates the boundary between the two.

Hila

Blood and lymph vessels make up the hilar shadows, the left being slightly higher because of the heart. Hila are abnormally pulled up if there is UL fibrosis, atelectasis or lobectomy, and pulled down by LL atelectasis. Ring shadows near the hilum are normal large airways seen in cross-section. Bilateral enlargement of hilar shadows could be due to pulmonary hypertension. Unilateral enlargement raises suspicions of malignancy.

Diaphragm

Height. On full inspiration, the diaphragm should be about level with the 6th ribs anteriorly, 8th laterally and 10th posteriorly. The right side is about 2 cm higher than the left because it is pushed up by the liver while the left is pushed down by the heart. A low flat diaphragm suggests hyperinflation (Fig 2.17). An elevated diaphragm could be:

- positional as in an AP film
- physiological due to lack of a full inspiration

FIGURE 2.18 A large pleural effusion in the left chest is obliterating the L lung and pushing the mediastinum away from the effusion

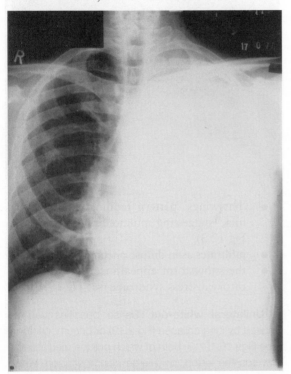

FIGURE 2.19a Atelectasis of the R lung, showing the mediastinum pulled towards the opacity, representing the collapsed lung, on the patient's right. The R main bronchus was blocked by a tumour

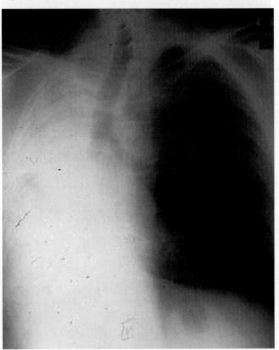

- pathological due to pressure from below, e.g. abdominal distension, or a shrinking lung above, e.g. lung fibrosis (Fig 2.20).

If one side of the diaphragm is raised, this could be due to lower lobe atelectasis, pneumonectomy, paralyzed hemidiaphragm or, on the left, excess gas in the stomach.

Shape. The diaphragm should be dome-shaped and smooth. Hyperinflation flattens it, while fibrosis can pull it up upwards into two peaks (Fig 2.20). Loss of the smooth surface may be caused by lower lobe or pleural abnormality.

Costophrenic angles. These delineate the ribs and diaphragm, being of interest to the physiotherapist because they provide the first clue to problems lurking in the base of the lung behind the dome of the diaphragm. The normal acute angle may be obliterated by the patchy shadow of consolidation or the smooth meniscus of a pleural effusion. However, 200–300ml of fluid needs to accumulate in the pleura before blunting the costophrenic angle.

Subphrenic area. Air under the right hemidiaphragm is expected after abdominal surgery. If it persists for more than a week, or appears spontaneously, it may indicate a subphrenic abscess or perforated gut. An air bubble under the left hemidiaphragm, sometimes containing fluid, is usually in the stomach and therefore normal.

Lung fields

Lungs that are too white usually indicate infiltrates. Lungs that are too dark suggest hyperinflation. Generalized hyperinflation is normally due to lung disease, and localized hyperinflation may be due to over-expanded lung adjacent to lobar collapse. Other observations are below.

Vascular markings. The fine white lines fanning out from the hila are blood vessels, which should be:

- larger in the lower zones to reflect the greater perfusion
- visible up to 2 cm from the lung margin
- more prominent with poor inspiration.

FIGURE 2.19b Atelectasis of the RLL, showing shift of the mediastinum towards the lost lung volume on the patient's right

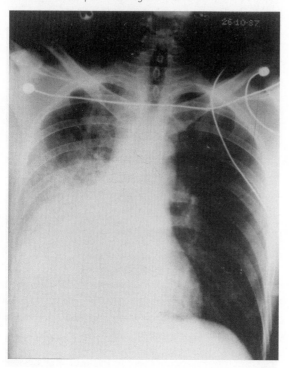

FIGURE 2.20 Diaphragm pulled up by the contracting lung tissue of fibrosing alveolitis

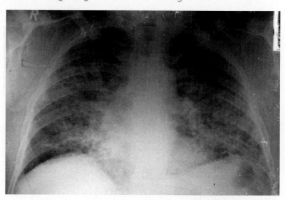

- 'batswings' pattern fanning out from the hila, suggesting pulmonary oedema (see Fig 12.3)
- infiltrates as in diffuse pneumonia (App. D)
- the snowstorm appearance of acute respiratory distress syndrome (see Fig 19.10).

Unilateral white-out. Dense opacities can be caused by lung collapse (Fig 2.19) or pneumonectomy (see Figs 16.12/13) both of which pull the mediastinum towards the lesion, or a large pleural effusion, which pushes the mediastinum away (Fig 2.18).

In conditions which reduce ventilation to the bases, hypoxic vasoconstriction squeezes blood upwards in order to match the better ventilated upper lobes, causing upper lobe diversion of vascular markings (see Fig 12.3).

A black non-vascular area demarcated medially by the white line of the visceral pleura indicates a pneumothorax (Fig 2.21). A small pneumothorax is easier to see on an expiratory film and a tiny pneumothorax may be seen in a lateral decubitus view (patient side-lying). Reversing black/white by changing from positive to negative may also be helpful.

Horizontal fissure. This is a thin white line visible in 60% of normal films, from the right hilum to the 6th rib in the axilla. It is pulled up by UL collapse and down by LL collapse.

Diffuse shadowing, e.g.:

- ground glass appearance indicating alveolar pathology such as inflammation
- reticular or a coarser honeycomb pattern, representing progressive damage, e.g. inflammation progressing to fibrosis in interstitial disease (Fig 2.20)

FIGURE 2.21 Large R pneumothorax, showing no lung markings in the dark area

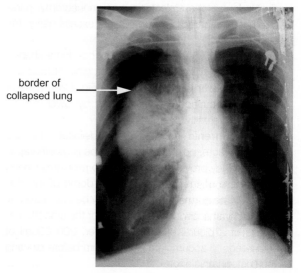

border of collapsed lung →

FIGURE 2.22 PA and lateral films showing a lung abscess in the middle lobe

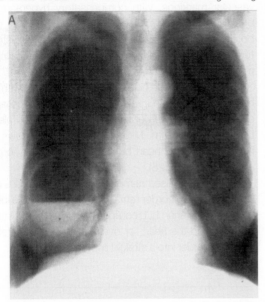
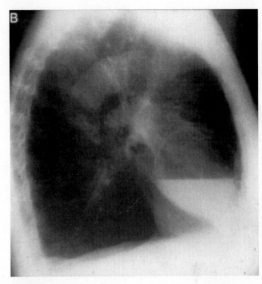

Ring shadows. These represent:
- bullae which have hairline borders, are air-filled and usually associated with emphysema (App. D)
- a cyst, with wall thickness >1 mm, often associated with bronchiectasis or cystic fibrosis
- a thick-walled abscess, often containing a fluid level (Fig 2.22).

Air bronchogram. Airways are visible if they are contrasted against an opacity such as pulmonary oedema or consolidation (Fig 2.23). If an area of collapse has no air bronchogram, the airway is obstructed.

Fluid line. This is a horizontal line, sometimes with a meniscus at the edge, atop a dense opacity. It may indicate the level of pus in an abscess (Fig 2.22), fluid in a stomach bubble under the left hemidiaphragm or, if it spans the width of the lung, a pleural effusion (Fig 2.24).

Opacities with no shift of adjacent structures. Consolidation is represented by a patchy opacity, often indicating pneumonia, frequently displaying air bronchograms and usually occupying a lobe or segment (Figs 2.23/3.21). Smaller opacities of about 3 cm diameter are known as pulmonary masses, those of 5–10 mm are called pulmonary nodules and those of

1–2 mm are miliary nodules. Bronchial tumours are usually located proximally, while metastases may be scattered.

Opacities with shift of adjacent structures. Collapse or loss of lung tissue causes shift of a moveable structure, e.g. the diaphragm (see Fig 16.20),

FIGURE 2.23 LLL pneumonia showing air bronchogram. Loss of R costophrenic angle suggests there is also some infiltration of his RLL. Patient is intubated, rotated to his left and has a kinked right apical chest drain

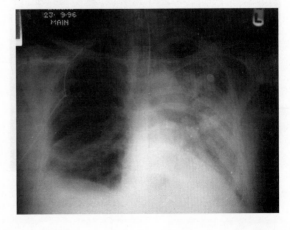

FIGURE 2.24 PA and lateral films showing the fluid line of a pleural effusion. The lateral picture shows fluid seeping up into the oblique fissure (which is invaginated pleura). Crossing this fissure can be seen the two borders of the scapulae, and anterior to these is the black trachea. The head and shaft of the humerus can also be seen.

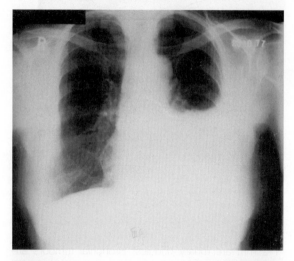

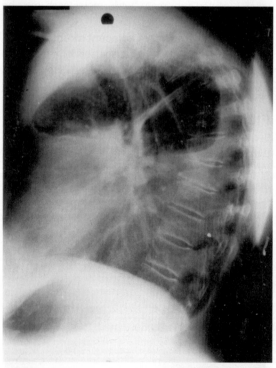

mediastinum (Figs 2.19), fissure or hilum, towards the area of lost volume. There may also be crowding of vascular markings, with compensatory hyperaeration of adjacent lung which appears darker, and loss of a border if the collapse is on the same plane as a structure such as the heart or diaphragm. A large collapse may cause rib crowding.

The RUL collapses into a triangular opacity, with the horizontal fissure migrating upwards. LUL collapse shows loss of the left upper cardiac border and elevation of the left hilum. Middle lobe collapse shows silhouetting of the R heart border but is more obvious in a lateral film (Fig 2.25).

A fuzzy and raised hemidiaphragm suggests LL collapse. The heart border remains clear because the lower lobes are posterior. LLL collapse may form a 'sail' shape either behind the heart, or overlapping and obliterating the heart border into a straight line (see Fig 3.11).

FIGURE 2.25 Lateral film showing dense opacity of a collapsed wedge-shaped middle lobe against the less dense opacity of the lozenge-shaped heart. The upper border of the wedge is the horizontal fissure and the lower border the oblique fissure. The patient is facing towards the left of the picture.

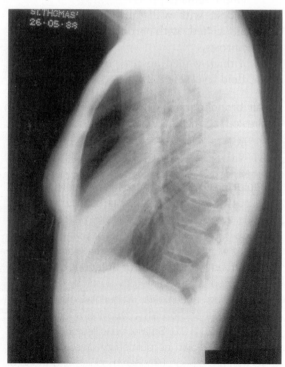

The following lobes may be collapsed or consolidated if these borders are obscured:

- LLL: L hemidiaphragm
- RLL: R hemidiaphragm
- LUL: aortic arch
- RUL: R upper mediastinum
- lingula: L heart border
- middle lobe: R heart border

Bones

The bones are examined with care following cardiopulmonary resuscitation or other trauma, or if the patient is suspected of having osteoporosis or malignant secondary deposits. A fresh rib fracture is seen as displacement of the border of the rib, which helps distinguish it from other overlapping structures. Old fractures are identified by callous formation. Bony secondaries may appear as densities.

If any positive pressure treatment is planned for a patient who has fractured ribs, a radiologist should be asked to check the film because a pneumothorax may be hiding, for example behind the cluster of rib shadows at the apex.

Artefact

Extrathoracic tissues cause shadows that may project onto the lung fields, e.g. rolls of fat or breast shadows. Hardware may also be apparent, e.g. the radio-opaque tip of a nasogastric tube in the stomach or a tracheal tube above the carina. Other tubes and lines are discussed in Ch. 18.

Lateral film

A lateral film (Fig 2.26) shows the lungs superimposed on each other. The different structures may be either

FIGURE 2.26 Lateral film of a normal lung. The aorta is seen arching above and behind the heart. Dark spaces anterior and posterior to the heart are where the two lungs touch each other. The vertical white borders of the scapulae and the dark outline of the trachea can be seen. The patient has a tracheostomy bib

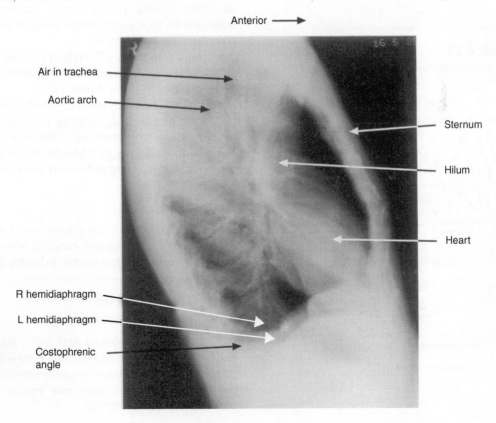

more or less distinguishable than on the PA film. Lesions that were concealed behind the diaphragm or heart may now be apparent, e.g.:

- LL collapse may appear as a white triangle at the costophrenic angle.
- A pleural effusion of just 50 ml can now blunt the costophrenic angle.
- If the oblique fissure is visible, any lesion behind it is in a lower lobe.

Fig 2.27 illustrates the different structures visible on a lateral film.

Other tests

Computed tomography (CT)

CT scans provide computed digital imaging from cross sectional films, viewed as if from a supine patient's feet (Fig 2.28). Manipulation of the data produces images in any plane, creating greater sensitivity to soft tissues than conventional x-rays and without interference from

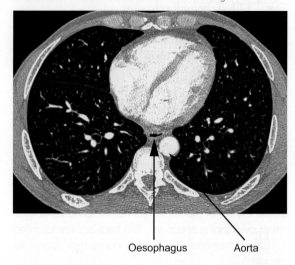

FIGURE 2.28 CT scan of normal lung

Oesophagus   Aorta

Normal heart and lungs, CT scan

overlying structures, at the cost of a greater radiation dose.

CT scans identify consolidation, atelectasis, abscesses, cavities, pleural effusion, pneumothorax, bullae and the thick walled dilated airways of advanced bronchiectasis. Variations are:

- high-resolution CT (HRCT) scans, which achieve greater sensitivity for diffuse lung diseases by using thinner slices
- spiral CT, which scans the whole chest with one breath-hold, reducing radiation exposure and motion artefact from breathing
- contrast agents to highlight blood vessels, e.g. for detecting pulmonary embolism.

Fluoroscopy

Fluoroscopy projects moving images onto a monitor, e.g. to identify diaphragmatic paralysis. Videofluoroscopy is a modified barium swallow to identify dysphagia (Park & Lee 2012).

Ventilation-perfusion imaging

$\dot{V}_A/\dot{Q}$ computed tomography (Bajc 2011) maps the distribution of ventilation and perfusion in the lung. Poor perfusion but good ventilation suggests pulmonary embolism, while poor ventilation may indicate airway obstruction (Mistry et al 2010).

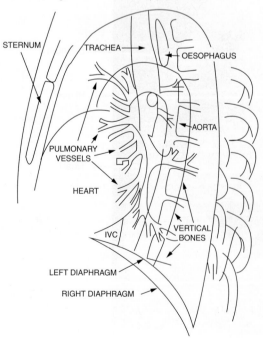

FIGURE 2.27 Representation of lateral film in a patient facing to the left of the picture

STERNUM
TRACHEA
OESOPHAGUS
AORTA
PULMONARY VESSELS
HEART
VERTICAL BONES
IVC
LEFT DIAPHRAGM
RIGHT DIAPHRAGM

Ultrasound

Ultrasound waves act as a visual stethoscope by reflecting off an air/tissue interface. They can help identify atelectasis, consolidation, pleural disorders, gas trapping (Lobo *et al* 2014), and even readiness to wean (Soummer 2012).

Ultrasound is also used to guide invasive procedures and reduce the pain of repeated arterial puncture (Haynes & Mitchell 2010).

RESPIRATORY FUNCTION TESTS

ERV expiratory reserve volume
FEV₁ forced expiratory volume in one second
FRC functional residual capacity
FVC forced vital capacity
IRV inspiratory reserve volume
PCF peak cough flow
PEFR peak expiratory flow rate (peak flow)
RR respiratory rate
RV residual volume
TLC total lung capacity
VC vital capacity
V_T tidal volume
V̇O₂ oxygen consumption

Respiratory function tests (RFTs) quantify lung function in order to:

- define an abnormality, e.g. distinguish COPD from asthma
- indicate the progress of disease or response to treatment
- provide risk assessment, e.g. before surgery.

Tests for airflow obstruction may detect an impending asthma attack or identify ventilatory failure in progressive neurological disease. However they bear little relation to quality of life (Fig 2.29), and are rarely affected by physiotherapy.

Measurements vary with posture, ethnic origin, stature, sex and age, the last two variables relating to muscle strength and therefore relevant to tests requiring effort. Some measurements depend on fitness and time of day or year.

Working definitions

If two or more subdivisions of lung volume are taken together, the sum is called a capacity. All values are approximate.

Peak expiratory flow rate or **peak flow** (PF) is the highest flow that can be achieved during a forced expiration from full inspiration. It is also one of the parameters measured on the flow-volume loop (Fig 2.33).

- Normal value: 300–600 l/min
- Severe airways obstruction: <100 l/min, or unrecordable.

Vital capacity (VC) is the volume of gas that can be exhaled after a full inspiration (Fig 2.30b) and represents the three volumes under volitional control: IRV, V_T and ERV.

- Normal: 3–6 litres, or approx 80% of TLC
- For adequate cough: >1 litre.

Forced vital capacity (FVC) is similar to VC but with forced exhalation (Fig 2.31).

- Normal: equal to VC
- COPD: less than VC if the manoeuvre causes airway collapse.

Forced expiratory volume in one second (FEV₁) is the volume of gas expelled in the first second by a forced exhalation from a full inhalation (Fig 2.31).

- Normal: 80% of VC, or 2–4 litres
- Severe airways obstruction: <30–50% predicted.

FEV₁/FVC expresses FEV₁ in relation to FVC and is more accurate than FEV₁ alone (Fig 2.31).

- Normal: 0.7–0.8, i.e. FEV₁ = 70–80% of FVC
- Moderate airflow obstruction: 0.5–0.6
- Severe airflow obstruction: 0.3 (both values reduced but with a greater dip in FEV₁)
- Restrictive disease: up to 1.0 (both values reduced but a greater dip in FVC).

Total lung capacity (TLC) is the sum of the four primary lung volumes (RV, ERV, V_T, IRV), i.e. the total volume of gas in the lungs after maximum inspiration (Figs 2.30).

- Normal: 3–8 litres.

FIGURE 2.29 Lack of correlation between FEV_1 and quality of life, as measured by the St George's Respiratory Questionnaire, in 800 patients

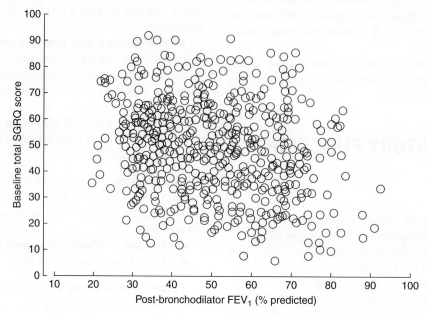

Functional residual capacity (FRC) is the volume of gas remaining at the end of a tidal exhalation (Fig 2.30a). It is a useful indicator of lung volume because it does not depend on effort, reflecting the resting position when inward and outward elastic recoil (p.8) are balanced. The reasons for the large volume of FRC is to dilute extreme changes in alveolar oxygen tension with each breath, and to protect the alveoli from collapsing at end-expiration. FRC is reduced with restrictive disorders and increased with lung hyperinflation.

- Normal in standing: about 40% of TLC, or approximately 2.4 litres
- Normal in supine: up to 2.2 litres
- COPD: up to 80% of TLC.

FIGURE 2.30a Volumes and capacities in standing and supine

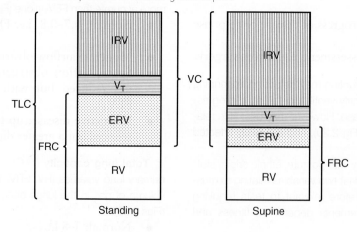

FIGURE 2.30b Pressure-volume curve (left) linking compliance to different volume levels on a normal spirogram. Also shown are spirograms for obstructive (middle) and restrictive (right) disorders

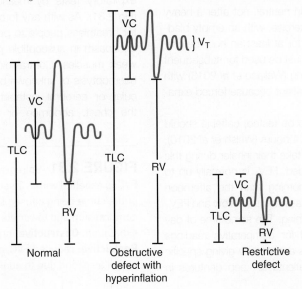

Normal   Obstructive   Restrictive
                        defect with   defect
                        hyperinflation

Tidal volume (V_T) is the volume of air inhaled and exhaled during one respiratory cycle (Fig 2.30). It mixes fresh gas with residual gas, as when the sea refreshes a tidal pool.

- Normal: 10% of VC, approx 300–800 ml, average 7 ml/kg body weight
- On exercise: up to 50% of VC.

Inspiratory reserve volume (IRV) is the extra volume of gas that can be inhaled voluntarily from end-inspiratory tidal volume (Fig 2.30a). It is normally kept in reserve, but is used during deep breathing exercises or with exertion. It is decreased in people with hyperin-flated lungs because it starts from a higher FRC. IRV is determined by inspiratory muscle strength, effort and size of the starting point (FRC + V_T).

- Normal: 3.1 litres

Expiratory reserve volume (ERV) is the extra volume of gas that can be exhaled forcefully from end-expiratory tidal volume (Fig 2.30a). It is decreased with obesity, ascites or after upper abdominal surgery.

- Normal: 1.2 litres

Residual volume (RV) is the volume of gas remaining in the lungs after maximum exhalation (Figs 2.30). It is inhaled with the first breath at birth and not exhaled until death because the outward recoil of the chest wall prevents the lungs emptying completely. RV prevents the lungs collapsing at low lung volumes and avoids the need for a mighty inspiratory effort for re-inflation. It is measured by gas dilution or body plethysmography. It is reduced with restrictive disease and increased with age or gas trapping, the ratio of RV to TLC being an index of hyperinflation.

- Normal: 20–30% of TLC, average 1.2 litres

Minute volume/ventilation is the volume of gas breathed in or out per minute, i.e. V_T x RR

- Normal: 5–7 l/min
- COPD: approx 9 l/min
- Acute respiratory failure: approx. 10 l/min, but the patient may not be able to sustain the work of breathing required, leading to ventilatory failure
- On brief maximum exercise: up to 150 l/min

Maximum voluntary ventilation is the volume of air inhaled and exhaled with maximum effort over 12–15 secs and relates to endurance, energy expenditure and functional performance (Cavalheri et al 2012).

- Normal: 50–200 l/min

Airflow obstruction

Measurements should be taken with the patient in loose clothing, their head in neutral, not after a heavy meal or recent vigorous exercise, with an empty bladder, and without smoking for at least an hour beforehand. The same position must be used for subsequent readings, preferably standing (Wallace *et al* 2013) with a stable chair behind the patient because forced exhalation can cause dizziness.

If bronchodilators are to be tested, caffeine should be avoided in the previous 4 hours (Welsh *et al* 2010), and if the patient needs to take their inhaler during this time, this should be recorded. FEV_1 is normally up to 0.15 litre higher in the morning than the afternoon (Lange *et al* 2009), but with asthma, peak flow and FEV_1 are lowest in the early morning. The same time of day should therefore be used for comparative readings when possible. Accuracy is assisted by giving specific instructions and asking patients to keep dentures in place.

Peak flow

The PF provides a quick and simple indication of airflow obstruction, but varies with effort and expiratory muscle strength. Three tests are performed, with a rest in between, and the best recorded. A 'windmill' trainer helps children, elderly people and those with learning disabilities to master the technique (Clare & Teale 2001).

Suggested technique is to:
- explain the purpose of the test
- check that the device is at zero
- demonstrate the technique with a separate device
- ask the patient to take a deep breath, then, with a firm seal on the mouthpiece, blow 'short, sharp and as hard as possible'.

Dependence on motivation means that it is inaccurate for children under four. It is also sensitive only to resistance in the large airways and is therefore invalid with COPD except to distinguish it from heart failure (Gough & Brewer 2012). PF is most usefully expressed as a percentage of the patient's previous best value, or if this is not available, as a percentage of that predicted for the patient's age and stature (as is spirometry, below). PF meters are available on prescription in the UK.

Spirometry

A spirometer measures volumes and is used for forced expiratory tests by measuring volume against time (Fig 2.31). As with any forced manoeuvre, it is difficult for breathless people to perform, may bring on bronchospasm in susceptible patients and is affected by weak muscles. Contraindications are pneumothorax, haemoptysis of unknown origin, aneurysm, cardiovascular or cerebral instability, and recent surgery to the chest, abdomen or eyes (Ranu *et al* 2011).

FIGURE 2.31 Spirograms. **Normal**: most of the FVC is expelled within 1 second, the decreasing slope of the curve being caused by progressive airway compression and lower elastic recoil during exhalation. **Obstructive**: prolonged exhalation. **Restrictive:** reduced FVC, all of which is expelled within a second due to augmented recoil

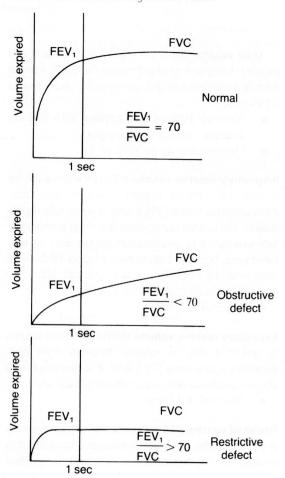

Spirometry can be performed in ventilated patients using an airtight connector.

FEV₁ is more tiring than PF but more accurate because the first second is the most sensitive to airway resistance. After a standardized inspiration (Centanni 2003), patients are exhorted to 'blast the living daylights out of the machine, and keep blowing until your lungs are empty'. When exhalation is nearly complete, it is best to emphasize continuing as long as possible rather than as hard as possible because forceful blowing can reduce expiratory time due to airway collapse. The recording needs to continue until a plateau is reached, which can take up to 15 seconds in someone with severe COPD. Much uninhibited encouragement is required, repeated on subsequent measurements.

Three technically satisfactory readings are required for accuracy, with at least two within 100 ml or 5% of each other. FEV₁ is subject to day-to-day fluctuations and declines with smoking (Fig 2.32) and age, normal lungs losing 25 to 30% of their FEV₁ over a lifetime (Washko 2012). It also declines with air pollution and some occupational exposures, including in New York fire-fighters after 9/11 (Holguin 2012).

Vital capacity is useful for measuring ventilatory reserve, indicating the ability to breathe deeply and cough. VC is sometimes reduced in obstructive disorders and always in restrictive disorders. It is also diminished with respiratory muscle weakness and is subject to day-to-day fluctuations. Measurement requires the patient to blow out from maximal inspiration but at a comfortable and sustained speed until no more can be exhaled. **Forced vital capacity** is done with maximal and forceful exhalation.

The **FEV₁/FVC** ratio is the standard diagnostic test for COPD (Ch. 3).

The **flow volume loop** is produced when a patient performs maximum inspiration followed by a maximum expiration (Fig 2.33). During inspiration, flow is dependent on effort throughout. During expiration, the highest flow occurs initially, where it is dependent on effort and represents large airway function. After a small proportion of VC has been exhaled, flow is independent of effort because increased driving pressure will not increase flow due to the small airways collapsing under the pressure of dynamic compression (p.229). Flow then depends solely on elastic recoil and small airways resistance.

In obstructive disease, expiratory flow shows a concave appearance representing attenuation of expiration as floppy airways collapse or narrowed airways obstruct. Restrictive disease shows a limited ability to generate flow.

'Lung age' can be identified from spirometry but this is a frightening concept for patients, who should be reassured that having '90–year-old lungs' is simply a technical term, that lungs have a large reserve capacity and that the septuagenarian Pope lost a lung in childhood and was in fine fettle at the time of writing.

Measurements independent of effort

Maximum mid-expiratory flow (MMEF, MEF₅₀) or the mid forced expiratory flow (FEF₂₅₋₇₅ or FEF₅₀), is the mean forced expiratory flow during the middle half of FVC, independent of effort, and is measured by the pneumotachograph, which detects the pressure drop across a resistance placed in the airstream (Groepenhoff *et al* 2011).

Lung volumes

Lungs cannot be completely emptied voluntarily and always retain their residual volume, so lung volumes are measured indirectly by one of the following:

- Plethysmography: the patient sits inside a sealed box in which the air is compressed, the resulting change in pressure enabling RV, FRC and TLC to be calculated. For more accurate results, e.g. prior to lung

FIGURE 2.32 Decline in FEV₁ with age in smokers and in those who have quit smoking, which can be used as a motivating tool for people who are still smoking

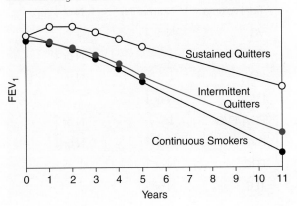

FIGURE 2.33 Flow volume loops. A dip in the effort-independent portion of the expiratory loop, above the line, indicates the obstructed airways of COPD and asthma. A restrictive pattern is represented by a small loop and rapid expiration.

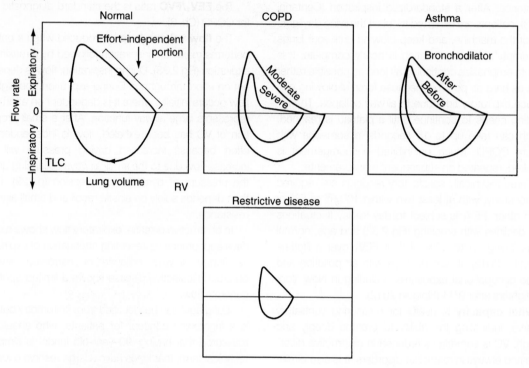

volume reduction surgery, HRCT is required (Garfield *et al* 2012).

- Gas dilution: air in the lungs is mixed with an inert gas such as helium, the dilution of which gives an indication of lung volume.
- Nitrogen washout: nitrogen comprises 80% air, so lung volume can be calculated by having the patient breathe nitrogen-free gas and measuring the expired nitrogen.

TLC and RV can also be measured by using one of the above plus spirometry.

Miller *et al* (2005) provide standardization for some lung function tests (LFT), and Table 2.8 compares results for obstructive and restrictive disease.

Tidal and spirometric volumes can also be measured by light plethysmography which shines a light on the patient and reproduces a 3D representation of chest and abdominal wall movement (Lunardi *et al* 2013). Unlike spirometry, effort is not required, and of interest to the physiotherapist is the real-time breathing pattern that is projected onto the screen, which can

identify right-left discrepancies and the relative contributions of chest and abdominal movement. It might also measure volume recruitment in ventilated patients (Fig 2.34).

TABLE 2.8 Effect of obstructive and restrictive disease on volume and flow measurements

	Obstructive	Restrictive
Tidal volume	Normal (N)	N or ↓
VC	N or ↓	↓
Peak flow	↓	N or ↓
FEV$_1$	↓	N
FVC	N or ↓	↓
FEV$_1$/FVC	↓	N or ↑
RV	N or ↑	N or ↓
FRC	N or ↑	↓
TLC	N or ↑	↓

FIGURE 2.34 Representation by light plethysmography of the chest and abdominal wall, with corresponding volume-time curve

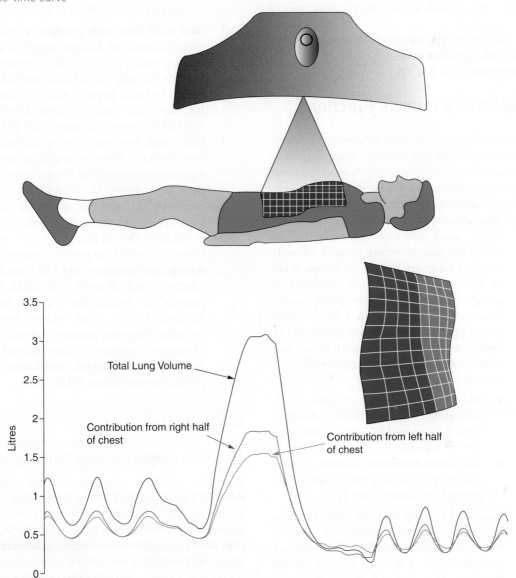

Total Lung Volume

Contribution from right half of chest

Contribution from left half of chest

Litres

Gas exchange

Pulmonary **gas exchange** is best evaluated by the alveolar-arterial gradient (p.20). The diffusion component of this reflects the integrity of the alveolar-capillary membrane and is monitored by gas transfer (transfer factor), identified as the total lung transfer capacity for carbon monoxide (TLCO). Normal values are 17–25 ml/min/mmHg. Reduced TLCO occurs with advanced age, heavy smoking, $\dot{V}_A/\dot{Q}$ mismatch (Nishimura 2011) or a thickened alveolar-capillary membrane, as occurs with fibrosis. However, even if TLCO is <50% predicted, there is enough reserve for diffusion to be adequate for normal metabolic demands (Hughes 2007).

Blood **oxygen levels** are measured by P_aO_2 or S_pO_2. Blood **CO_2 levels** are measured by P_aCO_2 or less painfully by capnography, which measures end-tidal CO_2 at the mouth as the patient exhales, normal levels being 4–6%.

A measure of **gas exchange at tissue level** is given by the saturation of haemoglobin with oxygen in the pulmonary artery (Ch. 17).

Respiratory muscle function

These tests need to be done in standard positions because of the effect of posture on thoracoabdominal kinematics (Gamna 2012). More than one test is advised because individual tests of respiratory muscle strength tend to overdiagnose weakness (Steier *et al* 2007).

1   **Vital capacity** is simple but relatively insensitive. Small pressures are required to inflate the lung, therefore reduced VC only occurs with severe muscle weakness. A fall of 25% or more in supine compared to upright may indicate diaphragmatic paralysis, and once it falls below 1 litre, ventilatory support may be required (Ranu 2011). Results are influenced by effort, fitness and compliance of the lung and chest wall.

2   **Mouth pressures** comprise:

   • Maximum inspiratory pressure (MIP), indicating diaphragmatic strength, measured from FRC and maintained for one second.
   • Maximum expiratory pressure (MEP), indicating expiratory muscle and cough strength, measured from TLC.

Keeping a firm lip seal, the patient inhales or exhales sharply against a blocked mouthpiece with a small leak to prevent pressure being generated by the mouth muscles. The best of three efforts is recorded. Technique must be meticulous and the patient's position standardized because values vary with effort, the initial lung volume, which affects muscle length, and a learning effect of the test. Values are:

   • Normal MIP: -100 cmH$_2$O.
   • Inspiratory muscle weakness: MIP below (less negative than) -80 cmH$_2$O.
   • Weaning failure: below -30 cmH$_2$O (Cairo 2012 p. 327).

   • Neurological patients at risk of ventilatory failure: <60% predicted (Mangera *et al* 2012) or below -20–30 cmH$_2$O (Cairo 2012 p.52).

3   **Sniff nasal inspiratory pressure** is easier for some patients and does not require a mouth seal, consisting of a short sharp maximal inhalation through one or both nostrils. Values should be more negative than -70 cmH$_2$O for men and more negative than -60 cmH$_2$O for women (Mangera *et al* 2012).

4   **Peak cough flow** is the velocity of air expelled from the lungs during a cough, measured by a pneumotachometer or, less accurately, by a peak flow meter. The patient is asked to inspire to TLC and then cough into the device via a face mask or mouthpiece. Normal is 720 l/min (Suárez *et al* 2002). At least 270 l/min is required to prevent complications during chest infections and 160 l/min for an effective cough (Bianchi *et al* 2012). Weak patients can precede the test with breath-stacking (Ch. 3). More invasive tests are transdiaphragmatic pressure and twitch diaphragmatic pressure. Non-volitional tests include cervical magnetic stimulation of the phrenic nerves (Fitting 2012).

Other tests

Maximum oxygen consumption ($\dot{V}O_2$max)

$\dot{V}O_2$ max quantifies maximum exercise tolerance, reflecting the integration of the central nervous, cardiopulmonary and metabolic systems. By measuring expired air while workload is increased, it identifies the point at which oxygen demand exceeds availability, the anaerobic threshold is reached and lactic acid is produced. It is a lengthy and exhausting test that is used for research or to assess a patient's suitability for lung resection. For clinical purposes it can be estimated from the six minute walk test (Ch. 9), but the correlation is less accurate for patients with COPD if peak exercise is limited by dyspnoea (Fregonezi *et al* 2012). Normal $\dot{V}O_2$max is >25 ml/kg/min, or 25 times the resting level.

Oxygen cost of breathing

This is assessed by determining the total $\dot{V}O_2$ at rest and the increased level of ventilation produced by hyperventilation, the added oxygen uptake being attributed to metabolism of the respiratory muscles. This is small at rest but can be 10% of total $\dot{V}O_2$ on exercise and up to 15% in endurance athletes (Dominelli & Sheel 2012).

Exhaled breath

An electronic nose provides distinctive smell-prints of volatile breath biomarkers for respiratory conditions such as COPD, asthma and lung cancer (Mazzatenta 2013).

CASE STUDY : Mr DT

Ms DT has late stage COPD and is visited at home.

Relevant medical history
- Depression

Social history
- Lives alone
- Help with shopping from son

Drug history
- Multiple COPD drugs, including oral steroids, on repeat prescription
- Sleeping tablets
- Long-term oxygen therapy

Subjective assessment
- Stopped going to shops since panic attack
- Can just manage stairs
- Use oxygen when I need it

Objective assessment
- Unable to speak in complete sentences due to dyspnoea
- Breathing pattern rapid and apical
- Thin
- S_pO_2 90% at rest, 87% on exercise

Question

What is your plan of action?

CLINICAL REASONING

Is this a suitable comparison group?

> ... we compared ... five subjects affected with chronic ventilatory failure due to Duchenne muscular dystrophy and treated with nasal intermittent positive pressure ventilation [with] an unventilated comparison group ... who refused long-term mechanical ventilation.
>
> Chest (1994), 105, 445–8

Response to Case Study

First visit

- Education on COPD to ensure that fears are addressed that might contribute to depression or panic attacks.
- Desensitization to breathlessness.
- Exploration with patient on when she feels that she 'needs' oxygen. Ms T says this is when she feels breathless or anxious. Explanation provided about (a) the limited association between breathlessness and oxygen, and (b) the need for oxygen at night and when possible in the day: 'the more the merrier'.
- Discuss how Ms T would like to address her depression, with suggested options being to talk to her son, talk to a counsellor and/or take anti-depressants.
- Breathing re-education.
- Initiation of sitting exercises and paced walking, with personalized tick chart for home practice.
- Provision of hand-held fan.
- Leaflets on COPD, sleep, panic attacks and breathlessness (App. B).
- Referral to community occupational therapist for management of panic attacks, insomnia and activities of daily living.
- Referral to community pharmacist for drug review and inhaler technique.
- Referral to dietician.
- Letter to GP requesting bone density scan and referral to respiratory consultant.

Plan for next visit

- Address end-of-life wishes.
- Further breathless management strategies (Ch. 7).
- Paced walking in garden.
- Stairs and progression of exercise programme.
- Assessment for ambulatory oxygen.
- Consider pulmonary rehabilitation.

Response to Clinical Reasoning

Patients unwilling to try non-invasive ventilation differ from those accepting the treatment and are therefore not a suitable comparison group.

RECOMMENDED READING

AARC (2013) Clinical Practice Guideline: blood gas analysis and hemoximetry. *Respir Care*; **58**(10): 1694–703

Armstrong LE, Johnson EC, McKenzie AL (2013) Body composition, energy expenditure and physical activity. *Eur J Clin Nutr*; **67**: 249–253

ATS/ERS (2005) Standardisation of lung function testing. *Eur Respir J*; (26): 153–61

Boros PW (2012) Reversibility of airway obstruction vs bronchodilatation. *COPD*; **9**(3): 213–15

Bruusgaard D, Tschudi-Madsen H, Ihlebæk C *et al* (2012) Symptom load and functional status. *BMC Public Health*; **12**: 1085

Cheuvront SN (2013) Physiologic basis for understanding quantitative dehydration assessment. *Am J Clin Nutr*; **97**(3): 455–62

Desborough MJ, Keeling DM (2013) How to interpret a prolonged prothrombin time or activated partial thromboplastin time. *Br J Hosp Med*; **74**(1): C10–C12

Foo JY, Chua KP, Tan XJ (2013) Clinical applications and issues of oxygen saturation level measurements obtained from peripheral sites. *J Med Eng Technol*; **37**(6): 388–95

Hansell DM, Bankier AA, MacMohon H *et al* (2008) Fleischner Society: Glossary of Terms for Thoracic Imaging. *Radiology*; (246): 697–722

Haroon A (2013) Differential diagnosis of non-segmental consolidations. *J Pulmon Resp Med*; **S8**: 001

Hughes JMB (2007) Assessing gas exchange. *Chr Respir Dis*; **4**: 205–214

Jain SN (2011) A pictorial essay: Radiology of lines and tubes in the intensive care unit. *Indian J Radiol Imaging*; **21**(3): 182–90

Lange NE (2009) Spirometry: don't blow it! *Chest*; **136**(2): 608–14

Mohrmann ME, Shepherd L (2012) Ready to listen: why welcome matters. *J Pain Symptom Management*; **43**(3): 646–50

Muñoz CX (2013) Assessment of hydration biomarkers including salivary osmolality during passive and active dehydration. *Eur J Clin Nutr*; **67**: 1257–63

Oikonomou A, Prassopoulos P (2013) Mimics in chest disease: interstitial opacities. *Insights Imaging*; **4**(1): 9–27

Rush EC (2013) Water: neglected, unappreciated and under researched. *Eur J Clin Nutr*; **67**(5):492–5

Singh V, Meena P, Sharma BB (2012) Asthma-like peak flow variability in various lung diseases. *Lung India*; **29**(1);15–18

Weiszhar Z, Horvath I (2013) Induced sputum analysis. *Breathe*; **9**:300–6

Wong CL, Holroyd-Leduc J, Straus SE (2009) Does this patient have a pleural effusion? *J Am Med Ass*; **301**(3):309–17

CHAPTER 3
Respiratory disorders

LEARNING OBJECTIVES

On completion of this chapter the reader should be able to:

- understand the pathological processes underlining obstructive and restrictive disorders, infections, lung cancer, the cardiorespiratory manifestations of systemic disease and respiratory failure

- identify the general management of these conditions

- use clinical reasoning to identify suitable strategies for the physiotherapy management of each disorder.

INTRODUCTION

Clinical medicine places too much emphasis on labelling disorders and too little emphasis on the integrative mechanisms which bridge these disorders

Killian 1998

Lung diseases are often slowly progressive, are usually incurable except for infections, and enjoy little media attention. Physiotherapy, however, can have a gratifying impact on a patient's quality of life (QoL).

The disorders are usually divided into obstructive and restrictive disease, both of which share an association with heart disease (Eriksson 2013), and disorders that fit neither or both categories.

Obstructive disease increases airway resistance and the work of breathing (WOB). Causes are:

- reversible factors, e.g. inflammation, bronchospasm or mucous plugging
- irreversible factors, e.g. fibrotic airway walls, or floppy airways due to loss of the elastic recoil that normally supports them
- localized lesions, e.g. upper airway tumour or foreign body.

Restrictive disorders reduce lung volume and compliance, increasing elastic resistance and WOB by means of:

- shrinking lung tissue, e.g. fibrosis
- compression from inside the chest wall, e.g. pleural effusion or pneumothorax
- compression by the chest wall, e.g. skeletal disorders

- reduced ability to expand the lung, e.g. neurological disorders.

Adverse conditions during foetal and early life contribute to lung disorders, along with the lung's vulnerability to the environment.

Medical management is in Chapter 5, and physiotherapy management in Chapters 6–9, but when specific to a disease, management is discussed in this chapter. Less common disorders are in the Glossary.

CHRONIC OBSTRUCTIVE PULMONARY DISEASE

The insidious onset, lacking the jolt of a first heart attack, may take away its ability to provide a sharp motivational shock
Jarvis 1995

Chronic obstructive pulmonary disease (COPD) is a group of disease subtypes characterized by airflow obstruction that is progressive and largely irreversible. It is associated with an abnormal inflammatory response to venal substances such as cigarette smoke and includes significant systemic effects, leading to disability from pulmonary and extra-pulmonary factors (Singer 2013). The clinical diagnosis of chronic bronchitis and the pathological diagnosis of emphysema usually occur together as COPD, with some patients having a preponderance for one or other disease entity.

Asthma and COPD are thought to be genetically related (Kaneko *et al* 2013) and can overlap (Fig 3.1), the combination increasing mortality (Kurai *et al* 2013).

COPD is suspected in smokers or ex-smokers aged over 35 who develop chronic productive cough, winter chest infections and shortness of breath (SOB). The diagnosis is confirmed by spirometry (Ch. 2), which is also used to stratify severity:

- Grade 1 or mild: FEV_1/FVC of 0.6–0.7, plus smoker's cough and little or no SOB
- Grade 2 or moderate: FEV_1/FVC of 0.5–0.6, plus SOB on moderate exertion
- Grade 3 or severe: FEV_1/FVC of 0.3–0.5, plus SOB at rest, hyperinflation and peripheral oedema
- Grade 4 or very severe: FEV_1/FVC <0.3.

FIGURE 3.1 Overlap of the common obstructive lung diseases

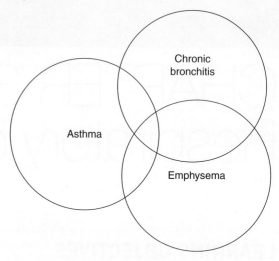

However, FEV_1 shows wide variability (Tashkin 2013) and is an unreliable marker of exercise limitation and health status (Vestbo *et al* 2013). Breathlessness, relates poorly to FEV_1 (Jones *et al* 2012a) and is the main concern of patients in both acute and chronic states (Kvangarsnes *et al* 2013). It is therefore the main focus of physiotherapy. The relevant ICF domains are severity of symptoms and functional impairment, which are also poorly related to physiological severity (Vercoulen 2012). Severe physical inactivity is the strongest independent predictor of mortality (DePew *et al* 2013).

COPD is laden with gloomy statistics:

- It kills as many people as lung cancer (Neerkin 2006), is the only chronic condition in the West for which mortality continues to rise (Young *et al* 2012) and by 2020 will be the third leading cause of death worldwide (Vlahos & Bozinovski 2014).
- Disadvantaged people are 14 times more likely to have COPD than rich people (DoH 2010a).
- Smoking is reaching 'epidemic proportions' in the Third World (Calverley 2000) as multinational companies offload their stocks of tobacco.
- Half of elderly smokers have the disease but only a third are diagnosed (Lindberg *et al* 2012).

The low rate of diagnosis is described as 'the silence of COPD', partly due to discrimination against smokers (Winstanley *et al* 2007) and partly due to patients' tendency to misattribute their symptoms to ageing (Pinnock 2012).

Once diagnosed, mortality can be reduced by pulmonary rehabilitation, smoking cessation, lung volume reduction surgery and some drugs (ZuWallack & Nici 2012).

Causes

Predisposing factors are:

- tobacco (John *et al* 2014) and genetics (Kaneko *et al* 2013)
- *in utero* exposure to smoking, and childhood respiratory illness (Soto-Martinez 2010)
- low birth weight and malnutrition (Duijts 2012)
- workplace exposure (Martin *et al* 2012) including hairdressing chemicals (Hashemi 2010), car emissions and the biomass fuel used by half the world's population (Miller 2013).

Patients are extra sensitive to cold air (Li *et al* 2014) and winter doubles the exacerbation rate (Jenkins *et al* 2012) and cold air may cause bronchospasm, while summer brings air pollution and sometimes a heavy heat that patients find difficult. People with COPD, like those with rheumatoid arthritis, are barometers for impending weather change.

Pathophysiology, clinical features and comorbidities

> *You're frightened about things, you get yourself worked up, then your breathing is worse*
> Patient quoted by Toms & Harrison (2002)

People with COPD tend to carry a burden of poorly controlled symptoms, possibly due to crisis intervention taking precedence over baseline functioning (Uronis

et al 2006). The natural history of the disease spans 20–50 years, with little or no symptoms until there is loss of up to 50% of lung function (Hodgkin *et al* 2009 p. 304) because airflow obstruction begins in the small airways (Martin 2013) where there is a wide total cross section.

Inhaled irritants stimulate epithelial cells (in chronic bronchitis) and alveolar macrophages (in emphysema) to release inflammatory mediators which damage airways and alveoli Inflammatory products disseminate around the body, where, along with other effects of the disease and its treatment, they predispose to conditions linked to inflammation such as bronchiectasis (Al-Kassimi 2013) and cardiovascular disease (Maclay & MacNee 2013). Other organs are affected by hypoxia due to impaired gas exchange (Gulbas 2013).

Chronic bronchitis

Chronic bronchitis is characterized by excess mucous secretion due to a rampant increase in the size and number of goblet cells. This causes a **productive cough**, first in the morning and then throughout the day. It tends to be dismissed by many patients as a smokers' cough but 20% of patients rate the cough as severe to extreme (Calverley 2013). The condition may be present without airflow obstruction at first (Kim & Criner 2013), but repeated irritation of the airways leads to inflammation, fibrotic changes and sometimes bronchospasm (Fig 3.2). Patients experience bronchospasm as **chest tightness** or a **wheeze**

Emphysema

Emphysema is primarily a disease of alveoli and the smallest airways, with secondary effects on larger airways. Repeated injury from cigarette smoke causes proteolytic degradation of the alveolar walls and destruction of elastic fibres (Martin 2013).

In the distal airways, bronchioles are destabilized by loss of the elastic recoil which normally splints them open, and the floppy airways collapse, trapping gas distally. In the alveoli, erosion of alveolar septa leads to enlargement of airspaces (Fig 3.2), sometimes breaking down into bullae, which are air-filled spaces with thin walls of attenuated emphysematous lung tissue.

Hyperinflation occurs when FEV_1 has declined to roughly half normal (Enright & Crapo 2000) and is caused by gas trapping and the following:

FIGURE 3.2 Airway and alveolus in normal lungs (top) and COPD lungs (bottom)

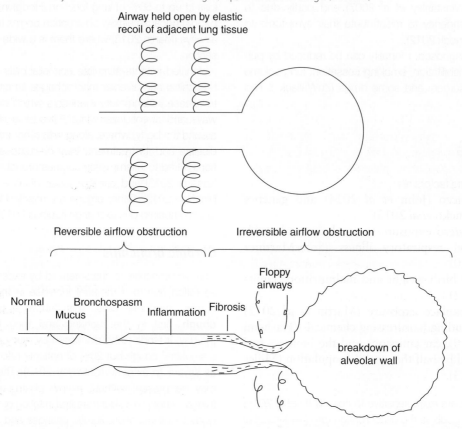

- Loss of elastic fibres reduces inward lung elastic recoil, which loses the fight to balance the outward chest wall recoil, leading to static hyperinflation.
- Active inspiratory muscle contraction is required to hold open the floppy airways, even during exhalation, leading to dynamic hyperinflation.

Hyperinflation worsens with exercise because the rapid respiratory rate makes it difficult for the lungs to empty (Cooper 2014), and is one of the main mechanisms of SOB (Lemyze et al 2012). It disadvantages inspiratory muscle function, already struggling with inflammation and sometimes malnutrition (Itoh et al 2013).

The flattened diaphragm inactivates the bucket handle action of the ribs and works paradoxically by pulling in the lower ribs on inspiration (**Hoover's sign**, Ch. 2), thus becoming expiratory in action. Dynamic

hyperinflation may prevent full expiration before the next inspiration starts, trapping more gas and leading to positive pressure in the chest known as intrinsic

FIGURE 3.3 Gas trapping, leading to increased resting lung volume, V_T being unchanged but FRC stabilizing at a higher volume. V_T: tidal volume, *FRC*: functional residual capacity

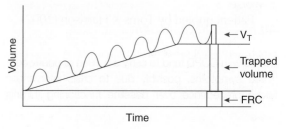

PEEP (Fig 3.3). This stabilizes on a higher, less compliant, portion of the pressure volume curve (see Fig 1.5), leading to the inspiratory muscles having to overcome an inspiratory threshold load of up to 6–9 cmH$_2$O, and sometimes working at near total lung capacity (Lahaije et al 2012).

Work of breathing is also increased by active exhalation if air needs to be forced out through obstructed airways, contributing to fatigue of the abdominal muscles on exercise (Hopkinson et al 2010). The effect of breathing with a hyperinflated chest contributes to musculoskeletal **pain** (Bentsen et al 2012).

Inefficient **abdominal paradox** (Ch. 2) may be evident (Kathiresan 2010) and some patients can only inhale by lifting up their entire rigid rib cage, leading to **hypertrophied accessory muscles**.

Breathlessness is the most disabling symptom (Calverley 2013), caused by airway narrowing, hyperinflation, muscle dysfunction and hypermetabolism, exacerbated on exercise by lactic acid production, which increases ventilatory drive (Jolley & Moxham 2009). **Exercise intolerance** is particularly troublesome during activities of daily living (ADL) (Castro et al 2012) when the accessory muscles of respiration may have to switch from assisting breathing to assisting upper limb activity. Other causes of exercise intolerance are cardiovascular impairment due to reduced venous return from the positive pressure created by dynamic hyperinflation (Tzani 2011) and deconditioning (Vogiatzis et al 2013). Physical inactivity is closely related to systemic inflammation and hospitalization, appearing to be a better predictor of mortality than clinical status (Lahaije et al 2012).

> ## KEY POINT
>
> Breathlessness affects the patient mostly as exercise intolerance.

Alpha$_1$-antitrypsin deficiency

Emphysema that develops in the 3rd to 5th decade of life may be due to a congenital lack of α_1-antitrypsin (AAT), a plasma protein which protects the alveoli from digesting themselves (p. 7). The disease takes an average six years to be diagnosed, especially as 50% of cases mimic asthma by showing reversibility to bronchodilators (Barker 2010), but it occurs in 1–5% of Caucasians who have COPD (Marciniuk et al 2012). Suspicions are raised if a non-smoker develops COPD symptoms or a smoker develops symptoms earlier than expected, especially if there is a family history of emphysema and/or liver disease (Sharp 2013). Diagnosis is by low serum AAT levels, protease inhibitor analysis or an electronic nose (Hattesohl et al 2011).

Treatment is by normal COPD management, especially smoking cessation, augmentation therapy with infusions of purified AAT (Wewers 2013), lung transplantation or, in the future, gene therapy (Mueller & Flotte 2013). There is a risk of cardiovascular disease and osteoporosis, which require prevention or treatment (Duckers et al 2010). Relatives planning parenthood are offered genetic counselling because of a 25% incidence in the children of two carriers.

Chronic bronchitis and emphysema

Whether either of these entities predominate, COPD inexorably progresses. Chronic hypoxia leads to compensatory proliferation of red cells (polycythaemia). This increases the oxygen-carrying capacity of blood and improves survival (Kollert et al 2013), but once packed cell volume (PCV) reaches 55%, the thickened blood impedes oxygen delivery, burdens the heart, causes pulmonary hypertension (Held 2013) and may lead to headaches.

Alveolar damage brings capillary damage. This combines with widespread hypoxic pulmonary vasoconstriction (p. 16) to augment pulmonary hypertension, increasing the load against which the right ventricle must pump, leading to hypertrophy and dilation of its ventricle, a condition known as cor pulmonale. When the myocardium can no longer cope, right heart failure develops, which is present in 20% of patients (Zeng & Jiang 2012), along with pulmonary oedema. Systemic BP rises in order to overcome the increased right atrial pressure, which strains the left ventricle and eventually leads to left heart failure. Lung damage continues (Fig 3.4), but patients die mainly from cardiovascular disease (Singh et al 2013).

Other features of COPD are below.

Fatigue is a problem in 90% of patients (Lewko et al 2009), worsened in the 33% of those who also have anaemia (Martinez-Rivera et al 2012) and linked to functional impairment and hospitalization (Paddison 2013). **Depression,** which has the greatest impact on QoL (Burgel 2013), has been found in 45% of patients

FIGURE 3.4 Progression of COPD to respiratory failure and heart failure. $\dot{V}_A/\dot{Q}$: ventilation/perfusion, DO_2: oxygen delivery to the tissues.

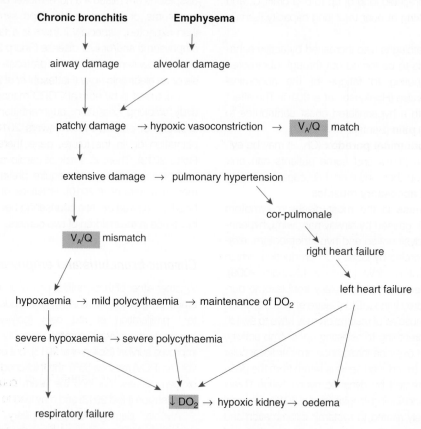

(Santus *et al* 2013) and **anxiety** in up to 75%, both of which are associated with poorer prognosis (Vestbo *et al* 2013). In only half of patients are these recognized and treated (Pommer *et al* 2012). **Frustration** is common, and COPD has been described as one of the most isolating of the chronic diseases (Toms & Harrison 2002). **Panic attacks** are ten times greater than in the general population (Livermore *et al* 2010).

Objectively, there is a rich tapestry of signs such as a plethoric **appearance, oedema** and a breathing pattern which may include **forced expiration, pursed lips breathing, prolonged expiration** with an inspiratory:expiratory (I:E) ratio of 1:3 or 1:4 and **soft tissue recession** (Ch. 2). Patients may lean forward on their elbows to force the diaphragm into a more efficient dome shape and stabilize the shoulder girdle for optimum accessory muscle action. Auscultation demonstrates the **crackles** of chronic bronchitis and/or the **quiet breath sounds** of emphysema.

Malnutrition, caused by excess energy demand, reduced energy supply and inflammation, has been reported in 26–52% of patients (Pirabbasi *et al* 2012). This predisposes to cachexia, dyspnoea, reduced exercise tolerance and cannibalism of the respiratory muscles for their protein (Lee *et al* 2013a).

Muscle dysfunction (Box 3.1) is reversible (Ribeiro *et al* 2013) but is a predictor of mortality, affecting respiratory and limb muscles, including weak quadriceps in a third of patients with even mild disease (Barreiro 2013), while upper limb muscles are often preserved because of their accessory role in breathing (Donaldson *et al* 2012). Exercise tolerance is often limited by lower limb weakness more than SOB (Vlist & Janssen 2010). The strength of the diaphragm may be preserved by working against obstructed airways, but its action is impaired by working at a mechanical disadvantage (Donaldson *et al* 2012), leading to functional muscle weakness (Lahaije *et al* 2012).

BOX 3.1

Skeletal muscle dysfunction in COPD.

Malnutrition
Cachexia
Hypoxia
Hypercapnia
Steroids
Deconditioning
Inflammatory mediators
Chronic heart failure

$\}$ ↓ lean muscle mass → respiratory muscle fatigue

SOB

respiratory failure

Muscle dysfunction contributes to a **risk of falls**, along with poor balance, some drugs and cognitive impairment (Roig *et al* 2012). **Cognitive impairment** is due to cerebral hypoxia secondary to hypoxaemia (Li 2013).

Hypoxaemia is greatest at night. Various studies have reported that 27–70% of patients who are not hypoxaemic when awake experience substantial desaturation at night, reflecting increased dependence on accessory muscles, which become hypotonic during sleep (Owens 2013). The resulting pulmonary hypertension may affect exercise tolerance independent of lung function (Cuttica *et al* 2011). Patients with severe disease may drop their S_pO_2 by 20% during non-REM sleep and 40% during REM sleep, which is greater than at maximal exercise (Ezzie 2011).

Hypoxaemia leads to **chronic renal failure** in a third of patients, which contributes to **oedema** and **cardiovascular disease** (Bruno & Valenti 2012), including hypertension (Vestbo *et al* 2013).

Hypoventilation at night, and sometimes in the day, causes **hypercapnia** in some patients (Donoghue *et al* 2003). **Sleep disturbance**, occurs in 78% of patients (Price *et al* 2013) and is the third commonest comorbidity, exacerbated by SOB, coughing, steroids (Greenberg 2009) and nocturnal oxygen desaturation, which predisposes to nocturnal cardiac dysrhythmias (Toraldo *et al* 2012). Cardiovascular complications are exacerbated by the combination of inflammation and smoking, which also contribute to **cancer**, **diabetes** and **osteoporosis** (Vestbo *et al* 2013). Osteoporosis is found in nearly half of patients (Silva 2011), especially in those who are inactive or on steroids. This worsens with an exacerbation (Kiyokawa *et al* 2012) and should not await fracture for diagnosis. Vertebral fractures have been found in 48% of patients never exposed to steroids, 57% of patients on

inhaled steroids and 63% of patients on oral steroids (Ionescu 2005).

Uncoordinated breathing combines with swallowing dysfunction (Cvejic 2011) to bring a risk of **gastroesophageal reflux**, which occurs in 37% of patients (Shimizu *et al* 2012) and predisposes to exacerbations (Terada 2010).

Tests

Screening is by **questionnaire** (Lyngso 2013) and diagnosis by **spirometry** but half of patients with obstructive findings on spirometry are not accurately diagnosed (Athanazio 2012). The test must be done after a bronchodilator so that COPD is not misdiagnosed due to the normal reduction of forced expiratory volume in one second (FEV_1) with ageing (Dyer 2012). Confirmation is by FEV_1/FVC of <0.70, along with relevant symptoms and/or a history of exposure to risk factors (Al-Kassimi 2013). Low **gas transfer** distinguishes emphysema from chronic bronchitis.

Radiology is unhelpful at first, except to exclude other smoking-related diseases such as cancer. Upper lobe diversion (p. 16) may then become apparent. Emphysema shows the signs of hyperinflation (see Fig 2.17) and sometimes bullae, while high resolution CT scan quantifies severity (Wang *et al* 2013a).

Oximetry may indicate whether **arterial blood gases** are required (Ch. 2). **Blood tests** include a full blood count to identify anaemia or polycythaemia. **ECG** (Warnier 2013), and **echocardiography** (Díez 2013) are advised. **Sputum induction** (Ch. 2) usually shows a high neutrophil count (Gupta 2013), but if eosinophils are present, the patient is likely to respond to steroids (Kitaguchi *et al* 2012). Neutrophillic inflammation is not controlled by steroids, which can actually prolong the survival of neutrophils (Barnes 2003). **Clinically** there may be hyperresonance to percussion, diminished breath sounds and wheezes (Oshaug *et al* 2013).

General treatment

> ## KEY POINT
>
> COPD is preventable and treatable but not curable.

Management should start at the Grade 1 stage (Maltais 2013), the main goals being to improve QoL and reduce the risk of exacerbations (Alifano *et al* 2010).

Multidisciplinary education is the first line treatment, and has been found to pay for itself nearly five times over (Gallefoss & Bakke 2002), partly by reducing admissions (Siddique 2012). This is best incorporated into a pulmonary rehabilitation programme, either in a group setting or at home (NICE 2012a). Telephone backup should be included (Franek 2012) as well as collaborative self-management to promote behaviour change (Benzo *et al* 2013). Anxiety and depression need to be addressed, which helps reduce the fear associated with exercise and so improves exercise tolerance (Nici 2000). Exercise itself reduces anxiety and depression (Hopkins *et al* 2012).

Smoking cessation is the only intervention which slows the progression of COPD, as well as reducing morbidity and mortality (Tønnesen 2013). Current smoking doubles the risk of death (Lindberg *et al* 2012) and without quitting, treatment is like running a bath without the plug.

Accurately-prescribed oxygen therapy for patients with chronic hypoxaemia has favourable effects on cognitive function, QoL, depression, exercise capability, frequency of hospitalization and survival (Katsenos 2011). Assessment should include 24-hour oximetry because of diurnal desaturations (Casanova 2006) and nocturnal oxygen therapy may be required for patients who would not otherwise qualify for home oxygen (Lacasse *et al* 2007). In the absence of hypoxaemia, dyspnoea is rarely an indication for oxygen therapy (Marciniuk *et al* 2011) but individuals vary (Uronis *et al* 2011).

The dietician may advise on nutritional repletion to improve exercise tolerance (Nici 2000), antioxidants to relieve symptoms (Tsiligianni 2010) and vitamin D to help prevent osteoporosis (Persson *et al* 2012).

Referral to the heart failure service may be required, and for patients with significant disability, referral to Social Services. Palliative care is associated with the end of life, but is suitable for COPD before this stage because palliation emphasizes the patient's goals, function and QoL (Reticker *et al* 2012).

Drug treatment

> *Participants reported great concerns over their use of multiple drugs. 'And slowly, you have to take more and more'*
> Boeckxstaens (2012)

Assessment of medication for airflow obstruction is usually based on spirometry (Fig 3.5) but for chronic disease, exercise tests (Sava *et al* 2012) can be included. Drug therapy fluctuates in its effect, partly due to the variable contributions of chronic bronchitis and emphysema (Lee *et al* 2011) and partly because only half of patients adhere to inhaled therapy (Cecere *et al* 2012). For hospitalized patients, hand-held inhalers allow earlier discharge than nebulizers (NICE 2010a) and are indicated unless nebulizers are objectively more effective (Smyth *et al* 2001).

Studies on airflow obstruction suggest the following:

- Combining different bronchodilators appear to be beneficial (Norman 2014) and are more effective than one bronchodilator and a steroid (Magnussen *et al* 2012).
- Short-acting β_2-agonists are for symptom relief, easing SOB by reducing hyperinflation and possibly respiratory drive (Gatta 2013). Long-acting β_2-agonists are for maintenance (Bollu 2013). The long-acting anticholinergics tiotropium and umeclidinium appear to reduce exacerbations (Tashkin *et al* 2012) and slow airflow obstruction (Decramer *et al* 2013) respectively. An ultra long-acting β_2-agonist called indacaterol can improve physical activity (Hataji 2013).
- Swift *et al* (2012) advise against using systemic steroids in the long term but different outcomes are reported for different subtypes

FIGURE 3.5 Inhaled drugs for COPD

p.r.n.: as required, i.e. according to symptoms; *LABA:* long-acting β_2-agonist bronchodilator; *ICS:* inhaled corticosteroid; *LAMA:* long-acting muscarinic antagonist (anticholinergic) bronchodilator.

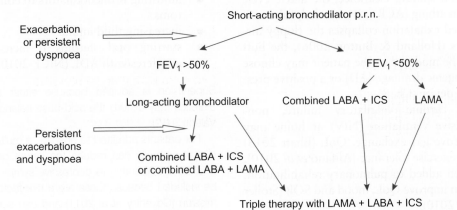

of the disease (Al-Kassimi & Alhamad 2013). Inhaled steroids also increase the incidence of pneumonia by 64% (Alifano *et al* 2010).

Other drugs include the following:

- Mucolytics such as carbocisteine (Mucodyne) or erdosteine (Erdotin) may reduce exacerbations (Poole *et al* 2012).
- Diuretics are widely used for peripheral oedema but may worsen hypercapnia, disturb acid base balance and upset electrolytes (Terzano *et al* 2012).
- β-blockers may benefit patients whether they have comorbid heart disease or not, and do not compromise the benefits of β_2-agonist bronchodilators (Matera *et al* 2013).
- Exercise capacity can be increased by udenafil (Park & Lim 2012).
- Breathlessness may be relieved by safely up-titrating opioids (Rocker & Cook 2013).

Surgical management

Surgery is occasionally indicated for symptom control in emphysema, varying from laser ablation of giant bullae to lung volume reduction (Cohen 2014). Lung transplantation for severe diffuse disease can lead to increased exercise tolerance, improved QoL and a longer life (Lahzami 2009), but comorbidity and organ shortage limit this option.

Physiotherapy

Exercise training is the most powerful intervention that is currently available to provide symptomatic relief in COPD.
                                    Ribeiro *et al* (2013)

Physiotherapy begins with information to reduce anxiety, continues with assistance to reduce WOB (Thomas *et al* 2010) and, when necessary, clear secretions, then builds up into pulmonary rehabilitation (PR) followed by a lifelong daily programme of activity that suits the individual's lifestyle (Ch. 9).
Research has identified the following:

PRACTICE TIP

Initial advice to patients: 'COPD does two different things to you: it lowers your oxygen and makes you breathless. Each of these need different treatments. Lack of oxygen is a chemical problem and requires oxygen therapy, which nourishes your brain and takes the strain off your heart. Breathlessness is a mechanical problem and requires physiotherapy . . .'

- To assist with ADL, regular exercise improves functional status and reduces the risk of hospitalization and mortality (Troosters *et al* 2013).
- To aid sputum clearance, the active cycle of breathing (ACBT) is often helpful, but if forced exhalation collapses the floppy airways (Holland & Button 2006), the huff can be modified or the patient may choose autogenic drainage (AD) or a positive pressure device (Ch. 8).
- For chronic ventilatory failure, non-invasive ventilation (NIV) at home may improve gas exchange, QoL (Bhatt 2013) and exercise tolerance (Alifano *et al* 2010). When added to pulmonary rehabilitation, it can improve QoL, mood and SOB (Stoller *et al* 2010).
- Some manual osteopathic techniques can reduce hyperinflation, increase thoracic mobility and improve exercise tolerance (Zanotti *et al* 2012).

Exacerbation

> *When it comes to breathing, fear is the worst enemy*
> Patient quoted by Kvangarsnes *et al* 2013

Worsening symptoms for at least 48 hours indicate an exacerbation, a distressing event for patients which reduces their longevity and QoL (Singh 2013). Symptoms are increased sputum volume, sputum purulence and lethargy, loss of appetite, poor sleep, SOB and fear (Kvangarsnes *et al* 2013). Rapid shallow breathing increases intrinsic PEEP so that 41% of inspiratory muscle effort may be required to overcome it (Peigang & Marini 2002). Between 24–50% of hospitalized patients also get panic attacks (Dowson *et al* 2010), which is a reminder of the importance of education.

Exacerbations are triggered by infection, pollution or unknown factors (Vestbo *et al* 2013). Myocardial damage may be evident by raised cardiac troponin levels in severe exacerbations (Søyseth 2013) and is a predictor of mortality (Chang & Robinson 2011).

A combination of antibiotics and steroids has shown short term benefit (Stefan *et al* 2013), and patients should have sufficient medication at home to begin self-management by:

- starting antibiotics if their sputum is purulent, if appropriate
- adjusting bronchodilators to control symptoms
- increasing fluid intake
- starting oral steroids if increased SOB interferes with ADL (NICE 2010a).

Supervision is advised because either steroids or diuretics may disturb the acid-base balance (Bruno & Valenti 2012).

For patients admitted to hospital, a multidisciplinary clinical pathway can reduce the length of stay (Ban *et al* 2012). Attention to depressive symptoms should be included because these are a risk factor for readmission (Coventry *et al* 2011) and can send patients into a downward spiral. As one patient said: 'the more you're housebound, the more depressed you get' (Gysels & Higginson 2009). Ventilatory failure occurs in a quarter of patients (DoH 2010a), for which non-invasive ventilation (NIV) is required if there is respiratory acidosis despite maximum medical treatment (RCP 2008). NIV reduces SOB and length of stay (Vestbo *et al* 2013), and a generous FiO_2 does not appear to upset the respiratory drive in hypercapnic patients (Savi *et al* 2013). If invasive ventilation is required, extubation straight to NIV reduces morbidity and mortality (Ornico 2013).

A multidisciplinary Hospital-at-Home service may reduce readmissions and mortality (Jeppesen *et al* 2012). Table 3.1 assists in the decision about home or hospital care.

Patients admitted to hospital must be card for by a respiratory team, have access to a specialist early discharge scheme with community support, and be reviewed within two weeks of discharge (DoH 2011a).

Physiotherapy involves sputum clearance with minimum effort from the patient. ACBT/AD may need to be modified (Ch. 8) and manual techniques may be preferable for those with significant breathlessness or fatigue, so long as there is no osteoporosis and percussion is rhythmic, steady and intermittent (Hill *et al* 2010).

Little-and-often quadriceps exercises should be started immediately, using an exercise diary for encouragement. An early exercise programme is usually well received and motivates patients to exercise after discharge (Tang *et al* 2013). Troosters *et al* (2010) found that a programme of 70% 1RM, using three sets of eight repetitions and Borg scores for dyspnoea and

TABLE 3.1 Factors to consider when deciding where to treat a patient (NICE 2012a)

Condition	Treat at home	Treat in hospital
Able to cope at home	Yes	No
Breathlessness	Mild	Severe
General condition	Good	Poor/deteriorating
Level of activity	Good	Poor/confined to bed
Cyanosis	No	Yes
Worsening peripheral oedema	No	Yes
Level of consciousness	Normal	Impaired
Already receiving home oxygen	No	Yes
Social support	Good	Living alone
Acute confusion	No	Yes
Rapid onset	No	Yes
Significant comorbidity (particularly cardiac disease and diabetes)	No	Yes
S_pO_2 <90%	No	Yes

fatigue, improved walking distance at discharge and was well tolerated by patients even with severe exacerbations. Some patients prefer electrostimulation, which may improve walking capacity (Chaplin 2013).

Written self-management action plans can reduce the duration of exacerbations, and patients are usually keen to follow them (Dhami 2012). They provide information on drugs, nutrition, exercise and emotional well-being, and can reduce health care utilization (Benzo 2012). A trip to the physiotherapy gym before discharge enables patients to feel and understand the degree of SOB on exertion that is required to build up and maintain exercise tolerance, e.g. 'breathless but not speechless'.

Premature discharge is associated with increased readmission and mortality (Reid *et al* 2012) but a managed discharge with follow-up visits and telephone contact has shown a dramatic reduction in re-admissions as well as reduced hospital-acquired infection, depression and deconditioning (Jones-Perrott *et al* 2004).

Following an exacerbation, there is an eight-week window of possible recurrence (Garvey 2012), but early PR has reduced readmission rates from 33% to 7% (Seymour 2010). Indeed, modified PR is now

recommended during an exacerbation (Blackstock 2012), but with the obvious need for adequate rest and sleep.

End stage disease

It is essential that advanced care planning and end of life discussions are initiated in advance of a life threatening situation
Lodewijckx *et al* (2012)

There is a striking difference between the management of people with end-stage COPD and those dying from cancer. COPD patients experience more anxiety, depression (Gore 2000) and dyspnoea but are prescribed less medication and have less access to comprehensive care (Marciniuk *et al* 2011) despite the UK guidelines stipulating that they and their carers should be offered specialist palliative care (DoH 2011a).

Physiotherapists can be instrumental in ensuring recognition of the patient's needs. This may include support of patients who prefer to die at home, which conveys less risk of cognitive disturbance and depression (Escarrabill 2009) and regular opportunities for discussion of prognosis, concerns and preferences for care (MacPherson et al 2013). Teamwork includes acute, community, respiratory and palliative care services (Crawford et al 2013).

Prioritizing palliation of symptoms does not preclude hospital admission or mechanical ventilation (Pinnock 2012). One of these milestones, or the initiation of home oxygen, or retirement on medical grounds, may provide the opportunity to initiate discussion on the patient's wishes. Patients usually die at night, which is thought to be due to the effect of nocturnal hypoxaemia on the cardiovascular system (Owens 2013).

Outcomes

What matters to most patients are exercise capacity, dyspnoea, exacerbations and QoL Glaab et al (2010). The following have been validated to assess these (Vestbo et al 2013):

- COPD Assessment Test (Jones 2013)
- Clinical COPD Questionnaire (Sundh et al 2012)
- BODE (body mass index, airflow obstruction, dyspnoea, and exercise capacity) scale (Glaab et al 2010)
- The 6-minute walk test, which also estimates prognosis (Holland & Nici 2013)
- Breathlessness, Cough and Sputum Scale (Leidy et al 2003)
- COPD Activity Rating Scale (Morimoto et al 2003)
- Postural control and fear of falling assessments using ICF links (Oliveira et al 2013a).

ASTHMA

Facilities for breathing retraining need to be available as part of the overall management of asthmatic patients.

Thomas et al (2001)

Asthma is a chronic inflammatory condition characterized by reversible and variable airflow obstruction caused by undue responsiveness to stimuli that are normally innocuous, a mechanism known as hyperreactivity. It is increasing in prevalence and severity, partly due to Westernized diets (Sismanopoulos 2013) and sedentary lifestyles (Dugger 2013). Mortality is low, but people die because they, their relatives or doctors do not see asthma as a potentially fatal disease, nor grasp the importance of prevention, nor recognize deterioration.

Asthma predisposes to COPD, both conditions being characterized by chronic inflammation and remodelling of the airways (Kaneko et al 2013) and its vasculature (Olivieri 2014). The two may be difficult to distinguish in later life, leading to under-diagnosis (Gillman & Douglass 2012) or over-diagnosis and unnecessary medication (Tzortzaki 2011). Differences are in Table 3.2.

Causes

Genetic, and environmental causes have been identified, with allergy involved in most patients (Dennis et al 2012a) and smoking sometimes implicated (Polosa et al 2013). Perinatal risks include maternal malnutrition or obesity, maternal smoking, prenatal stress (Khashan 2012), low birth weight, in vitrio fertilisation (Källén 2013a/b) and early antibiotics, possibly because these devour friendly gut flora which would normally help educate the immune system. Other risks are Caesarean delivery, due to lack of exposure to maternal microbes, and separation from the mother in the first weeks of life (Azad & Kozyrskyj 2012).

Other contributors include:

- in childhood, food allergy (Wang & Liu 2012), stress (Chida 2007), obesity (Black et al 2012) and fast food (Ellwood 2013)
- depression, anxiety (Bakal 2013)
- hyperventilation syndrome (HVS), which could be cause or effect, or which may be misdiagnosed as asthma (Meuret & Ritz 2010), studies finding that $1/4$ to $1/3$ of people treated for asthma have symptoms of hyperventilation (Bruton & Thomas 2011)
- vocal cord dysfunction, which may be simply mimicking asthma (Matrka 2014) or may relate to HVS; one distinction is that an expiratory wheeze often indicates asthma while an inspiratory wheeze is more likely a sign of vocal cord dysfunction

TABLE 3.2 Distinguishing features of asthma and COPD

	Asthma	COPD
Smoking history	Not necessarily	Usually
May start in childhood	Yes	No
Onset	Variable	Slow
Symptoms under age 35	Often	Rarely
Atopy	50% of patients	No
FEV_1	Variable	Reduced
TLCO	Normal	Reduced with emphysema
Corticosteroid trial	Responsive	Partial response in 10–20% of patients
Timing of symptoms	Episodic, diurnal, seasonal	Minor fluctuations only
Provocation of symptoms	Often weak stimulus, e.g. inhaled irritant	Often strong stimulus, e.g. infection.
Cough	Usually dry	Usually productive
Nocturnal cough	Patient wakes coughing	Wakes, then coughs.
Diurnal variability	Common	Uncommon
Breathlessness	Variable	Persistent and progressive
Induced sputum	More eosinophils	More neutrophils
Prognosis	Normal, except for refractory asthma	Progressive deterioration.

Note: *Atopy:* allergic hypersensitivity, *TLCO:* total lung transfer capacity for carbon monoxide (a measure of diffusion)

- house dust mite, and the damp homes which favour them (Kilpeläinen et al 2001)
- pollution (Chang *et al* 2012), poverty or stress (Koinis-Mitchell 2014).

The original cause of asthma may or may not be the same as the stimuli which typically trigger an asthma attack:

- allergic reaction to warm-blooded pets, pollen and some foods (Lee *et al* 2013b)
- car exhausts, pesticides and active or passive smoking (Butz *et al* 2012)
- change in temperature or thunderstorms, which sweep up pollutants (D'Amato *et al* 2013)
- chest infection, exercise without warm-up, certain drugs, such as aspirin, non-steroidal anti-inflammatories and some β-blockers (Mathew 2012).

Comorbidities include depression, diabetes and cardiovascular disease (Cazzola *et al* 2013).

Pathophysiology

Three phases of response take place (Fig 3.6):

1 *Sensitization* stage, which occurs in atopic people: exposure to allergens stimulates mast cells to release bronchoconstrictor mediators such as histamine. Over time, removal from the allergen does not prevent the development of asthma.

2 *Hyperreactive* stage, which occurs with or without an allergic component: continued exposure to allergens, or response to other stimuli, leads to release of inflammatory cytokines such as eosinophils, and sometimes secretion of excess mucus. Once asthma is established, inflammation is present even in the chronic state (Barbers *et al* 2012).

3 *Bronchospasm* occurs in response to various stimuli acting on hyperreactive airways.

FIGURE 3.6 Development of asthma, with the appropriate treatment on the left

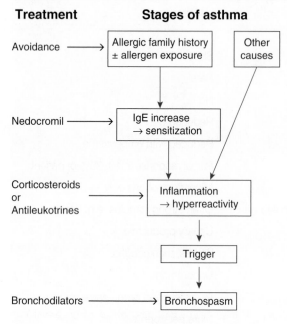

Classification and clinical features

Classic features are wheeze, chest tightness, dyspnoea and cough, particularly at night or in the early morning. Fatigue has been reported in 50% of patients, particularly in those with a perfectionist type A personality (Bakal 2013; Aguilar *et al* 2014). Allergic asthma, known as extrinsic, usually occurs in early life. Intrinsic asthma tends to develop in adulthood, and is more fulminant and less responsive to drug treatment. Variations are described below.

Chronic asthma, if well controlled, should cause no more trouble than an intermittent dry cough or occasional morning wheeze. Peak flow varies by <25%.

Severe chronic asthma causes frequent exacerbations and symptoms that significantly affect quality of life (QoL). Peak flow varies by >25% and patients tend to have a poor response to steroids, which paradoxically leads to higher doses being administered (Barnes 2011).

Refractory asthma is severe and unstable, occurring in less than 5% of patients (Bakal 2013). Patients have chaotic peak flows day and night, persistent symptoms despite multiple drugs, unpredictable dips in lung function and significant mortality (Dennis *et al* 2010a). They need individual arrangements for direct hospitalization if an attack occurs. The alternative term 'brittle' asthma is sometimes preferred by patients because it validates their experience. Another term 'Ferrari asthma' is not beloved by patients because it reminds them that they can go from 0 to intensive care in minutes.

Acute asthma reflects failure of preventive management or exposure to a specific stimulus. Work of breathing (WOB) is increased by bronchospasm of large airways and oedema of small airways. The associated hyperinflation may not increase WOB because increased inspiratory work is offset by greater airway patency (Wheatley *et al* 1990). There is chest tightness, wheeze and sometimes chest pain, which may cause diagnostic confusion and patient anxiety. Arterial blood gases are required if S_pO_2 falls below 92% (BTS 2012a). Nebulized treatment should be driven by oxygen, but if this is not available, an air compressor can be used with supplementary oxygen via nasal cannula (BTS 2008). A patient describes the experience as 'like being in the sea when you can't swim' (Casteldine 1993).

These may be modulated by psychological factors (Ritz 2012).

Airflow obstruction is caused by inflamed airways and, in the acute phase, by bronchospasm and sometimes mucous plugging (Dowell 2014). Persistent inflammation leads to remodelling, fibrosis and some irreversibility.

Heightened vascularity of the submucosa impairs humidification of the airway wall (Grainge 2011) and mucus is thicker and more difficult to clear than with other obstructive diseases (Donno *et al* 2000). This contributes to the plugging of small airways (Sivaprasad *et al* 2012); the airways of some people who have died of acute asthma may be so clogged with mucus on post-mortem that the lungs do not collapse when the chest cavity is opened (Wanner *et al* 1996).

Gastroesophageal reflux has been found in over 40% of patients (Tsikrika *et al* 2012), either because prolonged coughing and wheezing increase abdominal pressure or because oesophageal acid stimulated by steroid medication tips into the airways (Lazenby 2002).

A modest silver lining is that if the patient develops Alzheimer's disease, this might ameliorate their asthma because of progressive cholinergic failure (Ohrui *et al* 2002).

Severe acute asthma can present deceptively. The patient may have a blunted recognition of deterioration (Rubin & Pohanka 2012), and, if drowsiness develops, they may appear less distressed. High-dose oxygen must accompany the administration of salbutamol, because of potential interaction of the drug in the presence of severe hypoxaemia (Lipworth 2001). Hypercapnia indicates exhaustion and the need for mechanical assistance. Medical help should be sought immediately if the patient shows a reduced response to bronchodilator or the signs in Table 3.3.

If there are no breath sounds or wheeze on auscultation, the chest is too hyperinflated to transmit sound, an ominous sign known as the 'silent chest'. Dehydration, due to dyspnoea preventing fluid intake and causing loss of fluid from the respiratory tract, contributes to the mucous plugging (Fig 3.7) that is usually found in fatal asthma (Kuyper 2003).

> *All one's strength, that one feels becoming weaker and weaker, is concentrated into one last effort to take one slight breath that will allow the respiration to continue.*
>
> Ruiz 1993

Status asthmaticus describes an asthma attack prolonged over 24 hours and refractory to treatment,

FIGURE 3.7 Mucous cast of bronchial tree coughed up by an asthmatic patient during a severe exacerbation

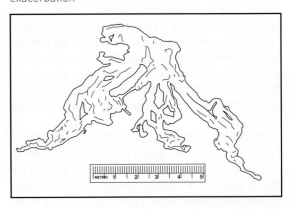

sometimes requiring extracorporeal support (Mikkelsen *et al* 2010).

Asphyxic asthma, also known as 'catastrophic asthma' or 'near fatal asthma', occurs when status asthmaticus progresses to respiratory failure (Louie *et al* 2012). If this occurs and the patient stops breathing before the crash team arrives, one person can administer assisted ventilation and, if the chest is dangerously hyperinflated, another can kneel astride the patient and squeeze the chest, either at end-expiration, or, according to Fisher *et al* (1989) at end-inspiration. Using this

TABLE 3.3 Some features of acute asthma
RR: respiratory rate; *HR:* heart rate, *BP:* blood pressure

	Severe	Life-threatening
S_pO_2	↓	<92%
P_aO_2	↓	<8 kPa (60 mmHg)
RR	>25	↓
P_aCO_2	↓	>6 kPa (45 mmHg)
HR	>110	↓
BP	↑	↓, or arrhythmia
Peak flow	< 50% predicted, or < 200 l/min	< 33% or unrecordable
Speech	Inability to complete sentence in one breath	Impossible
Auscultation	Wheeze	Silent chest
Colour		Any change
Consciousness		Any change

method, paramedics have managed to avoid out-of-hospital fatalities in patients who were asystolic on their arrival.

Exercise-induced asthma (EIA) is caused by mouth breathing cold dry air, leading to evaporation of airway surface liquid and bronchospasm. It occurs during or after exertion, with recovery about 30 minutes later. Preventive measures include training to improve physical fitness, warm-up and cool-down, a scarf over the mouth on cold days, anti-leukotrines (Kansra 2012) or a bronchodilator or nedocromil before exercise (BTS 2012a).

Nocturnal asthma, identified by a morning dip in peak flow of >20% compared to the previous evening, may be triggered by allergens in bedding, reflux in the supine position or an exaggeration of the circadian rhythm which sees airflow obstruction worst at 4 am and best at 4 pm (Durrington et al 2014)

Occupational asthma is usually diagnosed by a fall in FEV_1 of >20% over the working day or week, but may not become apparent for weeks or years.

'Difficult' asthma presents with symptoms that do not match up or respond to medication, especially if psychosocial factors are evident. This is sometimes because the symptoms mimic asthma (Aguilar et al 2014), the commonest misdiagnosis being HVS (Morice 1996). Patients should be under the care of a multidisciplinary difficult asthma service ((NICE 2013a).

Tests

Misdiagnosis may occur if a patient is given a bronchodilator because they feel breathless, then labelled as asthmatic because they have a bronchodilator. Accurate diagnosis should be in three stages (BTS/SIGN 2011):

1   Suspicions are raised by a history of acute attacks with wheeze, chest tightness, dyspnoea and cough.
2   FEV_1/FVC <0.7 indicates the likelihood of asthma.
3   A 15% increase in FEV_1 after a 14-day trial of prednisolone is confirmatory.

Other tests are on exhaled breath (Ricciardolo 2014), induced sputum (Kitaguchi 2012) or serum eosinophils (Yap et al 2013). Green or yellow sputum suggests the presence of eosinophils.

General treatment

Goals of treatment include minimal symptoms day or night, no limitation on physical activities, minimal use of short-acting bronchodilators and no adverse events from medication (Dowdell et al 2011). To achieve this, education should be at the heart of treatment, particularly as patients tend to tolerate unnecessary symptoms (Al Busaidi 2009).

Examples of prevention and education are:

- prenatal vitamin D for the mother (Carroll 2011) and breastfeeding after the birth (*Thorax* 2003)
- education that smoking reduces the efficacy of steroids (Braganza et al 2008)
- immunotherapy (desensitization), which is the only treatment that affects the mechanism of allergic disease (Compalati et al 2014)
- education for patients with associated panic disorder, which can halve panic symptoms, reduce medication and maintain asthma stability (Lehrer et al 2008)
- advice that air conditioners may be helpful (Boyle et al 2012) but not room humidifiers which can nurture house dust mite

Self-monitoring (Fig 3.8) and self-management programmes (NICE 2013a) improve adherence to medication, reduce the need for oral steroids (Clark et al 2012a) and help patients anticipate exacerbations (Honkoop et al 2013).

Medical treatment

Underuse, overuse and inappropriate use of medication is common. Patients are fond of their bronchodilators, and anxious patients tend to use them unnecessarily (Bakal 2013), but they do not prevent inflammatory damage to the airways. Except with acute asthma or brittle asthma, they should be used 'as required' only. Routine and unnecessary use of β_2-agonists may:

- reduce their effectiveness and increase airway hyperreactivity (Bakal 2013)
- encourage patients to rely on them when they should be seeking assistance

FIGURE 3.8 Peak flow information indicating (a) unstable asthma, (b) quick and slow response to triggers, (c) improved control with medication, (d) warning signs

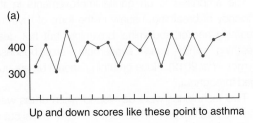

(a)

Up and down scores like these point to asthma

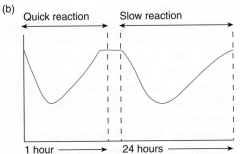

(b)

These scores show a quick reaction to cats and a slower one to flu

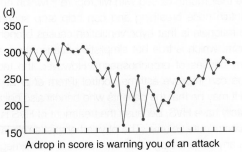

(c)

The less 'up and down' the score, the better the medicines are working

(d)

A drop in score is warning you of an attack

- worsen prognosis (Athanazio 2012) and increase the risk of death (Dennis *et al* 2012a).

The paradox is that β_2-agonists are often beneficial, even life-saving, but may be detrimental if not used accurately.

CLINICAL REASONING

Look out for bias when using research to support your practice, for example O'Byrne *et al* (2013) identified an article displaying benefits a-plenty from steroids for asthma, but not the detriments. The disclosures showed all the authors to be either employees of pharmaceutical companies or recipients of their generosity.

Drugs for chronic asthma

The principles of prevention should be considered at three levels (Warner & Warner 2000): the primary treatment (before sensitization), followed if required by secondary treatment (after sensitization but before disease development), then followed if necessary by tertiary treatment (of the disease itself). When possible, inhaled drugs should be by inhaler rather than nebulizer (Clark *et al* 2010), as in Fig 3.6 and Table 5.3.

This principle has been developed into a stepwise approach (App. C). People with mild disease can often be maintained at step one with a bronchodilator as required, but newly-diagnosed patients begin with a regular inhaled steroid to discourage them from the habit of grabbing their bronchodilator to relieve non-specific symptoms. If patients on step one need their 'rescue' bronchodilator more than three times a week, they should be under the care of a specialist (asthma nurse or physiotherapist, respiratory consultant or GP with extra training) (BTS 2012a). Stepping up or down can be instigated by patients online (Hashimoto 2011).

Drugs specific to asthma include omalizumab to dampen allergy and modulate immunity (Lommatzsch *et al* 2014), antileukotrienes, which mobilize inflammatory products to the circulation (Weir & Levine 2012) and nedocromil, which is no longer under patent and therefore of no interest to the pharmaceutical industry (Montuschi 2011). Nedocromil inhibits the release of inflammatory mediators and is one of the safest asthma drugs (Kewalramani *et al* 2008), but needs to be used regularly (Wills & Greenstone 2008). It is particularly useful for children (Korhonen *et al* 1999). It is inconvenient because of the need for four-times-daily dosing, and may take several weeks to show an effect.

Other options are biological drugs, nebulized heparin (Mathew *et al* 2012), coffee (Bara 2002), agents that act on taste receptors in the airways (Weaver 2013) and hookworms (Biggelaar *et al* 2004).

Drugs for acute asthma

High dose bronchodilators are required, preferably by inhaler with spacer (DoH 2010), or by nebulizer, sometimes continuously in the case of severe acute asthma (Dennis *et al* 2012a), or intravenously. Hypoxaemia is a major contributor to asthma deaths (Rubin & Pohanka 2012) and S_pO_2 should be kept above 94% (BTS 2012a). Steroids, antileukotrines (Zubairi *et al* 2013) or magnesium sulphate (Lalloo *et al* 2012) may be used, but antibiotics are not recommended without demonstrable bacterial infection. Sedatives can be dangerous in a severe attack (Singh 2011). Hospitalized patients must be followed up within two days of discharge (NICE 2013a).

Physiotherapy

Physiotherapy is most beneficial for people with severe chronic asthma (Bakal 2013). Patients who cannot clear their secretions during an acute attack may also require assistance. Benefits include improved QoL and exercise tolerance, and reduced symptoms and medication use (Bruurs *et al* 2013). Individual techniques are below.

Relaxation and breathing retraining

The following have been found helpful with chronic asthma:

- abdominal breathing: ↑ QoL (Prem *et al* 2013)
- relaxation with reduction of minute volume: ↑ QoL and peak flows, ↓ need for medication (Slader *et al* 2006)
- relaxation, reducing minute volume, abdominal breathing and nasal breathing: ↑ QoL and ↓ anxiety (Holloway & West 2007)
- reducing minute volume with capnography: ↓ symptoms, ↓ PF variability (Meuret 2007)
- pursed-lip breathing in a relaxed posture, manual reinforcement of exhalation,

abdominal breathing and posture correction: ↑ QoL, ↓ panic, agoraphobia and need for bronchodilators (Laurino *et al* 2012)
- relaxation: ↑ lung function (Huntley *et al* 2002).

The emphasis is on gentle improvements in the efficiency of breathing, usually in the form of rhythmic breathing and/or abdominal breathing, but not deep breathing which can exacerbate bronchospasm (Pyrgos *et al* 2012). Nose breathing should be encouraged throughout.

Two techniques were developed when drugs were less effective but can still assist patients who feel out of control of their breathing:

- Innocenti (1974) describes how patients can gain control by learning to change back and forth between abdominal and upper chest breathing, and to alter, breath by breath, the rate and depth of breathing.
- Weissleder (1976) describes teaching patients to first feel the quality of their breathing, then inhale through their nose slowly to eliminate any wheeze, then smoothly and slowly inhale in three different segments: abdominal, lateral costal and upper chest expansion, then exhale in reverse order. Muscle tension is controlled throughout.

The 'Buteyko' technique is based on reducing minute volume by slowing the respiratory rate, using breath-counting to build up CO_2, and rocking and walking as a distraction from the resulting air hunger. At night, patients may be asked to lie on their left side and/or tape their mouth closed with Micropore™ (which helps maintain nose breathing and can help stop snoring). The rationale is that hyperventilation causes bronchospasm, which is true but simplistic because there are many causes of bronchospasm. However, the technique can improve asthma control (Prem *et al* 2013) and it may be that the patients who benefit also coincidentally have HVS, because the treatment of HVS is to reduce minute volume. The physiotherapist's role is to give any patient diagnosed with asthma the Nijmegen questionnaire to identify HVS (Ch. 13), and if it is positive, either treat them for HVS or refer them to a respiratory colleague or Buteyko practitioner.

Other techniques are inspiratory muscle training (Weiner *et al* 1992), acupuncture (*Thorax* 2003), TENS on acupuncture points (Chan *et al* 2012) and yoga (Balaji *et al* 2012).

A dry cough can stir up bronchospasm and patients may need advice on cough control.

Exercise

Asthma and exercise have a curious relationship. Exercise can trigger an acute episode, but aerobic exercise with appropriate precautions has shown the following benefits:

- ↓ severity of asthma (Dugger 2013), ↑ exercise tolerance, confidence and independence (Emtner *et al* 1996)
- ↓ asthma symptoms and QoL (Eijkemans *et al* 2012)
- ↓ bronchospasm and morbidity in children (Philpott *et al* 2010).

Outdoor exercise is best taken in the least polluted areas and times of day. Asthma is the most common chronic medical condition in Olympic athletes, which may relate to inhaled pollutants (Kippelen *et al* 2012). Face masks protect against some pollutants but the filter must be changed regularly.

Validated outcomes include the Asthma Control Test, Asthma Control Questionnaire, the Royal College of Physicians 'three questions' (Scullion *et al* 2011) and the Asthma Quality of Life Questionnaire (Mathew 2012).

Physical assistance for acute asthma

Most conversations in A & E are directed over and about me, and rarely involve me in any meaningful way
Patient quoted by Carter (1995)

Some patients do not want to be touched during an attack but most do not want to be left alone. Some do not want to talk but all want to be consulted. Noise and crowding should be minimal. Medication, takes precedence over physical input.

Early attention to hydration may be required. Relaxed and rhythmic chest percussion may promote relaxation by input to receptors in the chest wall, with the added bonus of sometimes clearing secretions.

Some of the following advice may be beneficial for some patients.

- Sit upright, or lean slightly forward resting your arms on a table, or sit astride a chair

backwards with your arms resting on the chair's back.
- Keep warm.
- Sit near fresh but not cold air.
- Take sips of warm water (some prefer cold), though this should not be attempted in the throes of a bad attack.
- Breathe through the nose unless breathlessness makes this impossible.
- Dizziness with tingling hands or feet means that breathing is faster than it needs to be.
- Practice previously learned techniques of relaxation, abdominal breathing and control over breathing. These should be started at the first intimation of an acute episode.
- Cuddle a warm hot water bottle or vibrating pillow.
- Warm humidification or high-frequency oscillation may help clear secretions (Bose 2013).

Patients who continue to tire may need rehydration, and acidosis requires mechanical assistance. Continuous positive airway pressure at 3–8 cmH$_2$O relieves inspiratory muscles from their exhausting work of holding open the obstructed airways (Phipps 2003), but non-invasive ventilation (NIV) may be needed (Carson *et al* 2014). If positive pressure assistance is needed, the x-ray should be checked beforehand in case of pneumothorax. Unsuccessful NIV or deteriorating consciousness indicates the need for invasive mechanical ventilation. Children's asthma is discussed in Ch. 11.

BRONCHIECTASIS

Bronchiectasis is a chronic obstructive lung disease characterized by permanent distortion and dilation of the airway walls. This 'orphan disease' is underestimated in prevalence, incidence and morbidity (Goeminne 2010), probably because of a low level of clinical suspicion, or symptoms being ascribed to smoking (Smith *et al* 2010). Over one in 1000 Britons have the disease (Hill 2012), but it disproportionately impacts countries where children are not vaccinated against whooping cough and measles (Chang & Marsh 2012).

Causes

Bronchiectasis is not a final diagnosis as much as a common pathway of several acquired or congenital conditions predisposing to persistent lung infection. The cause is unknown in 50% of cases (Metersky 2012), but associated factors are in Box 3.2.

BOX 3.2

Conditions associated with bronchiectasis

- Congenital: cystic fibrosis or primary ciliary dyskinesia
- Infective: bacterial, viral or fungal, including lung tuberculosis and allergic bronchopulmonary aspergillosis
- Inflammatory: rheumatoid disease, inflammatory bowel disease, systemic lupus erythematosus
- Predisposition: immune deficiency, severe childhood respiratory infection
- Aspiration: foreign body or corrosive substance e.g. gastric acid.

A common process of inflammation or autoimmunity links the condition to inflammatory bowel disease, rheumatoid arthritis (Wilczynska et al 2013) and, in

29–50% of patients, COPD (Goeminne 2010). If no cause is found, patients should be tested for α_1-antitrypsin deficiency (Stoller & Aboussouan 2012).

Pathophysiology

Inflammatory damage to the bronchial walls stimulates excess thick mucus (Tambascio et al 2013) which may be focal or diffuse, the latter often accompanied by sinusitis or other comorbidity (Ramakrishnan 2013). The warm moist environment of the lung combines with the mucus to set up a vicious circle of infection, inflammation and further obstruction (Fig 3.9), compounded by oxidative stress (Olveira et al 2013). Thick mucus crushes the tender cilia and causes further damage (see Fig 8.1). An over-exuberant immune response to the colonizing microbes releases toxic inflammatory chemicals, particularly neutrophils. Persistent inflammation leads to fibrosis and sometimes sets off bronchospasm. Abscesses may develop in florid disease. The airways are chronically colonized in 60% of patients (Goeminne 2010).

'Traction' or 'dry' bronchiectasis is not actually bronchiectasis but an offshoot of pulmonary fibrosis in which lung tissue is pulled apart by scarring. It favours the upper lobes, which are more stretched, but does not produce excess mucus and physiotherapy is not indicated.

FIGURE 3.9 Vicious circle of the diseases of impaired mucociliary clearance

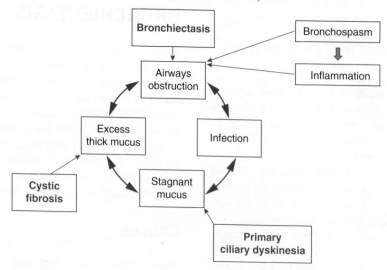

Clinical features

Voluminous quantities of sputum are produced but are inefficiently cleared because of corrugated airways and damaged cilia. Secretions cause coarse wheezes, crackles and squeaks on auscultation.

Respiratory and musculoskeletal factors contribute to exercise intolerance (Hill 2012). Muscle dysfunction is caused by inflammation, gas exchange abnormalities, inactivity, malnutrition, hypoxia and some drugs (Ozalp *et al* 2012). Dyspnoea on exertion is experienced by an average 75% of patients, chest pain by 50%, snoring by 44% and finger clubbing by 3% (Athanazio 2012). Fatigue can be disabling, caused by persistent cough, recurrent infection and dyspnoea (Hester *et al* 2012). Other features are loss of appetite, depression, anxiety, embarrassment, reduced confidence, altered relationships and social life and time off work (Tomkinson & Bruton 2009). Stress incontinence is a frequent result of excess coughing. Chest pain may reflect pneumonitis adjacent to the sensitive pleural surface and tends to lessen once the patient has an effective chest clearance regime.

Exacerbations occur several times a year and are identified by four or more of the following: change in sputum, ↑ dyspnoea, ↑ cough, fever >38°C, ↑ wheeze, ↓ exercise tolerance, fatigue, lethargy and radiographic signs of a new infection (Goeminne 2010). Acute infection can erode the airway lining and cause haemoptysis, leaving the airways more vulnerable to infection. Childhood exacerbations can be identified by specific clinical features and systemic markers (Kapur *et al* 2012).

FIGURE 3.10 Fluid levels in cysts behind the L breast shadow, indicating neglected bronchiectasis

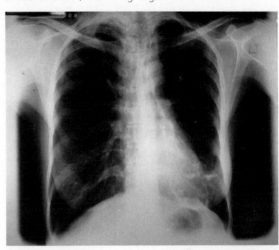

Tests

Spirometry usually indicates airway obstruction. If the disease progresses, a restrictive pattern may also develop (Athanazio 2012). However, neither lung function tests nor inflammatory markers appear to relate to quality of life (QoL) (Courtney *et al* (2008).

High-resolution CT scan is the gold standard for diagnosis and its sensitivity is thought to be the reason for a ten-fold increase in the rate of diagnosis (King & Daviskas 2010). It may show parallel tramlines, indicating thickened airway walls and ring shadows, which represent dilated airways seen in cross-section (Fig 3.10). Neglected disease shows 'glove finger

TABLE 3.4 Distinguishing features of bronchiectasis and COPD

	Bronchiectasis	**COPD**
Age	Varied	Older
Smoking history	Not necessarily	Usually
Auscultation	Noisy, may be localized	Diffuse crackles if chronic bronchitis
Sputum	Excessive, often thick and green	Moderate if chronic bronchitis
Haemoptysis	Sometimes	No
Finger clubbing	Sometimes	No
Imaging	Specific	Variable

FIGURE 3.11 Bronchogram illustrating the dilated airways of bronchiectasis in the R lower lobe. The straight L heart border ('sail sign') indicates previous L lower lobectomy

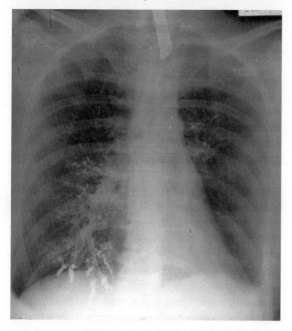

shadows' which are dilated bronchi full of solidified secretions, and the ring shadows may have fluid levels. A bronchogram outlines the dilated airways (Fig 3.11) but is rarely necessary.

Microbiology identifies the offending organisms during an exacerbation, and an annual sputum sample should be sent off when the patient is stable (BTS 2012b). Murray (2009) found a 5% incidence of bacterial colonization in mucoid sputum, 43.5% in mucopurulent sputum and 86.4% in purulent sputum. Patients should also be investigated for allergic bronchopulmonary aspergillosis, immune deficiencies (BTS 2012b) and comorbidities such as cardiovascular disease and osteoporosis (Gale *et al* 2012). Table 3.4 clarifies the difference with COPD.

Medical treatment

Disease progression can be avoided by ensuring that patients are under the care of a specialist centre, where education and systematic management are provided (French *et al* 2007).

Antibiotics are used as needed, alternating one or more antibiotics. For patients who deteriorate every winter, regular antibiotics can be taken in the cold months. Patients need a store of antibiotics specific to their usual organisms, to be taken at the first sign of colour change in their sputum. The macrolide erythromycin has antibiotic, anti-inflammatory and immunomodulatory effects (Figueiredo 2011). An exacerbation may require intravenous antibiotics, preferably managed at home. A blitz of oral, intravenous and nebulized antibiotics is sometimes able to eradicate the dreaded *pseudomonas* infection (White *et al* 2012a).

Antibiotics do not control the persistent inflammation which may be progressively damaging the airways, but inhaled **steroids** reduce inflammatory markers and sputum volume (Athanazio 2012). Also beneficial are the hyperosmolar agent **mannitol** (Bilton 2013), and **mucolytics**, have anti-inflammatory, antioxidant and mucoregulatory properties (Kim & Kim 2012a). Inflammation is exacerbated by lack of vitamin D, from which the majority of patients suffer (Chalmers *et al* 2013).

Bronchodilators are unhelpful unless hyperreactive airways are present (Athanazio 2012).

If medical treatment is unsuccessful or symptoms such as pain are intractable, surgical resection of nonperfused lung is occasionally indicated for localized disease. Transplantation may be possible in late stage disease (Mauchley *et al* 2012).

Physiotherapy

Bronchiectasis reduces mucociliary clearance to an average 15% of normal (Houtmeyers *et al* 1999). Untreated, patients will compensate with excessive coughing, which is antisocial, tiring and weakens the pelvic floor. Daily chest clearance improves QoL (Mutalithas *et al* 2008) and dampens down the vicious circle of secretions and inflammation (Volsko 2013).

Treatment begins with cough control (Chapter 8), patients being discouraged from coughing until they are ready to expectorate. A daily chest clearance programme is then required which is sufficient to eliminate coughing between sessions. Hydration, an exercise programme and ACBT/AD may be adequate. Some patients find home-based humidification helpful (Rea *et al* 2010) and regular inhaled 7% hypertonic saline may improve QoL (Kellett & Robert 2011). Other airway clearance techniques may be required (Ch. 8), and patients are the best judge of which suits them, but examples of objective studies are the following:

- The Flutter speeds sputum removal and may reduce airway resistance (Figueiredo *et al* 2012) but for some patients is less effective that ACBT (Eaton 2007).

- The Acapella increases sputum clearance, exercise capacity and QoL (Murray & Pentland 2009) and patients may find this more convenient than ACBT (Patterson *et al* 2005).
- Some patients benefit from intrapulmonary percussion (Paneroni *et al* 2011) or high-frequency chest wall oscillation (Nicolini 2013).

Pelvic floor exercises may be required, but stress incontinence usually needs referral to a continence physiotherapist. Pulmonary rehabilitation should be offered to those whose dyspnoea affects their activities of daily living (BTS 2012b), but patients must skip sessions when they have an infection in order to minimize cross infection. All patients must gel their hands, and equipment should be wiped down afterwards.

Outcome can be assessed by the St George's Respiratory Questionnaire (Smith *et al* 2010), reduced stress incontinence and improved QoL, especially fatigue.

CLINICAL REASONING

Look out for bias when using research to support your practice, for example ...

Article title: *Airway clearance in bronchiectasis: a randomized crossover trial of active cycle of breathing techniques (incorporating postural drainage and vibration) versus test of incremental respiratory endurance.*
Chron Respir Dis (2004) 1, 127

We need read no further: a technique aimed at clearing secretions is going to be more effective in clearing secretions than a technique that is not aimed at clearing secretions.

CYSTIC FIBROSIS

Cystic fibrosis (CF) is no longer a disease of childhood. The median age of predicted survival now approaches 40 (Flume 2012), and the number of adults with CF is expected to exceed the number of children in the next few years (Quon 2012).

CF is the commonest life-shortening recessively-inherited disorder in white populations and occurs wherever Europeans have settled, emerging in one in 3000 white births, 1:6000 Hispanic births, and 1:10,000 African-American births (Pletcher & Turcios 2012). The gene is carried by one in 25 Caucasians and comes to life when inherited from both parents. Two carriers have a 25% chance of each of their babies having CF and a 50% chance that each will be a carrier.

Despite the availability of both prenatal diagnosis and organ transplantation, improved survival is mainly due to advances in conventional treatment. This treatment takes on average 2 h per day (Peckham 2013), patients fitting their lives around chest clearance, inhaled and oral therapies and cleaning their equipment. As one patient responded when asked about her job: 'I'm a full-time cystic'.

Lung disease is the cause of death in 80% of patients (Flume 2012) and treatment is aimed primarily at improving quality of life.

Pathophysiology

CF is a chronic progressive disorder of the exocrine glands, manifesting mainly as an obstructive airways disease. In most cells the gene encoding CF is dormant, but in epithelial cells it is switched on, impairing ion and water transport across epithelial surfaces and obstructing various body lumens. In the gut, pancreatic insufficiency leads to malabsorption and fat intolerance. In the male reproductive system, blockage causes infertility in most patients (Hotaling 2014), but sexual function is not affected and fatherhood is possible artificially.

In the lungs, sodium and chloride ions cannot escape from the epithelial cells into the airways and maintain the salinity of mucus, reducing the volume of the liquid sol layer and thickening mucus so that an inviting medium for bacteria is created (Lai *et al* 2009). Mucociliary clearance is slowed and may come to a standstill with advanced disease (Sturm 2012). But the cough mechanism, now much needed, is compromised by the mucins in mucus becoming glued to the epithelium (Knowles & Boucher 2002). A neutrophil-dominated inflammatory response to pathogens releases DNA, whose strands bind together and thicken secretions further. As with bronchiectasis, inflammation disseminates systemically.

The lungs are structurally normal at birth, but intractable infection soon becomes established, even when the child is clinically well, leading to progressive damage and regular exacerbations (VandenBranden 2012).

Staphylococcus aureus is the commonest pathogen in infants and young children. Adults infected by the methicillin-resistant strain (MRSA) show double the rate of airflow obstruction (Vanderhelst *et al* 2012). *Pseudomonas aeruginosa* is the commonest bug in adults and has inherent antibiotic tolerance (Hurley & Prayle 2012). A minority of adults carry the feared onion rot organism *Burkholderia cepacia*, which increases the risk of pneumothorax (Mohan 2004), comes with up to 20% mortality (Dedeckova *et al* 2013) and requires segregation of patients, at great personal cost for those who have previously socialized freely. Even sibling separation is tolerated by some families. Respiratory equipment and treatment locations are also segregated.

Comorbidities

Gastroesophageal reflux disease (GORD) has been found in up to half of children over one year old (Fathi 2009), probably because of the abdominal pressure from frequent coughing. It should be treated with CF-specific medication rather than conventional drugs (Pauwels 2012).

Pneumothorax may occur in the later stages, possibly due to mucous plugging and gas trapping. High percentage oxygen assists reabsorption of gas from the pleura (ACPCF 2011). A chest drain may be required but the lung takes longer than average to re-expand (MacDuff *et al* 2010). Chest clearance should continue, but without unnecessary coughing.

Longer survival has given rise to new difficulties:

- **Osteoporosis** occurs in a quarter of adults due to malabsorption, delayed puberty, steroid therapy and, for some, immunosuppressive drugs after transplantation (Quon 2012).
- **Pain** can interfere with airway clearance (Kelemen *et al* 2012) and has been reported by 80% of patients, including headaches from coughing (Quon 2012), osteoporotic fractures and antibiotic arthralgia (Sandsund *et al* 2011).

- Pancreatic damage and steroid use predispose to **diabetes**, which is present in 20% of patients by age 15 (Balzer *et al* 2012) and exacerbates lung damage (Waugh 2010).
- **Liver disease** may lead to portal hypertension, coagulopathy and cirrhosis (Flass 2013). If complicated by ascites, sputum clearance is best done as upright as convenient for the patient.
- **Malnutrition** compromises respiratory defence and may be caused by liver disease, pancreatic insufficiency or inflammation (Kalnins 2012), sometimes contributing to **respiratory muscle fatigue** (Dassios *et al* 2013). The respiratory muscles themselves show normal or increased strength because of their work in breathing through obstructed airways (Heinzmann-Filho 2012) but other muscles may succumb to **peripheral neuropathy** (Chakrabarty 2013).
- **Cardiac dysfunction** may be caused by diabetes, pulmonary hypertension in response to prolonged hypoxaemia, myocardial fibrosis or systemic inflammation (Almajed & Lands 2012).
- Bronchial artery hypertrophy may lead to **pulmonary haemorrhage.**

Clinical features

It doesn't do too much for one's confidence to know that one has probably got halitosis, so I tend to talk to people sideways on.
Patient quoted by Hall (1984)

The antisocial nature of CF is due to delayed puberty, flatus, unrelenting weariness and incessant coughing, which occurs on average 20 times an hour (Dodd & Langman 2005). The fact that patients usually look well leads to misunderstandings about fatigue (Jarad *et al* 2012), a 20% incidence of anxiety and 10% incidence of depression (Peckham 2013). Objectively, wheezes and widespread crackles are heard on auscultation. Hyperinflation increases inspiratory work of breathing and is associated with reduced exercise capacity, but assists the airways to stay open and reduces expiratory resistance (Sovtic *et al* 2013).

Exacerbation is indicated by weight loss or worsening respiratory symptoms. If the cause is respiratory, secretions are thicker than normal and the patient may become less rather than more productive.

In the later stages, P_aO_2 falls and eventually P_aCO_2 rises. The inexorable deterioration is anticipated by patients, who each respond in their individual way. They often form strong attachments to each other, which provides comradeship but can be devastating when one dies.

Tests

Screening is possible at three stages:
1   Carrier screening has been found cost-effective (Norman 2012).
2   Prenatal diagnosis is available for pregnancies known to be at risk because of family history.
3   Neonatal screening improves survival for babies found to have CF (Dijk & Fitzgerald 2012).

After birth, the disease is suspected if an infant fails to thrive or has repeated chest infections. The skin tastes salty and confirmation is by a test for abnormally salty sweat at six weeks old. At puberty, lung function tests begin to show an obstructive pattern (Vermeulen *et al* 2014).

Radiography is normal in the early stages, then bilateral blotchy shadowing appears in the middle and upper zones. Later the signs of generalized bronchiectasis develop. High resolution CT scans may identify gas trapping and bronchial wall thickening (Flume 2012). Tomosynthesis reduces the radiation burden and shows up mucous plugging (Kim 2010).

General management

The aim is to reduce infections and prevent organ damage (Peckham 2013). Children and adults must be under the care of a multidisciplinary CF centre (Doull & Evans 2012). Passage from paediatric to adult care requires early preparation, autonomy for the patient including a flexible age of transfer, prior visits to the adult centre and good communication between all parties.

Education

When a baby with CF is born, education begins as soon as the parents have accommodated sufficiently to the diagnosis:
- CF children should, within their limitations, take part in normal physical activities.
- They should share with healthy siblings the disciplines and standards of the family.
- They are not infectious.
- No-one should smoke in the home, and infection control measures are required (Miroballi *et al* 2012).

Professional support reduces family isolation and improves attention for siblings. At adolescence, seven out of eight patients do not follow treatment recommendations (Ernst *et al* 2010), and self-help groups may be useful. Daily chest clearance is the greatest chore and time-related factors are the main reason for low adherence (Flores *et al* 2013).

Patients are advised to ask for annual bone density checks. Prevention of osteoporosis is by optimum nutrition in childhood, impact exercise and minimizing long-term steroids.

Nutrition

Optimum nutrition starts with breast feeding (Jadin *et al* 2011) and continues with lifelong enzyme supplements and a high calorie diet, sometimes assisted by nocturnal enteral tube feeding (Woestenenk *et al* 2013).

Medication

The backbone of medical management is an unremitting onslaught against bacteria. High doses of antibiotics are pumped into the body intravenously (IV) or by nebulizer (Naehri *et al* 2011). IV drugs are given either electively every three months or symptomatically (Breen 2012), delivered by a central line to avoid the complications of peripheral venous access, using a portacath which is a small reservoir implanted under the skin. This can be supervised at home, which avoids hospital infections, or in a specialist centre, which provides mutual support and family respite.

Recombinant human deoxyribonuclease (DNase) contains a clone of the gene responsible for breaking down DNA. When nebulized it may decrease sputum viscosity and improve pulmonary function (Bergin *et al*

2013) but it can overliquify secretions so that chest clearance is 'like eating soup with a fork', according to one patient. Assessment is complicated and requires a specialist centre.

Mucolytic drugs can loosen secretions so that they are easier to clear, e.g. mannitol, (Daviskas & Rubin 2013) or N-acetylcysteine (Bear 2013). Bronchodilators show objective benefit in a minority of patients but can paradoxically increase airway obstruction in as many (Dinwiddie 2000). The underlying cause of the disease can sometimes be treated by ivacaftor (Deeks 2013).

The inflammatory component of the vicious circle of airway damage can be ameliorated by anti-inflammatory drugs, but the side effects have limited their use (Flume 2012).

Assisted ventilation

Non-invasive ventilation (NIV) improves survival in critically ill patients, but invasive mechanical ventilation brings high mortality (Sheikh et al 2011). NIV can be used for acute decompensation or nocturnally for chronic respiratory failure, either as a bridge to transplantation or as palliation. Patients should be given the opportunity to discuss their preferences before the need arises.

Surgery

A patient who suffers a pneumothorax has a 50–90% chance of recurrence, and pleurodesis is often required: This does not contraindicate subsequent transplantation (Flume 2009).

Evaluation for transplant of heart, lungs and/or liver occurs when pulmonary hypertension supervenes (Damy et al 2012). Success can transform a chair-ridden invalid into an active person within weeks, with five-year survival at 50% (Flume 2012). Most of the pulmonary problems of CF are eliminated because donor lungs do not have the genetic abnormality, but bone loss is accelerated in the first year (Rosenblatt 2009). Ambulatory extracorporeal membrane oxygenation allows some patients to participate in physiotherapy and eat normally during their wait (Hayes et al 2012).

Obstacles to transplant are formidable, including the stress of waiting for donor organs, life long immunosuppressive drugs for the successful, and devastated families if the wait is too long or the transplanted organs rejected. A quarter of patients die while on the waiting list (Quon 2012), and the shortage of donors means that gentle palliative management may be supplanted by vigorous gastrostomy feeding, mechanical ventilation and other heroics to keep an increasingly desperate patient alive.

Future therapies

Gene transfer therapy is feasible because genetic material can be transferred by inhalation of a normal gene on a virus or other vector (Fitzgerald 2012). Stem cell therapies would target stem and progenitor cells in the lungs (Weiss et al 2011).

Physiotherapy

Long term trials of chest clearance are limited, possibly because it might be considered unethical to deprive a control group of a treatment that makes physiological sense. However, studies suggest that physiotherapy brings short term benefit (Rand et al 2013) and clinical reasoning suggests that this might be more prolonged.

Once CF has been diagnosed, chest clearance usually starts immediately in order to minimize chronic infection (Rand et al 2013). Adherence rates are well below 50% in the early years (Schechter 2007) and gruelling regimes produce no immediate improvement in well-being, with sputum quantity the only reinforcement. Goal setting, daily tick charts and a reward system can improve outcomes (Ernst et al 2010).

If convenient for the patient and family, chest clearance should be co-ordinated with nebulizer treatments, i.e. before antibiotics so that absorption of the drug is not hampered by mucus, and after bronchodilators or nebulized saline. Details of sputum clearance techniques are in Chapter 8, with aspects specific to CF below.

- Inhaled **hypertonic saline** improves mucociliary clearance (Fig 3.12) and works in a similar way to mannitol, but is time consuming and the side effects include the salty taste, bronchospasm and cough. Flume (2012) claims that twice daily use can reduce inflammation and exacerbations. Pezzulo et al (2012), found that once a day or less was equivalent to intensive rehabilitation and intravenous antibiotics. It is used before or during airway clearance and is usually preceded by a bronchodilator, then nebulized in concentrations of 3%–10%, in volumes of 3–10 ml (Rand *et al* 2013), depending on tolerance of the saltiness. Delivery under positive pressure may be beneficial (O'Connell *et al* 2011).

- **Exercise** has the advantage that most patients will do it, so long as they choose the type of exercise and it is started early, e.g. bouncing on a gym ball. Regular exercise reduces airflow obstruction (Kriemler *et al* 2013), enhances airway clearance and increases survival (Williams 2010). The six-minute walk test, although tedious for these busy patients, identifies those who might desaturate (Chetta 2001). Assessment and outcomes can be performed remotely, to save another trip to the clinic, using the three-minute step test (Cox 2013). Patients with advanced disease may be suited to muscle electrostimulation (Vivodtzev *et al* 2013).
- **Autogenic drainage** (AD) is popular with patients (Reix *et al* 2009) and if combined with hypertonic saline, reduces treatment time (Van Ginderdeuren *et al* 2011).
- The **active cycle of breathing** (ACBT) with **exercise** helps to improve aerobic performance, thoracic mobility and physical fitness in children (Elbasan *et al* 2012), but this study was unclear which modality was the effective one, or whether this enhanced chest clearance. For both AD and ACBT, the huff may need modification to avoid small airway closure (Kilpatrick *et al* 2001).
- **Positive expiratory pressure** (PEP) helps stabilize floppy airways in late stage disease and reduces exacerbations (McIlwaine *et al* 2013)
- Young children respond well to **blowing bubbles** and **bubble PEP.**
- **High-frequency chest compression** improves chest clearance and pulmonary function in the short term (Fainardi *et al* 2011) and **intrapulmonary percussive ventilation** has shown equivalent results to postural drainage (Varekojis *et al* 2003) (Ch. 8).
- If **postural drainage** is the chosen treatment, drainage time is about 15 minutes in younger children, but more in adolescents and adults, depending on patient preference, quantity of secretions and the effectiveness of other measures. **Manual techniques** are included if they produce more sputum or the patient finds them effective. This can be a burden for the family, but may reduce airflow obstruction when added to ACBT (Williams *et al* 2001). The patient's history should be checked for GOR and the head-down tip avoided if it brings on symptoms, although in young children this has not been shown to exacerbate the reflux (Doumit 2012).

The priority of patient choice is underlined by studies finding little difference in outcome between techniques (MAS 2009, Flume 2012). Chest clearance is usually done once or twice daily, or up to four times a day with an exacerbation, depending on the quantity of secretions. Treatment is continued until sputum is no longer expectorated or a rest is needed.

FIGURE 3.12 (a) normal mucus hydration, (b) CF dehydrated mucus, (c) restoration of hydration with hypertonic saline. *CF:* cystic fibrosis, *ASL:* airway surface liquid, *PCL:* periciliary layer

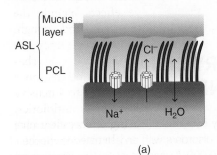
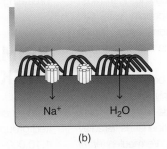
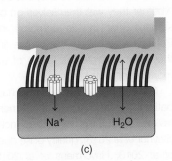

Musculoskeletal input helps ease stiffness in thoracic joints. In supine, for example, patients can breathe out and depress their shoulder girdles, then on breathing in raise their arms above their head, holding the stretch for a few seconds. Some gain benefit from a rolled up towel placed vertically under their thoracic spine. If this is done on waking or before sleeping it barely interferes with the patient's lifestyle. Hands-on input for non-inflammatory pain includes mobilizations to the ribcage and thoracic spine, and advice based on the Alexander technique (Sandsund *et al* 2011) and postural interventions (Massery 2005). Claims have been made that this can partially correct thoracic kyphosis and slow the decline in FEV_1 (ACPCF 2011). Precautions are to check for osteoporosis.

Early independence should be encouraged, with young children actively participating, and ten-year-olds able to do their own treatment during sleepovers. Older children are advised against cough suppression for social reasons, and reminded that clearing their chest before socializing reduces the need to cough.

Patients of any age may have difficulty expectorating, possibly because they don't like the taste. Children can be congratulated for coughing up anything, even saliva, with extra praise and stickers if they manage to produce 'froggies'. Swallowing large amounts of sputum can lead to vomiting up precious nutrition.

The 'optimum' programme is not always the most effective in the teenage years. Management is best negotiated, people with CF being particularly worth listening to because they are medically streetwise and understand much about their treatment. Motivation in hospitalized patients is enhanced by simple measures such as offering a choice of treatment times and techniques. Patients can also be invited to video their session, which helps them remember details of technique and which can be updated when required.

Patients will not always volunteer that they have stress incontinence, so they should be asked in private whether they wet themselves on coughing, with reassurance that this is common in people with CF. Patients may balk at the phrase 'incontinence', which they often interpret as floods of urine rather than the more acceptable leaking.

Once the optimum regime has been negotiated, patients usually require three-monthly physiotherapy reviews. Outcome measures include exercise tests (Saynor *et al* 2013), quality of life questionnaires (Bradley *et al* 2013, Havermans *et al* 2013, Vermeulen *et al* 2014), and for airway clearance, single-breath washout tests (Abbas 2013).

Precautions

Patients should not be asked to cough unnecessarily because excessive coughing can cause fatigue, stress incontinence (Dodd & Langman 2005) and collapse of central airways with impairment of sputum clearance (Zapletal 1983).

Haemoptysis occurs in 10% of patients, caused by hypertrophied bronchial arteries due to chronic airway inflammation (Fitzgerald 2012). Blood streaking of sputum is common and should be disregarded, but if >50 ml is coughed up in 24 hours, chest clearance, including exercise training, should be halted and the medical team notified. Frank haemoptysis usually indicates late stage disease and the patient will need hospital admission with sometimes bronchial artery embolization (Hurt & Simmonds 2012). Modified physiotherapy can continue once the patient is stabilized.

Measures to prevent cross infection include scrupulous hand washing, covering of sputum pots and single-patient use of all devices.

Patients with an FEV_1 <50% predicted are likely to show desaturation on exercise, which may be avoided by interval training (Ch. 9), a lower workload or supplemental oxygen. Fluids and sometimes extra salt are needed in hot weather because of the high salt content of sweat.

In advanced disease, physiotherapists should be alert to the breathlessness and pleuritic pain of a pneumothorax. CPAP does not appear to assist mucociliary clearance (Aquino 2012), but if this or NIV is used, high pressures should be avoided because of the risk of pneumothorax (Haworth *et al* 2000).

Anaemia may cause dyspnoea and reduced ability to exercise. Coagulopathy may contraindicate manual techniques. Oesophageal varices or haematemesis contraindicates all physiotherapy except abdominal breathing.

PRIMARY CILIARY DYSKINESIA

Primary ciliary dyskinesia (PCD) is a recessively inherited group of disorders with an estimated incidence of 1:10,000-1:40,000 (Lucas *et al* 2013). Disorganized motility of cilia leads to unco-ordinated mucociliary action similar to an escalator malfunctioning in rush hour, leaving the lungs vulnerable to airflow obstruction by the vicious circle on p. 92. There is virtually no mucociliary clearance and the patient compensates by coughing. Nearly half the patients have their middle lobe on the left and dextrocardia, indicating Kartagener's syndrome, a combination of bronchiectasis, situs inversus (mirror image of internal organs), and subfertility (due to dyskinetic cilia in fallopian tubes or on sperm tails) (Gupta *et al* 2013).

Clinical signs may be evident in the first year of life, but it is under-diagnosed because the syndrome shares similarities with bronchiectasis and CF (Kuehni *et al* 2010). The cilia are present from the middle ear to the conducting bronchioles, and PCD is suspected in children with glue ear, a perpetually runny nose, chronic sinusitis and frequent chest infections. Patients should be referred to a specialist centre, where diagnosis is by abnormal air flow mechanics (Knowles *et al* 2013) and genetic and cilia analysis (Pifferi *et al* 2013).

Selective antibiotics and daily chest clearance prevent the onset of bronchiectasis and progression of airway disease (Bush 2002). Chest clearance includes exercise, which improves lung function (Gokdemir *et al* 2013) and causes better bronchodilation than a β_2-agonist (Barbato *et al* 2009). Cigarette smoke exposure must be avoided to reduce the risk of sleep apnoea (Oktem *et al* 2013).

INHALED FOREIGN BODY

Inhaling an unwanted object usually occurs in children or in adults who are elderly, have neurological disease or drink excess alcohol. There is usually a history of paroxysmal coughing, followed by a relatively asymptomatic interval. Clinical signs may then arise, such as a localized wheeze, stridor, persistent cough, haemoptysis or non-resolving consolidation (Mishra 2013). Foreign bodies lodge preferentially in the right main stem bronchus because of its larger diameter and more vertical orientation than the left. This may lead to gas trapping initially and then gradual atelectasis over 18–24 hours as the trapped air is absorbed (Fig 3.13).

Small objects can be retained for months or, in the case of one patient who inhaled a whistle, 18 years (Wadhera 2009), causing a cough, wheeze or no symptoms. Many foreign bodies are made of vegetable

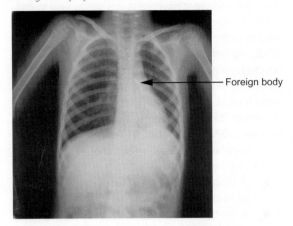

FIGURE 3.13 Left lower lobe collapse, with mediastinum shift to the left, following aspiration of a foreign body by a child

Foreign body

matter and do not show on x-ray. Most are capricious, and in young children difficult to diagnose.

Physiotherapy is contraindicated because of the risk of shifting the object to a more dangerous location (Naylor 2007). It is usually removed by bronchoscopy, following which there may be inflammatory secretions or a localized collapse that can require physiotherapy.

INTERSTITIAL LUNG DISEASE

Diseases that affect the parenchyma rather than the airways are covered by the umbrella term interstitial lung disease (ILD), indicating inflammation and fibrosis (Madhu & Hyun 2012). These shrink the lung, categorizing it as a restrictive disease. Causes include immune disturbance or exposure to toxic agents such as coal dust, cigarette smoke, stomach acid (Lee *et al* 2010) or asbestos (Frost 2013). Its incidence is rising (Akhtar *et al* 2013).

Pathogenesis

Macrophages attempt to engulf the inhaled particles, but the more toxic substances stimulate the macrophages to release inflammatory mediators. The resulting alveolitis may resolve but usually progresses to an aberrant repair mechanism and the remodelling of parenchyma into fibrosis (Fig 3.14). The differentiation of normal lung fibroblasts into myofibroblasts occurs by means of a 'Yin Yang' factor (Lin *et al* 2011), which is not as serene as it sounds and allows invasion of the damaged basement membrane in a similar way to metastatic cancer (Li *et al* 2011). This may explain why a third of patients develop lung cancer (Archontogeorgis 2012). As with all alveolar disorders, the capillaries are affected and pulmonary hypertension may develop, indicating the importance of cool-down after exercise to avoid a rapid fall in cardiac output and risk of syncope (Markovitz 2010). Other comorbidities are reflux, sleep apnoea, COPD (Raghu *et al* 2011) and a 21% incidence of coronary heart disease (Eriksson *et al* 2013).

The main effects are:

- ↑ lung stiffness, which increases the work of breathing (WOB)
- ↓ surface area of the alveolar-capillary membrane, impairing gas exchange
- skeletal muscle dysfunction (Dowman *et al* 2013).

Classification

Some of the 200 disorders (Spagnolo 2012) are the following.

Fibrosing alveolitis is the commonest and most devastating form of ILD. Causes include the drug amiodarone or occupational pollutants such as cement, metal or wood dust. Progression is relentlessly aggressive, with a median survival of two to three years (Rafii *et al* 2013). If there is no obvious cause, it is called cryptogenic or idiopathic fibrosing alveolitis (Hobbs 2014) and is probably the result of complex interactions between genetic and environmental factors, including tobacco smoke (Rosas 2013). If there is a known inhaled cause, it may be called extrinsic allergic alveolitis or hypersensitivity pneumonitis. The term fibrosing alveolitis can incorporate the end result of other disorders such as those described below, which may or may not be classified separately.

Bird fancier's and **farmer's lung** lead to fever and malaise four to eight hours after exposure to the organic dust. Lung fibrosis may develop if birds or farming cannot be kept at a distance.

The **pneumoconioses** are slowly-developing inhalation diseases (Mo *et al* 2014). The body reacts to each inhaled particle by creating an inflammatory wall of cells around it. Miners' lung and silicosis are forms of this occupational exposure.

Asbestosis is characterized by a delay of up to 50 years between inhaling asbestos dust and developing the disease (Wright *et al* 2002). Radiologically there is a

---

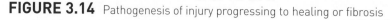

FIGURE 3.14 Pathogenesis of injury progressing to healing or fibrosis

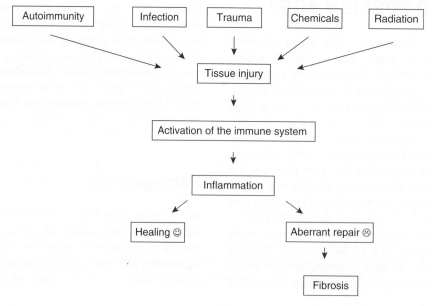

'shaggy heart' appearance and sometimes pleural involvement indicating mesothelioma (p. 118) or non-malignant pleural fibrosis (Dale *et al* 2013).

Rheumatoid disease is a systemic condition best known for inflamed joints, but in 10–15% of patients it also manifests as 'rheumatoid lung' which incorporates pleural, vascular, airway and fibrotic components, sometimes exacerbated by arthritis drugs (Diamanti *et al* 2011).

The following three conditions are connective tissue disorders which usually involve the lung and bring the added risk of bronchiectasis (Vij & Strek 2013).

Systemic lupus erythematosus (SLE) involves chronic inflammation of skin, nervous system, kidneys, blood vessels, joints and lungs, the latter causing pleurisy, pleural effusion and fibrosis. Complications include pneumonia due to treatment by immunosuppressive agents and a 50-fold increased risk of myocardial infarction (Goodman 2012).

Systemic sclerosis affects the skin and internal organs. It is characterized by altered microvasculature, disturbance of the immune system, deposition of collagen and sometimes a pulmonary vascular disorder (Hassoun 2012). If pulmonary hypertension develops, exercise training can improve quality of life (QoL) and possibly prolong survival (Grünig *et al* 2012). The alternative term **scleroderma** indicates that the skin is the most obvious organ involved.

Sarcoidosis is a chronic multisystem granulomatous disorder commonly presenting at ages 20–40, a third of patients being symptom-free but with radiological lymphadenopathy and sometimes infiltrates. Lung disease is the most common manifestation (de Boer & Wilsher 2010) but skin, eyes and joints may be affected. Granulomatous infiltration of the myocardium can affect the heart (Holland 2010) and exercise may be affected by peripheral muscle dysfunction. Causes are unknown but it is sometimes triggered by stress (Trombini 2012), and World Trade Centre dust has been identified in fire fighters who developed the disease after 9/11 (de Boer 2010). Sarcoidosis stabilizes or clears in the majority of patients, but others suffer irreversible fibrosis.

A 'double hit' condition has been identified in which the deranged remodelling of ILD is compounded by the tobacco-induced oxidative damage of COPD. Lung volumes are commonly within normal limits due to the opposing effects of fibrosis and hyperinflation, but the combination leads to premature lung ageing,

pulmonary hypertension and sometimes lung cancer (Chilosi *et al* 2012).

Clinical features

> **PRACTICE TIP**
>
> The rapid shallow breathing pattern that is adopted by most patients is probably the most efficient, so long as it is synchronous.

The lungs have a large reserve capacity and the following only emerge after considerable damage:

- progressive and unrelenting shortness of breath (SOB) due to damaged lung tissue stimulating afferent reflexes
- a tightly constrained breathing pattern, manifesting as shallow breathing to ease the elastic load and rapid breathing to maintain minute ventilation
- a dry cough due to lung distortion (Jones *et al* 2011)
- on auscultation, fine end-inspiratory 'velcro' crackles, caused by peripheral airways popping open (Flietstra 2011); these are unchanged by deep breathing, coughing or position change
- 'ground glass' radiological signs, representing the inflammatory exudate of alveolitis, progressing to reticular patterning and honeycombing, representing the fibrosis phase as alveoli are pulled apart to form cystic spaces (Fig 3.15), followed by extensive destruction
- $\downarrow P_aO_2$ and S_pO_2 due to $\dot{V}_A/\dot{Q}$ mismatch, $\downarrow P_aCO_2$ due to rapid breathing, and $\uparrow P_AO_2\text{-}P_aO_2$ due to a thickened alveolar-capillary membrane
- further hypoxaemia on exercise, not predicted by resting S_pO_2, and nocturnal hypoxaemia severe enough to affect QoL and physical functioning (Clark *et al* 2001)
- digital clubbing in three-quarters of patients (Oh *et al* 2012)
- fatigue and depression (Akhtar *et al* 2013)
- exercise limitation due to SOB in 65% of patients and leg fatigue in 35% of patients (Dale et al 2013).

FIGURE 3.15 Fibrosing alveolitis, showing reticular pattern in lung fields and blurred heart borders

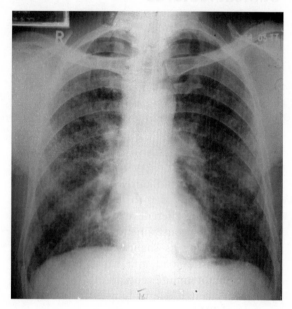

Tests

Suspicions are first raised by rapid shallow breathing following exercise. Respiratory function tests then show impaired gas transfer but do not quantify the extent of exercise limitation (Markovitz 2010). High resolution CT scan is often diagnostic, with transbronchial lung biopsy being confirmatory.

General treatment

Patients should be referred to a specialist multidisciplinary centre (Wells & Hirani 2008). Education includes information that smoking worsens outcome (Kropski *et al* 2013). An explanation of how scarring irritates nerve endings helps desensitize patients from the misconception that their SOB is causing damage.

Drugs are tricky. They may be beneficial if they dampen inflammation by inhibiting neutrophil infiltration and mediator release (Udalov 2010) but the side effects of steroids and other immunosuppressants can outweigh the benefits (Scullion 2011). Other drugs may have a moderate effect with some patients, e.g. N-acetylcysteine to protect tissues from oxidant-induced

damage (Gomer 2011), oral morphine or sildenafil for SOB (Ryerson *et al* 2012). Interferon may attenuate the fibrosis (Diaz 2012) as do two rather alarming drugs, thalidomide and carbon monoxide (Rafii *et al* 2013).

Oxygen is required in the later stages, usually at high FiO_2 (O'Driscoll 2011), and sometimes using a high flow nasal cannula, which can be run off one or two concentrators at home. This may reverse pulmonary hypertension, increase exercise tolerance and improve QoL (Criner 2013).

Lung transplantation offers hope for some patients (Rafii *et al* 2013), but for most, an end-of-life pathway needs to be negotiated. Mechanical ventilation usually fails (Güngör *et al* 2013).

Physiotherapy

> *Exercise training is one of the few treatments to induce positive changes in symptoms*
> Dowman et al (2013)

The patient's main problem is shortness of breath. Patients who are breathing irregularly may benefit from instruction in stabilizing their breathing pattern, but without slowing down the necessary fast respiratory rate. Deep breathing is likely to increase SOB; if a patient finds that it brings relief, they may also have hyperventilation syndrome, which is not uncommon with this condition.

Pulmonary rehabilitation can enhance functional capacity, dyspnoea and QoL (Dowman *et al* 2013), and should be started as early as possible (BTS/ACPRC 2009). Patients may prefer interval training, and rotation of exercises helps prevent fatigue of individual muscles (Elia *et al* 2013). Objective limitations to exercise are impaired gas exchange, pulmonary hypertension and muscle dysfunction (Holland 2010). Oxygen desaturation, which may be more severe than the degree of SOB indicates (Miki *et al* 2013), must be avoided, and ambulatory oxygen may increase walking distance even if patients do not require home oxygen (Hicks 2007).

Patients may respond to other measures (Ch. 7), including judicious use of non-invasive ventilation for those who find it brings relief (Braunlich *et al* 2013), but with close monitoring because stiff lungs risk causing a pneumothorax (Fukushima *et al* 2008).

Outcome measures include the MRC scale (Ch. 9), which correlates with physiological and functional parameters (Manali 2010) and, if not distressing for the patient, a six-minute walk test (Bois *et al* 2011), especially when combined with oximetry to measure the 'desaturation distance ratio' (Pimenta *et al* 2010).

PLEURAL DISORDERS

The pleural space normally contains <1 ml fluid, forming a film 10 µm thick (Davies *et al* 2010) but it is the conduit for 24 litres of fluid a day, secreted by the parietal layer and resorbed by the visceral layer (Peek *et al* 2000), suggesting that its function relates to fluid balance and the mechanics of breathing (Ch. 1).

Pleurisy

Pleurisy is inflammation of the pleural membranes and is sometimes associated with lobar pneumonia. It causes a pleural friction rub on auscultation (p. 52) and a savage localized pain because the parietal pleura is richly innervated. Pleurisy restricts expansion because of shallow breathing due to pain. If a pleural effusion develops, the pain dissolves as the raw pleural membranes are separated by fluid.

Pleural effusion

Pleural effusion develops when the pleural fluid filtration rate overwhelms the lymphatic removal rate. Excess fluid in the pleural cavity can be seen on x-ray (Fig 3.16, also Figs 2.18/24).

The effort of breathing against the wall of fluid increases the work of breathing (Leduc 2013) and the patient feels breathless. Objective signs include lack of breath sounds, a stony dull percussion note, reduced fremitus over the affected area and bronchial breathing just above the fluid level. Patients may have a dry cough, Ultrasound or a CT scan confirms the diagnosis.

Transudates are clear straw-coloured fluids caused by increased hydrostatic pressure or decreased oncotic pressure. They are characteristic of simple effusions caused by liver, kidney or the most common cause of pleural effusion, congestive cardiac failure (CCF, Puchalski *et al* 2013). **Exudates** are cloudy effusions which develop

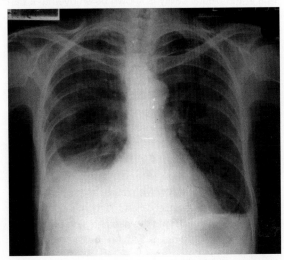

FIGURE 3.16 The patient's R side shows the dense opacity of a large pleural effusion, with a smooth horizontal border and meniscus laterally. The L shows a small effusion obliterating the costophrenic angle

by the passage of fluid through damaged capillary beds and into the pleura. They are associated with malignancy, pulmonary embolism or pneumonia. **Haemothorax** is blood in the pleura due to trauma or malignancy. Malignant pleural effusions may be secondary to a primary cancer or may relate to **mesothelioma** (p. 118).

Medical treatment is directed at the cause when possible. Symptoms can be alleviated by needle aspiration or thoracentesis, which must be done slowly in order to avoid rebound pulmonary oedema. If the effusion does not resolve, one-way valves or drainage tubes can be used. Surgery may be needed for a thickened restrictive pleura (Ch. 16). For relentless malignant effusions, pleuroperitoneal shunts or tunnelled pleural catheters can be used for palliation (Myers & Michaud 2013).

Physiotherapy is limited. Deep breathing exercises cannot expand lungs under pressure from fluid, but positioning may improve comfort and gas exchange. It is best to be guided by the oximeter, but people with a moderate unilateral effusion may benefit from side-lying with the affected side uppermost so that both ventilation and perfusion are greater in the lower lung and therefore better matched, while a large effusion may respond best with the patient lying on the affected side to minimize compression of the unaffected lung which may bring the added benefit of inhibiting a dry cough. Some patients require assistance with mobilization.

Empyema

Pus in the pleural cavity is known as empyema. It can complicate pneumonia, bronchiectasis, chronic aspiration, abscess or chest surgery, especially oesophageal surgery (see Fig 16.16), and brings a 20% mortality (Davies *et al* 2010). Radiologically it is similar to a pleural effusion but sometimes has a less clear horizontal line because the fluid is thick. The patient may be asymptomatic or toxic, depending on the organism and volume of pus. Treatment is by local and systemic antibiotics, with sometimes needle aspiration, lavage, prolonged tube drainage into a bag or with strong underwater seal suction, or surgery (Ch. 16).

Pus may break down the pleura, and the possibility of a fistula between pleura and lung means that the patient should not lie with the affected side uppermost in case infected fluid drains into the lung.

Pneumothorax

If either pleural layer is ruptured, air rushes into the pleural space, disrupting the negative pressure which normally keeps the lungs expanded. Causes include lung disease, overdistension of alveoli, trauma, including some medical procedures, and occasionally the production of gas-forming organisms through infection. The lung shrivels towards the hilum until pressure is equalized or the collapsing lung seals the hole. Presentation varies between chest discomfort to life-threatening cardiorespiratory collapse. Loss of volume >15% requires chest drainage (Ch. 16).

Clinical features are dyspnoea, pain, diminished breath sounds over the affected area and sometimes a hyper-resonant percussion note. Radiological signs are in Figs 3.17 and 2.21. For a large pneumothorax, the collapsed lung is seen shrunken around the hilum, sometimes with the mediastinum shifted away from the affected side, especially if the pneumothorax is under tension (see below).

Types of pneumothorax

The apex of the upright lung is subject to greater mechanical stress than the base because the weight of the lung pulls down on it. A **spontaneous pneumothorax**

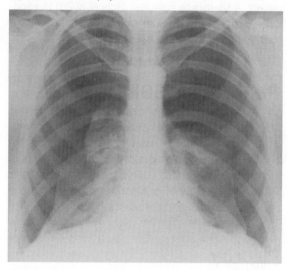

FIGURE 3.17 Large bilateral pneumothoraces in a patient with emphysema

usually occurs in this region, especially in tall thin young men (Pletcher & Turcios 2012) who are thought to grow faster than their pleura is able to keep up with. Although 'spontaneous', smoking increases the likelihood 22-fold in men and eight-fold in women (Wakai 2011).

A **secondary pneumothorax** may be caused by puncture from a fractured rib, inaccurate insertion of a cannula, high-volume mechanical ventilation, rupture of an emphysematous bulla or drug abuse with prolonged Valsalva breath-holds. It is termed an open pneumothorax if there is communication with the environment. A pneumothorax secondary to diseased lungs causes more severe symptoms and takes longer to heal. Rare precipitating factors are coughing fits, sneezing, breath-holding, loud music, playing a wind instrument and thunderstorms (Haga *et al* 2013).

A **tension pneumothorax** is an emergency which occurs if a tear in the visceral pleura acts as a valve so that air enters the pleural space but cannot escape, usually in mechanically ventilated patients. Progressive positive pressure thwarts cardiac output, and urgent action is required (Ch. 18).

Treatment

Medical treatment is aimed at expelling the pleural air, facilitating pleural healing and preventing recurrence. If small and symptomless, a pneumothorax can be left to resolve itself and the patient is usually discharged, with advice to return if dyspnoea worsens. A moderate first pneumothorax can be managed by needle aspiration. A larger pneumothorax can be treated with a Heimlich valve to enable air to escape but not re-enter, which may avoid hospital admission (Brims & Maskell 2013).

A chest drain is used if simpler methods are inadequate or the patient is on a ventilator. Suction is occasionally necessary, at low-pressure to avoid 'air-stealing', perpetuation of the air leak or re-expansion pulmonary oedema (MacDuff et al 2010). Once the air leak has sealed, i.e. when there is no more bubbling in the drainage bottle, the drain is clamped for some hours and then removed if imaging shows no recurrence.

Lying on the good side is often the most comfortable and is usually best for $\dot{V}_A/\dot{Q}$ matching, but lying on the affected side may speed absorption of air (Zidulka et al 1982). Patients may require assistance with mobilization. There is no evidence to link exertion with recurrence (MacDuff et al 2010), and exercise can be as vigorous as the patient is willing if the cause is traumatic, e.g. after stabbing, in order to encourage lung expansion (Senekal 1994). However, exercise should be moderate after pleural surgery in case the pleura comes unstuck again.

In the unlikely event that a patient is admitted but has no chest drain, high concentrations of inspired oxygen should be given unless contraindicated. This speeds resolution by increasing the absorption of air four-fold, the inert nitrogen being displaced by absorbable oxygen (Van Berkel et al 2010).

Surgery by pleurodesis (Ch. 16) is required if these measures fail, if the condition is recurrent or bilateral, or if the patient's occupation involves rapid changes in atmospheric pressure such as scuba diving or flying.

Precautions for an undrained pneumothorax include avoidance of positive pressure techniques (CPAP, IPPB, NIV or manual hyperinflation). Patients should also be advised to avoid paroxysm of coughing and intense yoga breathing techniques.

Once the pneumothorax has resolved, discharge advice is to avoid flying in the short term and avoid recreational diving for life, but physical exertion can resume so long as there are no symptoms (Eccles 2013).

NEUROMUSCULAR DISORDERS

Neurological conditions that cause generalized weakness usually cause respiratory muscle weakness. Weak inspiratory muscles cause a restrictive disorder by limiting lung expansion. Weak expiratory muscles impair the cough and hinder sputum clearance. The respiratory needs of paediatric and critically ill patients with neurological conditions are in Chapters 11 and 19.

Clinical features and monitoring

Any of the three physiotherapy problems may be present (Srour et al 2013):

1 Increased work of breathing (WOB) occurs if there are weak inspiratory muscles or a stiff chest wall.
2 Loss of lung volume results from limited expansion, a stiff chest wall or sometimes spasticity. Lack of alveolar stretch inhibits production of surfactant.
3 Sputum retention is likely if there are weak expiratory muscles and impaired cough.

Fatigue is ever present. If a chest infection occurs, hypercapnia may develop and patients usually have further difficulty clearing secretions (Homnick 2007). Chronic pain affects 20–40% of patients, caused by the centralization of pain and a vicious circle with depression (Borsook 2012).

Monitoring is required for progressive conditions. Respiratory muscle weakness may go undetected if limb weakness reduces activity, and ventilatory failure can arrive unexpectedly. Peak cough flow (PCF) assesses cough, while capnography and MIP (p. 68) provide warning of ventilatory failure (Kim et al 2011) (Ch. 2). Forced vital capacity (FVC) below 50% of normal requires assessment for non-invasive ventilation (NIV) (Carratù et al 2009). A suggested pathway for investigating and managing patients is in Fig 3.18.

The onset of hiccups, whose reflex arc is modulated by the central midbrain (Chang & Lu 2012) is a warning of potential brain stem dysfunction. Bulbar dysfunction is also associated with dysphagia, dysarthria, weak mastication, facial weakness, nasal speech, and/or a protruding tongue. Patients may need a face mask for spirometry (Wohlgemuth et al 2003).

Dysphagia is suspected by the signs in Table 3.5 and a low PCF. It may develop insidiously, but usually parallels or shortly follows the development of speech problems. Patients require speech-language therapy (SLT), and sometimes drugs such as botulinum (Lee et al 2009).

FIGURE 3.18 Pathway for monitoring and managing patients with neurological disorders and potential ventilatory failure

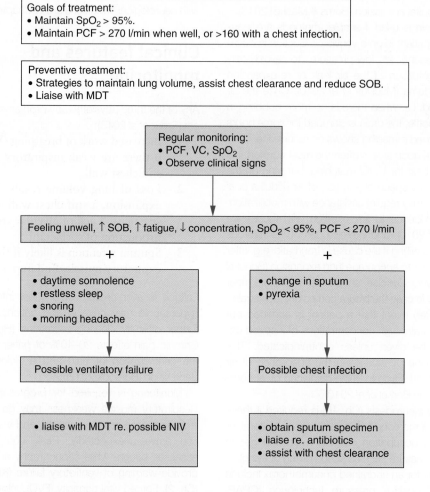

Goals of treatment:
• Maintain SpO_2 > 95%.
• Maintain PCF > 270 l/min when well, or >160 with a chest infection.

Preventive treatment:
• Strategies to maintain lung volume, assist chest clearance and reduce SOB.
• Liaise with MDT

Regular monitoring:
• PCF, VC, SpO_2
• Observe clinical signs

Feeling unwell, ↑ SOB, ↑ fatigue, ↓ concentration, SpO_2 < 95%, PCF < 270 l/min

+   +

• daytime somnolence
• restless sleep
• snoring
• morning headache

• change in sputum
• pyrexia

Possible ventilatory failure

Possible chest infection

• liaise with MDT re. possible NIV

• obtain sputum specimen
• liaise re. antibiotics
• assist with chest clearance

ADL: activities of daily living, *MDT:* multidisciplinary team including neuro-physiotherapist, *NIV:* non-invasive ventilation, *PCF:* peak cough flow, *SOB:* shortness of breath, *VC:* vital capacity

Dysphagia may lead to dehydration, which limits secretion clearance, and weight loss, which limits mobility. Other effects are aspiration, pneumonia, malnutrition and increased mortality (Macht *et al* 2011). If assistance with eating is not adequate, feeding can be by PEG (p. 160), or, so long as it does not cause feelings of choking, nasogastric tube. Monitoring dysphagia is by:

• water swallow test combined with oximetry (Connolly 2010)
• videofluoroscopy to identify delayed swallowing and reduced peristalsis, performed

by a radiologist and SLT, the physiotherapist standing by with suction equipment
• cervical auscultation to assess swallowing (Bergstrom *et al* 2014).

Classification

A weak cough is the main respiratory problem **in motor neurone disease** (MND), or its most common form **amyotrophic lateral sclerosis** (ALS). Patients

TABLE 3.5 Identification of a swallowing problem

Obvious indicators of dysphagia	Surreptitious indicators of dysphagia
• Difficulty with food or liquid in the mouth • Drooling • Difficulty swallowing • Coughing or choking before, during or after swallowing • Globus sensation ('lump in throat') • Hoarse voice • Feeling of obstruction • Regurgitation of undigested food • Nasal regurgitation • Unintentional weight loss	• Change in breathing pattern • Wet voice quality • Tongue fasciculation • Dry mouth • Heartburn • Change in eating e.g. eating slowly or avoiding social occasions • Frequent throat clearing • Recurrent chest infections or unexplained temperature spikes • Lack of elevation of larynx on swallowing

with bulbar onset ALS usually show dysarthria and dysphagia, with communication problems having a greater impact on the patient than loss of physical function (Mora *et al* 2012). Cortical atrophy predisposes to dementia (Schuster 2014), and patients with nocturnal hypoxia require oxygen at night to preserve cognitive function (Park *et al* 2014). In the later stages, NIV prolongs survival, improves quality of life (Baxter *et al* 2013) and can be managed at home (De Vito *et al* 2012), first at night and then continuously. Tracheostomy may be required if there is episodic stridor in the day and snoring at night, indicating intermittent adduction of the vocal cords (Shneerson 1996a). Dyspnoea may respond to some of the methods in Ch. 7, and can be relieved medically with diazepam or combined diamorphine/chlorpromazine/hyoscine. Excess salivation can be reduced by an anticholinergic such as atropine or hyoscine. Death occurs from respiratory failure, usually three to five years after onset of the disease; it may occur suddenly but is usually peaceful (Baxter *et al* 2013).

Expiratory muscles are disproportionately weak in people with **multiple sclerosis** (Klefbeck 2003), but bulbar dysfunction and abnormalities of breathing control can be significant. Inspiratory and expiratory muscle training may improve lung function (Srour *et al* 2013) and reduce fatigue (Ray 2013). Exercise has disease-modifying potential, but potential fatigue requires close adherence to the domains of the ICF, sometimes medication (Oral *et al* 2013) and always energy conservation (Blikman 2013).

Stroke with hemiparesis may increase CO_2 sensitivity and decrease voluntary ventilation on the weak side (Lanini 2003). Unilateral abdominal paradox on sniffing indicates unilateral diaphragmatic paralysis. Two thirds of patients harbour silent aspiration (Ratnaike 2002) and if they develop pneumonia, 20% die (Wilson 2012). Aspiration or reduced respiratory drive may cause hypoxaemia, especially at night (Roffe *et al* 2003) and supplemental oxygen should be given if S_pO_2 drops below 95% (Prasad *et al* 2011). Increased tone in any of the core muscles may increase WOB. Lung function may improve with manually-resisted inspiratory muscle exercise and pursed lips breathing but it is unclear whether this helped QoL (Seo *et al* 2013).

Myasthenia gravis is characterized by intermittent myasthenic crises which may cause upper airway obstruction, sleep apnoea or respiratory failure (Rassler *et al* 2011). Respiratory muscle training may reduce symptoms in mild or moderate disease (Rassler *et al* 2011).

Muscular dystrophy is a group of inherited disorders that involve progressive muscle weakness. Respiratory problems are the main cause of morbidity and mortality, most patients not realizing the extent of their respiratory muscle weakness until complications arise (ATS 2004). Respiratory function may improve with facilitation of respiration techniques (Nitz & Burke 2002). Survival can be prolonged by giving patients a pulse oximeter, and when S_pO_2 drops below 95%, using a regime of breath-stacking (p. 111), NIV and inexsufflation (AARC 2013a).

Post-polio respiratory syndrome may occur decades after the acute illness. Chronic overuse of weak muscles can lead to fatigue, respiratory distress, chronic pain (Werhagen *et al* 2013) and bladder symptoms (Kay 2013). 'Inspiratory muscle pacing' by inspiratory muscle training combined with part time NIV, can improve wellbeing (Klefbeck *et al* 2000). All physiotherapy must be modified to avoid fatigue.

Parkinson's disease is the second most common neurodegenerative disorder after Alzheimer's disease. Exercise improves gait (Ayán 2014), has a neuroprotective effect in reducing the risk of developing the disease or slowing its progression, and can improve cognition without excessive fatigue (Salgado *et al* 2013).

Diaphragmatic paralysis may be caused by MND, infection, trauma or malignancy. Nocturnal hypoxaemia sometimes occurs because of $\dot{V}_A/\dot{Q}$ mismatch in supine. Bilateral paralysis effectively removes a portion of the chest wall, obliging patients to exhale by contracting the abdominal muscles in order to push up the diaphragm, with passive inspiration possible in the upright position. Signs of bilateral paralysis or severe weakness are the following:

- orthopnoea unexplained by heart or lung disease
- accessory muscle activity unexplained by lung disease
- abdominal paradox during inspiration, especially in supine when the diaphragm is unable to counteract pressure from the abdominal contents
- postural fall in vital capacity (VC) of >50% in supine compared to upright
- symptoms of nocturnal hypoventilation, e.g. daytime somnolence, and hypercapnia, e.g. morning headache
- non-specific symptoms such as breathlessness or recurrent chest infections.

General management

Pulmonary complications are a well-known cause of morbidity and mortality (AARC 2013a). Oxygen is needed for hypoxaemic patients, but with a target saturation of 88–92% in case they have an inadequate hypercapnic drive (O'Driscoll *et al* 2011) especially in post-polio patients whose respiratory centres may have been damaged by the original viral infection. The multidisciplinary team includes SLT, occupational therapy and support groups (App B).

Management of chronic aspiration

Chronic aspiration is common in neurological disease if there is dysphagia or a poor gag reflex. A certain amount can be tolerated if mucociliary clearance is normal, but if symptoms are present, liaison with SLT, nursing staff and carers is required. Silent aspiration occurs without coughing but may cause any of the signs in Table 3.5 (p. 109).

Radiological signs can be regional or disseminated (Fig 3.19), which may progress to fibrosis (Lee *et al* 2010). Preventive measures are in App. C. 'Swallow rehabilitation' can take the form of isometric neck exercises to encourage laryngeal elevation (Logemann 1986) or neurostimulation (Michou & Hamdy 2013). The management of acute aspiration is on p. 114

FIGURE 3.19 Nodular shadows in the R lung, indicating chronic aspiration. The patient also has barotrauma on the L (pneumothorax in the upper zone and bulla in the lower zone) after prolonged mechanical ventilation, and scoliosis

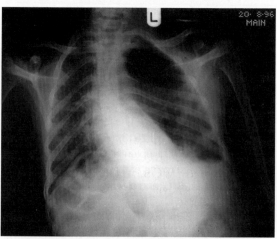

Respiratory physiotherapy

Some of the evidence-based techniques that have been found effective for specific disorders (above) may be beneficial for other neurological conditions. For assessment and outcomes, a neurological ICF Core Set has been validated (Bos *et al* 2013).

There are various studies showing that respiratory muscle training in the early stages of neurological disease improves respiratory muscle strength (Reyes *et al* 2013), but only research showing functional benefit has been discussed above.

Any of the three physiotherapy problems may be helped by the techniques in Chapters 6–8, outlined below in relation to neurological disease:

1   To assist sputum clearance, manual or mechanical support assists coughing for patients with PCF <270 l/min (AARC 2013a). The mechanical insufflator-exsufflator simulates a cough by applying positive and then negative pressure to the airway (Ch. 8). For patients with bulbar involvement, the insufflation phase should be avoided because patients can feel as if they are choking. The machine is not suited to patients without significant weakness because their muscles automatically resist.

2   To increase volume, breath-stacking or lung recruitment can be used. The patient takes a succession of deep breaths and stacks them behind their closed glottis. Assistance may be required by an in-exsufflator, a manual resuscitation bag and mask/mouthpiece, IPPB, or glossopharyngeal breathing (below). When done twice daily, breath-stacking can slow lung function decline and is particularly helpful before a cough (Srour *et al* 2013). Caution is required with fragile lungs because of possible barotrauma (Westermann 2013). Incentive spirometry and regular position change can also help maintain lung volume. If abdominal muscles show hypertonicity, inspiration may be facilitated by inhibitory postures.

3   To reduce WOB, a balance of rest and exercise is advised, avoiding the overuse of compensatory muscles and practicing interval training (Aboussouan 2009). Fatigue does not necessarily correlate with

disease severity and is partially reversible, e.g. by attention to hydration, nutrition and physical fitness, but is made worse by excess physical activity or distress (Lou *et al* 2010). Upright positioning may be more comfortable than other positions, and abdominal breathing enables some patients to use their muscles more efficiently. A useful side effect of in-exsufflation may be reduction of dyspnoea (Jones *et al* 2012b).

Patients with progressive disease are encouraged to make a decision on NIV before an acute episode precipitates action. They will need to know that if deterioration is progressive, weaning may be impossible. NIV can reduce a patient's dyspnoea, improve their quality of life and prolong survival (Jones *et al* 2012b). When used overnight it can improve sleep and prevent orthopnoea. The success of NIV can lead to loss of focus on the expiratory muscles, which may need to be strengthened by expiratory muscle training. Swallowing function can be enhanced by a bedside exercise programme (Kang *et al* 2012). An overview of respiratory physiotherapy for neurological patients is discussed by Jones *et al* (2012b).

Glossopharyngeal breathing is a technique that can be used to coax air into the lungs if FVC is <1 litre. Patients use their lips, soft palate and tongue to collect 30–200 ml mouthfuls of air into their mouth and throat, then after 6–30 mouthfuls, gulp it all into their lungs, using their tongue and pharynx, then hold it there by a closed glottis as the mouth is opened to collect the next bolus of air, building up to a single breath of up to 3 litres (Homnick 2007). Using a mirror, and in as upright a position as possible, training requires much concentration, with short daily sessions to avoid fatigue. A DVD is available (App. B). The following benefits have been demonstrated (Warren 2002, Filart *et al* 2003):

●   30 minutes' ventilator-free time
●   a safety margin in case of ventilator back-up failure
●   normalized speech, ability to cough, talk on the phone or call for help
●   easier defaecation
●   the ability to breath-stack independently
●   increased FVC.

Motivation is required to learn the technique, but some patients have been able to use it continuously, including at mealtimes when they briefly park the food at the side of their mouth.

SKELETAL DISORDERS

As with neurological disorders, some skeletal conditions restrict lung expansion even though the lungs themselves are usually normal.

Kyphoscoliosis

A distorted spine increases WOB because of reduced chest wall compliance, and a diaphragm forced to work from an inefficient configuration. Respiratory compromise may occur if the condition develops before adolescence (Fletcher & Bruce 2012). Exercise training can reduce dyspnoea and improve quality of life (Cejudo 2014).

Ankylosing spondylitis

This is a systemic disease which restricts breathing because of a rigid thoracic cage and kyphotic spine. X-ray signs include apparent hyperinflation because the chest wall becomes fixed in an inspiratory position. Lung involvement occurs in up to 30% of patients, including pleural thickening, upper lobe fibrosis and sometimes apical bullae (Maghraoui 2012). Attention to posture, thoracic mobility and exercise training are advocated (Halvorsen et al 2012).

CHEST INFECTIONS

Infection from viruses, bacteria or fungi can occur anywhere from the nose to the lung parenchyma. Chest infections are a common cause of exacerbation of lung disease and are the commonest acute problem dealt with in primary care (NICE 2008). They include anything from acute bronchitis, a common and usually self-limiting viral infection of the upper airways, to life-threatening pneumonia.

People at risk are those who are very old, very young, immunocompromised, stressed (Dhabhar 2009) or exposed to air pollution (Huang 2012). Physiotherapy may be required if patients are unable to clear secretions or need assistance with rehabilitation.

Respiratory tract infection

Upper respiratory tract infection covers pharyngitis, laryngitis, sinusitis, otitis media, the common cold and flu.

Physiotherapy beyond advice is not usually required. The **common cold** is an infection of the nose, throat, sinuses and upper airways, caused by 200 different viruses, of which rhinoviruses are the commonest. People with an inactive lifestyle are the most susceptible (Nieman et al 2010) and those with asthma or cystic fibrosis react strongly to the rhinovirus (Randell et al 2006). Patients are contagious two to three days before symptoms begin and remain contagious until symptoms have cleared.

The **influenza** virus can jump the species barrier and tends to occur in pandemics, including the 1918 episode which killed more people than the First World War (Rumschlag-Booms 2013). Flu reduces the speed of mucociliary clearance and increases susceptibility to secondary bacterial infections (Pittet et al 2010). Warm airways appear to have an antiviral effect and the patient's subjective need to keep warm should be encouraged (Bender 2000). A cough or sneeze propels droplets up to a metre, which is a reminder to take precautions when a patient coughs or is suctioned (Thompson et al 2013). Flu vaccination, if required, needs to be repeated annually because of virus mutation (Beck et al 2011).

Pneumonia

Pneumonia is caused by bacteria, fungi, chemical agents or viruses. These breach lung defences, inflame lung parenchyma and the smallest bronchioles, then fill and consolidate alveoli with fibrous exudate. Risk factors are stroke, poor nutrition, smoking, alcoholism, winter and the extremes of age. The pattern is altering as more critically ill patients survive, transplantation increases and antibiotic resistance grows. A quarter of hospitalized patients with pneumonia develop a major cardiac complication (Corrales et al 2013).

Clinical features include fever, shortness of breath (SOB) and tachycardia. If localized, the affected area is painful and may demonstrate a dull percussion note, pleural rub, decreased expansion and bronchial breath sounds or fine crackles on auscultation. Imaging often lags behind clinical presentation but tends to show a patchy opacity (Figs 3.20/21), which may not resolve for some weeks. Radiological signs are minimized in dehydrated patients (Goudarzi 2000).

A dry cough may later become productive of purulent or rust-coloured sputum as the consolidation resolves, but most of the exudate is removed by phagocytosis via

MINI CASE STUDY : MS TP

A 24 y.o. patient has been admitted with pneumonia.

Background
- Unemployed, mobile, independent.
- Heroin user.

Subjective assessment
- Well.

Objective assessment
- Patient in nightie, tucked up in bed.
- Apyrexial.
- Fluid balance normal.
- S_pO_2 normal.
- Auscultation – bronchial breathing left lower lobe, no crackles.
- Respiratory rate normal.
- Breathing pattern normal.

Questions
1. Identify the consolidation in Fig 3.20
2. Analysis?
3. Problems?
4. Goals?
5. Plan? Response on p. 115.

FIGURE 3.20 Ms TP

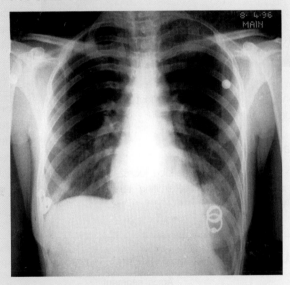

the blood stream. Sensitized nerve endings may leave a dry irritating cough for some time.

The structure of the lung is preserved and resolution is usually complete, but there is a legacy of increased risk of cardiovascular disease (Soto-Gomez 2013).

Medical treatment is by oral or intravenous fluids, antimicrobial drugs and oxygen if indicated. Physiotherapy is by positioning for ventilation/perfusion ($\dot{V}_A/\dot{Q}$) matching, CPAP if hypoxaemia persists despite optimum oxygen therapy (Liu *et al* 2010) and sometimes assistance with chest clearance. Early mobility shortens hospital stay (Mundy *et al* 2003), and rehabilitation helps reduce subsequent complications such as cognitive

impairment (Davydow *et al* 2013), falls and delirium (Mody 2012). Neuromuscular osteopathic techniques to relax the diaphragm and increase ribcage mobility have led to interesting reductions in hospital stay and the need for antibiotics (Noll *et al* 2010).

Pneumonia is known as 'community acquired' unless it develops in hospital. Subdivisions are below.

Bronchopneumonia

Bronchopneumonia is patchy and diffuse, often favouring the lower lobes and sometimes producing fine crackles on auscultation. It is most common in immobile or elderly people, over half of whom demonstrate

FIGURE 3.21 Consolidation of R upper lobe

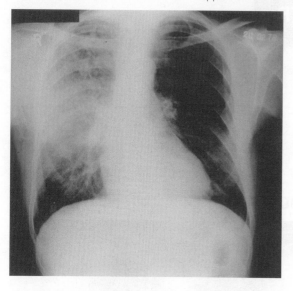

dysphagia (Cabre 2010). Complications include dehydration and confusion.

Lobar pneumonia

If pneumonia is confined to a lobe, localized pleuritic pain is a distinguishing feature, limiting tidal volume and mobility.

Aspiration pneumonia

Regurgitation: reflux of gastric contents into the oesophagus or oropharynx.
Aspiration: inhalation of foreign material into the airways beyond the vocal cords.
Microaspiration: repeated small episodes of aspiration that do not cause acute symptoms.

Acute aspiration may cause cough, SOB, tachycardia, wheeze and diffuse crackles, then within hours the development of aspiration pneumonia. It is based on inflammation rather than infection, with inflammatory mediators causing bronchospasm and sometimes a vicious pneumonitis which corrodes the alveolar-capillary membrane, depletes surfactant and causes chemical pulmonary oedema, haemorrhage and necrosis.

Radiological signs of consolidation are apparent within hours, then increase over one or two days, then either begin to resolve or show evidence of deterioration, e.g. acute respiratory distress syndrome or an abscess. The location of infiltrates helps identify the affected lobe (Fig 3.22) and therefore the postural drainage position to use, if appropriate.

Risk factors are:

* nasogastric tube or tracheal tube (Raghavendran *et al* 2012)

FIGURE 3.22 Pneumonia in different lobes caused by aspiration in varying positions

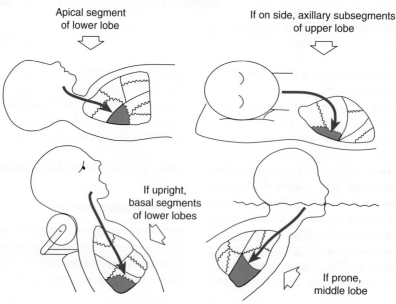

Apical segment of lower lobe

If on side, axillary subsegments of upper lobe

If upright, basal segments of lower lobes

If prone, middle lobe

- impaired mobility or poor dental hygiene
- old age, due to depression of the cough reflex (Yamanda *et al* 2008)
- altered consciousness, e.g. sedation, brain injury, alcohol intoxication, seizure, sleep
- pregnancy or obesity, due to increased abdominal pressure
- gastroesophageal reflux (Lee *et al* 2010)
- unexpected loss of consciousness.

If the cause is unexpected loss of consciousness, the patient and x-ray are checked for trauma, then immediate physiotherapy is required in the form of postural drainage, percussion, vibrations, shaking and cough or suction. If the patient aspirated in supine, positioning the patient prone may assist postural drainage, improve oxygenation and help prevent progression to established pneumonitis (Easby *et al* 2003). If the patient is able, other techniques to clear secretions can be used. If the cause is intubation, manual hyperinflation is usually required. Once consolidation has set in, as indicated by bronchial breathing, and if there are no crackles on auscultation, airway clearance techniques are ineffective, but positioning may assist $\dot{V}_A/\dot{Q}$ matching.

Pneumocystis pneumonia

The saprophyte 'pneumocystis' normally lives innocuously in human lungs, but in people whose defence mechanisms are weakened, they can become agents for opportunist infection. Invading fungal organisms damage the alveolar lining, causing hypoxaemia, SOB, chills, sweats, pleuritic pain and a dry cough. Auscultation may be normal or demonstrate fine scattered crackles. Imaging may be normal at first if immune deficiency delays the appearance of an inflammatory response, but later signs are disseminated reticular or granular opacities and air bronchograms (see Fig 2.23). Sudden deterioration raises suspicions of a pneumothorax. Physiotherapy may be required for acute SOB (Ch. 7).

Legionella pneumonia

Legionnaires' disease is a severe bacterial pneumonia which often leaves survivors with permanent lung fibrosis (Caterino 2013). When hospital-acquired, it is three times as fatal as the community-acquired variant (Jespersen *et al* 2010). It is not spread between humans but occurs in local outbreaks, especially near contaminated water

systems or inadequately-cleaned nebulizers (Mastro *et al* 1991).

BOOP or COP

Bronchiolitis obliterans organizing pneumonia (BOOP) or cryptogenic organizing pneumonia (COP) is characterized by granulation tissue becoming organized in the alveoli. It represents an indolent inflammatory extension of a primary process, e.g. bronchiolitis obliterans, cystic fibrosis, heart surgery (Sara 2008), cancer therapy or toxicity from medication (Camus 2004). It responds to steroids rather than antibiotics.

Hospital-acquired pneumonia

Pneumonia which develops more than 48 hours after admission to hospital is known as hospital-acquired or nosocomial pneumonia. It involves different pathogens to community-acquired pneumonia and brings higher mortality (Bargellini 2013). In the ICU, ventilator-associated pneumonia is the commonest infection (Meyer *et al* 2010) and the main cause of death (Khan *et al* 2009b). Cross-infection between patients is the likely offender, usually carried by staff, or infection from the patient's own colonized sites via invasive equipment or dental plaque (Ewan *et al* 2013). Nosocomial MRSA pneumonia is by definition difficult to manage, with airway secretions being a major site for infection (Laguna *et al* 2009).

Response to Case Study

1 **Consolidation**
   - Area of consolidation seen behind left pierced nipple.

2 **Analysis**
   - No accessible secretions. No atelectasis. No desaturation.
   - Bronchial breathing may linger but is not causing problems.
   - It is not necessary to 'treat the x-ray'.

3 **Problems**
   - No physiotherapy problems at present.

4 **Goals**
   - Self-rehabilitation.

5   **Plan**
   - Advise patient to get dressed and mobilize.
   - Liaise with team re. assistance for drug habit.

Pulmonary tuberculosis (TB)

TB is the world's most lethal infection, with nearly ten million new cases a year (Evans *et al* 2013). One third of the world's population is infected by the TB bacillus, which resides unobtrusively in immunocompetent hosts but may become active if defence mechanisms are impaired by poor living conditions, drug dependency or HIV infection (Gandhi *et al* 2010).

The lung is the commonest site of infection. Coughing disseminates infected aerosol, which can remain suspended in the air for some hours. Symptoms are fever, night sweats, cough, chest wall pain, weight loss, haemoptysis and SOB.

The tubercle bacillus is slow-growing and tough, responding only to six months' treatment with a combination of powerful antibacterial drugs. The patient is no longer infectious after two weeks' treatment, providing sputum is clear of the bacillus. 'Multidrug-resistant' TB requires second-line drugs for up to two years, bringing significant side effects and success rates of 65–75%. 'Extensively drug-resistant' TB may be incurable (Chaisson 2012).

The physiotherapist's role is usually confined to eliciting sputum specimens in a negative pressure room and devising ways to encourage exercise in an isolation cubicle. A high efficiency particulate air-filtering mask must be used throughout.

Aspergillosis

The aspergillus fungus lives in the soil, is ubiquitous, and inhalation is common. Allergic bronchopulmonary aspergillosis represents a spectrum of diseases resulting from impaired or excessive immune response to inhaling the fungus. It is found in 2–32% of people with asthma and 2–15% of those with cystic fibrosis (Agarwal *et al* 2012) and can occur opportunistically in people with neutropaenia, cancer, malnutrition, diabetes, TB or bronchiectasis.

Aspergillus spores germinate in the lung, forming a tangled mass termed a fungus ball or aspergilloma. Clinical features include malaise, weight loss, SOB, fever, haemoptysis and a cough productive of sputum containing brown plugs of the fungus. Diagnosis is by bronchoscopy, lavage or CT scan.

The condition may continue for years, sometimes leading to fibrosis and cor pulmonale. Treatment is by antifungal agents, sometimes reduction of immunosuppressive therapy and occasionally surgical or bronchoscopic removal (Stather 2013).

Abscess

A lung abscess develops when bacterial infection causes necrosis, producing pus-containing cavities in the lung parenchyma. Causes are aspiration of pathogen-laden material or a foreign body, or conditions such as an obstructing cancer or bronchiectasis.

Patients present with a spiking fever, night sweats, cough, putrid sputum, haemoptysis, pleuritic chest pain and fatigue. The x-ray shows an opaque lesion until communication with the airways is established, when drainage of the debris leaves a thick-walled ring shadow with a fluid line (see Fig 2.22). Prolonged antibiotics are required.

Physiotherapy is effective if the abscess is open to the airways, postural drainage being safe so long as the correct antibiotic is given and the posture is accurate and thorough to avoid dissemination of infection (App. F). Liaison with a radiologist is required to confirm the exact location of the abscess, but if there is doubt, the condition is best left to the antibiotics.

LUNG CANCER

Ageing has been described as the greatest of all carcinogens

Gems (2011a)

Precursors to cancer can be seen in most healthy people above middle age (Gøtzsche 2002), indicating the importance of keeping alert to suspicious signs. Most people with cancer now survive beyond five-years (McNeely 2012), but lung cancer kills more people (Wilcock *et al* 2013) and causes more distress (Ellis 2012) than other cancers. Smoking is the main culprit,

FIGURE 3.23 Turbulent airflow at branching of airway

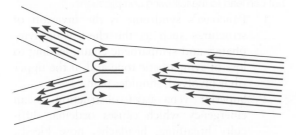

FIGURE 3.24

(Top) Dense opacity of L upper and mid zones partially obliterates a suspiciously-shaped 'aorta'. (Bottom) Darkened film shows 'aorta' to be a tumour squeezing the L main bronchus, reducing aeration of the L upper lobe.
Loss of volume is reflected in a raised L hemidiaphragm.

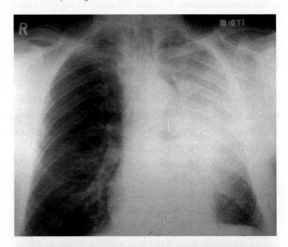

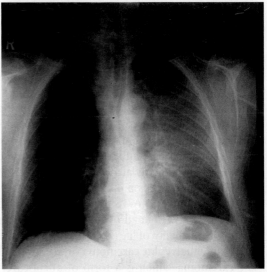

and most tumours arise in the large bronchi, whose bifurcations are the first to be hit by tobacco smoke (Fig 3.23). This also makes them amenable to diagnostic endobronchial ultrasound and bronchoscopy (Hennon *et al* 2013).

X-ray changes may be present for over six years without symptoms (Kahana 2000). A mass may hide behind the mediastinum, or a tumour in a main bronchus may not be obvious until the lung collapses (Figs 3.24, 2.19a). Early signs are unexplained cough or digital clubbing, recurrent pneumonia, and sometimes hypertrophic pulmonary osteoarthropathy, which causes pain and swelling of the wrists or ankles and may require bisphosponates for pain control (Kilaru *et al* 2012). The sensitivity of sputum cytology is 60% (Ammanagi *et al* 2012), and an 'electronic nose' can pick up the disease in exhaled breath (Dent *et al* 2013), as can dogs (Buszewski *et al* 2012).

Clinical features

The most distressing symptom is **shortness of breath** (SOB), caused by respiratory muscle weakness (Travers *et al* 2007), radiotherapy or the tumour itself. It occurs in up to 90% of patients and is less responsive to medication than is pain (Barton *et al* 2010). A persistent non-productive **cough** occurs in 40–70% of patients at initial presentation, caused by obstruction, pleural effusion, pneumonitis or comorbid COPD (Yorke *et al* 2012).

Cancer **fatigue** has been described as totally unlike even the most profound fatigue of an otherwise well person. This is not always understood by health staff, who tend to think that pain is a more disruptive symptom (Radbruch 2008). Fatigue is the symptom that most affects quality of life, affecting concentration (Borneman 2013) and sometimes continuing for months or years after treatment (Aynehchi *et al* 2013). It is not proportional to recent activity and is often not relieved by rest, so pacing needs to be incorporated into all physiotherapy interventions. In the final stage of life, fatigue has been described as a protective mechanism (Radbruch 2008). Causes are cachexia, anaemia, inflammation, deconditioning, sleep disturbance, pain, radiotherapy, chemotherapy or depression.

Depression is common, reduces adherence to treatment and increases mortality (Walker *et al* 2013). It tends to be undertreated because of an assumption, according to Weinberger *et al* (2012), that it is normal for cancer patients to be depressed. Normal does not mean OK.

Other clinical features are a diffuse or aching **chest pain**, **stridor**, a monophonic **wheeze**, **hoarseness** if the recurrent laryngeal nerve is involved, and sometimes **haemoptysis**. **Pleural effusion** is a poor prognostic sign.

Classification

The four main histologic subtypes are **adenocarcinoma, small-cell carcinoma, large-cell carcinoma** (also known as 'non-small-cell carcinoma') and **squamous cell carcinoma**. Less common are:

- **Kaposi sarcoma** (KS) which affects the skin, gut, connective tissue and lungs of immunocompromised people and is the most frequent AIDS-defining cancer (Dittmer *et al* 2012). Pulmonary KS affects the parenchyma, lymph nodes or pleura, manifesting as progressive SOB, cough and hypoxaemia.
- **Mesothelioma** which arises in the mesothelial cells of the peritoneum, pericardium or, most commonly, the pleura, where it is associated with malignant pleural effusion, finger clubbing and a chest pain 'like being encased in concrete'. It is caused by asbestos exposure and will increase by 5–10% per year in Europe over the next 25 years because of its decades-long latency period (Thompson *et al* 2014). It has a dismal prognosis and is normally fatal in 6–18 months (Zauderer & Krug 2012) but drugs and surgery can improve quality of life (Haas 2013).
- **Bronchoalveolar carcinoma** or **alveolar cell carcinoma** which is a form of adenocarcinoma and occasionally produces extreme quantities of watery sputum that sometimes responds to inhaled indomethacin (Tamaoki *et al* 2000). It is not caused by smoking and develops in peripheral lung tissue, manifesting as local or diffuse infiltrates on x-ray and causing SOB and a very productive cough.

Lung **metastases** are a poor prognostic sign requiring multidisciplinary teamwork (Koczywas *et al* 2013). They are sometimes resectable (Schlijper 2014) but can lead to the following complications:

1. Pancoast's syndrome is the invasion of structures such as the chest wall, lymphatics and sympathetic chain, leading to loss of sympathetic tone and, if the upper rib is involved, shoulder pain.
2. Superior vena cava obstruction is an emergency which causes oedema, difficulty breathing, headache, nose bleeds, haemoptysis, stridor and faintness on bending down. It requires radiotherapy, steroids, stenting (Duvnjak 2012) and raising the head of the bed.

Medical treatment

The aim is to inflict the greatest damage to the cancer with the least damage to the patient, but the disease is often disseminated at presentation. Chemotherapy may lead to 'chemo-brain', a form of cognitive decline which is often missed (Argyriou 2011), or 'chemo-lung', a form of lung fibrosis that can be aggravated by high concentration oxygen therapy (Allan *et al* 2012). Radiotherapy may cause rib fracture (Leprieur *et al* 2013).

Treatment of reversible factors includes palliation of upper airway obstruction by laser, stenting (which may cause a dry cough) or bronchoplasty (Juarez *et al* 2011). Immunotherapy assists the immune system to recognize and destroy residual cancer cells that conventional therapy misses (Heuvers *et al* 2013). The future holds promise with targeted aerosol chemotherapy (Zarogoulidis 2012).

Surgery is discussed in Ch. 16. The term 'resectable' indicates that the primary tumour can be completely excised, while 'operable' indicates that surgery brings an acceptably low risk of death or morbidity (BTS/SCTS 2010). Non-resectable tumours may respond to microwave ablation (Belfiore *et al* 2013). A third of patients have bone metastases which can cause pain, fractures and spinal cord compression, and surgery may be undertaken if life expectancy is long enough for patients to benefit from pain relief and improved mobility (Weiss 2011).

Most patients also have COPD (Ozalevli 2013), which requires treatment, and long-term survivors require ongoing care because of a heavy burden of continuing symptoms (Yang *et al* 2013). Undertreatment of lung cancer in elderly people is common, resulting in age-related survival variations (Peake 2003).

Physiotherapy

> *I came in a bent-over old man; I am leaving an upright, middle-aged gentleman*
> Patient quoted by McNeely (2012)

Physiotherapists may be involved at any stage including sputum induction, prehabilitation before surgery, postoperative management, relaxation, massage (Deng *et al* 2013), energy conservation, exercise and terminal care.

Moderate regular exercise induces cancer-preventive potential but a single bout of exhaustive exercise may increase the risk of some cancer development. In established cancer, after checking for anaemia, exercise, especially interval exercise (Ozalevli 2013) can improve fatigue, exercise capacity, and quality of life (Filaire *et al* 2013). It can enhance sleep quality (Sprod 2010). It should, however, include falls prevention strategies (Winters *et al* 2012) and pacing. Exercise is also beneficial after surgery (Garrod 2011) and during palliative chemotherapy (Henke *et al* 2014).

Spinal cord compression from metastases is always a risk so any new lower limb weakness must be reported. Occasionally a patient may cough up tumour tissue, so if a specimen has the appearance of a blood clot, it should be sent to cytology (Ochi *et al* 2012). Venous thromboembolism occurs in a third of patients (Connolly *et al* 2013).

Outcome measures include dyspnoea scales (Ahmedzai *et al* 2012, p. 100), functional scales (Dean 2013) and exercise tests (Henke *et al* 2014).

CARDIORESPIRATORY MANIFESTATIONS OF SYSTEMIC DISEASE

The cardiorespiratory system is influenced by most systemic disturbances. Oxygen delivery is impaired by anaemia, breathing is disrupted by acid-base imbalance and emotion, and the alveolar-capillary membrane is rendered leaky by sepsis. The conditions below are those with the most impact on cardiorespiratory function.

HIV, AIDS and immunosuppression

People with HIV (human immunodeficiency virus) are treated to prevent the development of AIDS (acquired immune deficiency syndrome). In countries where combination antiretroviral drugs are not available, the majority of deaths from AIDS are caused by conditions associated with immunodeficiency such as lung cancer (Winstone *et al* 2013) pneumocystis pneumonia (Sarkar 2013), abscess or TB.

The physiotherapist's role is to assess for mobility or respiratory problems. For people with HIV, thrice-weekly aerobic exercise can improve functional capacity while reducing fatigue and stress (Hand *et al* 2009), but prolonged intense exercise can further suppress the immune system (Fig 3.25).

FIGURE 3.25 Dose-dependent effect of exercise on risk and severity of respiratory tract infections

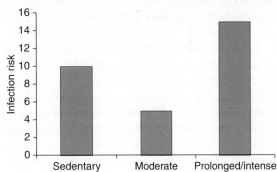

Sleep apnoea

> *I literally fell asleep into my plate*
> Patient quoted by Sims (2003)

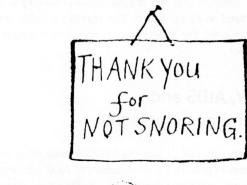

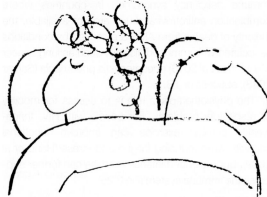

Approximately 15–20% of road accidents have been attributed to sleepiness and fatigue (Ftouni 2013), with fatality rates similar to alcohol-related crashes (Goel et al 2009). Sleep deprivation related to sleep apnoea has contributed to oil tanker spills, nuclear meltdowns and the Challenger space shuttle explosion (Howard 2005).

Sleep-disordered breathing occurs in 5–15% of the population (Punjabi 2013). Sleep apnoea occurs when breathing stops for more than ten seconds. Desaturation stimulates the respiratory centres, and the subsequent arousal may be accompanied by spectacular snoring. The patient is affected by daytime sleepiness, poor concentration, morning headaches due to CO_2 retention, memory loss and a disgruntled spouse. Hypoxaemia leads to cognitive decline, and sympathetic activation during arousal causes spikes in blood pressure, leading over time to cardiovascular disease and increased mortality. Even so, sleep apnoea usually goes undiagnosed (Carr 2012).

The risk of sleep apnoea is increased by smoking, excess alcohol, being male (because progesterone is a respiratory stimulant) and comorbid COPD, lung fibrosis or sickle cell disease (Owens 2013). It can worsen in hospital because of sedative drugs, the supine position and sleep deprivation. Diagnosis is made from symptoms, history and a sleep study.

Patients may misinterpret sleepiness as fatigue, and Devasahayam (2012) found sleep disorders to be the commonest misdiagnosis for people referred to a chronic fatigue clinic. Physiotherapists may be the first to suspect the condition.

Obstructive sleep apnoea (OSA) is due to nocturnal upper airway obstruction, leading to intermittent hypoxia which alters brain structure and function (Gozal 2013). It is often associated with obesity because a thick neck can choke patients in their own fat when muscle tone wanes at night. Childhood obesity has led to an increase in children with the condition (Yang 2012), who present with hyperactivity rather than sleepiness (Muzumdar & Arens 2013). Management is by weight loss, smoking cessation and avoidance of evening alcohol, exercise, stimulation of the genioglossus muscle, playing the didgeridoo (Chwiesko 2013) and avoiding sleeping supine, e.g. wearing a back-to-front bra with tennis balls in each cup. If lifestyle advice is not adequate, continuous positive airway pressure (CPAP) is used at night to pneumatically splint open the upper airway. This reduces the risk of cardiovascular disease (Phillips 2012), fatigue and sleep-related road accidents (Fig 3.26). Alternatives are high-flow nasal cannulae (Bräunlich 2013), contraptions to hold open the upper airway (Gakwaya et al 2014), surgery such as uvulopalatopharyngoplasty (Hou et al 2012), which is as complicated as it sounds, or tracheostomy.

Central sleep apnoea may overlap with OSA but involves no respiratory effort. It is associated with neurological disorders, heart failure or abnormal control of breathing (Malhotra & Owens 2010) including hyperventilation syndrome (Pevernagie 2012) and may require non-invasive ventilation (Delisle et al 2013). **Restrictive sleep apnoea** can occur with scoliosis, ankylosing spondylitis or diaphragmatic paralysis.

Regular exercise for people with sleep disorders can increase energy and reduce fatigue (Hargens et al 2013). Patients with a mixture of apneas may benefit from BiPAP (p. 213), using a timed back-up rate to counteract hypoventilation (Brown 2013).

Kidney disease

Kidney disease and its treatment may affect the cardiorespiratory system by causing:

- metabolic acidosis
- fluid overload, leading to pulmonary oedema and sometimes pleural effusion

FIGURE 3.26 Reduction in fatigue and number of road accidents in people with sleep-disordered breathing after a year of CPAP (Cassel 1996)

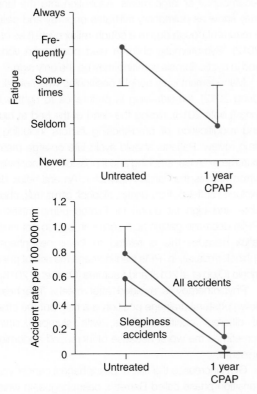

- breathlessness due to pulmonary oedema or to compensate for metabolic acidosis
- muscle wasting due to steroid treatment or uraemia.

Kidneys regulate the excretion of most drugs, and an adverse reaction to drugs is one cause of acute kidney injury, indicated by raised serum creatinine or reduced urine output. Treatment is by fluid management, renal replacement therapy if required (Ch. 19), discontinuation of nephrotoxic drugs and wary use of other drugs (Lapi et al 2013). Physiotherapy is based on exercise, including during dialysis (Orcy et al 2012).

Liver disease

The liver is the most metabolically active tissue by weight in the body, being served by two blood supplies and boasting over 500 functions. Most drug metabolism occurs in the liver, which complicates medical management when it malfunctions (Lin & Smith 2010). Predisposing factors of liver disease are alcohol misuse, malnutrition and some medications, more than 1000 drugs being associated with hepatic injury (Kim & Hattori 2010). If the cause of a liver problem is unknown, patients should be tested for alpha$_1$-antitrypsin deficiency (p. 77) (Pferdmenges et al 2013).

Complications relevant to physiotherapy are dyspnoea, which can be caused by hepatomegaly, ascites, pulmonary vascular complications (Fritz et al 2013) or cardiovascular disease (Perazzo et al 2014), and quadriceps weakened by 50% if alcohol misuse is the cause (Andersen et al 2012).

Precautions relevant to physiotherapy are the following:

- Tracheal suction is performed with caution if clotting is disturbed.
- Portal hypertension may cause oesophageal varices, in which case nasopharyngeal suction is contraindicated, unless essential, in case the catheter enters the oesophagus.
- Cerebral oedema can cause hyperventilation, which may require mechanical ventilation, and circulating toxins can cause encephalopathy, which reduces the patient's ability to co-operate.
- Bilirubin in the plasma of jaundiced patients limits the accuracy of oximetry.
- Following hepatic resection, blood glucose may be destabilized (Maeda 2010) which has implications for mobilizing patients.

Sickle cell disease

The pain of sickle cell crisis is one of the most intense in medicine.

Nagel 2001

Sickle cell disease is a genetic disorder occurring mostly in black populations and characterized by red blood cells crystallizing into a rigid sickle shape, rendering them unable to squeeze through small vessels. The result is vaso-occlusion, haemolytic anaemia and a disturbed immune system, leading to death at average age 45 (Adeniyi & Saminu 2011).

Intermittent sickling crises can be precipitated by nocturnal hypoxaemia (Owens 2013), pain, fatigue

(Panepinto 2014), dehydration, infection, extreme temperature change, smoking or sudden exercise. The ischaemic pain of a sickling crisis is notoriously undermanaged (Haywood *et al* 2011), particularly by staff who may suspect that African Americans misuse narcotics (Mossey 2011). This has been found with other conditions, Hispanics being twice as likely as whites to receive no analgesia after trauma, and black patients being 66% less likely to receive analgesia after leg fracture (Brockopp *et al* 2003). People with sickle cell disease must be under the care of a specialist unit where morphine is provided in doses sufficient to compensate for the drug clearing three to ten times faster than in the general population (Darbari *et al* 2012). Some patients carry a note from their specialist specifying the analgesia required.

When vaso-occlusion occurs in the pulmonary vasculature, an acute chest syndrome of pain, breathlessness, atelectasis and sometimes bronchospasm occurs (Hassan 2004). Pain causes diaphragmatic splinting and atelectasis, for which incentive spirometry has been found helpful (Adeniyi & Saminu 2011).

Patients benefit from advice on joint protection and pacing. Regular physical activity helps control endothelial dysfunction (Chirico *et al* 2012) but the disease is a risk factor for unexpected death with over-exertion (Key & Derebail 2012). Ice treatment should be avoided in case of rhabdomyolysis. Hypercoagulability is common and any sign of thromboembolism needs to be reported.

Gastroesophageal reflux (GOR) disease

GOR is the passage of gastric contents up into the oesophagus. This occurs in most people, but if frequent enough to damage the mucosa of the oesophagus or cause symptoms, it becomes a disease. Aspiration of this material can cause, trigger or exacerbate COPD, cystic fibrosis, asthma, sleep apnoea or interstitial lung disease (Fekri 2014). This association may relate to altered intrathoracic pressures or a shared vagal innervation by the oesophagus and bronchial tree (Caster *et al* 2011).

Risk factors are the extremes of age, intellectual disability (May & Kennedy 2010), smoking, alcohol, chronic aspiration and raised abdominal pressure e.g. obesity or frequent coughing.

Stomach acid outside the mucous-protected environment of the stomach causes heartburn, airway hyperreactivity, tooth erosion, nocturnal cough, morning hoarseness and a bitter taste in the mouth after recumbency or large meals. Aspiration into the lungs may show as pulmonary infiltrates on x-ray and cause a recurrent cough due to a cough-reflux cycle (Lee *et al* 2012). Symptomatic children feed poorly and vomit, and in cystic fibrosis vomiting may be the only sign.

Management is by upright positioning when possible (Jung 2012), left-side-lying in preference to right-side-lying (Loots 2013), raising the head of the bed at night and modification of predisposing factors including a drug review. Patients should avoid late or large meals, extreme exercise, smoking and if possible aminophylline which relaxes the cardiac sphincter. An anti-reflux diet excludes caffeine, fizzy drinks, alcohol, citrus fruit, chocolate and high fat products. Proton pump inhibitors (PPIs) decrease gastric acid secretion but do not inhibit reflux because this is related to lower oesophageal sphincter relaxation. PPIs also increase the risk of pneumonia (Ojoo *et al* 2013) and fractures (Ozdil *et al* 2013).

Physiotherapy is avoided after meals. The head-down postural drainage position is a risk, but the effect of different positions varies, with slumped sitting sometimes the worst because of increased abdominal pressure.

GOR increases the risk of oesophageal cancer via a transition phase called Barrett's oesophagus, in which metaplastic epithelium replaces the stratified squamous epithelium that normally lines the distal oesophagus (Coupland *et al* 2012).

Diabetes mellitus

The incidence of Type 2 diabetes is reaching epidemic proportions because of obesity and hypertension (Nisell 2013). Lung complications include collagen and elastin changes, acid-base disturbance and sometimes hyperglycaemia from steroids. Cardiac complications include coronary heart disease, which is the single most important cause of mortality and morbidity (Gheydari *et al* 2013). Other complications relevant to physiotherapy include fluid upset, hypotension, susceptibility to infection (Yende *et al* 2012), depression (Ernst 2012) and musculoskeletal complications (Baker *et al* 2012a).

With stable diabetes, regular exercise improves endothelial function (Golbidi & Laher 2012), increases insulin sensitivity (Jung & Han 2012), reduces stress

(Putiri *et al* 2012) and, when weight-bearing, increases exercise tolerance (Mueller 2013) so long as patients maintain hydration, look after their feet and when necessary increase their insulin or carbohydrates to avoid hypoglycaemic events. Warning signs of hypoglycaemia include light-headedness, rapid breathing, weakness and fatigue, and patients need to bring a glucose tablet to exercise sessions. Cardiac response to exercise is attenuated (Joshi 2010), and exercise capacity may be further impaired by orthostatic intolerance or autonomic neuropathy.

For surgical patients, major swings in blood sugar can occur, particularly with cardiothoracic surgery (Baynes *et al* 2001).

On the bright side, people with diabetes are less likely to develop acute respiratory distress syndrome (Barbas *et al* 2012).

Inflammatory bowel disease

Systemic dissemination of inflammation may occur from ulcerative colitis or Crohn's disease, predisposing to a selection of lung conditions such as bronchiectasis, interstitial lung disease, BOOP and asthma (Zgraggen 2013). Respiratory symptoms may appear years after the bowel disease (Mahadeva *et al* 2000) and the physiotherapist may be the first to make the connection.

Drug-induced cardiorespiratory disease

Adverse drug events are a significant preventable cause of hospitalization, especially in older people (Budnitz *et al* 2011). Cardiorespiratory examples are aspirin causing asthma, amiodarone causing fibrosis (Cott *et al* 2013) and cardiovascular drugs causing fatal bradycardias (Givens 2012). Exercise training can reduce drug misuse and decrease comorbid risk factors (Smith & Lynch 2012).

Reactions to illicit drug use depend on the substance, contaminants and route of administration. **Cocaine** can lead to strokes, myocardial infarction or multisystem failure (Zimmerman 2012). **Crack cocaine** can cause 'crack lung', encompassing fever, haemoptysis, dyspnoea, pulmonary edema, alveolar damage and the complications of its mode of delivery,

including necrosis of the nasal septum and barotrauma (Mégarbane *et al* 2013).

Cannabis can impair cognition (Battistella 2013), cause barotrauma (Golwala 2012) and bring complications related to the tobacco with which it is usually mixed (Tashkin & Simmons 2012). Prenatal cannabis exposure can have a long-lasting impact on the developing brain (Wu *et al* 2011). More optimistically, cannabis can reduce the pain of spasticity in multiple sclerosis (Corey-Bloom 2012), and non-psychoactive preparations have been used for nausea, neurodegenerative diseases, pain (De Vries 2012), bronchospasm, Alzheimer's disease, osteoporosis and some cardiovascular disorders (Kogan 2007).

RESPIRATORY FAILURE

The term **respiratory failure** (RF) is reserved for inadequate gas exchange as reflected in arterial blood gases, even though the process of respiration includes more than gas exchange in the lung. **Respiratory insufficiency** is a vague term that suggests adequate gas exchange but at some cost, and may presage respiratory failure.

Type I (hypoxaemic) RF is failed oxygenation, represented by P_aO_2 <8 kPa (60 mmHg). It is due to failure of the gas-exchanging function of the respiratory system and can be acute (e.g. pneumonia) or chronic (e.g. COPD).

Type II (hypoxaemic and hypercapnic) RF is failed ventilation, represented by P_aCO_2 >6.7 kPa (50 mmHg) as well as hypoxaemia (Fig 3.27). Raised CO_2 is caused by failure of the respiratory pump, e.g. impaired central respiratory drive or muscle weakness, and can be acute (e.g. severe acute asthma) or chronic (e.g. late-stage fibrosing alveolitis). Type II RF is also known as ventilatory failure and is accompanied by a fall in pH until renal compensation takes effect.

In the later stages of COPD, patients who develop chronic ventilatory failure have been called 'physiologically wise' because they are thought to protect their diaphragm from fatigue by hypoventilating, leading to hypercapnia (Bégin 2000), albeit unwittingly. They pay the price by more rapid disease progression. Patients with Type I RF keep their P_aCO_2 under control but at the cost of dyspnoea. The relevance to physiotherapists is that the latter group in particular responds to breathless management techniques.

FIGURE 3.27 Progressive changes in arterial blood gases during acute severe asthma

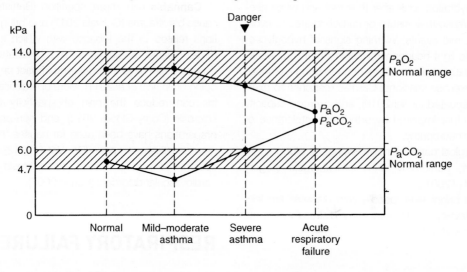

CASE STUDY : Mr MB

This 25 y.o. man from Nottingham has primary emphysema due to alpha$_1$-antitrypsin deficiency.

Background
- Recurrent childhood infections
- Unemployed, lives alone, 'finished with girlfriend because I'm too busy with hospital appointments'. Non-smoker

Subjective
- Grey sputum, cleared independently
- Shortness of breath worse since admission last April
- Watch TV much of the time
- Hoping for lung transplant

Objective
- Hyperinflation
- Breathing pattern normal
- ↑ respiratory rate on slight exertion
- Stooped posture
- Scattered crackles on auscultation.

Questions

1   CT Scan: evidence of emphysema (Fig 3.28)?
2   Analysis?
3   Problems?
4   Plan?

FIGURE 3.28a CT scan of Mr MB's chest

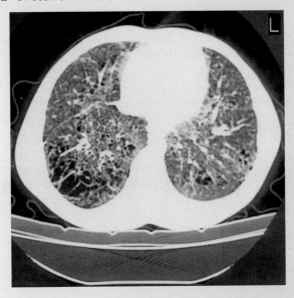

FIGURE 3.28b CT scan at diaphragm level

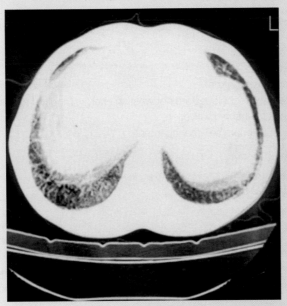

CLINICAL REASONING

The following study used lung inflation techniques to treat people with asthma. Has the correct problem been identified?

> *Lung inflation techniques such as incentive spirometry, voluntary deep breathing, intermittent positive pressure breathing and continuous positive airways pressure, are used to increase lung volumes during acute attacks and to reduce atelectasis, but published studies have failed to document their usefulness in the treatment of asthma.*
>
> *Eur Resp J (1993) 3, 353–5*

Response to Case Study

1   Scan
  - (3.28a) Black areas in the lung fields indicate breakdown of alveoli into large airspaces
  - (3.28b) 'Double border' of the diaphragm is due to MB being unable to hold his breath for the scan.

2   Analysis
  - Little ventilatory reserve
  - Previous fitness not regained since hospital admission
  - Inactive lifestyle
  - Poor posture contributing to inefficient breathing

3   Problems
  - Shortness of breath
  - ↓ Exercise tolerance

4   Plan
  - Educate on the relevance of exercise tolerance to eligibility for lung transplant
  - Educate on breathless management
  - Educate on posture correction
  - Assess exercise tolerance
  - Negotiate daily exercise programme
  - Check that chest clearance techniques are not wasting energy, modify if necessary
  - Follow up within a week to ensure motivation
  - Adjust programme until optimum self-management
  - Review three-monthly

Response to Clinical Reasoning

Is the patient's problem:
  - Loss of lung volume? No, acute asthma causes hyperinflation and 'lung inflation techniques' would be counterproductive.
  - Excess work of breathing? Yes, but the methods described would increase the work of breathing.
  - Sputum retention? Maybe, but these methods are not designed for sputum clearance.

This is the type of article that is interpreted as 'physiotherapy' being ineffective for people with asthma.

RECOMMENDED READING

Al-Dorzi HM (2013) Life-threatening infections in medically immunocompromised patients. *Crit Care Clinics*; **29**(4): 807–826

Aboussouan L (2013) Respiratory support in patients with amyotrophic lateral sclerosis. *Respir Care*; **58**(9): 1555–8

Bonavita J, Naidich DP (2012) Imaging of bronchiectasis. *Clin Chest Med*; **33**(2): 233–48

Bradley JM, Balp MM (2013) Quality of life and healthcare utilisation in cystic fibrosis. *Eur Respir J*; **41**(3): 571–77

Constantin D, Menon MK (2013) Skeletal muscle molecular responses to resistance training and dietary supplementation in COPD. *Thorax*; **68**(7): 625–33

El Maghraoui A, Dehhaoui M (2012) Prevalence and characteristics of lung involvement on high resolution CT in patients with ankylosing spondylitis. *Pulm Med*; **2012**: 965956.

Figueiredo D, Gabriel R, Jácome C (2014) Caring for people with early and advanced COPD: how do family carers cope? *J Clin Nurs*; **23**(1–2): 211–20

Fortun M (2014) Asthma, culture, and cultural analysis. *Adv Exp Med Biol*; **795**: 321–32

Garuti G (2013) Pulmonary rehabilitation at home guided by telemonitoring and access to healthcare facilities for respiratory complications in patients with neuromuscular disease. *Europ J Phys Rehab Med*; **49**(1): 51–7

Gerber LH (2014) Role of exercise in optimizing the functional status of patients with nonalcoholic fatty liver disease. *Clin Liver Dis*; **18**(1): 113–27

Jorine E (2013) Physical and psychosocial factors associated with physical activity in patients with COPD. *Arch Phys Med Rehabil*, **94**(12): 2396–402.e7

Hoffman LR, Ramsey BW (2013) Cystic fibrosis therapeutics. *Chest*; **143**(1): 207–13

Hu ST, Yu CC, Lee PS (2014) Life experiences among obstructive sleep apnoea patients receiving CPAP. *J Clin Nurs*; **23**(1–2): 268–78

Kaneda H, Nakano T, Taniguchi Y *et al* (2013) Three-step management of pneumothorax. *Interact CardioVasc Thorac Surg*; **16**(2): 186–92

Kline JN, Rose RM (2014) Central nervous system influences in asthma. *Adv Exp Med Biol*; **795**: 309–19

Louvaris Z (2013) Intensity of daily physical activity is associated with central hemodynamic and leg muscle oxygen availability in COPD. *J Appl Phys*; **115**(6): 794–802

McDonald VM (2013) Multidimensional assessment and tailored interventions for COPD. *Thorax*; **68**(7): 691–4

Meknes D (2012) Clinical effects of yoga on asthmatic patients. *Ethiop J Health Sci*; **20**(2): 107–112

Mogayzel P, Naureckas ET, Robinson KA *et al* (2013) Cystic Fibrosis Pulmonary Guidelines. *Am J Respir Crit Care Med*; **187**(7): 680–9

Murakami M (2013) Relationships between physical activity and pulmonary functions in Parkinson's disease. *Hong Kong Physiother J*; **31**(1): 51

NICE Guideline (2013) *Idiopathic pulmonary fibrosis (CG163)*

NICE Guideline (2013) *Acute kidney injury (CG169)*

Paratl G, Lombardi C, Hedner J *et al* (2013) Recommendations for the management of patients with obstructive sleep apnoea and hypertension. *Eur Respir J*; **41**(3): 523–38.

Penafortes JT, Guimarães FS, Moço VJ *et al* (2013) Relationship between body balance, lung function, nutritional status and functional capacity in adults with cystic fibrosis. *Braz J Phys Ther*; **17**(5): 450–7.

Rapin A (2013) Aerobic capacities and exercise tolerance in neuromuscular diseases. *Ann Physical Rehab Med*; **56**(6): 420–33

Reddy AP, Gupta MR (2014) Management of asthma: the current US and European guidelines. *Adv Exp Med Biol*; **795**: 81–103

Remels AHV (2013) The mechanisms of cachexia underlying muscle dysfunction in COPD. *J Appl Phys*; **114**(9): 1253–1262.

Schoos M (2013) Echocardiographic predictors of exercise capacity and mortality in COPD. *BMC Cardiovasc Dis*; **13**: 84

Spitzer C, Bouchain M, Winkler LY *et al* (2012) Childhood trauma in multiple sclerosis. *Psychosom Med*; **74**: 312–318

Tambascio J, de Souza HCD, Baddini M *et al* (2013) The influence of purulence on ciliary and cough transport in bronchiectasis. *Respir Care*; **58**(12): 2101–6

Terzi N (2007) Breathing-swallowing interaction in neuromuscular patients. *Am J Respir Crit Care Med*; **175**:269–76

Turcios NL (2012) Pulmonary complications of renal disorders. *Paed Respir Rev*; **13**(1): 44–49

Vianello A, Savoia F, Pipitone E (2013) "Hospital at Home" for neuromuscular disease patients with respiratory tract infection. *Respir Care*; **58**(12): 2061–8

Vitacca M, Vianello A (2013) Respiratory outcomes of patients with amyotrophic lateral sclerosis. *Respir Care*; **58**(9): 1433–41

Vreede KS (2013) Gait characteristics and influence of fatigue during the 6-minute walk test in patients with post-polio syndrome. *J Rehab Med*; **45**(9): 24–8

Wan ES, DeMeo DL, Hersh CP *et al* (2012) Clinical predictors of frequent exacerbations in subjects with severe COPD. *Respir Med*; **105**(4):588–594

Wedzicha JA (2013) Mechanisms and impact of the frequent exacerbator phenotype in chronic obstructive pulmonary disease. *BMC Med*; **11**:181

Yoo H (2013) Etiologies, diagnostic strategies and outcomes of diffuse pulmonary infiltrates causing acute respiratory failure in cancer patients. *Crit Care*; **17**:R150

CHAPTER 4
Cardiovascular disorders

LEARNING OBJECTIVES

On completion of this chapter the reader should be able to:

- identify risk factors for the development of cardiovascular disorders

- relate the pathological changes to the clinical features of hypertension, coronary heart disease and vascular disease

- outline the medical management of cardiovascular disorders.

INTRODUCTION

Neighbourly relations between heart and lungs are reflected in their integrated response to each other's disorders, especially when intravascular pressures are raised. Some heart and lung conditions also share aetiologies such as smoking (Dinas 2013), pathologies such as inflammation (Rommel 2013) and comorbidities such as diabetes and depression (O'Neil *et al* 2013). Neurological and mechanical coupling between the two systems help to maintain homeostasis (Shiogai *et al* 2010), but they can also affect each other negatively, e.g. myocardial damage can occur with exacerbations of chronic obstructive pulmonary disease (COPD) (Stone *et al* 2013) and a restrictive respiratory defect can be caused by the enlarged heart and pulmonary oedema of heart failure (Apostolo *et al* 2012).

Coronary heart disease has a prevalence similar to chronic lung disease (Enriquez 2013) but cardiovascular (CV) disease is the leading cause of premature death globally (O'Neil *et al* 2013). The incidence is decreasing in developed countries but this hopeful sign is now threatened by the rise in obesity, diabetes (Golbidi & Laher 2012) and inactivity (Vrdoljak 2014). Low-income countries are said to be 'drowning in a rising tide' of CV disorders due to tobacco and lack of public health preventive measures (O'Flaherty *et al* 2013).

Management is by:

- prevention and treatment through lifestyle change such as exercise (Golbidi & Laher 2012) from childhood onwards (IDEFICS 2013)

- early detection from biomarkers (Suzuki *et al* 2013)

- medication

- revascularization by angioplasty or bypass surgery
- implanted devices (Ottenberg *et al* 2013).

This chapter describes the pathophysiology and general management of these conditions, facilitating clinical reasoning so that problems requiring physiotherapy can be identified. Physiotherapy is by education and exercise, described in Ch. 12.

KEY POINT

'Fast food and slow motion' are the main avoidable contributors to cardiovascular disease.

HYPERTENSION

For some people with borderline hypertension, there is a choice. Lose weight and exercise and feel younger and better, or take tablets that might make you feel dreadful. It should be a no-brainer.

Bandolier (2003)

- **Systolic pressure:** pressure that the blood exerts on the blood vessels when the ventricles contract, normally 100–140 mmHg.
- **Diastolic pressure:** pressure that the blood exerts on the blood vessels when the ventricles relax, normally 60–90 mmHg.
- **Mean Arterial Blood Pressure (MAP):** cardiac output x peripheral vascular resistance, normally 80–100 mmHg.
- **Cardiac Output (CO):** volume of blood pumped by the left ventricle per minute, i.e. Stroke Volume (SV) × Heart Rate (HR), normally 5 l/min

- **Peripheral Vascular Resistance (PVR):** resistance to blood flow in the arteries.

The prevalence of **systemic hypertension** globally among adults aged >24 reached 40% in 2008 (Al-Ansary *et al* 2013). Systemic hypertension is a risk factor for cardiovascular disease and is present in 69% of patients with a first myocardial infarction (MI), 77% with a first stroke, in 74% with heart failure, and in 60% with peripheral arterial disease (PAD) (Aronow 2012a). It is also associated with impaired cognitive function (McCubbin 2012) and erectile dysfunction, the latter due to PAD or antihypertensive drugs (Javaroni 2012).

Pulmonary hypertension occurs when pressure is raised in the pulmonary circulation such that pulmonary artery pressure exceeds 25 mmHg at rest or 30 mmHg on exercise. Most cases are secondary to lung disorders (Weitzenblum 2013), left heart disease or sleep apnoea, but primary pulmonary hypertension may occur (Semenza 2014). The effect is pressure exerted on the right heart, leading to non-specific symptoms such as dyspnoea, chest pain or fatigue. Pulmonary vasodilator drugs help to control symptoms and slow progression of the disease. Exercise training can improve exercise tolerance and quality of life (Chan *et al* 2013), especially high-intensity interval training (Ciolac 2013).

Classification of systemic hypertension

Most common is **essential** or **primary** hypertension, which has no known cause. **Secondary** hypertension can result from vascular, endocrine or kidney problems (Loftus 2013). If the cause is corrected, blood pressure (BP) usually returns to normal.

Hypertension may also be classified according to its severity. **Benign** hypertension is asymptomatic but is not harmless because any sustained rise in BP carries the risks described above. **Resistant** hypertension is when BP is refractory to medication, occurring in 10–15% of the hypertensive population (Acelajado *et al* 2013). **Malignant** hypertension (also called a hypertensive emergency) occurs rapidly, with diastolic readings around 130 mmHg, causing damage to target organs such as the kidneys (Amraoui *et al* 2012) and requiring immediate medication.

Physiology

The driving force behind blood flow to the tissues is arterial blood pressure, regulated by PVR and CO. Fast acting neural mechanisms respond to changes in posture and activity (Fig 4.1a) and slow acting hormonal mechanisms respond by adjusting fluid balance (Fig 4.1b), both incorporating a negative feedback loop to maintain stability. BP increases during exercise and decreases during sleep.

Pathophysiology of systemic hypertension

Loss of elasticity in the large arteries and vasoconstriction of the smaller vessels drive up PVR and BP, inflammation (Schiffrin 2014) and blood viscosity playing a part and the kidneys responding by releasing renin and reducing sodium excretion (Mamenko *et al* 2013). The resulting hypertension can thicken arterial walls and damage the kidneys further. Genes and the environment contribute to the risk (Table 4.1).

FIGURE 4.1a Neural mechanism which controls cardiac output and BP

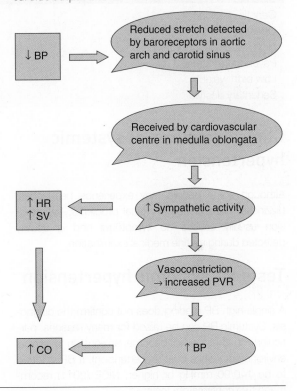

FIGURE 4.1b Renal mechanism which maintains BP and circulating volume, a negative feedback loop reacting to reduced BP and circulating volume

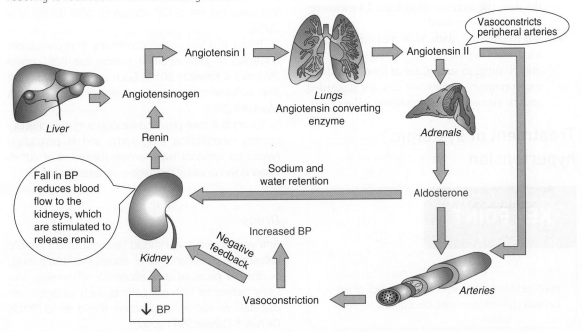

BP: blood pressure, *HR*: heart rate, *SV*: stroke volume, *CO*: cardiac output, *PVR*: peripheral vascular resistance

TABLE 4.1 Predisposing factors for systemic hypertension

Risk factors for essential hypertension	Causes of secondary hypertension
Genetic predisposition	Kidney disease
Obesity	Cushing's syndrome
High salt or alcohol intake	Adrenal gland tumour
Psychogenic stress	Coarctation of the aorta
Low birth weight	Corticosteroid medication
Sedentary lifestyle	Oral contraceptive pill

Clinical features of systemic hypertension

Although some people may experience headaches, dizziness, nose bleeds or visual problems, hypertension usually causes no symptoms and is usually detected during routine medical examination.

Tests for systemic hypertension

A single high BP reading does not confirm the diagnosis. Systemic BP can be raised for many reasons, particularly in those who become anxious in a clinical environment ('white coat' hypertension). If BP is found to be 140/90 mmHg or higher, NICE (2011) recommend two confirmatory tests:

- 24 hour ambulatory BP monitoring, with at least two measurements per hour during the day, the average of at least 14 measurements being required
- self-monitoring with two measurements at least one minute apart, recorded morning and evening, in sitting, for at least four days; measurements on the first day are discarded and an average of the remaining values used.

Treatment of systemic hypertension

KEY POINT

Education forms the basis of treatment because of the need for lifestyle change, the frequent lack of symptoms and patients' concerns about drug side effects.

Lifestyle

Lifestyle change can lead to significant reductions in BP (Robbins *et al* 2011), including:

- regular aerobic exercise for 20–30 minutes on most days
- weight loss for those with a BMI >25
- alcohol intake at no more than two units a day
- salt intake at no more than 5 grams a day (Strazzullo *et al* 2009).

More enjoyable lifestyle changes include dark chocolate, which improves endothelial function (Nogueira 2012). Gentle doses of wine have been advocated (Holahan 2012) but any benefit appears to be outweighed by increased risks of stroke, liver injury and some cancers (Krenz 2013). Avoiding meat may or may not be enjoyable, but vegetarians reduce their heart disease risk (Crowe *et al* 2013). Processed meat increases the risk of CV disease by 30% (Micha *et al* 2013).

Stress is a well-known contributor to hypertension, especially in jobs where a person has little control (Kivimäki & Kawachi 2013). Such patients may benefit from occupational therapy/relaxation or yoga (Mizuno & Monteiro 2013).

Exercise is best provided through a multidisciplinary cardiac rehabilitation programme and is particularly helpful for resistant hypertension (Dimeo *et al* 2012). Head-down postural drainage is contraindicated.

Drugs

Antihypertensive drugs should be considered if systolic pressure is persistently at or above 140–160 mmHg, or diastolic pressure at or above 90–100 mmHg, with lower targets for high risk patients such as those with diabetes or kidney dysfunction (Paiva *et al* 2012) DeTurk & Cahalin 2011 p.460.

Hypertensive people under age 55 are prescribed angiotensin-converting enzyme (ACE) inhibitors, which may bring the added benefit of improving muscle performance (Sayer 2013). Above this age patients are better managed with a diuretic or calcium channel blocker (Musameh *et al* 2013). Antihypertensive drugs are best taken in the evening (Mohandas & Ejaz 2012), but diuretics can be taken at a time to minimize the side effect of a need to pass urine. Some diuretics can also cause a metabolic acidosis and caution is advised for patients with comorbid COPD.

HEART FAILURE

- **Stroke volume:** volume of blood ejected by the ventricle in one contraction, normally about 70 ml.
- **End diastolic volume:** volume of blood in the ventricle at the end of filling, just before it contracts, normally 120 ml.
- **Ejection fraction:** stroke volume expressed as a percentage of end diastolic volume, normally >55%.
- **Systolic heart failure:** reduced or weakened pumping action of the heart, with ejection fraction <55%.
- **Diastolic heart failure:** low compliance of myocardium, but with normal contraction and normal ejection fraction.
- **Preload:** degree of stretch applied to the ventricle before contraction.
- **Afterload:** load that the ventricle must overcome to eject blood.

If the heart cannot pump all the blood returned to it, it is said to have failed. It is either unable to meet the needs of the body, or can do so only with elevated atrial filling pressures. Heart failure (HF) may be caused by coronary heart disease, hypertension, or, in 30% of patients, COPD (Vestbo *et al* 2013).

Acute HF is sudden and severe and requires urgent medical treatment to restore cardiac output. **Chronic** HF occurs gradually and is offset at first by compensatory mechanisms to maintain tissue perfusion, but eventually cardiac function declines and symptoms develop.

The prevalence of HF doubles with each decade of life (Strait 2013). It is the leading cause of hospitalization in the elderly population (Freitas *et al* 2012) and 50% of patients die within five years of diagnosis (Springer *et al* 2013).

Causes

Excess workload on the heart involves one or both ventricles and is thought to relate to oxidative stress and inflammation (Bhimaraj & Tang 2013), leading to one or more of the following:

- impaired contractility of the myocardium, e.g. after acute coronary syndromes (Kaul *et al* 2013)
- increased afterload, e.g. with hypertension or aortic valve stenosis
- increased preload, e.g. with mitral or aortic valve regurgitation.

Other risk factors are over- or under-weight (Kapoor 2010) and diabetes (Dhingra 2013).

Classification

Left ventricular failure (LVF)

LVF is the most common form of heart failure, gradually pushing up pressure in the left atrium and pulmonary vascular system. The resulting pulmonary hypertension may force fluid into the alveoli, creating pulmonary oedema.

The failing heart triggers compensatory mechanisms:

- Fast acting neural systems increase sympathetic activity, raising HR and myocardial contractility (Fig 4.1a).
- The slower response of the renin-angiotensin mechanism (Fig 4.1b) promotes the retention of sodium and water by the kidney, increasing preload and encouraging the myocardium to contract.

These raise the workload of the left ventricle further because angiotensin is an arterial vasoconstrictor and increases the afterload. Other factors that increase workload of the left heart are increased volume load, as in aortic valve regurgitation, or increased resistance to blood flow, as with systemic hypertension.

Right ventricular failure (RVF)

RVF occurs secondary to cardiopulmonary disorders such as pulmonary hypertension, right ventricular infarction, congenital heart disease, pulmonary embolism or COPD (Kevin & Barnard 2007). It is usually irreversible unless the ventricle is unloaded, e.g. by lung transplant for pulmonary hypertension (Drake *et al* 2011).

Enlargement of the right ventricle that has resulted from lung disease is known as **cor pulmonale**, caused by hypoxic vasoconstriction and pulmonary hypertension (p.16 and p.77).

Congestive cardiac failure (CCF)

CCF refers to combined LVF and RVF, with congestion in the pulmonary and systemic circulations.

Pathophysiology

In response to increased load, the left ventricular myocardium hypertrophies. The greater size and number of myocytes raises myocardial oxygen demand and increases the diffusion distance for oxygen. Some muscle fibres become ischaemic, leading to patchy fibrosis, stiffness and reduced contractility. The workload may cause the ventricle to stretch and dilate, leading to further force being required to maintain cardiac output. Systolic failure is by reduced ejection fraction and diastolic failure is by reduced end-diastolic volume. Metabolic effects include loss of bone mineralization, skeletal muscle and fat (Loncar *et al* 2013).

The stiffness and reduced contractility push up end-diastolic pressure, which is transmitted back along the pulmonary veins to the pulmonary capillaries, from which fluid is forced into the interstitial spaces and, if severe, into the alveoli, causing pulmonary oedema. The increased pulmonary vascular pressure raises the afterload of the right ventricle, in the same way as chronic systemic hypertension raises the afterload of the left

ventricle. Hypertrophy, patchy fibrosis, stiffness and reduced contractility of the right ventricular myocardium then ensues, as with the left ventricle, and CCF develops.

Clinical features

The main symptom is **shortness of breath** (SOB) due to pulmonary oedema, first on exertion and then at rest, which can be measured by a validated questionnaire (Parshall 2012). This combines with **fatigue** and **muscle weakness** to cause **exercise limitation**, which worsens prognosis and survival (Brandão *et al* 2012). These symptoms are often dismissed by the patient and medical staff as 'normal ageing' and it may fall to the physiotherapist to raise concerns so that a diagnosis can be made. **Sleep disturbance** occurs in 70% of patients, impairing quality of life (QoL) and reducing exercise tolerance (Andrews 2013). Irritation of lung parenchyma causes a **cough**.

Comorbidities include diabetes, sleep apnoea, obesity, depression and a 49% incidence of incontinence (Hwang *et al* 2013). About half of patients exhibit **cognitive impairment**, possibly due to cerebral oxygen deprivation (Alosco *et al* 2013) and some manifest a complex **pain** pattern (Light *et al* 2013).

Objective signs are **peripheral oedema** caused by venous congestion. Functional limitation at different levels of severity are in Table 4.2.

Pulmonary oedema

Pulmonary oedema is extravascular water in the lungs, caused by back pressure from a failing left heart. The main symptom is SOB, leading occasionally to a misdiagnosis of asthma, from which the confusing term 'cardiac asthma' arises. Dyspnoea due to pulmonary oedema is distinguished by **orthopnoea** and **paroxysmal nocturnal dyspnoea** (Ch. 2).

Interstitial pulmonary oedema barely affects lung function, but once the lymphatics become overloaded,

TABLE 4.2 Heart failure functional classification (New York Heart Association)

Class	Patient symptoms
Class I	No limitation of physical activity
Class II	Comfortable at rest, but ordinary physical activity results in fatigue, palpitations or dyspnoea
Class III	Comfortable at rest, but slight activity causes fatigue, palpitations or dyspnoea
Class IV	Symptoms at rest. If any physical activity is undertaken, symptoms increase

fluid squeezes into alveoli, causing alveolar oedema, a widened P_AO_2–P_aO_2 gradient and hypoxaemia. If alveolar fluid moves into the airway, it mixes with air and may be coughed up as white **frothy secretions**, becoming pink if blood is also squeezed out.

Radiology shows an enlarged heart, with bilateral fleecy opacities spreading from the hila due to fluid in the airspaces of the lung (see Fig 12.3). Fine crackles on auscultation may be heard over the lung bases, caused by the popping open of alveoli compressed by peribronchial oedema. Similar crackles can also be heard in immobile elderly patients without HF when they take a deep breath and their closed alveoli pop open.

Non-cardiogenic pulmonary oedema, distinguished by a normal-sized heart on x-ray, can be caused by fluid overload, systemic vasoconstriction, oncotic pressure changes (due to cirrhosis, malnutrition or nephrotic syndrome) or increased capillary permeability due to toxins or inflammatory damage.

Tests

Diagnosis may be challenging and the condition can be missed in up to 50% of patients, with the majority of those in residential care not being diagnosed (Hancock et al 2013). A blood test identifies raised levels of natriuretic peptide, a biomarker secreted by the ventricles in response to excessive stretch. An echocardiogram confirms the diagnosis by showing altered size, structure or function of the heart (Penicka 2014). Other tests are tissue oxygen utilization (Hogan 2012) and cardiac output recovery after exercise (Myers et al 2011). Cognitive screening is recommended (Alosco et al 2013).

Treatment

Patients with chronic disease should be under the care of a multidisciplinary heart failure team (Agvall et al 2013). Education is required to clarify terminology and help patients through the maze of their medication, salt and fluid management, which can be done without affecting thirst, appetite or QoL (Philipson et al 2013). This is best incorporated into a rehabilitation programme (Ch. 12). Home management and telemonitoring show promise (Bui 2013) and social support can reduce hospitalization, mortality, anxiety and depression (Årestedt et al 2013). Oxygen therapy does not make physiological sense because the problem is one of cardiac output rather than gas exchange, but it may be beneficial for patients with comorbid sleep apnoea (Criner 2013).

> ### KEY POINT
>
> Drug management is based on a 'start low, go slow' principle.

ACE inhibitors impede the conversion of angiotensin I to angiotensin II, and β-blockers reduce HR (Böhm & Reil 2013). Both drugs are up-titrated gradually over several weeks, balancing their beneficial effects on BP and HR with side effects such as cough, dizziness, hypotension or bradycardia (Strait 2013). Diuretics increase urine excretion and are considered if there is SOB or oedema. They are potent and non-selective, and over-enthusiastic use can lead to dizziness on standing, loss of calcium and potassium, weak grip strength (Ashfield et al 2010) and possibly distressing thirst (Waldréus et al 2013). Patients are often advised to reduce their fluid intake in order to reduce stress on the heart, but patients on diuretics may restrict it further if they have urinary incontinence or poor mobility. Anticoagulants such as warfarin reduce the risk of thromboembolism, stroke and myocardial infarct (MI) (Hopper et al 2013). Opioids can relieve SOB if given for several months, and can be administered safely (Oxberry 2013). Sildenafil may improve exercise capacity (Cooper et al 2013).

Implanted devices include biventricular pacemakers, defibrillators and left ventricular assist devices (Liu 2013), following which rehabilitation may be beneficial (English & Speed 2013). Some patients benefit from revascularization (Ch. 16). Transplantation may be considered if there are severe refractory symptoms or cardiogenic shock.

Patients with acute disease require assessment for risk before discharge (Stiell et al 2013). Palliative care is eventually required for most patients (Bekelman et al 2011).

CORONARY HEART DISEASE (CHD)

At 40 years old, the lifetime risk of coronary heart disease is one in two for men and one in three for women. If you still need a reason to pin the ten tips for healthy living on your fridge, surely this is it.

Bandolier (2007)

Mortality from coronary heart disease, also called coronary artery disease, is now falling, but it is still the leading cause of death in the developed world (Widmer 2014), with over half of patients being virtually asymptomatic until the first fatal presentation (Yang & Vargas 2012).

Causes

> *'Death by witchcraft' may relate to the effect of fear on the sympathetic and cardiovascular systems.*
>
> Flannery *et al* (2010)

The contribution of stress to CHD relates to hypercoagulation, cardiac electrical instability and coronary vasoconstriction, leading to US law recognizing the infliction of fright as a means of committing homicide (Flannery *et al* 2010). People who discuss their anger to resolve a situation have a reduced risk of CHD, but those who blame others appear to have an increased risk (Davidson & Mostofsk 2010). Other predisposing factors are sugary drinks (Ambrosini 2013), physical inactivity, visceral obesity, sleep disturbance, smoking tobacco (Cappuccio *et al* 2011) or marijuana (Thomas 2014), raised cholesterol, diabetes, kidney dysfunction (Baber *et al* 2013), rheumatoid arthritis (Sen 2014), diesel exhaust (Bradley & Cryar 2013) and cold weather (Xu *et al* 2013).

Pathophysiology

Atherosclerosis

Atherosclerosis underpins CV disease (Schiffrin 2014). Fatty streaks can form early in life but only become significant if they develop into atheromatous plaques. Plaques tend to develop where arteries branch because there is more stress on the vessel walls. Injured endothelium allows low density lipoprotein (LDL or 'bad cholesterol') to enter the vessel wall, where it is oxidized and attracts white blood cells which differentiate into macrophages. These ingest the LDL and become part of the atherosclerotic plaque. Inflammatory mediators released by the macrophages stimulate smooth muscle cells in the artery wall to migrate towards the damaged *tunica intima*. Here they multiply and synthesize collagen,

forming a fibrous cap on the arterial wall. This projects into the lumen of the artery and obstructs blood flow. Even at this stage, maintaining cardiovascular fitness by regular exercise helps to reduce LDL and strengthen the fibrous cap (Yoshikawa *et al* 2013).

The innate antithrombotic effects of normal vascular endothelium are disabled by atherosclerotic plaques. The damaged artery wall attracts platelets and triggers the formation of thrombi (blood clots). A small thrombus, or any material which leaks from the plaque, can be carried in the bloodstream as an embolus and block smaller vessels downstream, resulting in ischaemia of the tissues supplied by the artery.

Myocardial ischaemia

Much coronary blood flow occurs during ventricular diastole (relaxation), because the deep coronary arteries are compressed by ventricular pressures during systole. When exercising, increased HR raises myocardial oxygen demand while shortening diastole, leaving less time for myocardial perfusion. To meet the shortfall, the coronary arteries dilate in response to metabolites. In CHD, oxidized LDL molecules in atherosclerotic coronary arteries inhibit this vasodilation so that, on exercise or under stress, areas of myocardium may be deprived of oxygen.

Myocardial infarction (MI)

Severe or prolonged ischaemia leads to tissue death or infarction. Myocardial infarction is caused by blockage of blood flow through a coronary artery, usually caused by a thrombus in an artery narrowed by atherosclerosis, i.e. coronary thrombosis. One in four patients who have suspected coronary heart disease has unwittingly had a silent MI (Arenja *et al* 2013).

Classification and clinical features

Stable angina

Myocardial ischaemia leads to the crushing chest pain of angina pectoris. This is due to anaerobic respiration in ischaemic tissue releasing chemicals such as adenosine and lactic acid, sometimes worsened by vasospasm. It may be brought on by exertion, cold weather, stress or even eating, and can radiate to the neck, jaw and arms. Patients often describe the sensation as tightness or pressure rather than pain, and may use gestures such as clenched fists to help them explain. It resolves on rest.

Acute coronary syndrome (ACS)

ACS is triggered by rupture or erosion of an atherosclerotic plaque, leading to activation of the coagulation cascade and formation of a platelet-fibrin thrombus, which can grow rapidly and obstruct coronary blood flow, causing myocardial ischaemia or infarction. Chest pain which occurs at rest and is more severe and long lasting than stable angina indicates ACS. It may radiate from the chest but is not relieved by rest or medication. ACS is classified as follows:

- **Unstable angina,** caused by coronary occlusion but not associated with infarction. This is temporary but can progress to MI. Any new onset angina is considered unstable in the first few weeks since it suggests a new problem in a coronary artery.
- **Non-ST segment elevation MI** (NSTEMI), relating to the electrocardiogram (ECG) trace and caused by coronary occlusion sufficient to affect the innermost layers of the heart wall.
- **ST segment elevation MI** (STEMI), resulting from coronary occlusion which has caused full thickness cardiac necrosis.

In addition to chest pain, MI can cause dyspnoea, pallor, light-headedness, nausea, sweating and sometimes loss of consciousness. Elderly people may present more subtly with fatigue, nausea, sweating or syncope (Franken et al 2012). A 'silent MI' causes no symptoms and is only picked up if the patient has an ECG. Arenja et al (2013) found that one in four people with suspected coronary heart disease had already had a silent MI.

Complications include arrhythmias such as atrial fibrillation or AF (Chamberlain et al 2013a). Fatalities occur if a large proportion of muscle is damaged or if severe arrhythmias are triggered. Patients without hypoxaemia should not be given oxygen because it can cause coronary vasoconstriction (Decalmer & O'Driscoll 2013).

Ongoing fatigue can persist for months and is considered the most bothersome of continuing symptoms (Barnason et al 2008).

Tests

Acute chest pain requires a 12 lead resting ECG. Chest pain provoked by exercise requires an exercise ECG. In neither case does a normal ECG exclude ACS. A blood test can pick up biomarkers such as troponin, released by damaged myocardium within hours (Reiter 2013). This lingers for one to two weeks and helps to detect ACS, evaluate its severity and distinguish MI from angina. Computed tomography coronary angiography identifies patients likely to benefit from revascularization (Voros et al 2014), and other imaging technologies can detect subclinical atherosclerosis (Yang & Vargas 2012).

Prevention and treatment

> Interventions such as motorized scooters which reduce activity can increase cardiovascular risk.
>
> Zagol & Krasuski (2010)

Smoking cessation is recommended before any CV signs are evident (Talib 2014). For those with established CHD, exercise, diet, group support and stress reduction reduces hospitalization and may lower mortality (Zeng et al 2013). Major depressive disorder is present in approximately 20% of patients (Thombs 2013) and should be treated because it increases mortality (Stenman et al 2013).

Exercise training and drug management are considered superior to surgery for stable disease (Uhlemann et al 2012) and appear to mitigate disease progression (Boden 2013). Statins reduce LDL, and as a bonus reduce COPD exacerbations (Wang et al 2013b). Over half of patients hospitalized for CHD also have musculoskeletal problems, which places them at greater cardiovascular risk, so these will also need attention (Marzolini et al 2012).

Drugs

Aspirin inhibits the development of ACS. Statins reduce LDL, and as a bonus reduce COPD exacerbations (Wang et al 2013b). Stable angina is usually managed with nitrates. If ACS occurs, antiplatelets or

FIGURE 4.2 Angioplasty, showing (A) placement of deflated balloon, (B) balloon inflation, (C) stent in place after removal of balloon

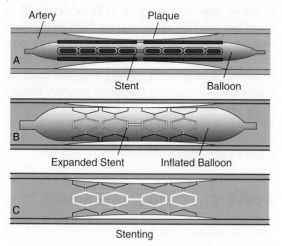

anticoagulants to reperfuse the myocardium are required, usually within hours, along with measures to prevent the side effect of bleeding (Bassand 2013). Beta-blockers benefit patients who are high risk (Nakatani 2013) or have a recent history of MI (Bangalore 2012); if these are not tolerated, calcium channel blockers may be given (Bruschke *et al* 2013).

Angioplasty

Coronary angioplasty, or percutaneous coronary intervention, involves the passage of a catheter, using a femoral or radial approach, into the blocked vessel, where a balloon at its tip inflates to crush the atheroma. A stent is usually left in place to keep it open (Fig 4.2.). Patients then lie flat for several hours to prevent bleeding, and after a period of observation are discharged with minimal activity restrictions. The procedure has shown better clinical outcomes than thrombolytic drugs (O'Brien *et al* 2013) and lower risk of stroke than bypass grafting (Palmerini *et al* 2013).

Surgery

Coronary artery bypass grafting (CABG) (Ch. 16) is used for multivessel disease or after failed angioplasty. A hybrid technique combines surgery and angioplasty (Repossini *et al* 2013).

PERIPHERAL ARTERIAL DISEASE (PAD)

> *About 80% of the patients whose legs or extremities I have to amputate are current smokers.*
>
> Surgeon quoted by ASH (2005)

Peripheral arterial disease, or peripheral vascular disease, is due to atherosclerosis of the arteries supplying the lower limbs. PAD may or may not be symptomatic, but about 20% of the UK population aged over 60 have evidence of the disease (NICE 2012b). It is not directly life threatening but is linked to ACS or stroke (Lau *et al* 2011). Management of PAD therefore helps reduce the risks of secondary events such as myocardial infarction or stroke (Muller *et al* 2013).

Causes

In common with CHD, modifiable risk factors include smoking, obesity, hypertension, diabetes (Sözmen 2014) and depression, the latter being partly explained by modifiable risk factors, suggesting that management of these factors could reduce the risk of PAD associated with depression (Grenon *et al* 2012).

Clinical features

Intermittent claudication, a fiendish cramp-like calf pain caused by ischaemia, occurs in 10–15% of patients, set off by walking and ceasing on rest. It may also occur in the buttock, thigh or arch of the foot, depending on the location of the blockage (Muller *et al* 2013). Pain at rest (Table 4.3) indicates progression of the disease towards critical ischaemia, and repeated ischaemic episodes damage the muscles and nerves (Hiat 2006).

Objective examination may reveal cool skin, altered skin colour, loss of hair and poor toe nail growth.

Tests

A comprehensive history is needed to exclude musculoskeletal causes of leg pain. Good foot pulses are

TABLE 4.3 Classification of peripheral artery disease (Norgren *et al* 2007)

Fontaine classification		Rutherford classification		
Stage	Symptoms	Grade	Category	Symptoms
I	Asymptomatic	0	0	Asymptomatic.
IIa	Mild claudication	I	1	Mild claudication.
IIb	Moderate to severe claudication	I	2	Moderate claudication.
			3	Severe claudication.
III	Ischaemic rest pain	II	4	Ischaemic rest pain.
IV	Ulceration or gangrene	III	5	Minor tissue loss.
			6	Major tissue loss.

insufficient to exclude PAD, and a specialist clinic is required to compare systolic pressures in the upper and lower limbs (Bundo 2013), apply walking tests and questionnaires, and sometimes administer a heel rise test (Monteiro *et al* 2013) or assess calf oxygenation (Miranda *et al* 2012).

To accurately localize the narrowed segments, non-invasive imaging such as ultrasound, CT angiography or magnetic resonance angiography may be used (Bosch *et al* 2013). The abdomen is palpated to check for a pulsatile abdominal mass that could indicate an aortic aneurysm.

Treatment

> **KEY POINT**
>
> The principles of management are stopping smoking and keeping moving.

Prevention is preferred because treatment of conditions such as hypertension may not change the course of PAD once it is established. Smoking cessation lessens the risk of critical leg ischaemia, MI and death. Control of diabetes and high cholesterol, if present, are required, as well as the sleep apnoea from which 85% of patients suffer (Utriainen *et al* 2013). Drugs include β-blockers, if not contraindicated (Aronow 2012b), and

antiplatelets, which also reduce CHD mortality (Wong *et al* 2013).

Revascularization by localized angioplasty or bypass grafting reduces pain and may improve lower limb function (Barbosa *et al* 2010). Patients who have had an aortofemoral graft should avoid hip flexion on the affected side for three days. They may get up before they are allowed to sit, and can start gentle mobilization two to three days postoperatively, depending on graft patency and the surgeon's instructions. Spinal cord stimulation is beneficial for late-stage disease (Deogaonkar 2014) but if critical limb ischaemia has developed, amputation is required. Gene therapy holds promise for the future (Jazwa *et al* 2013).

ANEURYSMS

An aneurysm is a permanently dilated section of a blood vessel to more than 150% of its normal diameter (Lavall *et al* 2012), caused by atherosclerosis and occurring most commonly in a cerebral artery or the aorta.

Causes

Weakness of elastin and collagen fibres in the vessel wall predispose to aneurysm. Abdominal aortic aneurysms are commonly related to atherosclerosis. Connective tissue disorders also pose a risk because of loss of elastic and muscle fibres, and hypertension can accelerate the process (Issenbacher 2005). Once formed, aneurysms progressively enlarge and the diameter is a strong predictor of rupture, which brings high mortality.

Clinical features

An intact aortic aneurysm is often asymptomatic and the first indication of its presence may be when it ruptures. Occasionally patients develop pain in the chest, back or abdomen. Aneurysm of the ascending aorta may cause aortic valve regurgitation which can progress to congestive heart failure.

Complications

Thrombus formation within the aneurysm is common and may be a source of emboli. Aortic dissection involves separation of the aortic layers longitudinally, progressing within the vessel wall in either direction, leading to pain, systemic ischaemia and sometimes rupture (Broder et al 2013). A ruptured aortic aneurysm presents with severe chest or abdominal pain, hypotension and tachycardia; rapid surgery or endovascular stent graft is required (Smith & Ramirez 2013).

Tests

Ultrasound MRI and CT scans can assess aortic diameter if an aneurysm is suspected (Stein et al 2014). Thoracic aneurysms might be detected on a chest x-ray. Risk scores and diagnostic algorithms are available for early detection of dissection (Suzuki et al 2013).

Treatment

Patients with a known aneurysm are advised on the management of risk factors, and antihypertensive medication and statins may be prescribed. Moderate physical activity is thought to reduce progression of atherosclerosis-related aneurysms (Lavall et al 2012) and may significantly improve fitness and quality of life (Tew et al 2012). It is considered safe if the aneurysm is <5 cm in diameter (Myers et al 2011).

If the aneurysm is <5.5 cm diameter, regular ultrasound screening monitors its growth. Once over 5.5 cm, elective surgical repair is considered because the likelihood of rupture begins to overtake the risks of surgery. Laparoscopy is possible, but open procedures are more common. Elective repair has an operative mortality of 1–5%, which contrasts with an 80% mortality associated with the emergency surgery that is required for a rupture (Gawenda 2012).

Aortic aneurysm is a contraindication for head-down postural drainage.

THROMBOEMBOLISM

Thrombosis is the development of a clot in the vascular system. Embolism occurs if this clot breaks away and is swept off in the blood stream.

Thrombosis

Arterial thrombosis is most commonly associated with atherosclerosis. Venous thrombosis is usually caused by Virchow's triad: slow blood flow, damaged or abnormal vessel walls and changes to blood chemistry. The veins of the legs are the most common site of deep vein thrombosis (DVT) which presents as pain, tenderness, swelling, redness, warmth, and sometimes pain on dorsiflexion (Homan's sign), any of which must be reported. Diagnosis is confirmed by ultrasound or D-dimer blood test (NICE 2012b). Predisposing factors include surgery and cancer, the combination causing DVT to be the most common postoperative cause of death for patients with cancer (Thai et al 2013).

Prevention of DVT is by adequate hydration, avoidance of immobility including prolonged sitting (Howard et al 2013), and the use of anticoagulants, pneumatic compression devices and compression stockings (NICE 2010c). Compression thrombo-embolus deterrent (TED) stockings promote blood flow from superficial to deep veins (Ebm et al 2012), so long as there is no peripheral arterial disease, neuropathy, leg oedema or skin disorder. They apply graduated compression that is greater in the lower calf and diminishes up the leg, and must be individually measured, fitted and monitored (Macintyre et al 2013). The physiotherapist's main task is to advise patients or their family to smooth out the omnipresent tourniquet-like wrinkles in TED stockings which reduce blood flow and can themselves cause thrombosis (Byrne 2001).

Pulmonary embolism (PE)

A fragment of a thrombus may escape to form an embolus which is carried in the circulation until it becomes lodged in a smaller vessel. The natural resting place of an embolus which has originated from a DVT is a pulmonary arteriole, where 90% reside (Lapner 2013). The relationship between DVT and pulmonary embolism has given rise to the term venous thromboembolism, which covers both conditions.

PE is a blockage in the pulmonary vasculature, usually by a blood clot. It is the leading preventable cause of death in hospital patients (Lapner 2013) and is commonly not diagnosed or even suspected until after the patient dies. Close to 40% of patients with a DVT have an asymptomatic PE (Berman 2003). Death occurs if the clot leads to pulmonary hypertension severe enough to cause unmanageable right ventricular afterload and right heart failure (Tapson 2012).

Suspicions are raised if a patient complains of dyspnoea and a sharp localized pleuritic pain, occasionally complicated by haemoptysis. Pallor may be apparent, S_pO_2 is usually reduced and a pleural rub can sometimes be heard on auscultation. D-dimer testing indicates fibrinolytic activity in the blood but is not specific for PE. Radiology may help exclude other disorders that mimic PE, but CT pulmonary angiography is required for confirmation. Less than a quarter of patients have symptoms or signs of DVT (Lapner 2013).

Prevention is by avoidance of DVT or by implanting a filter in the inferior vena cava in high risk individuals (Prasad 2013). Immediate management of PE is by giving oxygen and placing the patient supine, thus boosting venous return to the left heart which is deprived of pulmonary artery flow. Treatment is by thrombolytic therapy to dissolve the clot (Sharifi *et al* 2013), followed by heparin. If there is a reversible risk factor, treatment is continued for three months, but with active cancer or a second unprovoked PE, treatment is indefinite (Lapner 2013). Patients with chronic (Polastri 2013) or massive (Mazur *et al* 2013) PE may require embolectomy.

Mobilization is considered safe once anticoagulation has started. Indeed, outpatient treatment of PE is recommended for low-risk patients (Wells 2012).

CASE STUDY : Ms GF

Consider the management of this 87 y.o. patient from Muscat admitted with a chest infection and deteriorating mobility.

Background
- Lives alone
- Independently mobile prior to admission
- No relevant medical history

Nurse report
- Patient needs assistance to mobilize

Subjective assessment
- Pain in right leg

Objective assessment

- Calf swollen and hot
- Doppler ultrasound confirms DVT

Started on subcutaneous heparin and elastic compression stockings.

Questions

1   What is the most likely cause of DVT in this case?
2   Will mobilizing increase the likelihood of a PE?
3   Would bed rest prevent a PE?
4   Would bed rest or ambulation be more effective in reducing pain and swelling?
5   Goals?
6   Plan?

CLINICAL REASONING

Is this a sensible control group?

Postoperative non-invasive ventilation (NIV) was extolled in a study in which the active NIV group received 50% oxygen but the control group (without NIV) received unspecified oxygen using a 'venturi mask at an adjusted oxygen flow of 6 l/min'.

BMC Anesthesiol (2011) 11: 10

Response to Case Study

1   **Cause**
    - In this case the most likely cause of DVT is immobility.

2   **Mobilzation**
    - Early ambulation, combined with compression and anticoagulants, does not significantly increase the incidence of new PE with uncomplicated acute DVT (Pashikanti & Von 2012, Galanaud & Kahn 2013, Clark *et al* 2013).

3   **Bed rest**
    - Prescribing bed rest for patients with acute DVT does not reduce their risk of developing a new PE (Trujillo-Santos *et al* 2005).

4   **Pain and swelling**
    - Pain and oedema resolve faster in patients treated with early ambulation and compression than those 'treated' with bed rest (Blattler & Partsch 2003, Partsch *et al* 2004).

5   **Goals**
    - Relief of pain and swelling
    - Independent mobility and ADL.

6 Plan

- Education on hydration and exercise.
- Liaise with nursing staff re. hydration and mobility.
- Provide exercise tick chart and theraband.
- Mobilize frequently, with mobility aid at first if required.
- Encourage dressing in the daytime.
- Liaise with OT and domiciliary team.

Response to Clinical Reasoning

For the control group, there is no explanation of what the oxygen was adjusted for, and what was adjusted.

BMC Anesthesiol (2011) 11, 10

RECOMMENDED READING

Akiyode O (2013) Peripheral arterial disease. *Topics Geriatr Rehab;* **29**(3): 179–86

Al-Zaiti (2013) Syncope and cardiac rhythms. *Am J Crit Care;* **22**(4): 361–2

Alastalo H, Räikkönen K, Pesonen A-K *et al* (2012) Cardiovascular morbidity and mortality in Finnish men and women separated temporarily from their parents in childhood. *Psychosom Med;* **74**: 583–7

Alagiakrishnan K (2013) Medication management of chronic heart failure in older adults. *Drugs Aging;* **30**(10): 765–82

Berardi C (2013) Heart failure performance measures: eligibility and implementation in the community. *Am Heart J;* **166**(1): 76–82

Blazek A (2013) Exercise-mediated changes in high-density lipoprotein. *Am Heart J;* **166**(3): 392–400

Book WM, Shaddy RE (2014) Medical therapy in adults with congenital heart disease. *Heart Failure Clin;* **10**(1): 167–78

Buber J, Rhodes J (2014) Exercise physiology and testing in adult patients with congenital heart disease. *Heart Failure Clin;* **10**(1): 23–33

Chesbro SB (2013) Reliability of ankle-brachial index measurements. *Topics Geriatr Rehab;* **29**(3): 195–202

Choudhry NK, Glynn RJ, Avorn J (2014) Untangling the relationship between medication adherence and post–myocardial infarction outcomes: Medication adherence and clinical outcomes. *Am Heart J;* **167**(1): 51–8.e5

Curtis AB (2013) Practice implications of the Atrial Fibrillation Guidelines. *Am J Cardiol;* **111**(11): 1660–70

Fairbrother P, Ure J, Hanley J (2014) Telemonitoring for chronic heart failure. *J Clin Nurs;* **23**(1–2): 132–44

Forslund AS, Lundblad D, Jansson JH *et al* (2013) Risk factors among people surviving out-of-hospital cardiac arrest and their thoughts about what lifestyle means to them. *BMC Cardiovasc Dis;* **13**: 62

Lucchetti G (2013) Rare medical conditions and suggestive past-life memories. *Explore (NY);* **9**(6): 372–6

Miller NH (2012) Adherence behavior in the prevention and treatment of cardiovascular disease. *J Cardiopulm Rehab Prev;* **32**(2): 63–70

NICE Guideline (2013) Lower limb peripheral arterial disease (CG147)

NICE Guideline (2013) Venous thromboembolic diseases (CG144)

NICE Guideline (2013) Myocardial infarction with ST-segment elevation (CG167)

Perera P (2014) Cardiac echocardiography. *Crit Care Clinics;* **30**(1): 47–92

Pryor T, Page K, Patsamanis H (2014) Investigating support needs for people living with heart disease. *J Clin Nurs;* **23**(1-2): 166–72

Ravi B (2013) The relation between total joint arthroplasty and risk for serious cardiovascular events in patients with moderate-severe osteoarthritis. *BMJ;* **347**: f6187

Robinson LA (2013) Anemia treatment protocol for the HF patient. *Heart Lung;* **42**(4): 305

Siervo M, Fewtrell MS, Wells JCK (2013) Acute effects of violent video-game playing on blood pressure and appetite perception. *Eur J Clin Nutr;* **67**: 1322–4

Stansby G, Berridge D (2013) Venous thromboembolism. *Br J Surg;* **100**: 989–90

Tung A (2013) Critical care of the cardiac patient. *Anesthesiol Clin;* **31**(2): 421–32

White A, Broder J, Campo TM (2012) Acute aortic emergencies. *Adv Emerg Nurs J;* **34**(3): 216–29

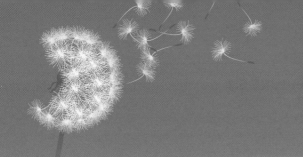

CHAPTER 5
General management

INTRODUCTION

Patients are managed by a multidisciplinary team, and physiotherapists will liaise with doctors for oxygen therapy, dieticians for nutrition, and pharmacists and nurses for medication. Physiotherapists' main input with patients is educational.

OXYGEN THERAPY

Oxygen is a colourless odourless drug with side effects and risks, but with rational prescription, precision of administration and objective monitoring, it can be a potent therapy for the respiratory patient.

Indications and limitations

> ### KEY POINT
>
> Oxygen is a treatment for hypoxaemia, not breathlessness.
>
> BTS 2008

The UK guidelines begin with the wise words above. Supplementary oxygen should normally be prescribed if resting P_aO_2 is <8 kPa (60 mmHg) or S_pO_2 <94%. This includes temporary hypoxaemia, e.g.:

- before and after suction
- during exercise, if demonstrable benefit is shown
- at night if desaturation is identified
- for specific patients peri-operatively.

Oxygen may also be required for potential hypoxaemia, e.g. after premedication for some cardiorespiratory patients and for first-time administration of bronchodilator drugs or hypertonic saline.

Giving oxygen to patients who are not hypoxaemic, e.g. following normoxaemic myocardial infarction or stroke, may reduce regional oxygen delivery because hyperoxia causes vasoconstriction (Decalmer & O'Driscoll 2013).

Assessment for both acute and long term oxygen includes nocturnal monitoring because of the risk of respiratory failure in some patients (Fig 5.1) and the lack of correlation between day and night requirements (Fig 5.2). Desaturation at night is associated with cognitive impairment (Yamout 2012).

Oxygen may reduce dyspnoea in the severely hypoxaemic individual but there is no evidence that supplemental oxygen reduces dyspnoea in the normoxaemic or mildly hypoxaemic patient (Decalmer & O'Driscoll 2013). Education is more helpful than the psychological crutch of an expensive drug. Most people cannot feel hypoxaemia, although some veteran patients know that a certain fuzzy feeling in their head indicates reduced oxygen levels (Uronis et al 2011), in which case this should be objectively confirmed by oximetry and supplemental oxygen titrated to their target saturation. Breathlessness and hypoxaemia often coexist, but they are caused by different mechanisms and require different management.

Other limitations are the following:

1 Directing oxygen into the throat does not guarantee its arrival at the mitochondria. Tissue oxygenation depends not just on inspired oxygen but also on gas exchange at the alveolar capillary membrane, lung perfusion, haemoglobin levels, cardiac output, vascular sufficiency and tissue perfusion.

FIGURE 5.1 Drop in mean P_aO_2 and rise in mean P_aCO_2 during sleep stages in patients with severe stable COPD, showing damaging episodes of ventilatory failure. *II:* stage II, *III:* stage III, *REM:* rapid eye movement stage

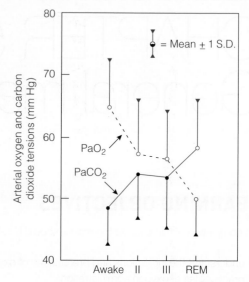

2 If hypoxaemia is due to a large shunt, benefit is limited because shunted blood does not 'see' the added oxygen (Ch. 1).

Complications

1 For patients depending on their hypoxic drive to breathe (p. 7), high concentrations of inspired oxygen can impair this drive. These patients should carry their own Venturi mask and an 'alert card' (Fig 5.3) which provides information on their target saturation for ambulance and other health staff (DoH 2010).

2 Discomfort can be caused by dry mucous membranes, eye irritation, a sense of being smothered, difficulty expectorating or excess work of breathing (WOB) due to inadequate flow. A patient oxygenating their forehead is a familiar sign of this problem. Aqueous cream may help dry lips, increased flow rate may reduce WOB

FIGURE 5.2 S_pO_2 in people with COPD: (a) linear relationship between rest and exercise, (b) lack of relationship between rest and sleep (modified from Schenkel 1996)

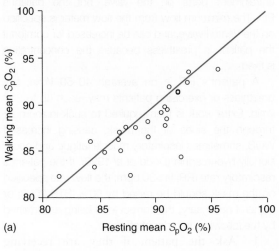

(a)

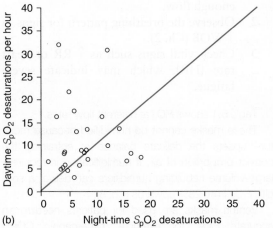

(b)

FIGURE 5.3 Oxygen alert card

OXYGEN ALERT CARD

Name: _____

I am at risk of type II respiratory failure with a raised CO_2 level.

Please use my _____ % Venturi mask to achieve an

oxygen saturation of ____ % to ____ % during exacerbations.

Use compressed air to drive nebulisers (with nasal oxygen at 2 l/min). If compressed air not available, limit oxygen-driven nebulisers to 6 minutes.

---

and 110 hours at 100% oxygen, but for patients it is difficult to distinguish the effects of the disease, the oxygen and other treatments (Kallet & Matthay 2013). High concentrations should not be withheld from patients who are critically hypoxaemic (Crooks *et al* 2012).

5   Oxygen creates a fire hazard by supporting combustion. Smoking is banned, and home equipment must be kept away from heaters and open flames (Litt *et al* 2013).

6   For neonates, high concentrations can cause blindness (Ch. 10).

7   'Absorption atelectasis' can occasionally develop if high concentrations of oxygen replace inert nitrogen (the main constituent of air) so that alveoli are no longer held open by a cushion of gas. This can occur in mechanically ventilated patients receiving more than 70% oxygen at low tidal volumes (Cairo 2012, p. 339), e.g. those with ARDS (Derosa *et al* 2013), but is not usually significant if a high fraction of inspired oxygen (F_iO_2) is required, e.g. during general anaesthesia (Staehr *et al* 2012, O'Brien 2013). Absorption atelectasis can be used positively when oxygen is used to increase absorption of gas from a pneumothorax or subcutaneous emphysema (p. 107).

8   Tubing can be a trip hazard.

9   Individual devices may create their own complications, as discussed below.

or a different device may be indicated. Humidification is required if the patient has thick secretions or feels uncomfortably dry, which often occurs at over 4 l/min (Chidekel *et al* 2012).

3   Oxygen is not physically addictive, but dependency occurs when patients rely on it unnecessarily.

4   Prolonged exposure to pure O_2 may cause inflammatory lung toxicity. This has been demonstrated in animals and healthy volunteers, who have experienced substernal pain, cough and sore throat after between 4

FIGURE 5.4 Dilution of oxygen by room air

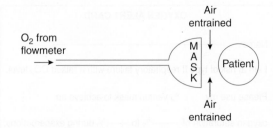

Delivery devices

Oxygen emerges from the flow meter at 100% but is diluted by entrainment of room air (Fig 5.4). After dilution, **high flow** systems deliver a flow to the patient that usually matches their own inspiratory flow rate and so are often preferred by breathless patients. **Low flow** systems deliver oxygen to the patient at a lower flow than their own. High and low flow systems relate to high and low accuracy, not to high and low concentration, as described below.

Low flow (variable performance) mask

These simple masks deliver a flow that is less than the patient's own peak inspiratory flow (PIF), with room air sucked in through entrainment ports and sides of the mask or cannula. The more breathless the patient, the more room air is entrained and the lower the F_iO_2 they receive. F_iO_2 therefore varies with the patient's own breathing pattern, as well as the flow selected on the flow meter. Low flow masks provide uncontrolled oxygen because of the variable F_iO_2, but they are suitable for patients who do not require an exact concentration, e.g. during suction or after surgery.

The flow rate should be maintained above 5 l/min to avoid rebreathing CO_2 (BTS 2008). This flow can be marked on the flow meter with tape to remind staff of the correct setting.

High flow (fixed performance) mask

Known also as Venturi masks (Fig. 5.5) these deliver a controlled oxygen concentration by forcing a jet of oxygen through a narrow orifice before entering the mask, causing a shearing effect which draws room air into the

gas stream through fixed-size entrainment ports. The speed of the resulting flow virtually abolishes the rebreathing of room air via the mask, even if it is loosely fitted. It delivers the F_iO_2 specified on the colour-coded Venturi valve. This F_iO_2 depends on the size of the entrainment ports on the valve, not the patient's PIF. The minimum flow from the flow meter is specified on the Venturi valve, and can be increased for comfort if the patient is breathless because the concentration is fixed.

A patient's PIF is on average 40–50 l/min, but breathless or exercising patients may reach up to 200 l/min. Extra work is then required to suck in room air through the sides of the mask, causing increased WOB, sometimes inspiratory muscle fatigue and occasionally hypercapnia (Dodd *et al* 1998). If the patient's respiratory rate (RR) is >30 bpm, the flow rate specified on the mask should be raised by 50% (BTS 2008) or higher if necessary, the correct level being ascertained by the following, in order of efficacy:

1 Ask the patient if they are receiving enough flow.
2 Observe the breathing pattern for signs of ↑ WOB (Ch. 2).
3 Check vital signs such as ↑ RR or heart rate (HR), which may indicate severe fatigue.

Table 5.1 shows F_iO_2 at different flow rates.

These masks cannot be humidified because moisture upsets the delicate balance of entraining the correct proportion of air. If humidification is required, large-volume nebulizing humidifiers can deliver a specific F_iO_2 from 28% upwards (Ch. 8).

Venturi masks are used for patients needing an accurate F_iO_2, for example, hypercapnic COPD patients who are dependent on their hypoxic drive to breathe, and for breathless patients whose PIF is too high to tolerate a low flow system. High capacity masks are available which can maintain a steady percentage even with very breathless patients.

Reservoir systems

Reservoir masks deliver high percentage oxygen by means of a reservoir bag (Fig 5.6). During exhalation, oxygen fills the bag instead of being lost to the environment, then during inhalation this oxygen enriches the inspired gas. A **partial-rebreathing** bag receives

FIGURE 5.5 High flow Venturi system: (a) colour-coded valves with fixed-size entrainment ports, (b) blue 24% valve fitted to mask, (c) oxygen delivered from the left, driven through the narrow orifice and then drawing in room air through entrainment ports

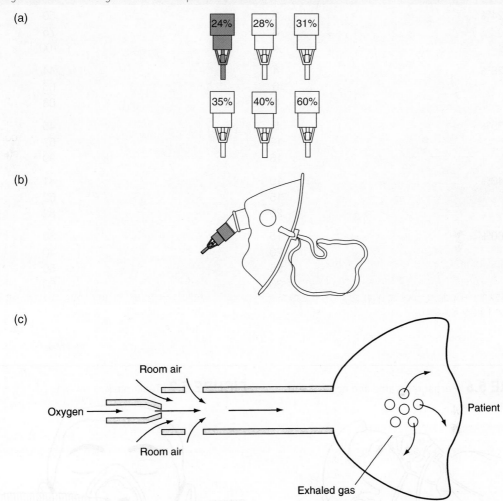

oxygen plus exhaled gas equivalent to the patient's anatomic dead space, delivering approximately 35–60% oxygen on the next breath. A **non-rebreathing** system has valves at the reservoir bag and one side vent of the mask to prevent the mixing of exhaled gases with the fresh gas, delivering up to 90% oxygen (Garvey *et al* 2012).

Before applying the mask, the reservoir bag must be filled with oxygen by occluding the valve between the reservoir and the mask. The flow rate must be at least 15 l/min, or high enough to keep the bag inflated throughout the respiratory cycle, however breathless the patient. Reservoir masks cannot be humidified.

Tusk mask

High F_iO_2 can be achieved by creating reservoirs out of two 20 cm lengths of wide-bore corrugated tubing which are inserted into each exhalation port of a simple mask (Fig 5.7) or partial rebreathing mask (Hnatiuk *et al* 1998).

Nasal cannula

These cannulae deliver oxygen into the nostrils so that patients can talk, cough, eat and drink unhindered. They are low flow systems and the F_iO_2 is not accurate, rapid breathing increasing the F_iO_2 because less room

TABLE 5.1 Oxygen concentrations delivered from high flow systems, showing how flow from the flow meter can be altered for different total flows to the patient according to need, while maintaining F_iO_2

Concentration	Oxygen flow (l/min)	Flow to patient (l/min)
24%	2	50
	3	75
	4	100
28%	4	44
	6	66
	8	88
35%	8	45
	12	67
	16	90
40%	10	41
	15	62
	20	82
60%	15	30
	20	40
	25	50
	30	60

FIGURE 5.6 Partial rebreathe and non-rebreathe reservoir masks

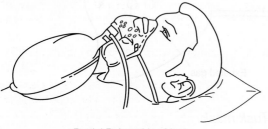

Partial Rebreathing Mask

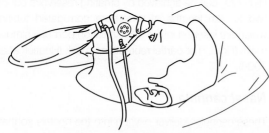

Non-Rebreathing Mask

FIGURE 5.7 Tusk mask

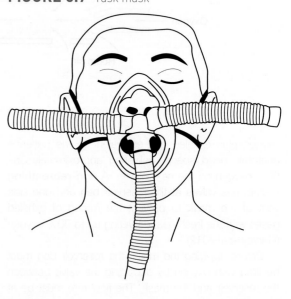

air is entrained. Nose breathers do not receive a higher F_iO_2 because the pharynx acts as a reservoir for oxygen during expiration, which is drawn on during inspiration (Wettstein *et al* 2005). High flow from the flow meter may cause irritation and sometimes nose bleeds. Nasal discomfort can be eased by humidification (Miyamoto 2008) or aqueous cream, but not lanolin in case of allergy, and not petroleum jelly (Vaseline) which is petrol-based and reacts with oxygen.

Indications for nasal cannulae are:

- home oxygen
- patients who find masks uncomfortable
- confused patients, especially if high concentrations are needed, when cannulae can be used with a mask in case the mask is pulled off
- hypoxaemic patients using an incentive spirometer, inspiratory muscle trainer, ultrasonic nebulizer and, for certain patients, a nebulizer (p. 168).

High flow nasal cannula

Figure 5.8 shows the Optiflow high-flow system. This system is more comfortable than normal nasal cannulae (Cuquemelle *et al* 2012), delivering oxygen through a heated humidifier and air/oxygen blender via medium-bore tubing with flow rates of 15–40 l/min (Ward 2013). Advantages are:

1   The high flow can reduce dyspnoea (Lenglet *et al* 2012).
2   It delivers higher F_iO_2 than a simple mask at flows of 6–10 l/min, and equal F_iO_2 at 12 l/min.
3   It delivers higher F_iO_2 than a non-rebreathe system at flows of 6 l/min, and equal F_iO_2 at 8–15 l/min.
4   Modest continuous positive airway pressure (CPAP) is generated (Parke *et al* 2007), which increases functional residual capacity (Wettstein 2013) and may reduce the WOB (Bräunlich 2013).
5   It can decrease the need for non-invasive ventilation (Peters *et al* 2013).

Disadvantages are that it delivers a more variable F_iO_2 than a simple or non-rebreathe mask (Garcia *et al* 2005) and has been reported to cause barotrauma in children (Hegde 2013).

Of particular interest to physiotherapists is the increased lung volume that can be achieved (Corley *et al* 2011) and the claim that it can increase exercise tolerance in people with advanced COPD when using an exercise bike or treadmill (Chatila *et al* 2004).

Nasopharyngeal catheter

A specialized low flow catheter can be lubricated and inserted into a nostril to reach just behind the uvula, then taped to the face. Several holes near the tip diffuse the flow, but patients often complain of a sore throat. These catheters are unsuited to infants because they occlude most of the nasal airway, and they are often not tolerated by children. They are sometimes used for short periods when a device is needed that must not become dislodged. A flow of 3–4 l/min usually delivers inspired concentrations of 30–40%, but high flows have been known to cause barotrauma (Alifano 2010).

Transtracheal catheter

A small hole can be surgically created into the trachea, percutaneously or through a tunnelled route, through which a small transtracheal catheter (Fig 5.9) can be introduced to deliver long term oxygen therapy. The system suits patients who prefer it for cosmetic reasons, who can undertake protocols to prevent encrustation and infection, and who find the reduced flow requirements convenient (Shih 2011). High flow

FIGURE 5.8 Optiflow high-flow system

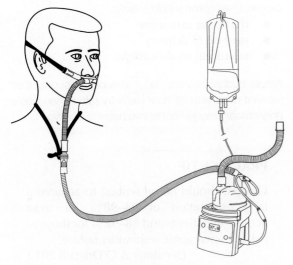

FIGURE 5.9 Oxygen delivery systems. From left: simple mask, nasal cannula, transtracheal catheter

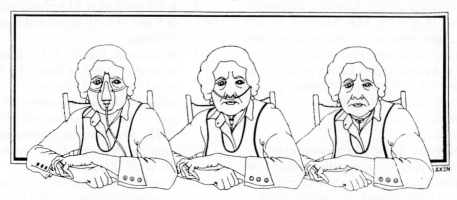

transtracheal catheters may also reduce WOB and augment CO_2 removal (Garvey *et al* 2012). Disadvantages relate to the need for surgical placement, with the accompanying risks of infection or subcutaneous emphysema.

Head box and oxygen chair

Clear plastic boxes over the heads of babies deliver high flow humidified oxygen (Ch. 10). The flow must be directed away from the baby's face and care taken to ensure that the edges of the box do not rub the skin. Oxygen chairs incorporate a plastic canopy or hood over an upright infant. Both need gaps to avoid CO_2 rebreathing.

T-piece

A T-piece delivers oxygen to an intubated spontaneously breathing patient via the tracheal tube. Humidified oxygen is delivered through one end and exhaled gases leave through the other. So long as the flow rate is greater than the patient's PIF, it acts as a high-flow device.

Acute oxygen therapy

In the acute setting, oxygen must be administered continuously (AARC 2002a) unless hypoxaemia has been demonstrated only in specific situations such as sleep or exercise. Patients should be informed that oxygen is not addictive, and some patients need reassurance that an oxygen mask is not a sign of terminal illness. Patients on acute oxygen therapy should only have their mask removed for expectoration or other brief reason.

> ## KEY POINT
>
> Prescription 'as required' is never appropriate.
> BTS 2008

The UK guidelines stipulate that the target saturation should be prescribed on the drug chart and monitored on the observation chart (BTS 2008). All team members need to be involved because both prescription and monitoring are notoriously neglected (Decalmer & O'Driscoll 2013), and lack of prescription is defined as a drug error in the UK. Inadequate oxygenation is not obvious because the brain is the most vulnerable organ (Karakontaki 2013). Some local protocols enable physiotherapists to prescribe oxygen. Prescription should specify:

- the target saturation
- method of delivery
- nocturnal modifications.

Astute budget holders find it cheaper to supply their relevant beds with 24-hour oximetry rather than waste unnecessary oxygen or deprive patients of oxygen.

> ### PRACTICE TIP
>
> Oxygen should be prescribed to achieve a target saturation of **94–98%** for most acutely ill patients and **88–92%** for those at risk of hypercapnic respiratory failure.
> Decalmer & O'Driscoll 2013

Patients with COPD

People with hypercapnic COPD vary in their response to oxygen. The major risk is giving too little oxygen, which leads to cardiac arrhythmias and tissue injury including damage to brain cells (Murphy et al 2001). However, nearly half of patients retain CO_2 during an exacerbation (Decalmer & O'Driscoll 2013) because sustained hypercapnia has left them dependent on hypoxia rather than hypercapnia as their chemoreceptor ventilatory stimulus. Uncontrolled oxygen may therefore knock out their respiratory drive, leading to hypoventilation, drowsiness and respiratory acidosis which can be lethal. Normocapnic COPD patients are not at risk, but occasionally a similar reaction has been found in people with other hypercapnic conditions such as neurological or sleep disorders, asthma, cystic fibrosis, bronchiectasis, chest wall disorders and obesity hypoventilation (Decalmer & O'Driscoll 2013).

For these patients, a simple low flow mask is inadequate, and nasal cannulae are unsatisfactory because exhausted patients may hypoventilate, entrain little room air and receive dangerously high F_iO_2 levels (Davies & Hopkin 1989). If nasal cannulae are necessary for patient comfort, monitoring of blood gases is required until it is known whether or not they are retaining CO_2.

These patients require controlled oxygen therapy titrated to their individual response in order to preserve respiratory drive while nourishing brain cells (BTS 2008):

- If the patient has acute hypercapnia, or if they have a history of hypercapnia when acutely unwell, or if they habitually retain CO_2 in the chronic state, or if none of this is known, controlled oxygen is delivered by Venturi mask, starting at 28% and titrated upwards or downwards to maintain S_pO_2 at 88–92%. If a nebulizer is needed, this should be driven by compressed air with supplementary oxygen given concurrently by nasal cannulae, using oximetry to maintain the target S_pO_2.
- If a normocapnic patient is not drowsy and is known not to have had previous episodes of hypercapnia, oxygen should be given to a target S_pO_2 of 94–98%.
- If the patient has severe hypoxaemia and their response to oxygen is not known, the target saturation should be 94–98%, but the patient kept under constant observation until blood gases are obtained.

Sometimes the F_iO_2 required to correct hypoxaemia still affects the respiratory drive. If P_aCO_2 rises above 10.6 kPa (80 mmHg) or pH falls below 7.35, or if the patient becomes drowsy or fatigued, non-invasive ventilation should be initiated. If P_aCO_2 still continues to rise and pH to fall, a decision is required on whether to instigate mechanical ventilation and/or decrease F_iO_2 further, bearing in mind that hypercapnia may not be a response to high F_iO_2 but due to a deteriorating condition.

Worse than too high or too low F_iO_2 is intermittent oxygen (Nadal 2013), which stirs up inflammation (Douglas et al 2013) and is like intermittent drowning (Fig 5.10c). Oxygen stores less than those for CO_2 because abundant CO_2 is needed for acid-base balance. If F_iO_2 is allowed to fall, CO_2 crowds out oxygen and causes a sharp drop in P_aO_2 (Collins 1976).

After F_iO_2 has been changed, oxygen equilibration requires 10 mins following an increase and 16 mins following a decrease, after which blood gases can be reassessed (Weinreich 2013).

A smart flow meter which automatically titrates oxygen flow to the target S_pO_2 is available for acute patients (Lellouche & Erwan 2012) and for exercising patients (Cirio et al 2011).

Patients with other conditions

Patients with pneumonia or acute asthma may need generous levels of oxygen because they are often severely hypoxaemic. This needs to be delivered at high flows because they are often severely breathless. Postoperatively, hypoxaemia may be transient and low risk patients usually require only a few hours' oxygen after surgery, but for people with lung disease or those undergoing heart, lung or other major surgery, several days and nights of supplementary oxygen may be required (Ch. 16).

Home oxygen

It's a fine line between helping me and being a blinking nuisance.
Patient quoted by Pugh & Enright (2012)

Long term oxygen therapy (LTOT)

Only smoking cessation and LTOT can extend survival in COPD patients with severe hypoxaemia (O'Driscoll

FIGURE 5.10 Potential effects of oxygen administration on arterial blood gases (in kPa) for COPD patients in ventilatory failure: (a) continued deterioration, (b) excessive F_iO_2 leading to ↓ respiratory drive, hypoventilation and further ↑ P_aCO_2, (c) intermittent removal of O_2, (d) normalization of blood gases

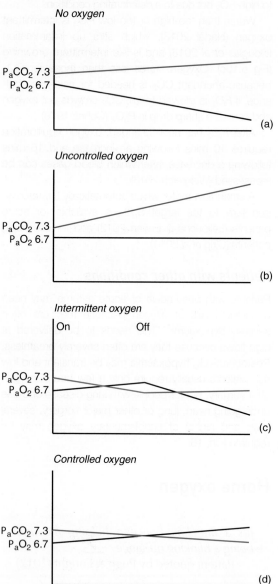

As well as prolonging life, accurately-prescribed LTOT has shown the following benefits with COPD:

- ↑ exercise capacity cognition and quality of life (Hodgkin *et al* 2009)
- ↑ P_aO_2, ↓ P_aCO_2, ↑ haemoglobin and possibly ↓ systemic inflammation (Howard 2012)
- ↓ exacerbations and hospital admissions (Dunne 2009)
- ↓ pulmonary hypertension, ↑ cerebral blood flow, alertness and motor speed (Criner 2013).

People with chronic hypoxaemia due to other diseases may also benefit (NHS 2011), including improved oxygenation with nocturnal oxygen for people with cystic fibrosis (Elphick & Mallory 2013).

Assessment for LTOT is mandatory, with the patient's condition stable and using the equipment that is planned for their home. After resting for 30 minutes, S_pO_2 is assessed. If it is >92% the patient is sent home and will be monitored at six-monthly intervals. If it is <92%, a capillary or arterial blood gas (CBG or ABG) is taken on room air. LTOT is indicated if any of the following apply:

- chronic stable hypoxaemia with P_aO_2 <7.3 kPa (55 mmHg) breathing air, on two samples taken at least three weeks' apart
- hypoxaemia <8 kPa (60 mmHg) if there is nocturnal hypoxaemia, peripheral oedema or pulmonary hypertension
- disabling dyspnoea in terminal respiratory disease (NHS 2011).

To assess flow rate, the patient rests for 30 minutes on 1–2 l/min and their CBGs/ABGs monitored. These may need to be repeated with increasing flow rates every 30 minutes until a P_aO_2 at or >8 kPa (60 mmHg) is achieved. If this is not possible without a rise in P_aCO_2, home non-invasive ventilation is considered. Any symptoms of CO_2 retention (headache, warm hands, flapping tremor) are noted so that the patient is aware of these.

Several nights' oximetry recording is required because of night-to-night variability (Lewis 2003) and the inability of predicting nocturnal requirements from daytime levels (Krachman *et al* 2008 and Fig 5.2). If this is not possible, nocturnal oxygen requirements can be identified by CBGs/ABGs taken at 0700 (Tárrega *et al* 2002) or, less accurately, by the daytime S_pO_2 (NICE 2010). Even less accurately, but better than nothing, is

2011). Clinical reasoning and good communication are needed to ensure accurate assessment and prescription.

FIGURE 5.11 S_pO_2 during sleep without added oxygen (hatched bars) and with oxygen (open bars) in a patient with severe COPD *SWS:* slow wave sleep; *REM:* rapid eye movement sleep

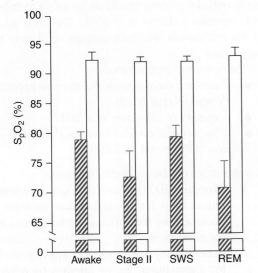

the flow rate at night being increased by 1 l/min (Rees & Dudley 1998). The value of nocturnal oxygen therapy is shown in Fig 5.11.

Oxygen should not be prescribed on hospital discharge unless hypoxaemia is severe, in which case it can be supplied temporarily, then assessed objectively when the patient has stabilized. Once prescribed, ongoing support and S_pO_2 monitoring should be maintained and the requirement for LTOT verified annually. Different activities may require different flow rates, e.g. eating, digesting, having sex and travelling (Nava 2011).

Patients are advised that oxygen should be used for as long as they can manage without unnecessary disruption to their lifestyle. 'The more the merrier' is their maxim. The minimum prescription is throughout the night, but >15 hours per 24 is preferable (Katsenos 2011), and near-continuous oxygen is ideal (Hodgkin *et al* 2000 p. 135), one study reporting an increase in pulmonary vascular resistance when oxygen was stopped for just three hours a day (Criner 2013). The goal is to achieve a P_aO_2 of at least 8.7 kPa (65 mmHg) without a rise in P_aCO_2 by more than 1.3 kPa (10 mmHg). The flow rate for this is generally 1.5 to 2.5 l/min, which can be increased by 1–2 l/min during exercise if indicated.

Three systems are available (Fig 5.12):

1 Oxygen cylinders contain compressed oxygen, delivered through a regulator valve. They run out of oxygen rapidly and the pressure is inadequate for driving a nebulizer or if long tubing is required. They deliver cold dry oxygen.

FIGURE 5.12 Home oxygen systems. From left: cylinder, portable liquid oxygen, concentrator

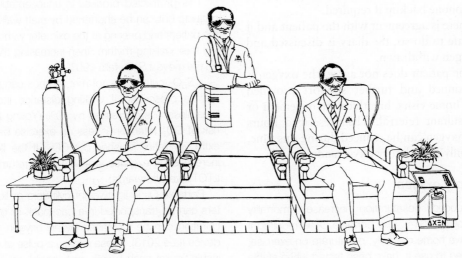

2   Oxygen concentrators separate oxygen from room air and deliver it at atmospheric temperature and humidity. Their noise can be reduced by putting the machine on a towel and in a separate room. Small devices can be powered from a car battery.

3   Liquid oxygen is stored at near absolute zero in thermos containers. Advantages are that electricity is not required, and light portable canisters can be filled from the container for easy mobility. Disadvantages include evaporation over time.

Domiciliary oxygen means that the disease is visible and can no longer be denied. Veteran patients on LTOT are often willing to talk to new patients and their carers, who may feel dismayed at the prospect of life spent tethered to bulky equipment.

Occasionally a patient stops needing their LTOT, either because it was mis-prescribed or occasionally because their condition has improved. In this case, they may find the prospect of losing their reassuring oxygen worrying. A suggested protocol for discontinuing LTOT is below (NHS 2011):

- 1st assessment: if S_pO_2 is >94% after 15 minutes without oxygen, a further assessment is arranged in 1–2 weeks.
- 2nd assessment: if S_pO_2 is >94% after 1 hour without oxygen, the patient is given a diary to be kept for the next week. They record when and where they have used or felt they needed to use their oxygen, with telephone backup if required.
- If there is agreement with the patient and it is safe to do so, the diary is discussed and oxygen withdrawn.
- If the patient does not agree, the oxygen is continued and further support provided e.g. home visits, breathless management or consultant referral. The prescribed hours on oxygen can be reduced during this time, or only ambulatory oxygen advised.

Ambulatory oxygen

Exercise-induced desaturation increases mortality (Andrianopoulos 2014), and portable O_2 is required if patients leave home regularly, desaturate on exercise, are motivated to use it, have been tested when stable and, if possible, have completed a pulmonary rehabilitation programme.

Exercise desaturation is not accurately predicted by baseline oxygen saturation but is likely if resting S_pO_2 is <95% (Andrianopoulos 2014). Ambulatory O_2 (Ambox) is prescribed if patients desaturate by 4% or to below 90% exercise (LeBlanc et al 2013). This may occur in the first minute and then stabilize, or it may be progressive.

The benefits of Ambox include:

- ↑ cerebral oxygenation and exercise capacity (Vogiatzis et al 2013)
- ↑ quality of life (Dyer et al 2012)
- ↓ hyperinflation and exertional breathlessness (O'Donnell et al 2007).

Disadvantages can be avoided by education:

1   Morgan (2009) found that some patients reduce their activity rather than increase it because they feel anxious or hampered by the equipment.

2   Patients may use Ambox inappropriately for short bursts in an attempt to relieve breathlessness (Young 2005).

It is handy to combine assessment for Ambox with assessment for pulmonary rehabilitation. The endurance shuttle walk test (ESWT) may be more responsive for detecting walking improvements than the six-minute walk test (6MWT) (Revill et al 2010). Ear oximetry is sometimes more accurate than finger oximetry due to movement artefact, so long as the ear is pink and well-perfused (Barnett 2012). Assessment is in Table 5.2.

This protracted process is unacceptable to many patients but can be shortened by staff walking behind the patient and peering at the oximeter without disturbing their walking rhythm, then increasing the flow rate on the move if S_pO_2 falls <90%.

If S_pO_2 criteria are not met, Ambox can sometimes still be prescribed if walking distance increases or breathlessness decreases by 10% (Young 2005). The risk of CO_2 retention is less on exercise because the extra ventilation washes out CO_2. If the flow rate is increased on exercise, patients must return it to their LTOT level afterwards.

Portable O_2 in lightweight cylinders or liquid canisters can be transported in a backpack or on a trolley. Duration can be increased by an oxygen-conserving device (Lee 2013). These release a pulse of oxygen on inspiration at each breath and should not be used at

TABLE 5.2 Assessment for Ambox

1	Rest for 30 minutes on room air or on added oxygen at the patient's resting O_2 prescription rate if they are on LTOT
2	Record Borg score and S_pO_2
3	Perform baseline walk test on room air, or at the patient's usual LTOT flow rate. Record distance, Borg and S_pO_2
4	Rest for 30 minutes (6MWT) or 40 minutes (ESWT) on room air or LTOT
5	If S_pO_2 is <90%, repeat walk test with an extra 2 l/min oxygen. Record distance, Borg and S_pO_2
6	If S_pO_2 is still <90%, rest, then repeat with an extra 2 l/min oxygen. Record distance, Borg and S_pO_2
7	Continue as above, adding oxygen until S_pO_2 is >90%
8	Record recovery time to baseline Borg and S_pO_2 levels

night when the breathing rate reduces, nor for breathless patients needing a high flow because their inspiratory flow will exceed the capability of the device. They are also less efficient for mouth breathers.

Flow from liquid oxygen is adequate with up to 200 feet of tubing, from concentrators with up to 100 ft, while cylinders can only deliver 1–2 l/min at up to 100 ft of tubing (Cullen & Koss 2005). These should be verified with the manufacturers.

Self-assessment while driving is advised. For flying, aircraft cabins contain the equivalent of 15% oxygen, so patients are advised to arrange for oxygen to be provided if their P_aO_2 is below 9.4 kPa (70 mmHg) on F_iO_2 of 0.15 (Dodd et al 1998). The battery life of portable concentrators varies (Fischer 2013) as do airline charges, and masks or nasal cannulae may not be provided.

Short-burst oxygen therapy (SBOT)

There is some evidence that SBOT reduces recovery time after activities of daily living in a selected group of patients with COPD (Quantrill et al 2007), but most studies find sparse evidence for this treatment (BTS 2006) and it is estimated that 75% of patients would be removed from SBOT if accurately assessed. At the same time, 25% of those who use only SBOT are thought to be candidates for LTOT. Short-burst oxygen is different from temporary oxygen (p. 146).

Hyperbaric oxygen therapy

Hyperbaric oxygen is 100% oxygen delivered at pressures greater than atmospheric. Once haemoglobin is fully saturated, the partial pressure of oxygen in the plasma rises, which increases the driving force of oxygen diffusion from blood into the tissues. Hyperbaric oxygen does not improve tissue oxygenation under normal circumstances but can stimulate healing in refractory wounds or irradiated tissues, and may reduce the risk of lower limb amputation 2–3 fold in people with diabetes (Thom 2011).

Beneficial effects have also been claimed for some sports injuries (Barata 2011), chronic ulcers (Kaur et al 2012), stroke (Zhang 2010), gas gangrene (in which the high PO_2 environment inhibits anaerobic organisms), carbon monoxide poisoning (Weaver et al 2002), crush injuries, ischaemia, burns, decompression illness, post-radiation damage, compromised skin grafts (Slotman 1998), acute brain injury (Huang 2011), chronic brain injury, autism (Rossignol et al 2009) and neurological damage in some neonates (Yin et al 2013). It is contraindicated if there is an undrained pneumothorax.

Heliox

Helium is an inert gas with $1/8$ the density of nitrogen. When blended with 21% oxygen it is called Heliox and can be used to bypass obstructed airways, e.g. with asthma (Dennis et al 2012a), COPD (Santus et al 2013) or patients requiring invasive or non-invasive ventilation (Kirkby 2013). Heliox can also relieve stridor and assist breathing through airways narrowed by tumours, burns or vocal cord paralysis (Khanlou & Eiger 2001).

NUTRITION

- **Anorexia:** reduced desire to eat, frequently accompanying illness.
- **Malnutrition:** lack of specific nutrients; accompanied by undernutrition or sometimes obesity.
- **Undernutrition:** inadequate intake of dietary energy, leading to <90% ideal body weight.
- **Wasting:** loss of fat and muscle.
- **Cachexia:** severe loss of fat and muscle, including respiratory muscle, caused by excess protein catabolism and leading to <80% of ideal body weight.
- **Sarcopenia:** loss of muscle mass and strength, caused by cachexia or ageing.

Nutrition and hydration are often neglected in all types of healthcare.

Leach *et al* (2013)

Breathing and eating are basic life processes that are intimately related in their mechanics, emotive associations and physiology. Air and food share common pathways for intake, then separate for processing, then their products join up in the blood for distribution to the tissues for the production of energy. Despite this interdependence, nutrition is still an overlooked area of respiratory medicine (Muscaritoli *et al* 2010). Malnutrition is the most common condition in hospitalized patients, which increases complications, readmissions and mortality (Frew *et al* 2010). For example:

1   Malnourished surgical patients have three times more postoperative complications and four times greater risk of death than well nourished patients having similar operations (Bairami *et al* 2012).
2   A third of patients admitted to UK hospitals are malnourished or at risk of malnutrition, and half of elderly patients do not have adequate access to fresh drinking water or assistance with eating (Leach *et al* 2013).

If malnutrition combines with disease and inflammation, it can reach the point of cachexia, which may be helped but is not reversed by nutritional support (Engineer & Garcia 2012) and possibly β_2-agonists (Joassard *et al* 2013).

Muscle accounts for 60% of the body's protein stores, and loss of muscle mass is directly responsible for reduced vital capacity, functional impairment, increased likelihood of falls and loss of autonomy (Muscaritoli *et al* 2010). For people with COPD, fatigue is a debilitating symptom, but Similowski (1991) found that well-nourished patients with stable COPD show no evidence of chronic fatigue.

KEY POINT

Physiotherapy may be nullified if a patient is malnourished.

Causes of poor nutrition in cardiorespiratory patients

- Eating becomes a chore rather than a pleasure for breathless people because the combined actions of eating and breathing are in competition.
- People with hyperinflated chests may feel full after a small meal, especially when accompanied by the air-swallowing associated with dyspnoea.
- Appetite can be reduced by smoking, depression, the taste of sputum and some drugs such as digoxin (Stajkovic *et al* 2011).
- Desaturation can be caused by the accessory muscles being diverted to assist eating, the breath-holding required for swallowing, and the extra metabolic activity of digestion and assimilation.
- Increased WOB raises calorie requirements.
- Exercise limitation and fatigue discourage the preparation of healthy food and predispose to excess fat stores (Stubbs 2004).
- Oxygen therapy or mouth-breathing can dry the mouth.

- 'Hospital malnutrition' is exacerbated by unappetizing food, missed meals due to tests or procedures, the traditional low priority given to nutrition, patients' loss of access to their own kitchen and long overnight fasts (Söderström 2013). Elderly patients may be unaccustomed to the processed high salt food that is common in hospitals, which may also increase thirst.
- Other contributions are dysphagia, poor cognition or feeling ill (Leach *et al* 2013).

Effects of poor nutrition in cardiorespiratory patients

Nutrition affects cardiorespiratory health from the womb onwards. Maternal malnutrition increases the risk of cardiovascular disorders in their offspring (Jackson *et al* 2011). A high sugar intake in youth predicts chronic disease risk (Hirshberg 2012) and caffeinated fizzy drinks are associated with fractures in teenage girls (Wyshak 2000). At all ages, excessive consumption of high calorie processed foods can lead to systemic inflammation (Alissa & Ferns 2012). A deficient diet increases susceptibility to the effects of tobacco smoke, air pollution and allergens, whereas a 'Mediterranean diet' is associated with cardiovascular health (Grosso *et al* 2014) and cognitive function (Kesse-Guyot 2013).

Poor nutrition erodes muscle (Kim *et al* 2008) impairs ciliary motility, aggravates the emphysematous process, depletes surfactant, increases WOB (DeMeo 1992), reduces exercise capacity (Roig *et al* 2012), increases infection risk (Smith *et al* 2012), slows wound healing, suppresses the immune system, increases mortality (Leach *et al* 2013) and reinforces the whole unhappy process by blunting hunger. Overfeeding can increase acidosis (Ayers & Warrington 2008).

Management

Attention to nutrition should be a routine preventive measure for preoperative patients and for those with acute or chronic illness, especially those with COPD, cancer or conditions associated with dysphagia. Nutritional supplementation can improve quality of life and respiratory muscle strength in malnourished people with COPD (Ferreira *et al* 2012) and should not be left until protein has been cannibalized from their respiratory muscles.

Education for breathless patients includes the following:

1 Eat multiple small meals.
2 It may be helpful to clear secretions before meals, and teeth-cleaning or using a mouth wash can reduce the bad taste of inhaled drugs or sputum.
3 If breakfast is difficult, try liquidizing it.
4 Have prepared meals ready in the fridge, to microwave when feeling too breathless to cook.
5 Ensure adequate vitamin C, which is needed daily because it is poorly stored. This vitamin speeds mucus transport (Behndig *et al* 2009), dampens down infection (Hernandez *et al* 2011), improves mood (Wang *et al* 2013c), helps preserve muscle strength (Cesari 2004) and may slow the decline in lung function (McKeever 2002). When taken with vitamin E, Fillmore (1999) claims that cardiovascular mortality is reduced by 53%. Intake is often reduced during hospitalization (Hughes 2003).
6 Ensure adequate vitamin D, whose anti-inflammatory properties benefit people with respiratory (Iqbal 2012) cardiovascular (Correia *et al* 2013) and critical illness (Amrein 2012), and lack of which is associated with infection (Lange *et al* 2013), osteoporosis, diabetes, cancer, rheumatoid arthritis and multiple sclerosis (Hirani *et al* 2010). Adequate vitamin D can be obtained from exposure of the hands and face to 10 minutes' strong sunlight for light skin, or 60 minutes for dark skin (Love 2003).
7 The antioxidant effects of garlic ('Russian penicillin') are said to help prevent chest infections, COPD, cardiovascular disease, aid expectoration and stop hair loss (Petrovska 2012). Combining its ingestion with milk reduces the antisocial after effects (Persson & Persson 2012).
8 Make use of homemade drinks such as milk shakes and, if there is no sensitivity to the acid, fresh fruit juice, but avoid

energy drinks if there is a risk of heart disease (Higgins *et al* 2010).

9   Try taking liquids separately from meals, to reduce satiety.

10 Avoid hard or dry food, or add sauces such as gravy or custard.

11 Avoid gas-forming foods.

12 Ensure meals are leisurely, enjoyable and taken sitting up with elbows on the table to stabilize the accessory muscles.

13 It may help to reduce dairy foods if secretions are a problem, because they can increase the viscosity of mucus (Enderby 1995), possibly because of the adhesive characteristics of lactobacilli (Van Tassell 2011). It may be necessary to try this for a month to identify if it is helpful, in which case adequate substitutes for calcium will be required.

Supplementary feeds provide concentrated nutrition orally or nasogastrically (NG). For patients with dysphagia who are intolerant of an NG tube, or for those requiring long term supplementary feeding, percutaneous endoscopic gastrostomy (PEG) directly into the stomach is advised (Fig 5.13). Oral feeds should be taken with a glass rather than through a straw, to avoid excess WOB, and are supplementary to meals, not a replacement. Enteral feeds are best given at night to encourage daytime eating, with the head of the bed raised. For patients at risk of desaturation, insertion of NG or PEG tubes should be accompanied by oximetry (Rowat 2004). Both NG and PEG tubes have been associated with suffocation in elderly patients hospitalized with pneumonia (Komiya *et al* 2013), but the two were not distinguished in this study and it is difficult to identify whether the cause was mechanical interference from an NG tube or the pathology itself.

For surgical patients, malnutrition affects morbidity and mortality, and patients at risk require preoperative immune-enhancing nutritional support (Kuppinger *et al* 2012). Some surgical cancer patients benefit from probiotics (Liu *et al* 2013b) and fish oil dampens inflammation in bypass patients (Berger 2013).

For medical patients, nutrition screening should take place on admission, especially for cardiorespiratory patients who may show a complicated pattern of weight loss, fluid retention, obesity and masked malnourishment (Frew *et al* 2010). Patients encumbered by non-invasive ventilation need extra attention (Reeves

et al 2013). Physiotherapists may be the first to identify the need for nutritional support and request a dietician referral.

Nutrition and physical activity are highly interrelated, complementary and synergistic.
Franklin *et al* 2013

RESPIRATORY DRUGS

One of the first duties of the physician is to educate the masses not to take medicine.
William Osler

● *Agonists* activate a receptor response.
● *Antagonists* block a receptor response.
● *β₁ receptors* stimulate heart rate and contractility.
● *β₂ receptors* stimulate bronchodilation.
● *Half-life* indicates the time for plasma levels to drop to 50%. A drug is eliminated after five half-lives.
● *Drug metabolism* is determined by patient age, size and the drug's route of excretion. The very young and very old are slower to metabolize drugs. Drugs metabolized by the liver or excreted by the kidney are affected by liver or kidney dysfunction.

Diseases such as COPD are largely irreversible, but despite this (or maybe because of it) patients tend to be subjected to blind polypharmacy, the risk of adverse side effects increasing exponentially with the number of agents prescribed (Green & Maurer 2013). 'Advanced' countries tend to show a bias towards over-treatment (Katz 2013). Other possible problems are that:

● patients may be prescribed drugs when in hospital which are then continued by repeat prescription after discharge without a drug review
● Up to 50% of patients are non-adherent with their drugs, which Darbishire (2012) found accounted for more than 10% of older-adult hospital admissions and 20%

FIGURE 5.13 Flow chart for patients at risk of malnutrition. *NG:* nasogastric, *PEG:* percutaneous endoscopic gastrostomy, *PICC:* peripherally inserted central catheter

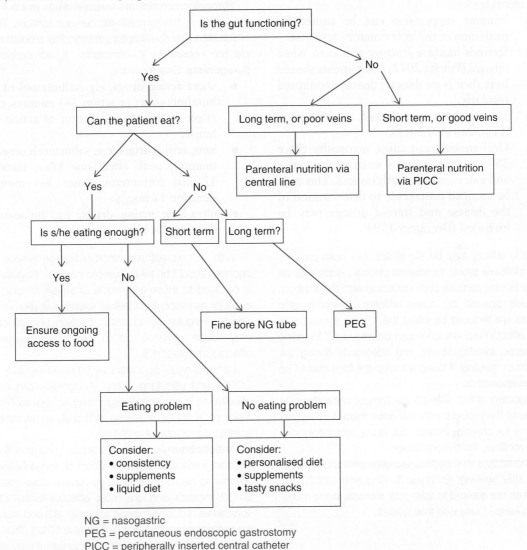

NG = nasogastric
PEG = percutaneous endoscopic gastrostomy
PICC = peripherally inserted central catheter

of preventable adverse drug reactions among ambulatory elderly patients.

It may be the pharmacist or nurse who educates the patient about their medication, but this is reinforced by the physiotherapist, who needs to understand the indications, side effects and delivery systems of different drugs. Domiciliary physiotherapists need to check the drugs of patients returning from hospital with their discharge summary and ensure that these are kept under review (Milos *et al* 2013).

Medication for specific diseases is described in the relevant chapter and for different problems below.

Drugs for inflammation

Glucocorticosteroids (also called corticosteroids and shortened to the term steroids here) are potent and non-specific anti-inflammatory agents. In the airways, they reduce the inflammation that can set off bronchospasm, oedema and mucous hypersecretion. They improve symptoms and reduce exacerbations in COPD and asthma but do not slow progression of disease (Raissy 2013). Side effects are listed in Table 5.3, with details below:

1   Immune suppression can be caused by mediation of the inflammatory response.

2   Steroids increase fracture risk even when inhaled (Putcha 2012) and patients should have their bone mineral density monitored regularly.

3   Steroids have been linked to depression (Lehmann *et al* 2013).

4   Oral steroids can cause myopathy (Shee 2003) which reduces exercise tolerance and can increase breathlessness. This may be ascribed mistakenly to deterioration of the disease and steroid dosage may be increased (Decramer 1994).

Side effects may be significant, but both patients and staff are prone to 'steroid phobia', especially as patients may confuse corticosteroids with the anabolic steroids abused by some athletes. Systemic side effects are reduced by using the inhaled route. Local side effects from inhalation can be minimized by using a spacer, inhaling slowly, and afterwards rinsing the mouth or gargling. If using a mask, the face should be wiped afterwards.

Concern about side effects tempts prescribers to nibble at the problem with low dose therapy. This may be fine for chronic asthma, but acute respiratory disease requires short sharp doses.

The body's own cortisol secretion peaks an hour or two after waking (Primhak & Kingshott 2012) and patients are advised to take their steroids in the morning to keep in tune with their bodies.

Drugs for bronchospasm

Response to bronchodilators is usual in asthma, less frequent in chronic bronchitis and less so in emphysema. However, long-acting bronchodilators have been found beneficial for people with COPD and asthma, sometimes in combination (Spina 2014).

Reversibility to bronchospasm is defined as improved FEV_1 or FVC by 12–15% after a bronchodilator trial (Hanania *et al* 2011). Measurements are taken 20 minutes after a β_2-agonist or 40 minutes after an anticholinergic.

Both sympathetic (adrenergic) and parasympathetic (cholinergic) receptors have been identified in bronchial smooth muscle.

Sympathomimetics are versatile drugs which mimic the action of the sympathetic nervous system. Those which stimulate β_2-receptors in bronchial smooth muscle are known as β_2-stimulants, β_2-adrenergics or **β_2-agonists**. Examples are:

●   short acting drugs, e.g. salbutamol or terbutaline: onset of action 3–5 minutes, peak effect 20 minutes, duration of action 3–5 hours.

●   long acting drugs, e.g. salmeterol: onset 15 minutes, peak effect one hour, duration 12 hrs; formoterol: onset 3–5 minutes, duration 12 hrs.

●   ultra-long acting drugs, e.g. indacaterol: duration 24 hours.

With chronic asthma, short-acting or 'rescue' β_2-agonists should be taken symptomatically. Regular use is confined to those with acute or severe chronic disease, or as prophylaxis before exercise or allergen exposure. Regular β_2-agonists, if taken unnecessarily, may induce tolerance to their own bronchoprotective effects (Cazzola 2013).

Long acting β_2-agonists may be taken regularly with COPD, and ultra-long acting β_2-agonists can be as effective as the anticholinergic drug tiotropium (Vogelmeier *et al* 2010) or a long acting β_2-agonist/steroid combination (Cope *et al* 2011).

Anticholinergic (antimuscarinic) bronchodilators such as tiotropium block the effect of acetylcholine on autonomic nerve endings. They have a slow onset of 20–30 minutes and are most effective with COPD, sometimes reducing exacerbations (p. 80) and increasing exercise tolerance (Yoshimura *et al* 2012). They can be used in combination with β_2-agonists if they show an additive effect. Individuals show different response patterns and may react better to β_2-agonists, anticholinergics or both. Side effects include cardiovascular events (Singh *et al* 2013a) and, with the nebulized drug, glaucoma if a mouthpiece is used.

Theophylline and its derivatives such as aminophylline and caffeine are part of the methylxanthine group of drugs which can bronchodilate, stimulate respiration, enhance respiratory muscle function (Schumacher 2004), improve exercise capacity (Voduc *et al* 2012) and reduce inflammation (Akram 2012). Side effects are legion, including interactions with other drugs and suicidal thoughts in some asthma patients (Favreau *et al* 2012). Precise dosage is required, usually with a slow-release preparation, and blood levels are checked regularly.

If an inhaled bronchodilator and steroid are prescribed, it is best to take the bronchodilator first to assist penetration of the steroid, but complicated instructions can demotivate patients, and it is more important that the drugs are taken than a sequence adhered to.

Details are in Table 5.3.

Drugs for breathlessness

Sometimes the cause of shortness of breath (SOB) can be treated, for example by diuretics, bronchodilators or steroids. For a direct effect on the symptom itself, the following have shown varying degrees of efficacy:

1   Morphine is the mainstay (Fig 5.14), working on opioid receptors throughout the respiratory tract (Mahler *et al* 2010). The side effect of respiratory depression does not appear to affect gas exchange except in severe cases (Boland *et al* 2013), and it must be given in sufficient dosage (Uronis *et al* 2006). The skills of a palliative team may be required.
2   Fentanyl is an opioid that can relieve SOB in as little as five minutes when given

transmucosally as 'lollipops' (Hallenbeck 2008).
3   Bronchodilators may reduce SOB in some patients independent of their bronchodilating effect, probably by reducing hyperinflation.
4   Buspirone is an anxiolytic which can reduce breathlessness and increase exercise tolerance without causing sedation (Argyropoulou 1993, Gokben *et al* 2012).
5   Sildenafil (Viagra) may reduce SOB in pulmonary fibrosis by relaxing vascular muscles and decreasing pulmonary hypertension (Ryerson *et al* 2012) but tends to worsen gas exchange and quality of life with COPD (Lederer *et al* 2012).
6   SSRI antidepressants either lift the depression that increases SOB, or the serotonin acts directly on the brainstem respiratory centres (Uronis *et al* 2006).
7   Inhaled furosemide may ameliorate SOB in people with acute COPD (Vahedi *et al* 2013).

Drugs to help clear secretions

If mucoactive drugs are needed, they should improve mucus transport rather than irritate the airways because irritation simply creates more secretions. They should also optimize viscosity rather than over- or under-hydrate the mucus because cilia prefer a viscoelastic gel rather than either loose or thick mucus.

The following may be beneficial for some patients (Balsamo *et al* 2010):

1   Mucolytics such as carbocisteine (Mucodyne), acetylcysteine or erdosteine reduce viscosity by degrading polymers in mucus. They also have anti-inflammatory and antioxidant properties (Zheng 2013).
2   Mucoregulatory agents include anti-inflammatories, e.g. indomethacin or anticholinergics, some macrolide antibiotics, e.g. erythromycin, or drugs which decrease mucus hypersecretion, e.g. atropine.
3   Methylxanthines and β_2-agonists are mucokinetics, which increase ciliary beat frequency and mucus hydration (Kim & Criner 2013).

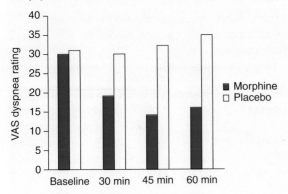

FIGURE 5.14 Effect of subcutaneous morphine on dyspnoea in cancer. *VAS*: visual analogue scale

TABLE 5.3 Medication for airways obstruction. (Generic names start with lower case letters and brand/trade names (in brackets) with upper case.)

Drug	Delivery	Side effects
Cromones to prevent inflammation (asthma only)		
nedocromil sodium (Tilade)	Inhalation	
Corticosteroids to treat inflammation		
beclometasone (Qvar, Clenil) budesonide (Pulmicort) fluticasone (Flixotide) Mometasone Ciclesonide	Inhalation	Hoarse voice, oropharyngeal candidiasis, dysphonia, pharyngitis, osteoporosis
prednisone prednisolone hydrocortisone	Intravenous Oral	Weight gain, muscle atrophy, infection risk, peptic ulceration, fragile skin, bruising, hyperglycaemia, diabetes, hypertension, mood change, adrenal suppression, delayed healing, retarded growth in children
Antileukotrienes to treat inflammation (asthma only)		
montelukast (Singulair) zafirlukast (Accolate)	Oral	Headache
Bronchodilators to treat bronchospasm		
Short acting β_2-agonists:		
salbutamol (Ventolin) terbutaline (Bricanyl)	Inhalation Oral Intravenous Subcutaneous	Tremor, tachycardia, agitation, atrial fibrillation, muscle cramps and (with high doses) 'inner restlessness'
Long acting β_2-agonists:		
salmeterol (Serevent) formoterol (Foradil) bambuterol (Bambec) indacaterol (Ombrez)	Oral Inhalation	
Anticholinergics:		
tiotropium (Spiriva) ipratropium (Atrovent)	Inhalation	Dry mouth, blurred vision, constipation (or diarrhoea from laxatives), urine retention, glaucoma, possible cardiovascular risk
Methylxanthines:		
theophylline aminophylline	Oral Intravenous	Headache, gastric ulcer, insomnia, nausea and vomiting, arrhythmias
Combined bronchodilators		
ipratropium and salbutamol (Combivent)	Inhalation	
Combined steroid and bronchodilator		
fluticasone and salmeterol (Seretide) budesonide and formoterol (Symbicort) beclometasone and formoterol (Fostair)	Inhalation	

4   The effectiveness of nebulized saline in speeding mucociliary clearance (Ch. 8) can be doubled by pre-treatment with the diuretic amiloride (Sood *et al* 2003).

5   Mannitol is a diuretic, but inhaled as a dry powder it creates an osmotic drive for water to move into the airway lumen. It is less irritating than hypertonic saline and can benefit people with bronchiectasis, asthma and cystic fibrosis (Daviskas & Rubin 2013).

Mucolytics have produced minimal impact on airway diseases (Randell *et al* 2006) but patients may find them subjectively beneficial.

Drugs for smoking cessation

Nicotine replacement is available as patches, chewing gum, lozenges, inhalators and nasal sprays (Scherphof *et al* 2014). Medication includes Bupropion (Zyban) and Varenicline (Champix), the former having some agreeable side effects such as increased libido and reduced weight, but the latter bringing disagreeable cardiovascular (Kuehn 2013) and psychological side effects (Aschenbrenner 2012). Nicotine vaccines offer promise (Lisy 2013).

Drugs for infection

The 'war on antimicrobial resistance' by escalation is about as likely as the chance of winning the 'war on terror'

Isaacs & Andresen 2013

An antibiotic is indicated if a patient's condition is caused by bacterial infection, if the organism responsible is sensitive to the antibiotic prescribed and if the infection is unlikely to resolve without assistance. It is administered orally, intravenously or by nebulizer.

Antibiotics often have to be given blind at first because 24 hours are needed for microbiological results. Thereafter antibiotics should be specific and time-limited to inhibit the emergence of resistant organisms. The 'revenge of the microbe' has led to organisms becoming resistant to antibiotics faster than new drugs are created, with some infections now untreatable

(Sandora 2012). Causes of a potential post-antibiotic era include antibiotics in agriculture (Fang *et al* 2014) and waste water (Wang *et al* 2014) as well as in medicine (Kuehn 2014). For mild disease, antibiotics sometimes maintain a cycle of 'medicalizing' a self-limiting illness in which patients attribute resolution to their antibiotics (NICE 2008). Prophylactic antibiotics are reserved for people with chronic sepsis such as cystic fibrosis.

Interesting alternatives are some essential oils (Yap 2013), probiotics for ICU-acquired pneumonia (Barraud *et al* 2013), maggot therapy for antibiotic-resistant wound infections (Sherman 2009) and, possibly more pleasingly, plenty of hot tea and coffee for MRSA infection (Matheson *et al* 2011).

Drugs to inhibit coughing

To suppress a non-productive and irritating cough, medication is available if physical means (Ch. 8) are to no avail. The efficacy of drugs is limited (Dicpinigaitis 2011), and protocols have been developed (Ojoo *et al* 2013, Shimizu *et al* 2013). Centrally-acting agents are gabapentin (MacKenzie 2014), dihydrocodeine, dextromethorphan (Irwin *et al* 2006), morphine and nicotine replacement, the latter explaining the temporary increase in coughing on smoking cessation (Bolser 2010). Baclofen works at spinal and supraspinal sites, and can also be used to treat hiccups. Peripherally-acting cough suppressants include benzonatate which reduces the sensitivity of stretch receptors in the lung. Benefit may also be found with antihistamines (Ojoo *et al* 2013), ipratropium, acetylcysteine or erdosteine (Bolser 2010). A cough caused by asthma or ACE inhibitors can be reduced by theophylline or indomethacin, and a post-infection cough may be helped by ipratropium (Irwin *et al* 2006). 'Cough mixtures' may contain both expectorant and suppressant, but are strong placebos and the sugar content is thought to briefly soothe irritated airways.

Drugs to improve ventilation

Respiratory stimulants should be used with caution if the respiratory muscles are already labouring because further stimulation may override the protective function of fatigue. Respiratory stimulants do not reverse the underlying cause of ventilatory failure.

Doxapram drives ventilation via chemoreceptors and the respiratory centres, but at the cost of central nervous system stimulation, agitation, shaking, hallucinations, increased WOB, dyspnoea and sometimes panic attacks (Wemmie 2011). An infusion is sometimes tolerated by drowsy patients if they hypoventilate following surgery, drug overdose, or if they are in ventilatory failure and awaiting noninvasive ventilation (Golder *et al* 2013).

Drugs to improve sleep

Behavioural treatments are preferable (Buysse 2013) and traditional sedatives and hypnotics tend to suppress the respiratory drive, but drugs which may be suitable for respiratory patients are zolpidem (Krachman *et al* 2008) or melatonin receptor agonists (Greenberg & Goss 2009).

KEY POINT

Drugs are tested by the people who manufacture them ... in such a way that they exaggerate the benefits of treatments ... Sometimes whole academic journals are owned outright by one drug company.

Goldachre (2012)

Delivery devices

Are respiratory drugs best ingested or inhaled? Aerosolized medication was being delivered directly to the respiratory tract in 1500 BC (Colice 2009), and its advantages are the same today:

- rapid onset of action
- local delivery to maximize positive effects and minimize side effects
- delivery of drugs that are inactive by other routes.

Disadvantages are:

- less effective lung deposition with airflow obstruction, turbulent airflow and mucous plugging, leading to patchy and mostly central distribution in people with advanced COPD or acute severe asthma (Laube *et al* 2011)
- loss of much of the drug to the atmosphere, stomach and pharynx, although high doses compensate for this

- deposition in the upper airways causing localized side effects, especially with steroids (Nave & Mueller 2013)
- with nebulizers, infection risk (AARC 2002a).

Inhalers

Pressurized inhalers (Fig 5.15) such as the metered dose inhaler (MDI) deliver an aerosol by suspending an active drug in a propellant. The traditional MDI is portable and cheap, but inhaler technique is said to be poor in 50% of people with asthma, and somewhat embarrassingly, only 5% of junior doctors were found to use it correctly (Price *et al* 2013). Slow deep breathing facilitates peripheral deposition (Sanchis *et al* 2013), but specific instruction is cost-effective, reducing exacerbations and SOB, and improving QoL (Göriş 2013). Breath-actuated inhalers such as the Autohaler or Easi-Breathe co-ordinate drug release with inhalation.

A **spacer** (Fig 5.15) is a chamber between the patient and inhaler which acts as a reservoir from which the patient inhales the aerosol. Advantages are the following:

1. Propellants and large particles drop out in the chamber and aerosol momentum is slowed so that less is lost by impaction on the back of the throat, thus reducing local side effects and doubling pulmonary deposition (Vincken *et al* 2010).
2. Less co-ordination is required because the drug remains suspended in the spacer until the patient inhales, although early inhalation is advised.
3. High doses can be delivered during acute episodes.

Spacers should be used when possible for metered dose inhalers, and always for children taking steroids. Infants can use a soft face mask attached to the spacer. The large pear-shaped spacers such as the Volumatic are cumbersome but efficient, simulating the aerosol cloud from an inhaler. Tidal breathing is recommended, and the Aerochamber gives a warning whistle if used incorrectly. Large spacers should be washed with detergent once a month without rinsing, and then air-dried, in order to reduce static charge which attracts the drug to the walls of the spacer rather than the lungs (NICE 2012a).

Dry powder inhalers such as the Turbohaler, Handihaler and Accuhaler require less co-ordination, and 75% of patients have been found to use them

FIGURE 5.15 Inhalers (top) and spacers

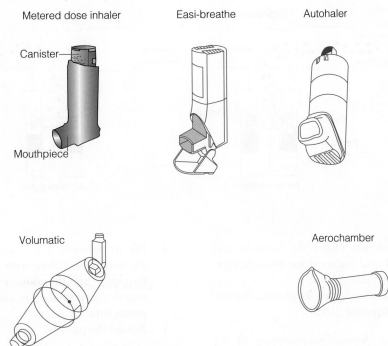

Metered dose inhaler   Easi-breathe   Autohaler

Canister

Mouthpiece

Volumatic   Aerochamber

correctly (Fink 2000). They draw air through powder to create an aerosol which is released on inspiration. Disadvantages are that children under six, breathless people and those with bronchospasm may be unable to generate sufficient inspiratory flow. The powder is sensitive to moisture, so it is either stored in foil blisters or patients are warned against exhaling into the device. Tiotropium delivered via the Respimat inhaler has been associated with higher mortality than when delivered by the Handihaler (Jenkins & Beasley 2013).

Problems for all inhalers are:

• the need for co-ordination and/or manual dexterity

FIGURE 5.16 Dry powder inhalers

Handihaler   Accuhaler   Turbohaler

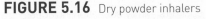

• confusion about when to use which inhaler, or forgetting the number of puffs (patients can lift a finger as they take each puff)
• difficulty in understanding instructions, e.g. mistaken spraying of the drug up the nose, onto the chest, into the armpits or, after one patient was told that her asthma was caused by her cat, onto the unfortunate pet.

Patients need the opportunity to try out and choose which inhaler suits them. Instructions and inhaler identification charts are in App. B.

Small-volume nebulizers

Nebulizers deliver solutions of a drug dissolved in a liquid or suspensions of drug particles in a carrier liquid, using compressed air, oxygen or ultrasonic power.

Jet nebulizers (Fig 5.17) run on air or oxygen and use the Venturi principle (p. 148), which creates a variety of droplet sizes:

• large particles impact on a baffle and fall back into the nebulizer chamber
• particles >6 μm diameter are lost in the upper airways

FIGURE 5.17 Small volume jet nebulizer for delivery of saline or medication

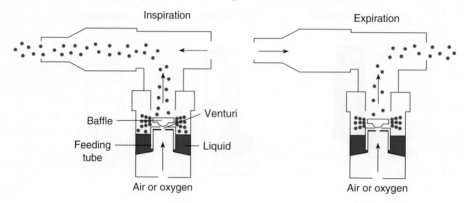

- particles 2–6 μm target the bronchi and bronchioles and are used for bronchodilators and steroids
- particles <2 μm deliver antibiotics to the alveoli (Darquenne 2012).

Breath-synchronized devices reduce some of the wastage.

The following technique is suggested:

1   The driving gas should be prescribed on the drug chart (Satya 2004). Acutely hypoxaemic asthmatic patients require high F_iO_2 levels, which, paradoxically, may be best delivered by air-driven nebulization combined with nasal cannulae (Caille *et al* 2009). People with acute hypercapnic COPD require the same combination but with monitoring of S_pO_2, close observation with the first dose and patients asked to report any symptoms of CO_2 retention. If an air compressor is not available, oxygen-driven nebulization should be limited to six minutes for people with COPD (BTS 2008).

2   Select a mouthpiece if possible, unless patient preference or excessive dyspnoea precludes this. Nose breathing filters the drug and reduces lung deposition by a quarter (Salmon *et al* 1990) and aerosol escaping from a mask can affect the eyes.

3   If possible, have the patient sitting upright in a chair. Ensure breathless patients have support for their elbows.

4   Fill to between 2.5–6 ml, depending on the nebulizer. Dilute with normal saline if required. Set the flow rate to 6 l/min, unless a compressor is used, which has a preset flow rate.

5   Advise the patient:
- to mouth-breathe if possible
- to intersperse tidal breaths with some slow deep breaths and some end-inspiratory holds to improve deposition (Bauer *et al* 2009)
- if using a mouthpiece, not to obstruct the air port
- to allow ten minutes for completion
- after each use to empty and dry the nebulizer with a paper towel, or when in hospital, follow infection control protocol
- once a day to wash the nebulizer in hot soapy water, rinse and dry with air from the compressor or oxygen supply, or follow local protocol; drying is the most important part of the cleaning process (Dodd 1996).

For home nebulizers, family education includes:
- the importance of cleaning the equipment
- regular servicing: the compressor becomes less effective even though it continues to produce a mist
- '4-hourly nebs' does not mean during the night.

Some nebulizer solutions should not be mixed, and the pharmacy will provide up-to-date information. Tapping the nebulizer when the liquid is beginning to fizz is useful for antibiotics when exact dosage is required. When nebulizing via a tracheostomy, the inner tube should be removed (Pitance *et al* 2013).

Ultrasonic nebulizers are popular with patients because the density of the mist speeds up the process, but they do not suit all drug suspensions.

For patients with chronic disease who remain symptomatic despite inhaler use, a nebulizer trial can be performed, with the first dose administered in hospital in case of side effects such as cardiac arrhythmias. Drug trials for home use should not be undertaken during acute illness. If patients use nebulizers at home, they require adequate advice and back-up servicing.

Positive expiratory pressure (p. 235) may be combined with nebulizers but the dose may need adjustment (Berlinski 2013)

Inhaler or nebulizer?

Patients tend to prefer nebulizers even when equivalent doses are delivered (Smyth *et al* 2001), possibly because they are automatically given nebulizers when admitted to hospital, so nebulizers 'must be best', or perhaps because nebulizers create an impressive mist and do not demand respiratory gymnastics for co-ordination. However, nebulizers come with disadvantages:

1   People at home with severe acute asthma may be over-reliant on repeated use when their airways are dangerously obstructed and they need to get themselves to hospital (Heslop & Harkawat 2000).
2   Nebulizers are expensive and require servicing and cleaning (Yawn *et al* 2012) but 'horrifying tales' of contamination have been reported, both in hospital (Botman 1987) and at home (Lane 1991).
3   Patient adherence may be hindered by the lengthy time for completion.
4   Less drug reaches the lung (Fig 5.18), although a higher dose compensates.

NICE (2012a) stipulates that nebulized therapy only be prescribed at home if it leads to one or more of the following:

● ↓ symptoms
● ↑ ability to undertake activities of daily living

● ↑ exercise capacity
● ↑ lung function.

The following may be suited to nebulizers:

● people who are too breathless or confused to use an inhaler
● people who need large doses rapidly
● antibiotic, antifungal or local anaesthetic drug delivery
● patients in whom assessment has shown improved outcome compared to inhalers.

The task of assessment for delivery systems, patient education and periodic checks (Ari *et al* 2012) may fall to the pharmacist or physiotherapist. Deposition of the drug is improved by chest clearance beforehand if required (Wolkove *et al* 2001).

> *The young physician starts life with 20 drugs for each disease, and the old physician ends life with one drug for 20 diseases.*
>
> William Osler

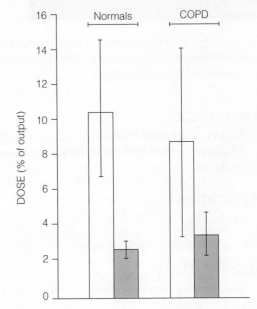

FIGURE 5.18 Dose of drug delivered by metered dose inhaler (open columns) compared to nebulizer (shaded columns)

BRONCHOSCOPY AND LAVAGE

Access to the bronchial tree for diagnostic or therapeutic purposes is achieved with a fibre optic bronchoscope, a thin flexible instrument passed through the nose and down into the subsegmental bronchi, using local, nebulized or general anaesthesia. Complications include discomfort, laryngospasm, bronchospasm, bleeding, arrhythmias, nausea/vomiting, infection, hypoxaemia (AARC 2007) and the complications of the suction pressure that is usually applied (Palazzo & Soni 2013). Prolonged hypoxaemia is reduced by using high-flow nasal oxygen (Lucangelo et al 2012).

Diagnostically, bronchoscopy can be used for:

- observation
- biopsy, e.g. to identify a malignant lesion
- brushings, e.g. obtaining lower airway microbiology samples in patients with pneumonia or to identify parenchymal lung disease, using a protected specimen brush to avoid contamination by upper airway flora (Kang & Kim 2012)
- lavage, which involves wedging the scope into a bronchus, washing 120–200 ml warmed saline through a separate channel, then aspirating this along with fluid and cells from the lower respiratory tract and alveoli for diagnosing parenchymal lung disease.

Therapeutically, bronchoscopy can be used for placing stents (Hürtgen & Herber 2014), identifying and resecting tumours, palliating upper airway cancers or removing foreign bodies. It may substitute for physiotherapy in clearing secretions if there is intractable sputum retention with no air bronchogram on x-ray, i.e. with blocked central airways. To re-expand atelectatic areas, it can be combined with selective insufflation of air, which needs to be followed by physiotherapy to prevent recurrence (Jelic et al 2008).

Patients are usually told the 'why' of bronchoscopy, but not always the 'how'. Physiotherapists can check that patients understand the procedure and that they feel able to ask questions of their bronchoscopist who tends to underestimate patients' level of tolerance (Hadzri et al 2010).

CASE STUDY : MR FJ

A 32 y.o. father from Eastbourne has been referred for 'twice weekly percussion and postural drainage'. He has polychondritis (chronic inflammation of the cartilage, including in the tracheobronchial tree) which has led to collapse of his tracheal and bronchial cartilages.

Background

- Surgery on deformed chest and formation of tracheostomy 15 years ago.
- Discharged with instructions to change and clean tracheostomy tube twice-weekly.

Medication

- Prednisolone

Social history

- Lives with wife and three children, started office job two months ago, non-smoker.

Subjective assessment

● Occasional chest infections, last one six weeks ago which has never quite resolved.
● Always have a bit of phlegm, usually no problem clearing it but more difficult over the last six weeks.
● Change tracheostomy tube nine-monthly.
● Slightly breathless on exertion but not bothersome.
● Tracheostomy tube sometimes causes a dry cough.

Objective assessment

● Abnormal chest shape (Fig 5.19).
● Respiratory rate normal.
● Breathing pattern slightly laboured.
● Clinically well hydrated.
● Posture: round shoulders.
● Auscultation: scattered crackles.

Questions

1 Why might Mr J have chest infections?
2 What could have prevented the last chest infection from being fully resolved, and what could be causing the difficulty in clearing his chest?
3 Is the breathlessness on exertion a problem?
4 Is the dry cough a problem?
5 Analysis?
6 Problems?
7 Goals?
8 Plan?

FIGURE 5.19a Mr FJ

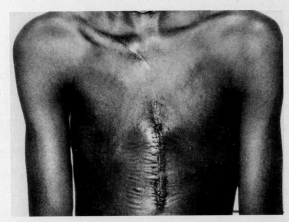

FIGURE 5.19b   Mr FJ

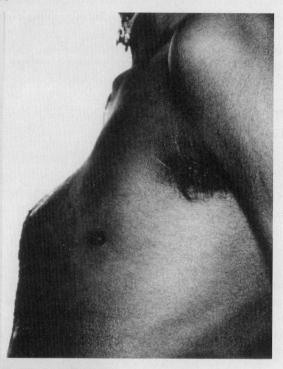

CLINICAL REASONING

The following study investigated chest physiotherapy (CPT) for people with pneumonia. There was no mention of crackles on auscultation.

- Does the physiotherapy fit the pathology?
- What of the stated complications of CPT?

> *Inclusion criteria ... comprised the presence of unilateral pneumonic infiltrates on chest X-ray ... we found no statistically significant short term therapeutic benefit from percussion or vibration ... CPT can cause ... barotrauma, bended endotracheal or ventilation tubing.*
>
> *Acta Anaesth Belg (1991) 42, 165–70*

Response to Case Study

1 **Reason for infections**
   - Tracheostomy bypassing upper airway defences
   - Infrequent tube changes

2 **Non-resolution of infection and difficulty clearing chest**
   - Change in job two months ago

- Inactivity
- Dry office atmosphere

3 Breathlessness on exertion

- It is not bothersome at present but may become so as Mr J ages and loses respiratory reserve.

4 Dry cough

- It depends on whether it worries the patient.

5 Analysis

- No major disruption to lifestyle at present, but potential for deterioration over time if chest infections recur.

6 Problems

- Risk of chest infections
- Some sputum retention
- Mild increase in work of breathing, probably due to chest shape
- Potential for reduced exercise tolerance

7 Goals

- Reduce risk of infection
- Increase exercise tolerance

8 Plan

- Negotiate more frequent tube changes. Twice weekly changes are unlikely to be adhered to and are probably not necessary at home (which is safer than the infection-prone hospital atmosphere). Motivate Mr J by explaining that a clean tube might reduce his dry cough.
- Negotiate lifelong and achievable programme to prevent chest infections and maintain exercise tolerance, preferably based on enjoyable exercise, e.g. football with children, but offer variety of techniques for mucous clearance (Chapter 8).
- Discuss possible effects of office atmosphere.
- Posture correction with advice on reminders, e.g. stickers on fridge.
- Advise patient to ask GP's advice on bone mineral density scan to check for steroid-induced osteoporosis.
- Review six-monthly by phone and yearly face-to-face.

Response to Clinical Reasoning

A passing acquaintance with the pathology of pneumonia would have saved the researchers the trouble of beginning the study.

Physical treatment cannot influence inflammatory consolidation.

Imagination boggles at the image of CPT causing barotrauma and bending an endotracheal tube.

RECOMMENDED READING

Blakeman TC (2013) Evidence for oxygen use in the hospitalized patient: is more really the enemy of good? *Respir Care;* **58**(10): 1679–93

Braillon A, Bewley S, Herxheimer A *et al* (2012) Marketing versus evidence-based medicine. *Lancet;* **380**(9839): 340

Bossard MK (2013) Help with metered dose inhalers. *J Asthm Allerg Educ;* **4**(5): 237–9

Cates C (2013) Inhaled corticosteroids in COPD: quantifying risks and benefits. *Thorax;* **68**(6): 499–500

Chang J, Erler J (2014) Hypoxia-mediated metastasis. *Adv Exp Med Biol;* **772**: 55–81

Chikhani M, Hardman JG (2013) Pharmacokinetic variation. *Anaesth Int Care Med;* **14**(3): 126–128

Dai B, Kang J Yu N *et al* (2013) Oxygen injection site affects F_IO_2 during noninvasive ventilation. *Respir Care;* **58**(10): 1630–6

Delvadia RR, Longest PW, Hindle M *et al* (2013) In vitro tests for aerosol deposition. *J Aerosol Med Pulm Drug Deliv;* **26**(3): 145–156

Domenico S (2014) Current and novel bronchodilators in respiratory disease. *Curr Opin Pulm Med;* **20**(1): 73–86

Dyer F, Callaghan J, Cheema K *et al* (2012) Ambulatory oxygen improves the effectiveness of pulmonary rehabilitation in selected patients with COPD. *Chron Respir Dis;* **9**(2): 83–91

Fink JB (2013) Inhaler devices for patients with COPD. *COPD;* **10**(4): 523–35

Gariballa S, Alessa A (2013) Sarcopenia: prevalence and prognostic significance in hospitalized patients. *Clin Nutr;* **32**(5): 772–776

Gomes CA Jr, Lustosa SA, Matos D *et al* (2012) Percutaneous endoscopic gastrostomy versus nasogastric tube feeding for adults with swallowing disturbances. *Cochrane Database Syst Rev;* **14**,3: CD008096.

Heunks MA, Abdo WF (2012) Oxygen-induced hypercapnia in COPD: myths and facts. *Crit Care;* **16**:323–6

Kamin W (2013) Inhalation solutions – which ones may be mixed? *J Cystic Fibr,* Oct 2013

Kane B, Decalmer S, O'Driscoll R (2013) Emergency oxygen therapy: from guideline to implementation. *Breathe;* **9**: 246–53

Longest PW (2013) High-efficiency generation and delivery of aerosols through nasal cannula during noninvasive ventilation. *J Aerosol Med Pulm Drug Deliv;* **26**(5): 266–79

Morley JE (2014) Cognition and nutrition. *Curr Opin Clin Nutr Metab Care;* **17**(1): 1–4

Myers TR (2013) The science guiding selection of an aerosol delivery device. *Respir Care;* **58**(11): 1963–73

Olivieri D, Chetta A (2014) Therapeutic perspectives in vascular remodeling in asthma and chronic obstructive pulmonary disease. *Chem Immunol Allergy;* **99**: 216–2

Parke RL, Mcguinness SP (2013) Pressures delivered by nasal high flow oxygen during all phases of the respiratory cycle. *Respir Care;* **58**(10): 1621–4

Peel D (2013) Evaluation of oxygen concentrators for use in countries with limited resources. *Anaesthesia;* **68**: 706–712

Pitance L, Reychler G, Leal T *et al* (2013) Aerosol delivery to the lung is more efficient using an extension with a standard jet nebulizer than an open-vent jet nebulizer. *J Aerosol Med Pulm Drug Deliv;* **26**(4): 208–214

Sanford AM, Flaherty JH (2014) Do nutrients play a role in delirium? *Curr Opin Clin Nutr Metab Care;* **17**(1): 5–50

Schols AM (2013) Nutrition as a metabolic modulator in COPD. *Chest;* **144**(4): 340–5

Spina D (2014) Current and novel bronchodilators in respiratory disease. *Curr Opin Pulm Med;* **20**(1): 3–86

Vargas O (2013) The use of metered-dose inhalers in hospital environments. *J Aerosol Med Pulm Drug Deliv;* **26**(5): 87–296

PART II
PHYSIOTHERAPY

CHAPTER 6
Physiotherapy to increase lung volume

LEARNING OBJECTIVES

On completion of this chapter the reader should be able to:

● understand the influence of decreased lung volume on respiratory function

● evaluate the benefits and complications of mobilization, positioning, breathing exercises and mechanical aids to increase lung volume, and explain the clinical reasoning underlying each technique

● evaluate the outcome of interventions and ensure that benefits are maintained.

INTRODUCTION TO CARDIORESPIRATORY PHYSIOTHERAPY

> When applying evidence-based care, clinicians should ensure that each of their individual patients is involved in decision-making.
>
> Lodewijckx (2012)

What is cardiorespiratory physiotherapy? And does it work? The aims are to facilitate oxygen delivery to the tissues and improve a patient's quality of life. Methods to achieve this include education, manual and mechanical techniques, accurately-targeted exercise, reflective practice and response to patients in distress. It is ineffective to intervene with a process as personal as breathing without attention to the person as a whole.

Patients have described a physiotherapist's sensitivity and attentiveness as the most important part of the intervention, including praise, honesty and encouraging patients' own ideas (Wood *et al* 2013). Involving patients in goal-setting improves outcomes (Arnetz *et al* 2004), and Mansfield (2013) found that asking open-ended questions and listening to patients saved time. Humane care is compatible with evidence-based practice (Box 6.1).

BOX 6.1

Challenging dogma (1)

- 'Suffering, apparently, is not evidence based.
- Does this mean that we should discourage or shun evidence-based studies? Certainly not.
- Does it mean that it is so impossible to understand the subjective experience of another person that we shouldn't try? Absolutely not.
- It does mean that evidence-based methodologies are just one set of tools, useful for understanding certain aspects of reality, but not necessarily the best for understanding others.'

A suggested approach is to:
- assess the patient
- identify problems
- clarify expectations and negotiate SMART goals (below)
- agree a management plan and time frame
- apply education and treatment
- re-assess
- discuss and modify the plan according to ongoing assessment
- check if goals are met.

Using the above and the ICF (Ch. 2), education is best reinforced in writing. Patient handouts should be explicit, short, clear and copied for the physiotherapy notes. For hospital patients, these can be kept on memory sticks and slotted into ward computers to be individualized for each patient. In the community, standard handouts (App. B) may be used, or they can be individualized back in the office and sent to patients, to include their name, exercises to suit the home environment, and advice on where to put reminder post-its or tie the stretchy elastic.

Autonomy is facilitated by working with patients to set their own SMART goals, which are:
- Specific
- Measurable
- Achievable
- Relevant
- Time-based.

These should be regularly reviewed, and involve the family if appropriate.

Evidence-based practice is facilitated by Fig 6.1. This is a reminder that, for a profession backed by limited research, 'absence of evidence is not evidence of absence'. An example of the physiological reasoning component is in Box 6.2.

The next three chapters facilitate accurate treatment by distinguishing the three respiratory problems of reduced lung volume, increased work of breathing and sputum retention. They include the experience of patients so that empathy can be nurtured, without which the effectiveness of physiotherapy is limited.

FIGURE 6.1 Hierarchy of evidence

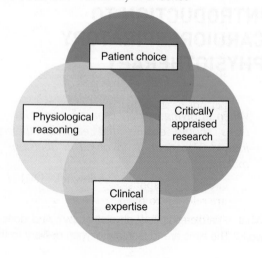

BOX 6.2

Challenging dogma (2)

Is IPPB a useful modality or a dangerous weapon in CF? We are told that IPPB is contraindicated in CF for risk of causing a pneumothorax. Is this a real or theoretical risk? Does anyone have proof of pneumothorax? The intrathoracic pressures generated during coughing (a frequent forced expiratory manoeuvre in CF) must surely exceed the pressures produced by IPPB? I have used IPPB, cautiously, and have found it invaluable when the patient is exhausted during chest infection and finding it difficult to co-operate. I would like to hear a well-reasoned argument against this practice and if one cannot be produced perhaps we should remove it from the contraindications and place it among the precautions.

IPPB: intermittent positive pressure breathing, *CF*: cystic fibrosis

---

Science is validating what humans have known throughout the ages: that compassion is not a luxury; it is a necessity.

Halifax 2011

WHAT IS LOSS OF LUNG VOLUME AND DOES IT MATTER?

The following conditions involve a degree of lost lung volume, anatomically or functionally or both, and with varying degrees of responsiveness to physiotherapy.

1   Atelectasis is collapse of anything from a few alveoli to the whole lung. Segmental, lobar and lung collapse (Figs 2.19, 6.16, 20.2, 20.2) are evident on X-ray (Cortés & Martínez 2013), or by reduced breath sounds/bronchial breathing, depending on size (Ch. 2). Causes include prolonged periods of shallow breathing, pleural disorder, bronchial obstruction, surfactant depletion and diaphragm dysfunction due to poor positioning, pain or compression from abdominal distension. Some of these causes are responsive to physiotherapy. All are relevant to physiotherapy. Hypoxic vasoconstriction (p. 16) can compensate for a degree of atelectasis, but significant lost volume decreases lung compliance (see Fig 1.5), impairs oxygenation (Aswegen & Eales 2004), risks lung injury (Duggan 2005) and, if due to a blocked airway, interrupts mucociliary clearance and facilitates bacterial growth distal to the blockage (Wanner *et al* 1996). Physiotherapy is indicated to treat or prevent atelectasis if it is caused or anticipated by immobility, poor positioning, mucous plug or diaphragm dysfunction, especially in non-alert patients.

2   Consolidation, shown by opacity on x-ray and bronchial breathing, reduces functioning lung volume. Physiological reasoning indicates that it is not possible to break down this inflammatory process by physical means, but progression of the process may be prevented by positioning or mobilization.

3   Pleural effusion, pneumothorax and abdominal distension compress the lung but are themselves inaccessible to physiotherapy. Positioning may improve comfort or gas exchange, and sometimes the patient may need assistance to re-expand the lung after the cause has been resolved.

4   Other restrictive disorders of the lung or chest wall reduce lung volume. The conditions themselves may not respond to physical treatment, but physiotherapy will usually be required for the patient as a whole.

Does any of this matter? Loss of lung volume is a problem if it causes a significant degree of:

- ↓ surface area for gas exchange, leading to ventilation/perfusion ($\dot{V}_A/\dot{Q}$) mismatch and ↓ S_pO_2
- ↓ lung compliance
- ↑ work of breathing.

Choice of technique to resolve these, as with other problems, is best achieved by reflective practice, listening to the patient and clinical reasoning, the latter incorporating practical, intuitive and ethical reasoning (Jensen & Greenfield 2012).

CONTROLLED MOBILIZATION

The most fruitful technique for increasing lung volume is getting up and walking (Dean 2006). When accurately targeted, this combines the upright posture, which reduces pressure on the diaphragm, with natural deep breathing. It is the first-line treatment for patients who can get out of bed.

To ensure accuracy, the level of activity is controlled so that patients become slightly breathless, but not enough to cause muscle tension. They are then asked to lean against a wall to get their breath back, while being discouraged from talking which would upset the breathing rhythm. Relaxing against a wall minimizes postural activity of the abdominal muscles, allowing the diaphragm to descend more freely. The controlled 'slight breathlessness' can then become deep breathing, rather than wasted as shallow apical breathing. Non-surgical patients can hold their hands behind their back while leaning against the wall, which stabilizes their chest and facilitates diaphragmatic descent. Patients who are not able to walk can use controlled activity by simply transferring from bed to chair, then getting their breath back by relaxing against the back of the chair. Even less ambitiously, when bed-bound patients have rolled onto their side, they can be encouraged to relax with their non-dependent arm rested on a pillow, which facilitates deep breathing as they recover their breath.

Once patients understand these principles and can identify the feeling of 'slight breathlessness' and 'getting your breath back', they can practise on their own, using walking and their normal functional activities as a medium for improving lung volume. Regular graded exercise can then be facilitated.

The body's reaction on moving from supine to standing (Ch. 1) is slowed after prolonged immobility, requiring a longer time sitting over the edge of the bed before standing up. Other safety precautions when mobilizing patients are the following:

- Check the patient's notes for precautions, e.g. if haemoglobin is low, this may be a contraindication to walking, but usually patients can be mobilized with caution if they are asymptomatic and are not to be transfused
- check brakes on beds, chairs and wheelchairs
- place chairs strategically in advance, supported against a wall
- if anticipating stairs, place chairs on landings
- safeguard intravenous lines
- avoid holding any arm that is using a walking aid
- ensure patients keep their hands out of their pockets; if dyspnoea obliges them to facilitate accessory muscle function by stabilizing their arms, they can hook just their thumbs into their pocket or a belt
- for the first 24 hours after surgery, watch the patient's face for colour change which might indicate postural hypotension caused by preoperative fluid restriction and perioperative fluid shifts
- discourage breath-holding
- when sitting a patient in a chair or wheelchair, add stability by tucking a foot behind the chair leg or wheel
- stand below the patient when going up or down stairs.

For patients who are unstable or have been immobile for an extended period, further safety precautions are in Ch. 18.

POSITIONING

Positioning is incorporated into the treatment of patients with any of the three respiratory problems. It can be used in its own right or in conjunction with other techniques.

This chapter covers patients who have lost lung volume, and, as this affects ventilation, how mismatch with perfusion affects gas exchange. Other aspects of positioning are mentioned when relevant.

PRACTICE TIP

No treatment should be carried out without consideration of the position in which it is performed.

The physiology of positioning for lung volume

- Functional residual capacity (FRC) increases progressively from supine, to half-lying, to sitting, to standing (Fig 6.2). Overall it doubles from supine to upright (Harris 2005). This is due to less pressure from the viscera against the diaphragm and reduced thoracic blood volume as gravity draws blood away from the chest.
- FRC increases from supine to side-lying (Fig 6.2b) or prone (Fink 2002).
- Slumped lying (Fig 6.3a) can be worse than supine due to pressure from the abdominal contents (Olsén 2005).
- Lung compliance increases and work of breathing (WOB) decreases progressively from supine, to sitting, to standing. WOB is 40% higher in supine than sitting (Wahba 1991), partly because of the load against the diaphragm and partly because small airways collapse and push the lungs down the compliance curve (see Fig 1.5).
- Compliance, FRC and S_pO_2 tend to be higher in side-lying than supine. (Frownfelter & Dean 2006 p. 316).
- In side-lying, the upper lung has the greatest volume (Duggan 2005) because it is pulled open by the weight of the mediastinum and the other lung dragging down on it (see Fig 1.8c). Although lungs are mostly air by volume, they are relatively heavy because of the weight of their circulating blood.

Positioning for lung volume

The following principles apply to immobile or relatively immobile patients who have atelectasis or potential atelectasis:

FIGURE 6.2 (a) Functional residual capacity (FRC) in different positions (Lumb 2000), (b) FRC as a percentage of the sitting value. 'Sitting' means sitting upright with legs dependent

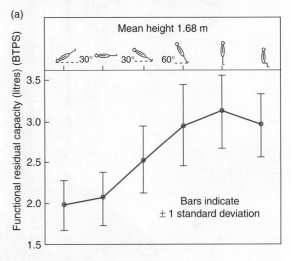

(a)

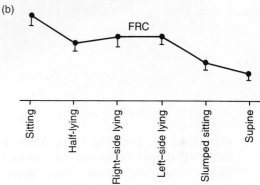

(b)

1 Sitting upright in a comfortable chair improves lung function (Nielsen 2003), so long as the patient is relaxed, which allows the diaphragm to descend freely. A foot stool tends to encourage the slumped position, but some patients need it for comfort, ankle oedema or a recent vein graft. Sitting for prolonged periods risks pressure sores (Stockton *et al* 2009), especially with feet up because this tilts the pelvis backwards onto the sacrum, but patients will be uncomfortable long before this and need to be returned to bed when they ask.

2 Half-lying in bed rapidly becomes the slumped position for most patients as they

FIGURE 6.3A The slumped lying position

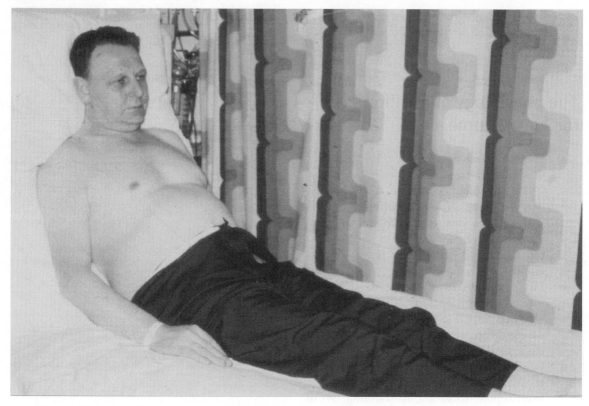

slide down the bed (Fig 6.3a). Time in half-lying should be limited for patients with reduced lung volume, unless necessary for a specific medical reason, or to minimize pain, or the patient finds it the most comfortable position.

3   Time should be spent in side-lying, well forward so that the diaphragm is free from abdominal pressure (Fig 6.3b). Side-lying can also be encouraged for sleeping. Relatively immobile patients should turn, or be turned, two-hourly in order to maintain comfort, lung volume and skin integrity.

4   Supine is unhelpful for gas exchange (O'Driscoll *et al* 2008), and lying down for lengthy periods is best avoided, especially for patients who have a high closing volume, e.g. people who smoke or are obese. Obese people lose 50% of their vital capacity in supine (Allman & Wilson 2011), and McCallister *et al* (2010) describe improved lung function with the bed head tilted up by 45°.

5   Walking about is ideal.

PRACTICE TIP

Compare breath sounds over your patient's lower lobes in different positions.

Positioning for gas exchange

Positioning for lung volume and for gas exchange usually go hand in hand, but to optimize $\dot{V}_A/\dot{Q}$ matching in people with unilateral lung disorders, specific considerations apply. Reduced ventilation on the affected side overrides any physiological ventilation

FIGURE 6.3B Side lying. The patient has an acutely distended abdomen, but his diaphragm is relieved of pressure by his rolling well forward

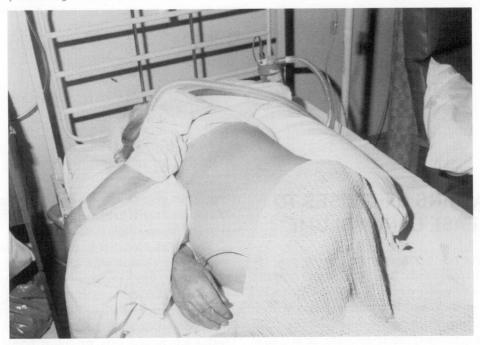

gradient (Ch. 1) and lying with the affected lung uppermost leads to better ventilation of the dependent normal lung, which is matched with its better perfusion (Fig 6.4).

However, patients vary, and clinical reasoning suggests the following order of preference when positioning patients for optimum lung volume and gas exchange:

1   Patient comfort (patients do not breathe well if uncomfortable).
2   Oxygen saturation (this may take precedence over patient comfort if S_pO_2 is compromised).
3   The physiological reasoning above.

As well as optimizing gas exchange, the 'affected lung up' rule promotes comfort following thoracotomy or chest drain placement, facilitates postural drainage, and helps improve lung volume when atelectatic lung is positioned uppermost to encourage expansion (Tucker & Jenkins 1996).

Exceptions to the 'affected lung up' rule are:
● recent pneumonectomy (Ch. 16)
● large pleural effusion (Ch. 3 and Fig 2.18)

● bronchopleural fistula in case unsavoury substances drain into the unaffected dependent lung
● occasionally if there is a large tumour in a main stem bronchus (Fig 6.5), because, with the affected side uppermost, the tumour may obstruct the bronchus and cause breathlessness
● any situation in which the oximeter or patient comfort contradicts the above.

These are guidelines only and patients need individual assessment. For people without unilateral disease, prone delivers the most homogenous ventilation (Riera et al 2013) which is normally impractical except for some people with acute respiratory distress syndrome.

After treatment, the physiotherapist should clarify to nursing staff why the patient has been left in a specific position, explaining that this should be maintained until the patient wants to move or it is time to turn. Night staff should be included in training on positioning. Oximetry is useful to demonstrate the effectiveness of positioning to both patient and staff.

FIGURE 6.4 Effect of positioning with one-sided pathology, e.g. thoracotomy or unilateral pneumonia. With the affected lung dependent (a), the better-ventilated upper lung does not match the better-perfused lower lung. With the affected lung uppermost (b), the lower lung is both better ventilated and better perfused. $\dot{V}$: ventilation, $\dot{Q}$: perfusion

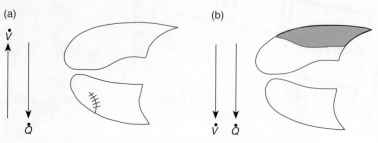

BREATHING EXERCISES TO INCREASE LUNG VOLUME

Deep breathing to increase lung volume may be required for patients who have demonstrable atelectasis and are relatively immobile. There is no evidence for a preventive effect, but clinical reasoning suggests that regular deep breathing may be beneficial for high risk patients, e.g. following oesophagectomy, so long as it is done accurately. It should be performed in cycles of no more than 3–4 breaths so that maximum effort is put into each breath, dizziness from over breathing is avoided and shoulder tension inhibited.

The term 'thoracic expansion exercises' is synonymous with deep breathing but care must be taken to ensure that more than the thorax is expanding. The art of deep breathing is to allow the abdominal muscles to relax and the diaphragm to descend.

Once inflated, alveoli stay open for about an hour so long as tidal breaths are maintained, and 10 deep breaths every waking hour are considered necessary to maintain lung volume (Bartlett *et al* 1973). This is a tall order for those who are distracted by the events and uncertainties of hospital life, and a tick chart is helpful, with patients using the nurses' hourly observations as reminders.

Deep breathing

FIGURE 6.5 Tumour in left main bronchus, which may obstruct the airway if the patient is positioned with this side uppermost

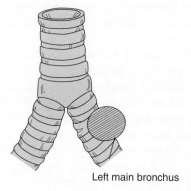

Left main bronchus

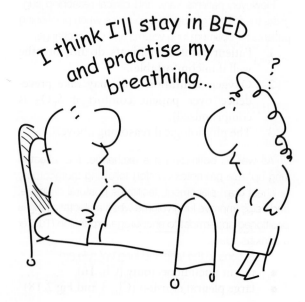

I think I'll stay in BED and practise my breathing...

Optimum conditions are needed to ensure that the deep breaths reach peripheral lung regions, i.e.:

- minimum pain, nausea, dry mouth, discomfort, fatigue, anxiety or tension
- accurate positioning, usually alternate side-lying-inclined-towards-prone, to facilitate expansion of the base of the uppermost lung
- avoidance of distractions
- minimum breathlessness, e.g. patients having time to get their breath back after turning
- taking a slow steady breath to maintain laminar flow (Fig 6.6).

Breathless people should not be asked to breathe slowly.

If side-lying is undesirable, upright sitting is the next option. Long-sitting might be necessary in some circumstances but limits diaphragmatic descent.

When patients are relaxed and have got their breath back, they are asked to breathe in through their nose, deeply and slowly to ensure optimal distribution of ventilation, then sigh out. A demonstration is usually required. Breathing through the nose warms and humidifies the air but doubles resistance to airflow, and patients may need to mouth-breathe if they are breathless or have a nasogastric tube. Some respond better when asked to take a long breath rather than a deep breath, or when asked to 'breathe in your favourite smell'. Monitoring is by observation that abdominal and ribcage excursion are maximal but without counterproductive tension. Subtle changes in instruction can help this balancing act of a breath that is both deep and relaxed.

FIGURE 6.6 Top: a slow smooth breath facilitates laminar flow and peripheral distribution of inhaled gas. Bottom: a fast breath encourages unhelpful turbulence

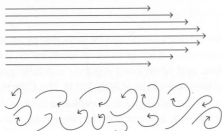

Distribution of ventilation is related to position, flow and pathology. The physiotherapist's hands may be placed over the basal area for monitoring purposes and for patient reassurance, but not with any assumption that this magically redistributes ventilation to the underlying lung. Similarly, 'localized' breathing exercises do not make physiological sense because humans are unable to deform individual portions of the chest wall. However, patients can still be found obediently performing 'unilateral breathing' and 'basal costal breathing'. Even if localized breathing were physically possible, as in some yogi masters, the way in which the two layers of pleura slide on each other means that the lung responds generally rather than locally to a deep breath.

After every few breaths, the patient should relax and regain their rhythm. Breathing rate and pattern should be observed at this time, and the patient may need praise or a change in instruction before proceeding. Patients should not be engaged in conversation between cycles.

> **PRACTICE TIP**
>
> Sometimes patients are more relaxed and breathe more effectively between a cycle of breaths than during the deep breathing itself, in which case attention should be paid to minimizing tension during the next cycle.

Deep breathing has shown the following benefits:
- ↑ diaphragmatic displacement and basal ventilation (Brasher *et al* 2003)
- ↑ lung volume, lung compliance and $\dot{V}_A/\dot{Q}$ matching (Agostini & Singh 2009)
- ↑ airway resistance and upper airway patency (Hillman 2013)
- ↑ oxygen saturation (Manzano *et al* 2008)
- bronchodilation, except for people with asthma (Hulme *et al* 2013)
- ↑ surfactant secretion (Melendez 1992)
- ↑ mucociliary clearance (Button & Boucher 2008)
- preferential gas distribution to dependent regions (Schnidrig *et al* 2013)
- with slow deep breathing, greater alveolar stability (Tomich *et al* 2010).

The benefits for postoperative patients are in Ch. 16.

The resulting increased tidal volume, as opposed to the increased respiratory rate that is achieved with mobilization, suggests that some patients need deep breathing as well as mobilization (Durrant & Moore 2004).

End-inspiratory hold

Air can be coaxed into poorly-ventilated regions by including a breath-hold for a few seconds at the end of a full inspiration. This boosts collateral ventilation, distributes air more evenly between lung segments and is thought to be as important as inspiratory volume (Tomich et al 2010). Observation will identify if the end-inspiratory hold is effective, comfortable, or, conversely, disturbs the breathing pattern. Accurate instruction is needed to prevent shoulder girdle tension. The end-inspiratory hold is unsuited to breathless people as it upsets their breathing pattern.

Abdominal breathing

When used in an appropriate position, abdominal breathing (Ch. 7) can increase lung volume if used with an emphasis on the depth of breathing.

Sniff

Even after a full inspiration, it is often possible to squeeze in a wee bit more air and further augment collateral ventilation by taking a sharp sniff at end-inspiration, which facilitates diaphragmatic action (Cahalin et al 2002). Sceptical patients can be won over by a reminder that however packed a rush-hour underground train is, an extra person can usually squeeze in.

Neurophysiological facilitation of respiration

Lung volume can be increased by cycles of:
- perioral stimulation, applied for 10 seconds just above the top lip (Fig 6.7a)
- intercostal stretch, applied unilaterally or bilaterally on exhalation (Fig 6.7b).

The mechanism of these techniques may relate to stimulation of the suckling reflex and intercostal muscle stretch reflex respectively (Chang et al 2002).

Other effects are yawning, coughing, swallowing and abdominal contraction (Jones 1998). Some patients vary in their response from breath to breath and day to day. It is worth trying slightly different finger positions and pressures, and sometimes finger vibrations. Effects may be cumulative.

The technique is useful for some drowsy patients, those with neurological conditions, in whom excess tone may become relaxed (Bethune 1994) and patients on assisted ventilation, especially if they are unable to turn.

Rib springing

Rib springing is chest compression during expiration, with overpressure downwards and inwards in the bucket handle direction of rib movement, then a quick release at end-expiration. This may cause a deeper subsequent inspiration.

INCENTIVE SPIROMETRY

CLINICAL REASONING

Is there logic in the following arguments?

There is little evidence to support the use of incentive spirometry in airway clearance …
Eur Respir J (1999), 14, 1418–24

Incentive spirometry is not a sensitive method for the study of pulmonary function.
Am Ass Osteopathy J (1995), Fall, 9–13

Incentive spirometry is not intended for airway clearance or for pulmonary function testing.

A sustained deep breath can be facilitated by an incentive spirometer, which gives visual feedback on volume and flow, and when used regularly can both prevent and reverse atelectasis (AARC 2011). The Coach, Voldyne and Respivol (Fig 6.8) are **volume** devices which encourage slow and controlled inhalation by maintaining a marker (indicating flow) between two marks, and

FIGURE 6.7 Neurophysiological facilitation of respiration. (a) Perioral stimulation: moderate pressure inwards and downwards. (b) Intercostal stretch: firm pressure downwards on ribs 2 and 3. (c) Co-contraction: pressure against lower ribs and pelvis, applied at right angles on alternate sides and maintaining pressure for up to 2 minutes or until desired effect. (d) Vertebral pressure: finger pressure against vertebrae between T2 and T10 (Bethune et al 1975)

(a)

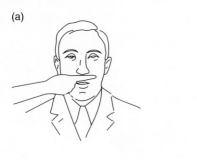

(b)

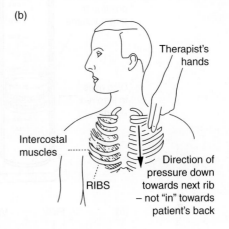

(c)

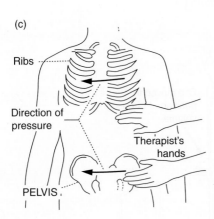

(d)

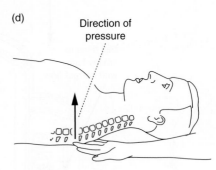

encourage a deep breath by raising a disc (indicating volume). The end-inspiratory hold is maintained while the disc descends. These devices impose half the work of breathing of the other devices, encourage abdominal rather than ribcage motion (Agostini & Singh 2009), lead to slower deeper breathing (Tomich et al 2010) and increase chest wall volume (Paisan 2013).

Flow devices are slightly less patient-friendly. The Triflo (Fig 6.9a) controls flow by the patient inhaling so that two out of three plastic balls are raised, the third being a control which should not move because this indicates excess flow and therefore turbulence. An end-inspiratory hold is maintained for 3–5 seconds while the balls are suspended. It is possible to cheat by taking short sharp breaths, and some patients enjoy turning it upside down and blowing.

The Mediflo Duo (p. 236) is cheap and cheerful, and can also be used as a PEP device (Ch. 8). For incentive spirometry, the tubing is inserted into the side and the top hole is blocked. The pointer is turned to the target number on the blue scale and the patient breathes in until the ball floats, then holds their breath for the end-inspiratory hold by keeping the ball floating.

Suggested technique is the following:

1 A demonstration is given using a separate device.

2 Patients should be relaxed and positioned as for deep breathing, either side-lying (particularly if extra volume is required for one lung) or sitting upright, preferably in a chair with their feet down.

FIGURE 6.8 Volume incentive spirometers: (a) the Coach, the disc on the left indicating volume, and the marker on the right indicating flow, (b) Voldyne, (c) Respivol

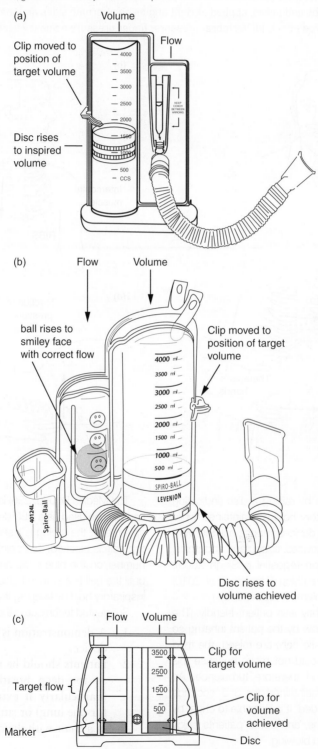

FIGURE 6.9 Flow incentive spirometers: (a) Triflo and (b) Mediflo

(a)

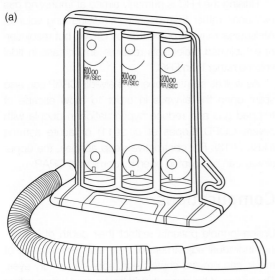

(b)

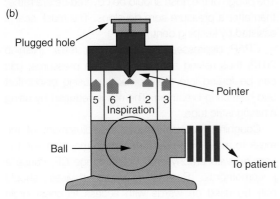

3   With lips sealed around the mouthpiece, the patient inhales slowly and deeply. The patient watches the flow indicator while the physiotherapist monitors the patient's breathing pattern.
4   An end-inspiratory hold is sustained if possible.
5   After exhalation, normal breathing is resumed and shoulder girdle relaxation is rechecked.

Patients are advised to take ten incentive spirometry breaths per waking hour. Those on oxygen can use nasal cannulae or an incentive spirometer which entrains oxygen. People with tracheostomies can use a connecting tube.

The same effect can be obtained by deep breathing without the incentive spirometer, but the incentive of using a device often creates greater inhaled volume, a more controlled flow and more enthusiasm to practise. However, individuals vary, as does the research, which is either positive (Wren *et al* 2010) or neutral (Makhabah *et al* 2013). Observation of expansion and breathing pattern is therefore required to identify whether the patient takes a deep breath more effectively with or without the device.

Incentive spirometry is suitable for children and those with learning difficulties because it can be learnt by demonstration. It is not suited to breathless people, and those with fragile lungs should not use it too vehemently because a pneumothorax has been recorded in a person with emphysema (Kenny 2013).

CONTINUOUS POSITIVE AIRWAY PRESSURE (CPAP)

For spontaneously breathing patients who cannot muster the breath for incentive spirometry, functional residual capacity (FRC) can be improved by a device which delivers continuous positive pressure by face mask. This improves gas exchange by pneumatically splinting open the alveoli. The same effect is achieved with the grunting adopted by infants in respiratory distress and with the yelp used by some tennis players.

Compared to non-invasive ventilation, CPAP delivers the same flow of gas throughout inspiration and expiration, exceeding the flow rate of patients even when they are breathless. It is like putting their head out of the window of a speeding car, and, along with the tight-fitting mask (Fig 6.10), is not always comfortable. A full face mask or a helmet (Ch.7) may be better tolerated (Belchior *et al* 2012). Alternatively, modest positive pressure can be achieved by a high flow nasal cannula (Lucangelo *et al* 2012) or a cheap 'bubble-CPAP' device (Brown *et al* 2013a).

Effects and indications

When comfort is optimized, CPAP increases FRC (Fig 6.11), improves gas exchange and has been found useful for:

FIGURE 6.10 CPAP mask

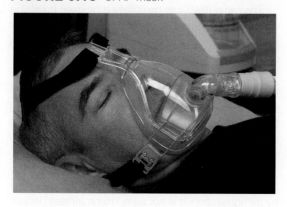

FIGURE 6.11 Effect of CPAP on lung volumes. V_T: tidal volume; FRC: functional residual capacity

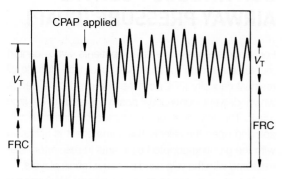

- pneumonia (Lim *et al* 2007) or pulmonary oedema (Keenan *et al* 2011)
- flail chest (Gunduz *et al* 2005) which can be stabilized more comfortably with the steady pressure of CPAP than with the varying pressures of assisted ventilation (Fig 6.12), so long as there is no barotrauma

- postoperative patients (Almutairi *et al* 2012).

Raising the FRC is primarily aimed at improving gas exchange rather than directly increasing lung volume. Atelectasis may be prevented by CPAP, but resolution of established atelectasis requires an increase in tidal volume rather than FRC.

As well as splinting open the alveoli, CPAP can also splint open the airways in order to allow escape of trapped gas and reduce hyperinflation in people with severe COPD (Lopes *et al* 2011) or acute asthma (Busk 2013). For obstructive sleep apnoea, the upper airway can be splinted open by domiciliary CPAP.

Complications

Uncomfortable patients restrict their depth of breathing. Individual adjustment of the mask, or a change of mask, can prevent chafed skin, sore ears or dry eyes. The bridge of the nose should be covered before rather than after a pressure sore develops. The mask seal is assisted by keeping dentures in.

CPAP depresses the swallowing reflex (Nishino 2012) thus risking aspiration. At high pressures, gas can be forced into the stomach, causing discomfort and restricting breathing. The risk is reduced by using a nasogastric tube.

Coughing requires removal or adjustment of the mask to avoid high pressures which may damage the ears or, with emphysema or late-stage CF, cause a pneumothorax. Positive pressure devices should only be used on wards with access to chest drain equipment.

High pressures may compress alveolar vessels, redistribute blood from chest to abdomen, increase right ventricular afterload and reduce cardiac output.

CO_2 retention can occur if a hypercapnic patient breathes with a small tidal volume against a high pressure setting.

FIGURE 6.12 Pressure-time waveforms for CPAP (left) and non-invasive ventilation which delivers less pressure on expiration (right). P_{AW}: airway pressure

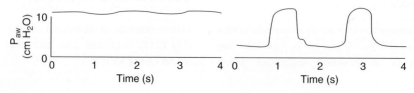

Contraindications and precautions

CPAP should not be used in the presence of:

- barotrauma: undrained pneumothorax, subcutaneous emphysema or large bulla
- inability to protect the airway from aspiration
- facial trauma including surgery (Chebel 2010)
- excessive secretions
- haemoptysis of unknown cause
- Type II respiratory failure.

It should be used with caution in the presence of:

- major haemodynamic instability
- intracranial pressure >15 mmHg
- bronchopleural fistula
- large tumour in the proximal airways, because inspired gas under pressure may be able to enter but not exit past the obstruction.

A nasogastric tube is required if CPAP is used:

- following oesophageal surgery, to prevent positive pressure jeopardizing the anastomosis
- in the presence of nausea because vomiting into a sealed mask against a rush of positive pressure is an unhappy experience and risks aspiration.

Technique

The high flows of CPAP require an efficient heated humidifier to safeguard the cilia (Sommer *et al* 2013), but a heat-moisture exchanger may be adequate for short periods.

The suggested procedure is the following:

1 Patients should be in a high dependency area or close to the nurses' station on a dedicated respiratory ward.
2 After explanations and consent, a pressure is chosen that is low enough to be tolerable but high enough to maintain adequate gas exchange, usually 5–10 cmH$_2$O.
3 The flow is turned on.
4 The patient assists with putting on the mask in order to reduce anxiety. The mask should not be strapped on until the patient has felt the flow and is ready.
5 Flow, pressure and F_iO_2 are re-adjusted for patient comfort and the target S_pO_2.
6 Regular checks are required on S_pO_2 and the comfort and seal of the mask.
7 After use, the mask should be removed before turning off the flow.

INTERMITTENT POSITIVE PRESSURE BREATHING (IPPB)

The slings and arrows of fashion have not been kind to IPPB, and attitudes have oscillated between hero-worship and ostracism. The technique has been scrutinized mercilessly in the literature and found wanting, usually because it has been used in the wrong way for the wrong patients. IPPB is simply pressure-supported inspiration without positive end-expiratory pressure (PEEP) (Fig 6.13) using a machine such as an in-exsufflator (Ch. 8) without the expiration component, or the Bird (Fig 6.14).

Unlike CPAP, positive pressure is intermittent and triggered by the patient, followed by passive expiration.

Indications

IPPB is theoretically non-invasive ventilation but is not normally referred to in this category because it is not used to rest the respiratory muscles. Patients with atelectasis who are drowsy, weak or exhausted may benefit from IPPB. Patients who are unwilling, restless or in pain do not. Pain is not a contraindication in itself, but if atelectasis is caused by pain, it is best to deal first with the pain because muscle splinting may prevent the

FIGURE 6.13 The pressure-time waveform of IPPB, showing the negative pressure of each patient-triggered breath

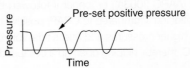

FIGURE 6.14 Bird ventilator and circuit

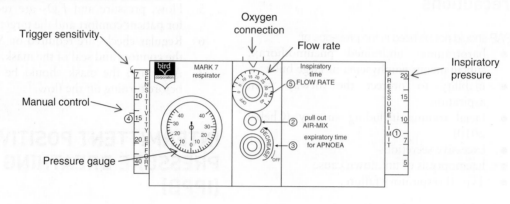

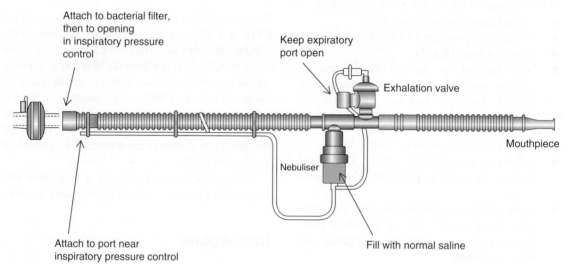

patient accepting the positive pressure. Sputum retention may also be an indication in the case of drowsy, weak or exhausted patients, e.g. those with neurological problems.

Effects

If the patient is relaxed, comfortable and well positioned, with controls accurately adjusted, IPPB increases lung volume, this increase lasting for about an hour (AARC 2003a), or longer if followed by accurate positioning. Compared to CPAP, positive pressure reaches higher pressures and raises tidal volume rather than FRC, thereby helping open up a collapsed lung. In

practical terms, IPPB is best for opening up collapsed alveoli, and CPAP for maintaining the increased volume.

IPPB is less effective than spontaneous deep breathing in patients able to do so. As with other positive pressure devices, the extra air is delivered less homogenously to diseased lungs (Banks *et al* 2010).

Complications

With the Bird, it is possible that hypercapnic COPD patients may lose their hypoxic respiratory drive because 40% oxygen is delivered by most machines. This may not be a problem if adequate tidal volumes are delivered (Starke *et al* 1979), but it would be advisable for patients at risk to be kept under observation after treatment. An option is to use air as the driving gas instead of oxygen, with supplemental oxygen added via either a nasal cannula (if a mouthpiece is used), or entrained directly into the tubing. More accurate adjustments are achieved with machines that have an oxygen blender.

Air swallowing may occur, especially if bulging cheeks are noticed or the patient burps.

A side effect that can sometimes be used to advantage is that techniques such as IPPB, incentive spirometry or deep breathing can make patients slightly breathless, even though this is not the aim. These patients can then be positioned for optimum distribution of ventilation and allowed to get their breath back. If undisturbed, this encourages comfortable deep breathing using the same 'slight breathlessness' as used with controlled mobilization.

Contraindications and precautions

These are similar to CPAP, except for Type 2 respiratory failure, which is not a contraindication for IPPB.

Technique for the Bird

Patients are normally positioned comfortably in side-lying with the affected lung uppermost. If the aim is to increase lung volume, this directs the positive pressure preferentially to this non-dependent lung (Guérin *et al* 2010). If sputum retention is the problem, this acts as modified postural drainage which does not load the diaphragm.

The machine is plugged into the oxygen outlet. The **apnoea switch** should be kept off to prevent automatic triggering. The **nebulizer** is filled with sterile isotonic saline and tested by activating inspiration with the red manual button.

The **air-mix switch** is maintained in the out position by a clip, which ensures that air is entrained to dilute the oxygen. For occasional patients who require high levels of oxygen, 100% is delivered by pushing in the air-mix button. For Entonox, the air-mix knob is pushed in to ensure the patient receives all the gas. The flow may need to be increased with these modifications.

The inspiratory **sensitivity** determines how much negative pressure the patient must generate in order to trigger a breath, a low number indicating that little effort is required. It is set so that the patient can trigger inspiration with ease ('Is it easy to breathe in?').

The **flow rate** determines how fast the gas is delivered, a low number being used for a slow long breath and a high number for a fast short breath. It is set as low as comfortable to encourage laminar flow and optimum distribution of ventilation (Fig 6.6). Breathless patients need a high flow for comfort ('Is that enough air?').

The **inspiratory pressure** is set according to patient comfort ('Is that blowing too hard?'). The pressure dial should show a smooth rise to the pre-set pressure at each breath to indicate patient coordination with the machine. It may be helpful to start with sensitivity, flow and pressure all at no. 10.

The patient then takes a small breath in to trigger the Bird and the machine does the rest, so long as the patient does not prematurely stop inspiration by active exhalation. The flow and pressure dials may need adjusting until the patient's breathing pattern settles ('allow all that fresh air to fill your lungs'). Then:

1   If volume loss is the problem, the pressure is gradually increased until maximum expansion is obtained without disturbing the breathing pattern; these increases may need to be in tiny increments, and stopped as soon as the breathing pattern looks the slightest upset, then turned down marginally until the breathing pattern settles.

2   If sputum clearance is the aim, it is less important to maximize lung expansion with the inspiratory pressure button and the aim is optimum comfort.

Percussion may be included for chest clearance if it does not upset the breathing pattern, but measures that decrease lung volume, such as the head-down tip or vibrations, may distract the patient from the delicate process of allowing the air in.

The physiotherapist's job is to:

- adjust the pressure, and occasionally adjust the flow rate to compensate because flow governs the speed with which the pre-set pressure is reached
- reassure and advise the patient to allow the air to fill the lungs and not to blow out
- observe the abdomen for unwanted active expiration
- observe the face for discomfort

- observe ribcage and abdominal movement to ensure that expansion is improving.

Usually the objective is achieved within 5–10 minutes for lung volume and 5–15 minutes for sputum clearance. If there is no change in auscultation or sputum production in this time, it can probably be judged ineffective, though another attempt later may be successful. The patient should be positioned appropriately afterwards, to maintain any benefit. The nebulizer is then cleaned according to hospital policy.

Occasionally well-practiced and alert patients can use IPPB independently and are sometimes reassured by having it available by their beds at night.

Options include a retard cap to create a slight positive end-expiratory pressure, which the manufacturers claim might prevent recollapse of alveoli. A mouth flange can be used to assist the mouth seal. A mask can be held on the face of semiconscious people, but can be frightening and patients need explanations and the freedom to say no. IPPB can also be used via a tracheal tube with inflated cuff; this might suit spontaneously breathing patients with a tracheostomy, but for ventilated patients, manual hyperinflation is more flexible.

Fig 6.15 shows how IPPB increases lung volume. It also shows how the sitting position does not facilitate ventilation to the lower lobes.

CLINICAL REASONING

Do we need to read further than the title of this article?

Efficacy of chest physiotherapy and intermittent positive pressure breathing in the resolution of pneumonia.
    New Eng J Med (1978), 299, 624–7

Neither 'chest physiotherapy' nor IPPB could logically influence the pathology of pneumonia, which is an inflammatory process and not amenable to physical intervention.

Trouble shooting

1 Prolonged inspiration, and pre-set pressure not reached: check for leaks in the circuit or at the mouth. If these are not the cause, try reducing pressure and/or increasing flow. If unsuccessful, try a nose clip.
2 Pre-set pressure reached too quickly: check that the patient is not actively breathing out, blocking the mouthpiece with their tongue or letting pressure generate in their mouth only. If a semi-conscious patient blocks their airway, the head should be slightly extended and the jaw protracted.
3 Machine triggers into inspiration too early: turn up the sensitivity, check that the apnoea knob is off.
4 Machine repeatedly triggers during inspiration: check that servicing is up to date.

IPPB will become obsolete as non-invasive ventilators evolve, but at present it is very useful for a very small number of acutely unwell patients.

Table 6.1 compares the different mechanical aids to increase lung volume.

FIGURE 6.15 Increased volume with tidal breathing, deep breathing and IPPB in sitting, showing preferential ventilation to the anterior (ventral) lung compared to the dorsal (posterior) lung, which contains mostly the lower lobes (Banks et al 2010). *Electrical impedance tomography:* measurement of lung volume. *Tidal:* tidal volume breathing, *D.Br:* deep breathing

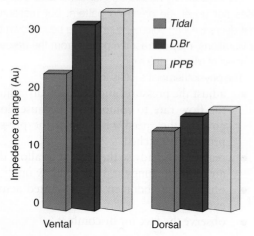

TABLE 6.1 Characteristics of devices to increase lung volume

Incentive spirometry	CPAP	IPPB
• Full patient participation • End-inspiratory hold • Physiological distribution of ventilation • Minimal supervision • Minimal infection risk • Quiet • Cheap	• Positive pressure is continuous • Face or nasal mask • Can accommodate breathless or tired patient • Usually uncomfortable • Used for raising FRC and increasing gas exchange	• Positive pressure on inspiration only • Mouthpiece or face mask • Can accommodate breathless or tired patient • Can accommodate semiconscious patient • Used for raising tidal volume and opening collapsed alveoli. • Used for sputum clearance

FRC: functional residual capacity

OUTCOMES

Success in the treatment of patients with reduced lung volume can be identified by the following:

- ↑ breath sounds or elimination of bronchial breathing
- resonant percussion note
- opacity cleared radiologically (see Fig 20.2)
- ↑ chest expansion
- ↑ S_pO_2, with allowance for other variables which affect oxygenation, e.g. increased F_IO_2
- lung ultrasonography or electrical impedance tomography (Wallet *et al* 2013)
- achievement of SMART goals and ↑ function, e.g. stair climbing or activities of daily living.

CASE STUDY : Ms MB

Identify the problems of this 72 y.o. postoperative patient from London, then answer the questions.

Social history
- Sheltered accommodation, walks with frame

History of present complaint
- OA knee → total knee replacement
- Two days later: transferred to intensive care due to respiratory distress, disorientation and sputum retention; intubated and ventilated
- One day later: extubated and returned to ward

Subjective

- Sleepy, wakeful night
- Little pain

Objective

- Apyrexial
- Good fluid balance
- Obese
- Slumped in bed
- Restless
- Rapid asymmetric breathing pattern
- Feeble non-productive coughs
- Frequently falls asleep → mask slips → S_pO_2 drops
- PN dull both lower lobes
- Auscultation: ↓ breath sounds RLL, ML and LLL; scattered coarse crackles
- S_pO_2: 52% on air, 60% on F_IO_2 of 0.6
- Radiograph as in Fig 6.16.

FIGURE 6.16 Ms MB

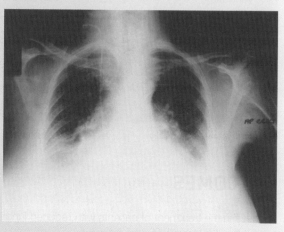

Questions

1 Analysis?
2 Problems?
3 Goals?
4 Plan?

ABGs: arterial blood gases, F_IO_2: fraction of inspired oxygen *HPC:* history of present complaint, *LLL:* left lower lobe, *ML: middle lobe, OA:* osteoarthritis, *PN:* percussion note, *RLL:* right lower lobe.

CLINICAL REASONING

Comment on the physiology and logic of the following:

. . . in patients with suspected pulmonary emboli there is no evidence that IPPB would increase alveolar ventilation more than deep breathing . . .
From the term 'deep breathing', it is understood that by voluntarily moving regions of the wall of the thoracic cage, underlying lung tissue is appropriately aerated.

S Afr J Physiother (1991) 41, 63–7

Response to Case Study

1 **Analysis**
   - Radiograph indicates ↓ lung volume bibasally.
   - Possible causes of disorientation: hypoxia, intensive care experience, lack of sleep.

- Immobility, poor position and shallow breathing exacerbating ↓ lung volume.
- Disorientation and immobility exacerbating sputum retention.

2 Problems

- Inability to fully co-operate
- Poor gas exchange
- Atelectasis
- Sputum retention
- Knee weak and immobile

3 Goals

- Short term: orientate, optimize gas exchange, mobilize
- Long term: rehabilitate for sheltered accommodation

4 Plan

- Liaise with team about obtaining ABGs and increasing gas exchange; consider CPAP if oxygen therapy inadequate, or non-invasive ventilation (NIV) if ventilation inadequate.
- Communicate with patient, family and health team to assist orientation.
- Liaise with team about optimizing environment for autonomy, familiarity, rest and sleep.
- Position for gas exchange, mobilization of secretions, knee comfort and function.
- Attempted deep breathing (ineffective).
- Attempted ACBT/AD (ineffective).
- IPPB.
- Percussion and vibrations.
- Daily written programme of knee exercises, plus maintenance trunk and arm exercises, communicated to relatives.
- Progress to incentive spirometry and ACBT/AD as patient becomes more alert.
- Sit out, mobilize with walking frame, progress.

(Neither CPAP nor NIV were needed due to success of orientation, positioning and IPPB.)

ABGs: arterial blood gases, *ACBT/AD:* active cycle of breathing and/or autogenic drainage, *NIV:* non-invasive ventilation.

Response to Clinical Reasoning

- The physiology defies logic. Increasing alveolar ventilation would not break up a pulmonary embolus.
- The logic defies logic. The only way of 'moving regions of the wall of the thoracic cage' is to fracture the ribs.
- The premise defies logic. IPPB is not intended to increase alveolar ventilation more than deep breathing. It is for patients who are unable to deep breathe voluntarily.

RECOMMENDED READING

AARC (2003) Clinical practice guideline: Intermittent positive pressure breathing. *Respir Care*; **48**(5): 540–6

Agostini P, Naidu B, Cieslik H *et al* (2013) Effectiveness of incentive spirometry in patients following thoracotomy and lung resection including those at high risk for developing pulmonary complications. *Thorax*; **68**(6): 580–585

Bott J, Blumenthal S, Buxton M *et al* (2009) Guidelines for the physiotherapy management of the adult, medical, spontaneously breathing patient, Joint BTS/ACPRC Guideline. *Thorax*; **64**(Suppl.1): i1–i52

Cammarota G, Vaschetto R, Turucz E *et al* (2011) Influence of lung collapse distribution on the physiologic response to recruitment maneuvers during noninvasive continuous positive airway pressure. *Int Care Med*; **37**(7): 1095–102

Chung L, Tsai P, Liu B *et al* (2010) Home-based deep breathing for depression in patients with coronary heart disease: a randomised controlled trial. *Intern J Nurs Studies*; **47**(11): 1346–1353

Kalisch BJ, Dabney BW, Lee S (2013) Safety of mobilizing hospitalized adults: review of the literature. *J Nurs Care Qual*; **28**(2): 162–8

CHAPTER 7
Physiotherapy to decrease the work of breathing

LEARNING OBJECTIVES

On completion of this chapter the reader should be able to:

- understand the causes and mechanisms of breathlessness

- enable patients to reduce their perception of breathlessness

- demonstrate strategies to improve a patient's efficiency of breathing, build up their exercise tolerance and integrate these into their daily life

- recognize the need for non-invasive ventilation and implement the procedure safely and effectively

- identify the outcomes of treatment and modify actions accordingly.

INTRODUCTION

There is nothing worse than not being able to breathe.
> Patient quoted by Simon *et al* (2013)

Increased work of breathing (WOB) may be manifest objectively by a disturbance in the breathing pattern (Ch. 2) and subjectively by breathlessness. Breathing normally occurs subconsciously, but **breathlessness** occurs when there is awareness of the intensity of breathing (Fig 7.1). **Dyspnoea** is breathlessness that is distressing and occurs at a level of activity where it would not normally be expected. In practice, the words

FIGURE 7.1 Breathlessness

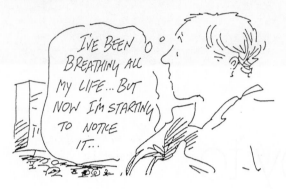

Increasing energy supply requires multidisciplinary teamwork. Reducing energy demand is the domain of physiotherapy and occupational therapy.

There is overlap between this chapter and Chapter 9. Assessment for breathlessness is on p. 254.

BREATHLESSNESS

> *It's very difficult not to panic when you're fighting for breath … you feel as if a vacuum is sucking the air out of you … you're quite literally fighting for your life.*
>
> Patient quoted by Williams (1993)

breathlessness and dyspnoea are used interchangeably, along with **shortness of breath** (SOB). These should be distinguished from the objective terms:

- **tachypnoea:** rapid breathing
- **hyperpnoea:** increased ventilation in response to increased metabolism
- **hyperventilation:** ventilation in excess of metabolic requirements.

Breathless patients are caught in a pincer of decreased ventilatory capacity and increased ventilatory requirements. The basic principle of reducing WOB is therefore to balance supply and demand, as summarized in Table 7.1. Training and rest, whether systemic or limited to the inspiratory muscles, are not mutually exclusive, indeed they are complementary. The principles of training and rest form the basis of clinical reasoning when treating the breathless patient.

Breathlessness is one of the most frightening and distressing symptoms that a person can experience. It is associated with anxiety, panic, helplessness and fear of dying (Simon *et al* 2013) and affects all domains of the ICF, including isolation for the family (Bausewein 2012). Like pain, SOB shows wide variation between individuals because it includes reactions to the symptom as well as the symptom itself. Like pain, it has affective (emotional) and sensory (intensity) mechanisms and shares four components of physical, psychological, interpersonal, and 'other distress' (Kamal *et al* 2012). Unlike pain, it commonly goes untreated (Mahler *et al* 2010), and the experience is difficult for others to fully understand because normal breathlessness such as running for a bus is of known duration, under control and without the fear component.

TABLE 7.1 Measures to optimize the balance between energy supply and demand

Measures to ↑ energy supply	Measures to ↓ energy demand
<ul><li>Oxygen therapy</li><li>Nutrition</li><li>Fluid and electrolyte balance</li><li>Optimum cardiac output</li><li>Vascular sufficiency</li><li>Adequate haemoglobin</li></ul>	<ul><li>Stress reduction</li><li>Sleep, rest and relaxation</li><li>Positioning</li><li>Breathing re-education</li><li>Paced exercise</li><li>Inspiratory muscle training and rest</li></ul>

Causes

> ## KEY POINT
>
> Breathlessness is a major link between disease and disability.

Dyspnoea is prevalent across acute, chronic, critical and terminal illness. Two thirds of the causes are cardiorespiratory (Lai 2011), and the symptom occurs in over 90% of patients with advanced COPD and over 60% of patients with advanced heart disease (Mahler *et al* 2010). Other causes are neuromusculoskeletal disorders, hyperventilation syndrome, hyperthyroidism, anxiety, anaemia, cancer, a distended abdomen and pain (Gui 2012). Dyspnoea may also occur towards the end of life, in healthy individuals who are deconditioned, and in 30% of elderly people during their activities of daily living (ADL) (O'Donnell *et al* 2007). The quality of SOB may help to identify its cause (Table 7.2).

'Air hunger' describes an uncomfortable urge to breathe, as if at the end of a long breath-hold. Patients may describe not getting enough air, or use emotionally charged descriptors such as a fear of dying.

Physiology

> *A respiratory physiologist offering a unitary explanation for breathlessness should arouse the same suspicion as a tattooed archbishop offering a free ticket to heaven.*
> Campbell & Howell 1963

Dyspnoea cannot be predicted from physiological data (Ambrosino 2004). The experience is a private phenomenon, inaccessible through the traditional understanding of physiology. It incorporates both sensory physiology and perceptual psychology, with the mechanics and emotional experience being inseparable (Mahler 1990). Like pain, it varies with the meaning of the sensation to the individual (Parshall *et al* 2012) and shares afferent pathways and cortical regions, but the respiratory motor system is unusual in having both automatic (brainstem) and voluntary (cortical) sources of motor command.

TABLE 7.2 Some characteristics of dyspnoea with different disorders

Disorder	Breathlessness	Other signs & symptoms
COPD	Slow onset	Sometimes productive cough Fatigue
Asthma	Episodic Especially on exhalation	Chest tightness Wheeze
Interstitial lung disease	Progressive Especially on inhalation	Rapid shallow breathing Dry cough
Pneumonia	Exertional	Sometimes pleuritic pain
Pneumothorax	Sudden	Pleuritic pain
Hyperventilation syndrome	Air hunger Not relieved by rest	Symptoms of $\downarrow P_aCO_2$
Pulmonary oedema	Positional Suffocating	Bilateral crackles on auscultation
Myocardial infarction	Sudden	Pain Nausea
Neuromuscular	Exertional	Rapid shallow breathing

Breathing is monitored by multiple sensory systems, e.g. muscle afferents, lung receptors, airway receptors and chemoreceptors (Fig 7.2). When excessively stimulated, these provide sensory feedback via vagal, phrenic and intercostal afferents to the medulla and central nervous system (CNS) (Ambrosino 2004), which processes it as a sense of effort, perceived as dyspnoea (Parshall et al 2012). This perception incorporates both intensity and distress, the latter processed in the prefrontal cortex and mid-brain (Horton 2010). Mechanical, cortical and chemical inputs are involved.

Mechanical inputs

Activation of proprioceptive pathways may be caused by an increase in workload or drive to breathe:

- ↑ WOB: mechanical abnormality such as hyperinflation is sensed by receptors in the joints and muscles of the chest wall (Ahmedzai et al 2012, p. 84)
- ↑ drive: peripheral receptors respond to stimuli from the lung parenchyma, e.g. in

pneumonia, or receptors in the airway respond to inhaled irritants, e.g. in asthma.

In health, the perception of increased effort does not usually elicit distress, the extra respiratory drive being rewarded by increased mechanical output and ventilation. However, when increased inspiratory muscle force exceeds 10–20% of the muscle force needed for normal unloaded inspiration, a mismatch between medullary respiratory motor discharge and peripheral afferent feedback gives rise to SOB (Burki & Lee 2012). This mismatch is described mind-numbingly as an 'inappropriate length-tension relationship' (change in respiratory muscle length not equating with tension developed by the muscle), 'efferent–afferent mismatch', 'neuroventilatory dissociation' or 'neuromechanical dissociation'.

Examples of this mismatch between incoming information and outgoing motor control are:

- ↑ resistive load, e.g. airflow resistance caused by obstructive airways disease
- ↑ elastic load, e.g. reduced compliance caused by a rigid chest, distended abdomen,

---

FIGURE 7.2 Mechanism of dyspnoea. If input and output are balanced, whether at rest or on exercise, there is neuromechanical coupling and no shortness of breath. If the system is out of balance, there is neuromechanical dissociation and the patient feels breathless

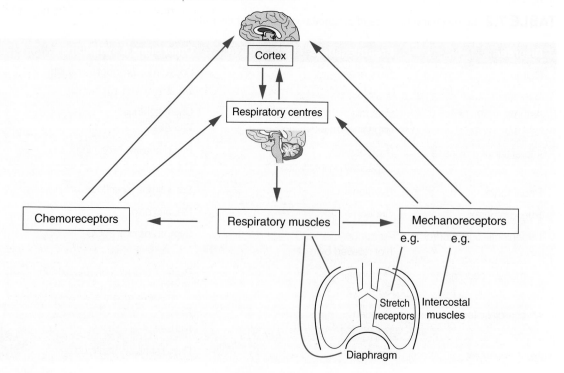

fibrotic lungs or increased alveolar surface tension from surfactant depletion due to pulmonary oedema

- ↓ energy supply, e.g. malnutrition or shock states in which perfusion to the diaphragm is impaired
- ↑ drive to breathe, e.g. parenchymal disorders such as fibrosis or pneumonia (which stimulate nerve impulses from interstitial receptors), acidosis or anaemia
- ↓ power, which reduces the ability to cope with normal WOB, e.g. neuromuscular deficiency, disadvantaged diaphragm due to hyperinflated lungs, or fatigue.

Respiratory muscle fatigue increases central motor command to the respiratory muscles and magnifies the perception of effort in the same way that a weight feels heavier the longer it is carried.

Cortical inputs

Past and present experiences will shape an individual's understanding and it is important to be able to piece together with the patient what meaning the symptom holds for them.

Syrett & Taylor 2003

Cortical and subcortical inputs affect any subjective sensation, and the wide variation in the experience of SOB relates to interactions between physiological, psychological and behavioural responses, in particular anxiety (Leivseth 2012) and, via the limbic system, fear (Kuroda 2012). These feed into a vicious circle:

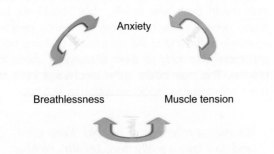

Other factors which exacerbate SOB are frustration and lack of social support (O'Donnell *et al* 2007). Hence the variation in the experience between

individuals, and the reason for education being the first step in treatment, especially by reattribution using desensitization (p. 205).

My anxiety had taken away any power that I might have to cope with my breathlessness.
Patient quoted by Syrett & Taylor 2003

Chemical inputs

Central chemoreceptors are limited in their contribution (Mahler *et al* 2003), as illustrated by some patients with abnormal arterial blood gases (ABGs) not feeling breathless, and many dyspnoeic patients having normal ABGs (Uronis *et al* 2006). The chemical contribution is mostly through sensing a rise in P_aCO_2 mediated through pH. Reduced P_aO_2 plays little part in the drive to breathe and contributes only slightly to SOB, which explains the limited effectiveness of oxygen therapy for dyspnoea. Excess stimulation of chemoreceptors can also result from lactic acidosis (O'Donnell *et al* 2007).

The above mechanical, cortical and chemical processes send afferent impulses to the respiratory centres, from where a deluge of efferent impulses are discharged to the muscles, perceived as a sense of effort:

- Receptor (mechanoreceptor or chemoreceptor)
  ↓
- Afferent impulse
  ↓
- Integration in the CNS, including contextual and cognitive influences
  ↓
- Efferent impulse
  ↓
- SOB

Effects on the patient

It's the worst feeling in the world ... it's like smothering to death ... to lose control of your breathing.
Patient quoted by DeVito 1990

The conscious experience of excess respiratory motor output can vary from feeling that breathing is no longer automatic, to total preoccupation and unremitting fear. Fear itself makes breathing more difficult, and mechanical loads stimulate neural fear centres (O'Donnell *et al* 2007). Patients may feel that they have lost control of their most basic physiological need. This is often compounded by social isolation for the patient and family, especially when SOB limits the patient's ability to converse (Michaels 2008). Carers themselves have reported feelings of helplessness, isolation and frustration (Bailey *et al* 2010).

Breathlessness has been described as invisible because of the lack of attention it receives from health services (Bailey *et al* 2010). A degree of imaginative skill is needed when working with people who are breathless in order to identify with the experience of, for example, spending night after night in a chair unable to sleep, or dreading the effort of going to the toilet, or anticipating the inexorability of death.

PRACTICE TIP

Hold your nose and breathe through a straw rapidly until you feel breathless. Then discuss with others your experiences, which will vary widely.

Management

Treatment is by addressing the cause when possible, using medication when suitable (Ch. 5), multidisciplinary care through pulmonary rehabilitation for people with chronic SOB, and a breathlessness clinic for end-stage disease (Bausewein 2012). Physiotherapy management in this chapter covers both acute and chronic SOB.

HANDLING BREATHLESS PEOPLE

At every breath I felt: was it going to be enough? I thought life was over, even though I knew that was irrational. I didn't want to have to be polite, I didn't want the effort of please and thank you. I didn't mind how much phlegm was there, it could just

stay there. The thought of a physio coming near me made me feel even more ill.

Clare is a physiotherapist whose description, above, of the dyspnoea that she experienced during pneumonia is a reminder of the sensitivity with which breathless people must be handled.

Most patients need acknowledgement of the reality of their experience, not empty phrases like 'don't worry' which can be counterproductive (Booth *et al* 2008). If patients know that we are aware that dyspnoea is frightening or even panic-making, this can be affirming and enables them to feel that we have some understanding of their experience.

PRACTICE TIP

More than with any other respiratory problem, patients who are breathless need some control of their treatment.

For severely breathless people, questions should require only a yes/no answer, or a thumb up or down. It is best not to pretend to understand if we do not, and patients should not have their sentences finished for them unless we know that this is what they want. They need to take their time and not be expected to talk unless they want to. For long term breathless patients, as with anyone who is chronically disabled, it is important to respect their knowledge. They know more than we do about the experience of their disease, and we learn much by listening to them.

The physical handling of acutely breathless patients requires maximum support, minimum speed and a rest between each movement. When patients are getting their breath back after activity, they should not be asked questions. Some severely distressed people, especially at the end of life, are relieved by being held and rocked, so long as there is plenty of space to breathe. This may initiate some mechanical input to chest wall receptors. Neck massage may also help.

It's such a relief not to be told 'Keep calm' and 'Just take a really deep breath'. Neither works when I panic.
Patient quoted by Syrett & Taylor 2003

Desensitization to breathlessness

> *Will I get much shorter of breath? Can I manage it? Is something terrible going to happen?*
>
> Patient quoted by Booth *et al* 2008

To reduce the anxiety that may inhibit activity and contribute to panic (Parshall *et al* 2012), patients are encouraged to detach the fear from their dyspnoea. First and foremost, they are told that breathlessness itself is not harmful. This is a revelation to some patients, who feel that it must be causing damage and that every breathless attack further progresses their disease (Stent 2001). They are more likely to believe us if we acknowledge that the disease itself is harmful, but that breathlessness is a symptom of the disease and not damaging in itself.

Once this is understood, patients are encouraged in activities that increase SOB in a way that they control, and then gently regain their breath, no longer fearful that they are damaging themselves. Patient and physiotherapist start by walking together, at a speed to cause a slight increase in SOB but not distress, the patient being reminded to maintain relaxed rhythmic movement, relaxed rhythmic breathing, a good posture and to stop to get their breath back whenever they want. Patients who are deconditioned and fearful might simply walk round the bed and sit down. They are then praised for their success in increasing and controlling their breathlessness, and desensitization is reinforced by reminders that they have done themselves good rather than harm. This encourages them to switch from fear of SOB to confidence in their ability to control it.

Desensitization is progressed by the patient being exposed to gradual increases in SOB on exertion, then integrating this with other activities, using the same rhythmic breathing, steady movement and reinforcement of the message. Attention to pacing is required for those who tend to rush at activities.

Fan

Dyspnoea may be reduced by a fan (Booth 2013), its mode of action being via trigeminal nerve receptors sending information to the sensory cortex (Ahmedzai

FIGURE 7.3 Hand held fan which can sit on a table or be kept on a loop around the neck

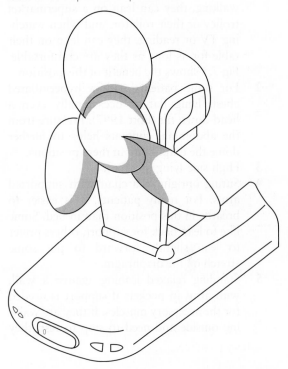

et al 2012, p. 81). Patients with sensitive airways may fare best with a bladeless fan (App. B). A small portable fan is also useful (Fig 7.3), preferably with a strong flow rate and soft blades because patients like to hold it close to their face.

Positioning

Many breathless people automatically assume a posture that eases their breathing, but others need advice to find the position that best facilitates their inspiratory muscles. Patients with a flat diaphragm may benefit from forward-lean positions which create pressure from the abdominal contents to dome the muscle and provide some stretch to its fibres so that it can work more efficiently.

Patients may find the following helpful:

1   Forward-lean-sitting (Fig 7.4) or forward-lean standing, e.g. with elbows on a mantelpiece. The arms should be relaxed and supported to stabilize the accessory

muscles. When out shopping, patients can lean on a freezer while taking plenty of time to choose their special offers. For walking, they can lean on a supermarket trolley or their rollator, and when watching TV or reading, they can lean on their table for as long as they are comfortable. Fig 7.5 shows the benefit of this position.

2   For some patients with a hyperinflated chest, lying flat or occasionally even a head-down tilt (Bott 1997). Pressure from the abdominal contents helps to further dome the diaphragm in these positions.

3   High-side-lying (Fig 7.6).

4   Sitting upright in a chair with supported arms. For many patients, it is easier to breathe in this position than in bed. Some like to lean back for support, others prefer to lean slightly forward to put some stretch on the diaphragm.

5   Standing relaxed leaning against a wall, with arms in pockets if support is needed for the accessory muscles. If they are walking outside and need to stop to rest, they

FIGURE 7.5 Proportion of patients finding benefit in forward-lean-sitting

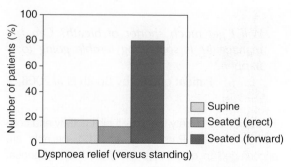

Dyspnoea relief (versus standing)

can put their phone to their ear so as not to feel self-conscious about standing still.

6   For patients who are breathless due to pulmonary oedema or a distended abdomen, upright positions are usually preferred.

Individuals can experiment with different positions. Some find the forward-lean positions claustrophobic, others unpredictably desaturate in different positions. Oximetry is useful as biofeedback and reassurance.

Mechanical input

Vibration over the chest appears to reduce breathlessness by stimulating receptors in the chest wall. Burki & Lee (2012) suggest that this is best done in phase with breathing, i.e. over the external intercostal muscles during inspiration and the internal intercostals during expiration, but this may be fiddly and the patient will say what is effective. Vibrations can be manual or with a mechanical vibrator, both being applied more gently than when clearing secretions so that they do not disturb the breathing pattern. The family can be shown this technique, as well as gentle rhythmic percussion.

Neuromuscular electrical muscle stimulation can reduce dyspnoea and assist ADL in patients with COPD (Bausewein et al 2008). It can also increase muscle strength and endurance (Al-Gibouri et al 2013).

Quality of movement

Patients can be advised that breathing is affected by talking, eating, posture and muscle tension. Many know this, but it is difficult for some to adapt if, e.g. they have

FIGURE 7.4 Relaxed forward-lean sitting, suitable for most patients with a hyperinflated chest and for some other patients with respiratory disease

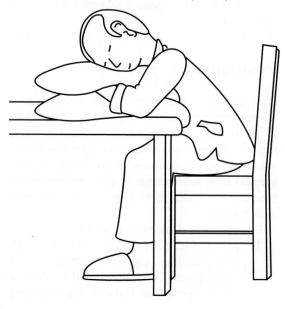

FIGURE 7.6 High-side-lying. The head rest is relatively low to prevent the patient slipping down the bed and to avoid kinking the spine

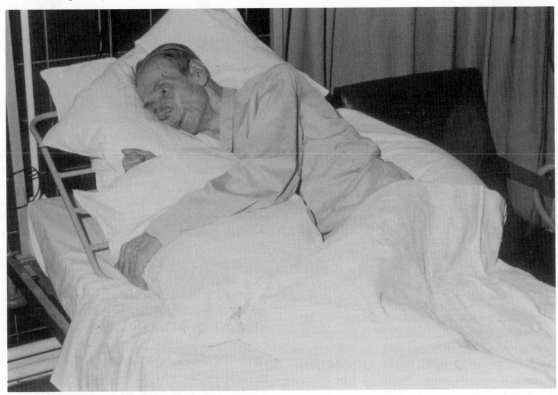

spent a lifetime of hyperactivity. Regularly pointing out how this disturbs their breathing, with reminders from carers to reinforce the message, enables patients to pace themselves and modify their quality of movement.

Thoracic mobility

Thoracic mobility may be impaired by chronic muscle tension, shortened anterior chest and shoulder muscles, abnormal mechanics of breathing, a forward head posture or tension due to a misplaced attempt to 'store' air. This can add a restrictive element to an obstructive condition and cause pain, sometimes misdiagnosed as pleurisy.

The following may improve posture, increase mobility or ease pain:

- in forward-lean-sitting: mobilizations to vertebral and scapular joints (Jones & Moffat 2002)

- sitting astride a chair to fix the pelvis: active or passive thoracic rotation
- crook-lying with a roll under the thorax: thoracic extension assisted by passive arm elevation
- for some participants who have developed a stiff hyperinflated chest: manual compression on exhalation in a bucket-handle direction
- muscle stretches (Carr 1993) which can increase vital capacity, reduce SOB (Kakizaki *et al* 1999) and decrease hyperinflation (Matsumoto 2004).

Precautions include checking for steroid-induced osteoporosis, and handling and positioning must not exacerbate dyspnoea. Patients are encouraged to do their own stretching exercises, including side-flexion, rotation and hand-over-head exercises.

Other respiratory problems

Loss of lung volume

If a breathless person also has a problem of reduced lung volume, e.g. postoperative atelectasis, positioning is the first-line treatment because it is least disruptive to the breathing pattern. So long as patients are relaxed, lung expansion will be facilitated as they get their breath back after turning to a position that facilitates both lung expansion and efficient breathing, e.g. high-side-lying.

If further measures such as deep breathing are necessary, the respiratory rate should be maintained throughout. When asked to take a deep breath, breathless patients sometimes respond by holding their breath. This can be avoided by advising them to 'keep breathing in and out', or telling them when to breathe in and out, until they find their own rhythm. No more than two deep breaths should be taken at a time.

Sputum retention

If a breathless person has a problem of sputum retention, the vibrations from oscillatory PEP devices (Ch. 8) are transmitted into the airways and can help reduce SOB (Fridlender et al 2012) as well as clearing the secretions. If manual vibrations are used, they should not disturb the breathing pattern. Percussion can be relaxing if a slow rhythmic technique is used. The head-down postural drainage position is relatively contraindicated for breathless people, except occasionally for those with a flat diaphragm.

SLEEP, REST AND RELAXATION

> There's no peace, no let up with this thing, it's with you 24 hours a day.
> Patient quoted by Williams (1993)

The only treatment for acute fatigue is rest. This can be achieved most satisfactorily by sleep. One of the cruel ironies of SOB is its effect on sleep. Fragmentation of sleep brings complications (Ch. 17) and tips patients into another vicious circle:

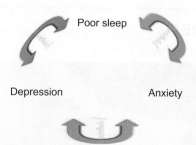

Sleep deprivation in respiratory patients may be due to SOB, coughing or anxiety, aggravated in hospital by noise, an unfamiliar environment and being woken for nebulizers.

Physiotherapists should avoid waking patients unnecessarily, ensure that their treatment does not cause excess fatigue, and contribute to, or initiate, the teamwork required for a good night's sleep (Ho et al 2002). It is a continuing puzzle that there is so little emphasis in the health care system on promoting the healing power of sleep.

Relaxation is facilitated by positioning, sensitive handling and information to reduce anxiety. Deeper relaxation may be achieved by using a relaxation technique. For this, patients should be warm, comfortable and have adequate fresh air. The physiotherapist's bleep should be re-routed and they should sit beside the patient rather than directly in front, to minimize self-consciousness. A technique such as the Mitchell method may be chosen which does not entail breath-holding or strong muscle contraction (Payne 2010). Other methods can be used which incorporate breathing itself, such as yoga techniques, which may also reduce stress and improve immune function (Zope & Zope 2013).

Patients should be reassured that there is no right or wrong way of relaxing, and that they can follow what feels right for them. Although it does not matter if they fall asleep (and relaxation can be a helpful technique for this when required), the purpose is to enjoy a hypometabolic conscious state and experience the tranquillity so that they can re-create it as desired and integrate it into their ADL.

The aim of relaxation is not to add another burden to the patient's daily routine, but for them to find brief moments in the day to check for tension and choose any aspect of relaxation that suits them.

The effects of relaxation are:
- ↓ SOB (Mahler et al 2010)
- ↓ anxiety and airway obstruction (Gift 1992)
- with meditation: ↓ respiratory rate, heart rate and BP (Melville et al 2012).

The key to relaxation is on going maintenance.

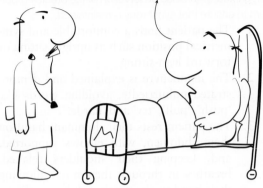

The last thing I want to know is that 30 different hormones are activated When I feel STRESSED...

BREATHING RE-EDUCATION

The measures described above may be adequate, but some patients find more structured breathing re-education helpful. The aims are to reduce WOB and give patients confidence in their ability to control breathless attacks.

When intervening in a person's breathing pattern, a minimalist approach is advised. Patients' individual compensatory mechanisms should not be interfered with mindlessly. Even if their breathing appears unnatural, it may be optimum for them. For example, if a patient relies on their accessory muscles to breathe, relaxing their shoulders may not be helpful. Hyperinflation increases SOB but may also be assisting the airways to stay open, so asking patients to reduce this by prolonging exhalation may or may not be helpful. If however, breathing is irregular, paradoxical or unnecessarily tense, re-education to improve breathing efficiency is often helpful.

There is no clear evidence that a voluntary act can become automatic, but practice can enable a breathing technique to be used more easily when required. Patients tend to find the techniques most useful when getting their breath back after exertion.

Preliminaries

Each of the following steps are best taken one at a time. Close observation will then determine whether this has been helpful, and/or if the next step should be initiated.

1   The position is chosen by the patient, but the physiotherapist might suggest any of the positions described previously.

2   Awareness of breathing is encouraged by bringing the person's attention to their breathing pattern. Are they breathing apically, abdominally, paradoxically, asynchronously, using pursed lips and prolonged expiration, breathing through their nose or mouth? The physiotherapist can sit in front of the patient and mirror their breathing pattern, then minor corrections can be suggested, but the aim is simply awareness at this stage.

3   If the patient manifests localized tension, e.g. with their hands or facial muscles, they can be advised to let that part feel heavy and relaxed.

4   Breathing patterns and body movements are contagious (Kuroda 2012) and the physiotherapist's own relaxed posture, steady breathing and quiet voice will help reduce the patient's tension.

5   Encouraging comments such as 'well done' and 'take your time' help facilitate relaxation.

Breathing then usually becomes slower and deeper naturally. Shallow breathing wastes energy because of ventilating dead space, and rapid breathing wastes energy because of turbulence. However, it may be counterproductive to encourage slow deep breathing beyond that developed naturally through the above because it can fatigue the diaphragm (Gosselink 2004). This is particularly relevant for people with interstitial lung disease, who tend to adopt rapid shallow breathing, a logical breathing pattern because of their high elastic recoil and low lung compliance.

Rhythmic breathing

If patients are not yet breathing rhythmically, they can be encouraged by demonstration, or by using hand movements as waves, or suggestions to 'breathe smoothly with a nice steady rhythm, in your own time'.

Breath-holding must be avoided. This is common in anxious people but increases tension and upsets the rhythm of breathing. It may be observed when patients are concentrating or making an effort. Its effect is to disorganize their WOB, as described by one patient: 'I walked a mile the other week without any problems, then over the weekend I got out of my car and immediately became breathless' (Simon *et al* 2013). If breath-holding is pointed out at each opportunity, with advice to 'keep the rhythm going', patients are often able to bring it under control. Patients find this habit easier to change than altering a life-time of rapid talking or body tension. The physiotherapist, patient and family members can compete to be the first to notice each instance of breath-holding.

A mirror may help, but with permission because some patients do not like mirrors. In patients without excessive SOB, nose breathing can be facilitated by suggesting they keep their lips together.

Once breathing is rhythmic, patients may be able to gently develop an abdominal pattern of breathing, as described below.

Abdominal breathing

An emphasis on abdominal movement during inspiration may lead to naturally slower deeper breathing, less turbulence, reduced dead space and shoulder girdle relaxation. The term 'diaphragmatic breathing' is sometimes understood by patients, even though it is not strictly accurate because, in the absence of phrenic nerve malfunction, all breathing patterns involve some diaphragmatic activity (Bruton *et al* 2011). The term 'breathing control' is abdominal breathing at tidal volume. The depth of the abdominal breath is immaterial (unless the aim is to increase lung volume) and the focus should be on a relaxed efficient breathing pattern.

Abdominal breathing may visibly break through a patient's wall of tension and has shown the following benefits:

- ↓ oxygen consumption ($\dot{V}O_2$) (Hodgkin *et al* 2009 p. 51)
- ↑ gas exchange (Cahalin *et al* 2002)
- ↑ functional capacity and exercise tolerance (Yamaguti *et al* 2012).

However, patients vary in how they respond and Fernandes *et al* (2011) found that for patients with asynchronous thoracoabdominal motion, who are dependent on their upper chest accessory muscles, abdominal breathing can increase SOB.

Clinical reasoning therefore suggests that the breathing pattern should be stabilized beforehand by facilitating rhythmic breathing. The following is then suggested, with close observation of the breathing pattern to ensure that synchrony is maintained.

1   The patient finds a comfortable and symmetrical position such as upright sitting or forward-lean-sitting.
2   The manoeuvre is explained and demonstrated unhurriedly, avoiding words like 'push', 'pull', 'try' and 'harder'.
3   The patient rests their dominant hand on their abdomen, with elbows supported, and, keeping their shoulders relaxed, breathes in through their nose, allowing their hand to rise gently, while visualizing air filling their abdomen like a balloon (the word 'stomach' can be substituted for abdomen).
4   They then sigh the air out.
5   They check that their shoulders remain relaxed and heavy, unless this upsets their breathing pattern.
6   If appropriate, they progress to forward-lean-standing and other positions.

Patients may respond to the physiotherapist's hands placed on their lower abdomen to encourage breathing 'in and down', but over-pressure does not appear to increase abdominal displacement (Tomich *et al* 2010) and may inhibit abdominal relaxation.

Variations include:

- putting the other hand on the quiet upper chest to compare it with movement of the abdomen
- advising the patient to imagine a piece of elastic round their waist which stretches as they breathe in
- trying a sniff at end-inspiration, which specifically recruits the diaphragm (Cahalin *et al* 2002) so long as this does not destabilize the breathing pattern
- if supine, placing a box of tissues on the abdomen to visually reinforce the movement
- incorporating incentive spirometry to encourage a steady flow
- reminding patients that when filling a kettle, they don't fill the top half first.

Some patients find that other positions facilitate abdominal movement, e.g. 4-point kneeling or standing with their hands on the back of their hips and elbows pushed backwards.

Efficacy is not always identifiable subjectively because of the unfamiliarity of a different way of breathing. If observation of the breathing pattern indicates that it appears more efficient, then the patient can be advised to practise at home. Subsequently, if the patient finds it helpful, they will be motivated to continue. If they do not find it helpful despite mastering the correct technique, then it is not worth persisting.

Square breathing

As both distraction and an aid to steadying the breathing, patients can focus on an imaginary square, or on a real square such as a window, picture or (off) TV screen. They breathe in (through the nose if possible) as they focus on the corner of the square and breathe out (through pursed lips if required) as they move along the edges. A few minutes morning and evening may enable them to feel more in control and then use it as required.

Yoga breathing

'Grounding the energy' is the simplest and quickest of relaxation techniques. Patients sit with their feet flat on the floor and visualize breathing air 'in through your head and out through your feet into the floor'. This is not exactly anatomical but usually facilitates relaxation during exhalation. Patients are encouraged to maintain a steady breathing pattern, and to 'sink into the chair' on the out-breath.

Prolonged exhalation

A reduction in the inspiratory:expiratory (I:E) ratio may help to reduce lung hyperinflation, which may reduce SOB. This can be assisted by counting, e.g. 'in/one, out/one/two/three', sometimes integrated with walking, so long as this does not stiffen the gait.

Pursed lips breathing (PLB)

Prolonged exhalation is incorporated into PLB, which involves breathing out actively through pursed lips,

keeping other facial muscles relaxed if possible. With the floppy airways of emphysema, the positive pressure reduces airway collapse (Jiang et al 2008). Patients who have not learnt it spontaneously (Spahija 2010) may benefit, and it can be taught via Skype (Nield & Hoo 2012). The following effects have been identified:

- ↓ dyspnoea (Nield & Hoo 2012)
- ↓ gas trapping, ↑ exercise capacity (Bhatt et al 2013)
- slower deeper breathing, speedier recovery after exercise, ↑ S_pO_2 (Garrod & Mathieson 2013)
- ↓ air trapping and panic attacks (Uronis et al 2006).

Increased expiratory resistance means that PLB is unlikely to help people with normal lungs at rest (Jiang et al 2008).

EXERCISE AND PACING

KEY POINT

Exercise is at the heart of dyspnoea management

Exercise can itself improve the breathing pattern (Collins et al 2001), especially in relation to spinal stability (Kweon 2013). It is discussed with patients at the first encounter, along with desensitization to breathlessness and the link to their SMART goals and ADL. Exercise should be simple and written down on tick charts (App. B), along with advice to exercise little and often.

For chronic dyspnoea, exercise is best developed within a pulmonary rehabilitation programme. Patients who prefer to stay home can put a static bike in front of their TV, using it just thrice weekly being sufficient to increase exercise tolerance (Guzun et al 2012). For acute dyspnoea, quadriceps exercises or T'ai Chi (Leung 2013) are beneficial. However breathless a patient, there is always a brief exercise that they can do, before building it up into exercise training.

Patients who have not learnt to pace themselves may rush at their exercise, which can be counterproductive. Walking alongside the patient, steadily and sometimes more slowly than they are used to, enables them to achieve control, stop when they need to and understand the relevance of energy conservation. Recreating and managing situations that typically increase SOB for each individual will improve confidence.

NON-INVASIVE VENTILATION (NIV)

NIV provides inspiratory muscle rest for people in ventilatory failure. Problems include reduced mechanical efficiency from a hyperinflated chest, increased load from obstructed airways or decreased force from depleted muscles.

NIV delivers a predetermined pressure or volume in response to patient effort. This is delivered via mask (Fig 7.7) or other interface. Compared to continuous positive airway pressure (CPAP), it is used for ventilatory (Type II) failure rather than oxygenation (Type I) failure. Compared to invasive mechanical ventilation (MV), NIV brings less complications, reduced mortality (Baird 2012) and is usually more comfortable. Intensive care is not required and patients can participate in their own management. However, NIV does not protect the airway, allows no direct access to the trachea for suction and cannot provide complete inspiratory muscle rest (Kallet & Diaz 2009).

NIV for acute disorders

For acutely ill patients, NIV can unload the inspiratory muscles, relieve SOB (Mahler *et al* 2010), reduce the need for intubation and improve outcomes (Chandra *et al* 2012). Patient handling skills are required to talk anxious patients through the process and enable them to allow the machine to assist their breathing.

Benefits have been found for:

- ventilatory failure with COPD, whether acute (Credland 2013) or chronic (Bhatt 2013); cystic fibrosis; pneumonia (Bargellini 2013) and postoperative patients (Calvo *et al* 2012)
- patients declining or considered unsuitable for MV (Bülow & Thorsager 2009); those requiring assistance with weaning or to prevent reintubation (Ornico *et al* 2013)

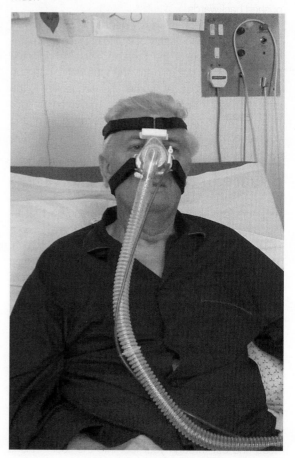

FIGURE 7.7 Non-invasive ventilation by nasal mask

- people with pulmonary oedema, if CPAP is not suitable (Keenan *et al* 2011)
- patients needing controlled oxygen therapy when the target S_pO_2 cannot be maintained without hypoventilation and acidosis.

High concentrations of oxygen can be entrained if necessary, even with hypercapnic COPD patients if there is a safety backup of mandatory breaths irrespective of respiratory drive.

A plan is required which addresses how potential failure of NIV will be dealt with, i.e. whether NIV is the ceiling of treatment or whether treatment will be escalated. If the latter is likely, the patient should be in a high dependency area where intubation is available. Otherwise a respiratory ward is acceptable.

NIV for chronic disorders

> *From our very first night she made a quite startling difference to my life. Just one night converted me to the joys and thrills of home ventilation. For the first time in months I felt reasonably clear-headed, I no longer fell asleep in mid-sentence, my headaches disappeared … my posture and balance noticeably improved.*
>
> Brooks (patient) 1990

NIV should be considered for people with symptoms of hypercapnia (Ch. 1). Benefits include:

- ↑ gas exchange, QoL and exercise tolerance for people with COPD (p. 82)
- ↓ WOB for people with fibrosis (p. 104)
- ↑ wellbeing and survival for people with neurological disease (p. 107) or cystic fibrosis (p. 98).

Patients who cannot get comfortable with a mask or other interface may prefer a tracheostomy. Long term ventilation often requires assistance with communication, which involves the family and is integral to the participation concept of the ICF framework (Laakso 2009).

Criteria

The following indicate the need for acute NIV:

- pH <7.35, P_aCO_2 >6kPa (RCP 2008)
- glottic control adequate to prevent aspiration.

Mixed acid-base and lactate disorders during hypercapnic COPD exacerbations are a strong indication for NIV (Terzano *et al* 2012).

Patients with chronic disease may benefit if they have advanced COPD, scoliosis, neuromuscular disease or are awaiting transplantation (Riha *et al* 2012).

Contraindications, precautions and complications

Exclusion criteria are the following (BTS/RCP/ICS 2008):

- life threatening hypoxaemia, i.e. the patient needs to go straight to intubation

- haemodynamic instability requiring inotropes or vasopressors (unless in the ICU)
- confusion or agitation
- upper gastrointestinal surgery or bowel obstruction, in case of air swallowing
- as with CPAP and IPPB: barotrauma, inability to protect the airway, risk of vomiting, excessive secretions, facial trauma, copious respiratory secretions or haemoptysis of unknown cause.

People with lung fibrosis have the highest risk of barotrauma (Fukushima *et al* 2008).

Discomfort and mask leaks are modified by trying different sizes and types of mask. Pressure sores may be avoided with forehead spacers or changing the interface (Fig 7.9). Other options are customized masks or different masks used in rotation. Some masks contain an inner lining which improves the seal by inflating on inspiration and lessens skin pressure by deflating on expiration. Skin irritation is also reduced by daily washing of the mask, spacer and the patient's skin, and using minimal strap tension. If the straps feel too tight, a smaller mask may allow them to be loosened, or a skull cap can be used.

Gastric distension sometimes occurs with volume-controlled machines or in patients with low chest wall compliance. Options are:

- experimenting with different positions
- considering a nasogastric tube
- using the lowest effective pressure
- changing from volume to pressure control (Ch. 17), or trying a different ventilator.

Nasal dryness may be helped by nasal drops. Mouth dryness usually responds to reducing air leaks through the mouth. Some machines have a button to switch off insufflations during swallowing (Terzi 2014).

Mode of action

NIV is more comfortable than CPAP because of individually controlled inspiratory and expiratory pressures superimposed on the patient's spontaneous breathing, i.e. bilevel positive airway pressure (BiPAP). The pressures are termed IPAP (inspiratory positive airway pressure) and EPAP (expiratory positive airway pressure) (Fig 7.8). In relation to the terminology of invasive ventilation:

- EPAP is equivalent to PEEP (p. 426)
- IPAP minus EPAP = pressure support (pp. 420 and 421).

FIGURE 7.8 BiPAP waveform

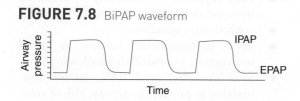

The term 'BiPAP' has been patented as a brand name for the Respironics models. The word is therefore synonymous with either the Respironics machine or this mode of ventilation on any machine. Other manufacturers may use different terms for the BiPAP mode, but it is used here in its generic sense.

Most machines are flow-triggered, flow-cycled and pressure-controlled (Ch. 17), the latter providing the comfort of a limited peak pressure, reducing the risk of pneumothorax and compensating for minor leaks so that ruthless tightening of headgear is not required. Volume-controlled machines may be suited to people with high or fluctuating airway resistance or lung compliance. The feel of different machines varies and patients have their own preferences.

The spontaneous mode relies on the patient to trigger every breath. The spontaneous/timed mode adds mandatory breaths if the patient does not breathe after a set time interval, with the back up respiratory rate (RR) set at about ten breaths/min. A timed mode is fully controlled ventilation for patients who have central sleep apnoea, or for some exhausted and sleep-deprived patients during their first night when they may fall into a deep sleep.

The 'rise time' is the time taken to reach the IPAP, and needs to be high for breathless patients. A neurally adjusted ventilatory assist mode (p. 421), improves patient-ventilator synchrony (Bertrand et al 2013).

Although the natural airway is intact, the high flows may overwhelm the usual airway humidification mechanism, and active humidification is advised (AARC 2012), especially if there is a mouth leak. The heated wire is best built into the tubing wall or wrapped around the outside so that it does not interfere with the flow. Passive humidification by heat-moisture exchanger (HME) may increase resistance, impair CO_2 elimination in hypercapnic patients (Lellouche et al 2012) and can interfere with patient triggering (Cairo 2012 p. 388), but low dead space models may be suitable (Boyer et al 2010). Some patients may be happy without humidification (Branson & Gentile 2010).

Acute patients normally need entrained oxygen titrated to their target S_pO_2. Both oxygen flow and humid-ification may affect the pressure settings. A nasogastric tube is required if the patient is at risk of vomiting or if high IPAP is used, using a fine bore tube to minimize mask leakage.

Interface

Oronasal or full face masks (Figs 7.9, top) are useful for the first 24 hours when patients are likely to be breathless and mouth-breathing. If nasal masks are used, they should be small enough to fit from half-way down the bridge of the nose to just below the nose, without impinging on the nostrils; a mask sizing gauge is helpful. A helmet (Ferrone et al 2013) needs a double-size minute volume to compensate for the extra dead space (Nava et al 2009) and is less effective at unloading the respiratory muscles due to trigger delays (Moerer et al 2009), but it is preferred by some patients (Rodriguez 2013). Devices that cover both nose and mouth require quick-release straps that the patient can use, and anti-asphyxia valves in case of ventilator malfunction. Some ventilator-dependent people prefer a mouthpiece in the daytime and customized mask at night. All interfaces affect nutrition, for which protocols are advised (Reeves et al 2014). Characteristics are in Table 7.3.

Technique

Patients need to be told the rationale of NIV and, when obtaining consent, other options, including intubation or palliation. The following is suggested:

1 An arterial line is advisable if local anaesthesia is not habitually used for arterial blood gases (ABGs).
2 Exhalation ports are designed to exhaust CO_2 and must not be blocked. They should be directed away from the patient's face.
3 The patient takes up the position they prefer, within reach of their call bell.
4 IPAP is usually started at about 10 cmH_2O and titrated until a therapeutic response is achieved, using 2–5 cmH_2O increments every 10 minutes for acute patients. The maximum tolerated is normally 25 cmH_2O, but IPAP at 15 and EPAP at 5 brings most measures of WOB towards normal (Kallet & Diaz

FIGURE 7.9 Selection of interfaces. Clockwise from top left: oronasal mask (with spacers at forehead level to take pressure off the bridge of the nose), full face mask, nasal pillows and helmet (Respironics)

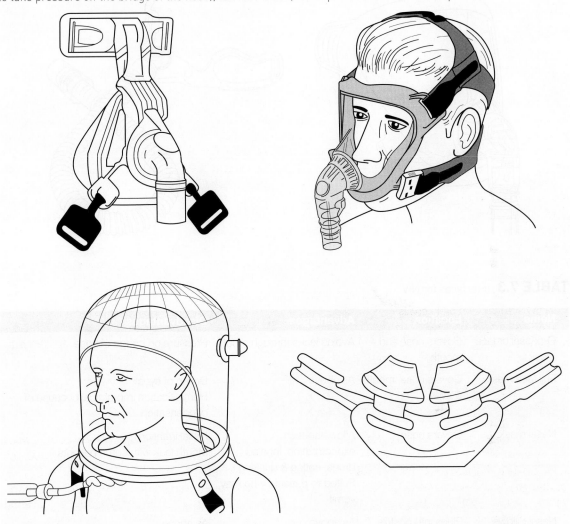

2009). If inspiratory and expiratory pressures are equal, CPAP is delivered.

5 The machine is turned on and the patient allowed to feel the air blowing against their hand, and then on their face, before it is strapped on. The straps should then be tightened equally on both sides and with enough space for two fingers under the straps in order to protect the skin (Nava *et al* 2009). If the patient cannot take off the mask independently they must be in a high-dependency unit.

6 Patients are asked to keep their mouth shut if they can. Some may voluntarily do this once they feel the relief of their breathing being supported, but others are committed mouth-breathers. If they do not want a chin strap or collar, side-lying with a pillow supporting the chin may help. Small leaks are acceptable with pressure-controlled machines so long as they do not interfere with triggering into inspiration or cycling into expiration, and so long as tidal volume and ABGs are adequate.

FIGURE 7.10 Full face mask (left) and nasal pillows (right)

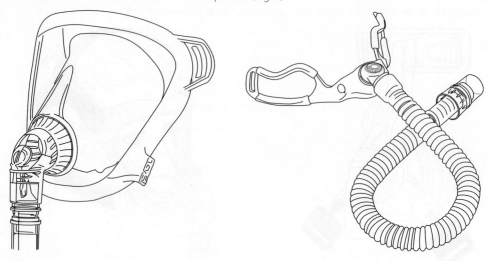

TABLE 7.3 Interfaces for NIV

Name	Location	Advantages	Disadvantages
Oronasal or face mask	Covers nose and mouth	Avoids leaks through mouth	Pressure on bridge of nose
Full face mask	Covers nose, mouth & eyes	As above	Drying of eyes Humidification impractical because of condensation
Nasal mask	Covers nose	Allows speech, expectoration, inhaled drugs, eating & drinking Suited to patients who may vomit	Nasal irritation Mouth leak with some patients
Nasal pillows	Plugs into nostrils	As above Avoids contact with the bridge of the nose or cheeks ↓ dead space Less claustrophobic Allows spectacles	As above Not tolerated by some patients
Mouthpiece	Held by patient's mouth	Useful if pressures >25 cmH$_2$O are needed	
Helmet	Covers head and neck	Less claustrophobic for some patients	Pressure in axillae due to armpit straps. Humidification impractical because of condensation May lead to CO$_2$ rebreathing

7   Improvement in RR and pH in the first hour is a predictor of success. If P_aO_2 does not rise adequately, IPAP and EPAP should be increased equally, and/or F_iO_2 increased. If P_aCO_2 does not reduce sufficiently, IPAP is increased, but P_aCO_2 should not be forced down too quickly if there is high bicarbonate, otherwise metabolic alkalosis may supervene. S_pO_2 should be checked after any alteration in IPAP or EPAP. A decision to proceed to intubation, if indicated, needs to be made within the first four hours (BTS/RCP/ICS 2008).

8   For acute patients, S_pO_2 is monitored continuously. One repeat ABG is required at 30–60 minutes. Vital signs, symptoms of hypercapnia, patient-ventilator synchrony (Hess 2011a) and mask comfort are monitored ¼-hourly for the first hour, then, if stable, hourly for 4 hours, then 2–4 hourly. Analysis of the waveforms helps optimize management (Di Marco *et al* 2011).

9   Acutely ill patients are best given continuous NIV for 24 hours, with a face mask if tolerated, removing the mask only to talk, drink, eat and use their nebulizer if required. Questions to the patient need to be specific and require a yes or no answer.

10 Weaning takes the form of increasing periods of daytime spontaneous breathing, then the same process at night.

11 The mask should be removed before turning the machine off.

Nebulizers and pressurized inhalers, but not dry powder inhalers, can be used with NIV, after removal of the humidifier or HME, and avoiding use of a full face mask or helmet (Soroksky *et al* 2013). The active cycle of breathing or autogenic drainage can be used during NIV, and in patients with sputum retention can shorten the time on NIV (Inal-Ince *et al* 2004). The mask is removed for the huff phase, and pressure or volume may need to be increased during the thoracic expansion phase.

Whether the NIV service is nurse-led, physiotherapist-led or doctor-led, relevant staff need to be trained, including the medical team to provide timely ABGs.

Other ventilators

Some ICU ventilators have non-invasive modes, but ventilators designed specifically for NIV have better leak compensation (Hess 2013).

Negative pressure ventilation entails the application of negative pressure externally via a machine which encloses part of the patient's body, sucking air into the lungs through the natural airway. Negative pressure ventilators are bulky but suit some individuals who require long term support. Advantages are avoidance of the complications of positive pressure or mask, easier communication and the opportunity to use glossopharyngeal breathing (Ch. 3). Disadvantages are the cumbersome machinery and risk of sleep apnoea due to upper airway collapse.

Options are the following:

- The **tank** ventilator encloses all the patient except the head in an airtight iron lung. Disadvantages are size, noise, discomfort from the neck seal, immobility and inaccessibility of the patient. If the patient vomits, pressure must be equalized immediately by opening a porthole because of the danger of aspiration.

- **Jackets** and the rigid shell-like **cuirass** apply negative pressure over the chest and abdomen, and may be preferred by patients at home without the manual dexterity to use a mask (Ho *et al* 2013).

- The **rocking bed** uses gravity-assisted displacement of the abdominal contents to augment diaphragm excursion, usually for people with isolated bilateral diaphragm weakness. For immobile patients, the variation in pressure reduces the risk of skin breakdown (Tsakiridis 2012).

- The **pneumobelt** is preferred by some wheelchair users but is not for use in supine. For expiration, it inflates a bladder around the abdomen at $50 \text{ cmH}_2\text{O}$ to push up the diaphragm. For passive inspiration, it deflates to allow diaphragmatic descent (Liu *et al* 2012).

- **High frequency oscillators** deliver bursts of gas either through a mouthpiece, or externally by generating an oscillating positive and negative pressure through a cuirass. They reduce WOB by overriding spontaneous ventilation and are expensive but comfortable. They may also assist clearance of secretions (Ch. 8).

MINI CLINICAL REASONING

Consider the logic of the conclusion of Shapiro *et al* (1992) that 'inspiratory muscle rest confers no benefit' after encasing patients in negative-pressure body suits overnight. Patients were too uncomfortable to sleep and found a visit to the toilet an ordeal.

Perhaps they should have tried positive pressure NIV.

OUTCOMES

Reduced work of breathing can be judged by the following:

- ↓ SOB
- ↓ fatigue
- ↓ RR
- more synchronous breathing pattern

- for patients with chronic disease, ↑ exercise tolerance and ADL.

Outcome measures for SOB are below.

1 The Baseline Dyspnoea Index or Transitional Dyspnoea Index (Crisafulli 2010) measure SOB directly.
2 Visual Analogue Scales can measure breathing effort and breathing distress (Meek & Lareau 2003).
3 The Chronic Respiratory Disease Questionnaire can be interview-administered or self-administered (Bausewein 2012).
4 A three-minute walking protocol identifies breathing pattern improvements (Sava *et al* 2012).
5 Computerized questionnaires can be self-administered (Mahler *et al* 2012).
6 The Severe Respiratory Insufficiency questionnaire is suited to patients using long term NIV (Laakso 2009).

Further breathless scales are described by Norweg & Collins (2013). Outcome measures for exercise tolerance and function are on pp. 256 and 269.

CASE STUDY : Ms AB

A 72 y.o. patient from Oslo, with a diagnosis of asthma and COPD, is referred with worsening respiratory status.

Relevant medical history

- Pneumonia aged 11
- Recently resected colon cancer

History of present complaint

- Asthma since flu aged 30, worse last few months

Family history

- Two brothers 'died of emphysema'

Social history

- Lives with husband
- Two flights of stairs, crawls up on all fours due to breathlessness
- Never-smoked

Subjective

- Can do shopping, nothing much else (I was able to do everything till last year)
- Headache on waking, sometimes at night
- Poor sleep, slide off pillows and wake with cricked neck, sleepy in daytime
- Coughing attack sometimes, frightened of choking, usually little phlegm
- Wet myself when coughing. Try not to drink too much
- Used to be hyperactive, difficult to be now, husband tells me to slow down
- Frightened of having emphysema
- Doctor says I don't have emphysema
- Breathlessness eased by nebulizer, neck massage, cup of tea

Objective

- Rapid talking
- Rapid moving
- Rapid shallow breathing
- Tense breathing pattern, mostly upper chest
- Clinically dehydrated
- Dry cough
- Auscultation: scattered faint crackles

Questions

1 Comment on the diagnosis
2 What could be the cause(s) of Ms B's headaches?
3 What could be the cause(s) of Ms B's insomnia?
4 Analysis?
5 Problems?
6 Plan?

CLINICAL REASONING

Comment on the connection between the following statements. Does the conclusion fit?

. . . perceived quality of life appears to be linked with peripheral muscle force in COPD patients . . . Consequently, peripheral muscle training may be an important tool in improving quality of life. . .

Eur Resp J (1996) 9, 23, 144s

Response to Case Study

1   **Diagnosis**
    ● SOB could be caused by asthma, cancer or COPD, possibly augmented by anxiety.
    ● Indirect questioning confirmed that patient had not asked about outcome of cancer surgery.

2   **Headaches**
    ● Possible causes are 'cricked neck' at night, poor sleep, anxiety, $\uparrow P_aCO_2$.

3   **Insomnia**
    ● Possible causes are anxiety, SOB, sleeping position, headaches.

4   **Analysis**
    ● Deterioration probably too consistent for asthma and too rapid for COPD, although there is a family history of COPD and maybe passive smoking. Possible return of cancer.
    ● Anxiety could be related to SOB, stress incontinence, fear related to coughing attacks, or linking brothers' deaths from a disease causing SOB to Ms B's own SOB.
    ● Hyperactivity is counterproductive.

5   **Problems**
    ● Ms B's lack of clarity about diagnosis
    ● Headaches
    ● Stress incontinence
    ● Inefficient use of energy by rapid talking, moving and breathing
    ● SOB and reduced exercise tolerance
    ● Possible sputum retention

6   **Plan**
    ● Obtain clarification of diagnosis, including RFTs, drug history, radiology and prognosis from cancer surgery.
    ● Explain COPD, emphysema and asthma to Ms B.
    ● Sleep – position, butterfly pillow, sleep hygiene (App.B).
    ● Discussion on relaxation strategies; Ms B chose sewing.
    ● Acknowledge difficulty of changing a lifetime's habit of a tendency to rush at things, provide advice.
    ● Exercise programme, energy conservation and pacing, including stairs.
    ● Breathing re-education, to be practiced at intervals during the day.
    ● Explain that likely reason for stress incontinence is unnecessary coughing, teach pelvic floor exercises, refer to continence physiotherapist.
    ● Discussion on fluid intake.
    ● Cough control, including differentiation between dry and wet cough.
    ● Ensure that Ms B has a selection of sputum clearance and effective cough techniques.
    ● Discuss pulmonary rehabilitation.
    ● Discuss future unless Ms B prefers not to.
    ● Follow up.

RFTs: respiratory function tests, *SOB*: shortness of breath.

Response to Clinical Reasoning

Chicken and eggs. The second statement may be a correct conclusion, but the first statement does not prove that weak peripheral muscles *cause* impaired quality of life.

Peripheral muscles may weaken as a *result* of exercise limitation or malnutrition. Both are common in COPD, as is impaired quality of life.

RECOMMENDED READING

Cano G (2013) Dyspnea and emotional states in health and disease. *Respir Med*; **107**(5): 649–55

Caroci AS. Lareau SC (2004) Descriptors of dyspnea by patients with chronic obstructive pulmonary disease versus congestive heart failure. *Heart Lung*; **33**(2): 102–10

Delzell JE (2013) Common lung conditions: acute dyspnea. *FP Essent*; **409**: 17–22

Dwarakanath A, Elliott MW (2013) Noninvasive ventilation in the management of acute hypercapnic respiratory failure. *Breathe*; **10**: 338–48

Gagliardi E, Innocenti Bruni G, Presi I *et al* (2014) Thoraco-abdominal motion/displacement does not affect dyspnea following exercise training in COPD patients. *Respir Physiol Neurobiol*; **190**: 124–30

Gimenez M, Saavedra P, Martin N *et al* (2012) Bilevel exercise training and directed breathing relieves exertional dyspnoea for male smokers. *Am J Phys Med Rehabil;* **91**(10): 836–45

Gregoretti C (2013) Choosing a ventilator for home mechanical ventilation. *Breathe*; **10**: 394–408

Keenan SP, Sinuff T, Burns KEA *et al* (2012) Clinical practice guidelines for the use of noninvasive positive-pressure ventilation and noninvasive continuous positive airway pressure in the acute care setting. *CMAJ*; **183**(3): E195–E214

Londner C, Al Dandachi G, Plantier L *et al* (2013) Cross-sectional assessment of the relationships between dyspnea domains and lung function in diffuse parenchymal lung disease. *Respiration*; Aug 27

Mularski RA, Reinke LF, Virginia Carrieri-Kohlman V *et al* (2013) An official American Thoracic Society Workshop report: assessment and palliative management of dyspnea crisis. *Am J Respir Crit Care Med;* **10**(5): S98–S106

Spahija J (2010) Factors discriminating spontaneous pursed-lips breathing use in patients with COPD. *COPD*; **7**(4): 254–61

CHAPTER 8
Physiotherapy to clear secretions

LEARNING OBJECTIVES

On completion of this chapter the reader should be able to:

- identify if a patient has excess secretions or sputum retention

- understand the effects, indications and contraindications of hydration, humidification, exercise, breathing techniques, manual techniques and mechanical aids to clear secretions

- select, with the patient, the most suitable strategies for their needs and teach them safely and effectively

- recognize when coughing needs to be facilitated and/or suppressed, and implement appropriate methods

- understand the indications and contraindications for suction and demonstrate safe, effective technique with minimal subjective or objective trauma

- evaluate the outcome of secretion clearance.

SPUTUM IN PERSPECTIVE

Airway mucus is normally swallowed once it reaches the throat. If expectorated, it is called sputum. **Sputum retention** is suspected in a patient with excess secretions who is dehydrated, semi-comatose or with an ineffectual cough due to weakness or inhibition. Sputum retention is considered a problem, by definition. **Excess secretions** are identified subjectively by the patient or objectively by crackles heard at the mouth or on auscultation.

Are excess secretions a problem?

The production of large amounts of sputum does not necessarily mean that the patient is experiencing difficulty clearing sputum.

Hess 2002

In the short term, if excess secretions are seen or heard to obstruct breathing, or if they cause distress or oxygen desaturation, they are a problem and need to be cleared.

In the long term, it is unknown whether excess secretions contribute to airflow obstruction (Hess 2002), including for people with COPD (Vestbo *et al* 2013), because, unlike inflammation or bronchospasm, excess mucus is patchy. People with non-acute COPD tend to complain more about breathlessness than sputum, and the evidence that excess secretions affect lung function in stable COPD is underwhelming, although they may predispose to infection (Vliet 2005). If patients are not troubled by a cough and are able to cough out their sputum when required, it is probably unnecessary for them to include routine chest clearance in their daily lives, but with an exacerbation they may need advice or assistance on chest clearance.

However, patients with bronchiectasis, cystic fibrosis (CF) or primary ciliary dyskinesia have a damaged mucociliary escalator (Fig 8.1) and are locked into a vicious circle of excess secretions and inflammation (see Fig 3.9). Excess secretions are assumed to be a problem for these patients in the long term, and they are therefore advised on a daily regime of chest clearance.

What is the specific problem?

1   Is mucociliary clearance the problem, which can be impaired by hypoxia, infection, damaged airways, dehydration, cigarette smoke, immobility, anaesthetic agents or pollution (Randell *et al* 2006, Houtmeyers 1999)?

2   Is coughing the problem, impaired by weakness or pain?

3   Is expectoration the problem, impaired by a dry mouth or embarrassment?

Once a technique has been found helpful, it is required p.r.n. for patients with an acute problem. People with chronic disease may find chest clearance in the early

FIGURE 8.1 Top: normal mucociliary clearance mechanism (see also Fig 1.1). Bottom: thick mucus impairing ciliary function

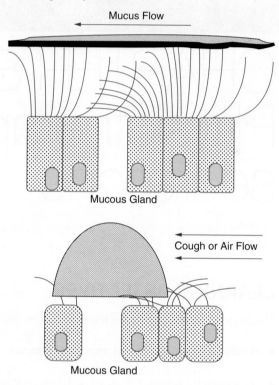

Mucus Flow

Mucous Gland

Cough or Air Flow

Mucous Gland

morning helps clear the night's accumulated secretions, and an hour before sleep reduces nocturnal coughing.

HYDRATION AND HUMIDIFICATION

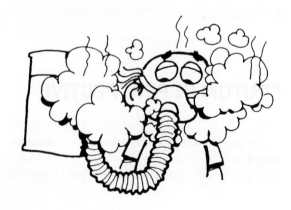

Normally the bronchial tree is fully saturated with water vapour from the fifth generation onwards (Cairo 2012 p. 106). From here to the alveoli, airway secretions are bathed in optimum humidity, with the temperature at 37°C and relative humidity at 100%. This 'saturation boundary' is moved deeper into the lungs by mouth breathing, rapid breathing, dry medical gases or bypass of the natural airway with a tracheal tube, making it more difficult to maintain the integrity of the mucous blanket. Systemic dehydration compounds this problem. Liquid added to airway surfaces selectively enters the mucous layer, causing it to swell and maintain the connection between cilia and mucus, thus increasing mucous transport rates (Randell *et al* 2006).

Classification

Hydration

The mucociliary escalator provides a frontier against the onslaught of 25 million particles inhaled per hour, or twice that for smokers (Rogers 2007), but its function relies on optimum viscosity of the mucus and optimum thickness of the sol layer so that the cilia tips can reach the mucus (Ch. 1). Water is the main constituent of the body, which is intolerant of even a 1% loss (Holdsworth 2012), and hydration is the dominant variable governing mucus clearance. It is more important than ciliary activity, as shown by the airway dehydration of cystic fibrosis leading to more rapid and severe airway destruction than the dysfunctional cilia of primary ciliary dyskinesia, and the difficulty of neutrophils in killing bacteria enmeshed in thick mucus (Randell *et al* 2006). Mucus has the viscoelastic properties of both liquids (viscosity) and solids (elasticity), and hydration optimizes this balance (Button & Boucher 2008).

Adequate daily fluid intake is thought to be approximately 2 litres, 80% of which comes from fluids and 20% from the water in food (Holdsworth 2012). Thirst is an adequate guide for most adults (Benton 2011), but elderly people and some patients need advice to drink their 1.5 litres a day (Fig 8.2), although requirements vary with ambient temperature, fever and exercise.

People normally drink because of thirst, for enjoyment, to keep cool or warm, or for a drink's energy content. Patients may restrict their intake because of anxieties about incontinence, frequency due to diuretics or, in hospital, not being near the toilet. One study found that over a third of hospitalized patients were unable to drink as often as needed, and over half were thirsty due to inability to reach their drink and unwillingness to bother busy staff (Blower 1997).

FIGURE 8.2 Recommended daily fluid intake for a healthy adult

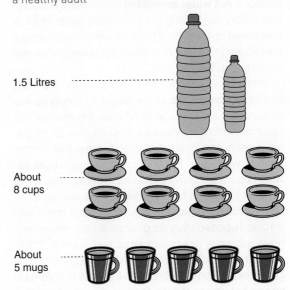

1.5 Litres

About 8 cups

About 5 mugs

There is no evidence that overhydration speeds mucociliary clearance, but a patient may need a trial of increased fluid to identify if this helps expectoration, in which case it can be incorporated into the daily routine. Juices and canned drinks are acceptable but not as efficient as water and should be taken with meals because of their acid content. Caffeine drinks such as tea, coffee and cola have some diuretic action but are adequate as fluid intake and preferred by some patients, preferably not taken with meals to prevent them binding with iron. Pineapple and papaya contain bromelain, a protein-digesting enzyme which some patients find helps to loosen their mucus. Milk may adversely affect mucus in some people (Ch. 5). Alcohol does not count as fluid intake (Mentes & Kang 2011).

Dehydration is also associated with urinary tract infection, unstable BP, coronary heart disease and venous thromboembolism. Fluid regulation may be complicated by acid-base or electrolyte disturbance, kidney dysfunction, pulmonary oedema or diuretic therapy (Popkin *et al* 2010).

PRACTICE TIP

A glass of water kept beside the patient, in hospital or at home, is a useful reminder to maintain hydration.

Hot water humidification

The capacity to hold moisture is increased when gas is heated. A **hot water humidifier** or hot water bath creates vapour by passing gas over sterile water which is maintained at 45–60°C. This is allowed to cool along a specific length of tubing to reach the patient at relative humidity of 100% and 37°C.

When used with non-intubated patients, the nose and larynx cause some of the vapour to condense into drops which are too large to navigate the airways. Hot water humidifiers are therefore most effective for intubated patients and for small children to keep their narrow upper airways clear. For adults with an intact airway, hot water humidifiers assist in moistening a dry throat, and enough humidity reaches the airways to be effective for some patients, e.g. for those at home with chronic hypersecretory lung disease, for whom two hours a day may reduce exacerbations (Rea et al 2010).

The humidifier should be heated continuously to minimize colonization with bacteria. If the wide-bore tube has no hot wire to reduce condensation, the humidifier should be kept below the patient to prevent condensed water tipping into their airway, and the tubing needs regular emptying manually or by water traps in the circuit.

A **steam inhalation** uses the same principle by delivering vapour from near-boiling water to the patient via a mouth piece or with a towel over the head. Some patients find it beneficial, but the temperature of the water is not controlled and the container is easily knocked over. It s contraindicated for hospitalized patients, and patients at home may prefer a steamy cup of tea or hot shower.

Cold water bubble humidification

Cold gas bubbled through cold water shows no objective benefit (Ward 2013) except as a placebo, and was condemned as 'dangerously inadequate' over four decades ago (Graff & Benson 1969). It carries the risk of infection (BTS 2008) possibly because it can render bacteria airborne (Rhame 1986). The untiring enthusiasm of sales representatives has kept up sales in the form of 'diffuser' humidifiers which create smaller bubbles, but research is still lacking.

Nebulized humidification

Large-volume nebulizers convert a sterile liquid into an aerosol whose droplets are small enough to navigate the nasal passages and vocal cords in order to reach the airways.

Large-volume jet nebulisers (Fig 8.3) commonly use sterile cold water because heat is not necessary for this mechanism, although heated nebulizers are available which combine both vapour and aerosol. When used continuously they increase mucus transport (Sood et al 2003).

Small-volume jet nebulisers, used periodically before physiotherapy, are the same as those used for drug delivery (Ch. 5). These 'saline nebs' deliver typically 2 ml normal saline, also known as physiological saline or isotonic saline and of the same osmolarity as the body. They wet the throat and upper airway, but efficacy has not been established (AARC 2003b) and neither research nor physiological reasoning has suggested that this small amount improves mucociliary clearance, nor that the benefit outweighs the infection risk. However, patients often find them helpful (Khan 2004), possibly because they contain saline rather than water, so they can be justified under the hierarchy of evidence (Ch. 6).

It is therefore suggested that:

- if the patient's problem is a dry mouth or throat, mouth care may be sufficient
- if the problem is thick secretions, a large-volume nebulizer is required
- if the patient finds a small-volume nebulizer helpful, or if it produces more secretions than the large-volume nebulizer alone, it can be used as often as required, but not in place of continuous large-volume nebulization.

Small-volume saline nebulizers may also be useful in the community, where bacteria are less vicious than the hospital varieties, but patients must still be given advice on infection control (Bonilla et al 2014).

An **ultrasonic nebulizer** is a self-contained electrical device which transmits vibrations through a liquid to atomize its particles. Oxygen can be added with a nasal cannula. Advantages are its silence, speed and efficiency. Disadvantages are expense and the density of the aerosol, which may cause bronchospasm in people with sensitive airways. For patients who have difficulty clearing their own secretions, a physiotherapist should be on hand because of the increased volume of secretions that may be produced.

Heat-moisture exchange

Heat-moisture exchangers (HMEs) (Fig 8.4) are usually used with a tracheal tube or non-invasive respiratory

FIGURE 8.3 Large-volume nebulizers incorporating a Venturi device to deliver fixed percentage oxygen. (a) The pickup tube is inserted into sterile water in a sterile jar (Henleys). (b) The system is screwed into a prefilled jar of sterile water (Intersurgical)

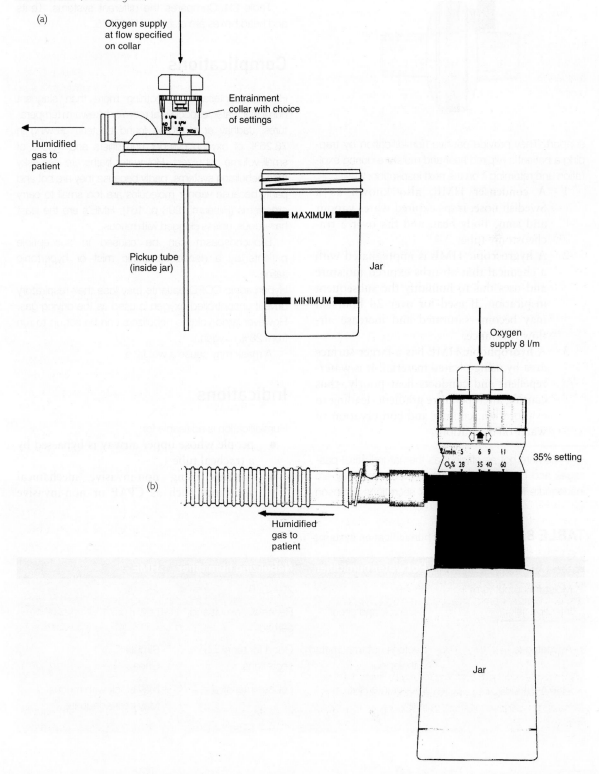

FIGURE 8.4 Heat moisture exchanger

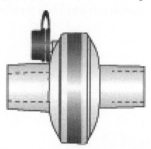

support. They provide passive humidification by trapping a patient's expired heat and moisture during expiration and returning it on the next inspiration:

1   A **condenser** HME, also known as a Swedish nose, traps expired water vapour and some body heat, and fits over a tracheostomy tube.

2   A **hygroscopic** HME is impregnated with a chemical that absorbs expired moisture and uses this to humidify the subsequent inspiration. If used for over 24 hours, it may become saturated and increase airflow resistance.

3   A **hydrophobic** HME has a larger surface area by using pleated material. It is water-repellent and conducts heat poorly, thus causing a temperature gradient, leading to evaporation, cooling and conservation of water on expiration.

HMEs are not as efficient as the natural nasal passages and become less effective over time. They are inadequate for patients with thick secretions (Branson 1996) but are convenient for mobile patients, for use with a manual ventilation bag (p.459) or for limited periods of assisted ventilation. They usually incorporate a bacterial and viral filter.

Table 8.1 Compares the different systems. Tents and head boxes are discussed in Ch. 5.

Complications

Hospital bacteria enjoy nothing more than stagnant humidifier water, especially at room or lukewarm temperatures. Jadhav *et al* (2013) found bacteria growing in 78.26% of oxygen cylinder humidifiers and 47.5% of small-volume nebulizers. Hot water baths are less risky than nebulizing systems, partly because they are hot and partly because vapour molecules are too small to carry organisms (Pilbeam 1998 p. 161). HME's are the least hazardous, unless clogged with mucus.

Bronchospasm can be caused in susceptible patients by a dense ultrasonic mist or hypertonic saline.

Hypercapnic COPD patients may lose their respiratory drive if uncontrolled oxygen is used as the driving gas. However large-volume nebulizers can be set up to run from 28% oxygen.

A mask may cause a wet face.

Indications

Humidification is advisable for:
- people whose upper airway is bypassed by a tracheal tube
- patients using non-invasive mechanical assistance such as CPAP or non-invasive

TABLE 8.1 Comparison of humidification systems

	Hot water humidifier	Nebulizing humidifier	HME
Moisture output (g/m³)	35–50	20–1000	25–35
Infection risk	Reservoir and circuit	Reservoir, circuit and aerosol	Low risk
Advantages	Bacteria not transmitted with vapour	Good for tenacious secretions	Simple Cheap
Disadvantages	Labour intensive Bulky	Labour intensive	May block with mucus May be inadequate

ventilation (an HME may be adequate if the patient is comfortable)
- people with thick secretions
- babies at risk of airway blockage with secretions
- people on oxygen therapy who (a) have hyperreactive airways (heated system required) or (b) are using a mask for prolonged periods with high flow rates and find this uncomfortable (BTS 2008) or (c) are mouth-breathing, nil-by-mouth or have a dry mouth and find expectoration difficult.

Humidification is not required for people with permanent tracheostomies because adaptation occurs over time (Shelly *et al* 1988).

Technique

A mask or mouthpiece can be used, depending on patient comfort. For a hot water humidifier, the manufacturer's instructions indicate the correct length of tubing, how to maintain gas flow and ensure the reservoir does not dry out.

Large nebulizers normally use sterile water to avoid salt deposition. Small nebulizers use isotonic saline. Hypertonic saline may be used diagnostically (App.C) or therapeutically (pp.94/98).

EXERCISE

Exercise can be an enjoyable and effective way to speed up mucociliary clearance (AARC 2013a). The increased minute ventilation augments shear stresses on mucosal surfaces and helps regulate mucus hydration (Kim & Criner 2013), and the accompanying catecholamine release stimulates cilia (Randell *et al* 2006). Benefits have been identified for people with CF (Hebestreit 2001) and COPD (Langer *et al* 2009). With primary ciliary dyskinesia, it has been found more beneficial than drugs in aiding bronchodilation prior to physiotherapy (Phillips *et al* 1998). It is used cumulatively with other techniques.

BREATHING TECHNIQUES

Both of the following techniques are flexible, efficient and effective when taught correctly. They foster independence because once taught they can be used without assistance. They are particularly suited to people with chronic lung disease, but are adaptable to those with acute conditions, autogenic drainage being preferable for fatigued patients. They are described separately but are based on the same principles and can be adapted or combined to suit each patient.

Active cycle of breathing techniques (ACBT)

ACBT consists of a cycle of huffs at various lung volumes interspersed with relaxed abdominal breathing and deep breathing. Relaxed abdominal breathing reduces the risks of bronchospasm, desaturation or coughing fits. Deep breathing counteracts airway closure, augmented by end-inspiratory breath-holds to further open airways via collateral ventilation.

Mechanism

Airflow from the huff interacts with the liquid-lined surface to develop a shear force which, if fast enough, propels mucus in the direction of flow (Graf & Marini 2008). The location at which this occurs depends on the lung volume at the start of the huff. During the huff, pleural pressure becomes positive and equals airway pressure at a point called the equal pressure point (EPP). Towards the mouth from this point, the normal pressure gradient is reversed so that pressure outside the airway is higher than inside, squeezing it by a process known as dynamic airway compression. This limits airflow, but the squeezing of airways mouthwards of this point mobilizes secretions. At low lung volumes, the EPP is furthest from the mouth because pleural pressure is higher and lung elastic recoil pressure lower, so that huffing facilitates more peripheral airway clearance. Huffing at higher lung volumes is thought to mobilize secretions from the more central airways nearer the mouth (Fig 8.5).

Technique

Patients take up their position of choice. This is often sitting, but some find postural drainage positions helpful, e.g. alternate side-lying or head-down if they are not at risk of a headache when they do the huff. If the patient is sitting, the following sequence is best demonstrated while facing them:

FIGURE 8.5 The equal pressure point (EPP) moving from distal airways (top) to central airways (bottom).
FRC: functional residual capacity

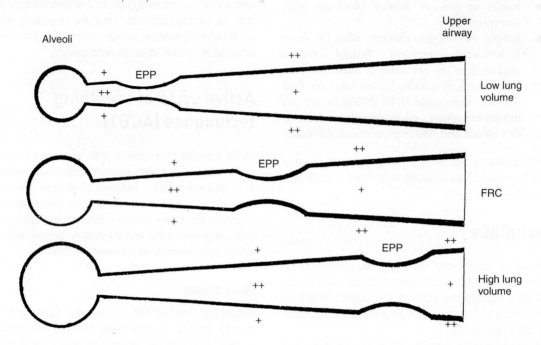

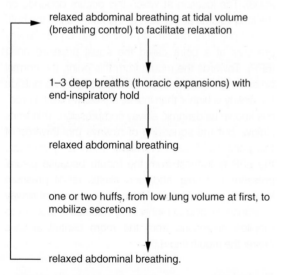

relaxed abdominal breathing at tidal volume (breathing control) to facilitate relaxation

↓

1–3 deep breaths (thoracic expansions) with end-inspiratory hold

↓

relaxed abdominal breathing

↓

one or two huffs, from low lung volume at first, to mobilize secretions

↓

relaxed abdominal breathing.

Cycles continue until the chest is subjectively or objectively clear, or the patient tires.

Huffing usually starts from low lung volume. Once the patient feels that their secretions have moved proximally, the huff starts from medium lung volume. When secretions are felt or heard to move to the central airways, higher lung volumes may be used. Many patients can identify when secretions are shifting, or they simply move the starting point of their huff from a low to higher lung volume after several cycles.

If secretions are heard or felt at the start, they should be cleared from the upper airway with a cough or huff from high lung volume, before beginning the cycle.

PRACTICE TIP

Huffing from low lung volumes may be easier for some patients if they take a normal breath in, partially breathe out, then huff near the end of the exhalation.

Maintaining an open throat during the huff is facilitated by patients keeping their mouth and throat relaxed, rolling their tongue in the direction of flow, imagining they are steaming up a mirror or pushing a tennis ball out of their open mouth, or huffing through a paediatric peak flow mouthpiece (so long as they know not to do the short sharp blow needed for a peak flow test).

Flexibility is encouraged. The number of deep breaths and huffs vary, and the force of the huff can vary greatly in order to balance efficacy with avoidance of adverse effects. Rests between cycles may be required, and for those who are tense or liable to bronchospasm, more abdominal breaths can be taken. The sequence can vary so long as the principle of alternate stretching and squeezing is maintained, interspersed with relaxed breaths. If patients cannot breathe abdominally then they can just allow their breathing to become relaxed and rhythmic during that part of the cycle.

The patient will make their own adaptations, and the physiotherapist can check whether these are helpful. Unhelpful examples include:

- huffing at too high a lung volume at first
- taking too sharp an inhalation, thus pushing the secretions back down or stirring up bronchospasm
- not relaxing between cycles
- coughing before secretions are accessible
- huffing without doing the full cycle, which can cause more airflow obstruction than coughing (Fig 8.6).

Patients with undiagnosed hyperventilation syndrome may develop symptoms when they take the deep breath, in which case the technique needs to be modified. Huffing should be delayed or modified if it causes bronchospasm, fatigue or spasms of coughing. Some patients prefer to do several cycles of deep and abdominal breathing before the huff. Technique must be checked regularly.

FIGURE 8.6 A section of the bronchial tree (a) at FRC, (b) at full inspiration, (c) at full expiration and (d) during coughing

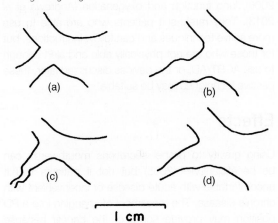

l cm

Patients often prefer ACBT to manual techniques (Syed 2009) but may find it complicated to learn three components, and the principles can be applied using two components only, i.e. the deep breath can be combined with the abdominal breath by taking 'a nice big comfortable relaxed sigh'. This stretches the airways but maintains relaxation.

Autogenic drainage (AD)

AD creates high airflow in different generations of bronchi without allowing airway collapse, using control of the rate and depth of the breath. This clears secretions from small to large airways by gradually increasing functional residual capacity (FRC) from low to high volume.

For people with CF or bronchiectasis, the full sequence can take 30–45 minutes, but it is less burdensome when combined with activities such as nebulizing drugs or watching TV. For other patients, the length of treatment is shorter and flexible. Control of the speed of inhalation and exhalation is the key.

Indications

AD is particularly suited to people with chronic hypersecretory disease, but selected components can be used, for example, with postoperative patients who are anxious about pain and stitches, people with haemoptysis or bronchospasm or those at risk of panic attacks. For breathless people, short sessions are required, with modifications to avoid upsetting the breathing pattern, e.g. no breath-hold, and maintenance of an adequate respiratory rate. Adolescents appreciate that AD may reduce their hyperinflated chests, so long as they do not start inhalation before fully breathing out.

Effects

AD improves airflow in the small airways, clearing secretions that are not easily accessible. Compared to ACBT, it may show faster mucus clearance (Miller *et al* 1995), a greater increase in S_pO_2, and, for chronically hypercapnic patients, a greater reduction in P_aCO_2 (Savci *et al* 2000). However, patients are best able to identify which suits them.

Technique

Patients choose their position. Most sit upright, though some prefer supine, and occasionally prone. Facial muscles, shoulders and arms should remain relaxed throughout, and the throat and glottis kept open, with the neck maintained in slight extension to avoid obstruction to airflow.

Patients may need to blow their nose if it is obstructed, and the upper airway cleared of secretions to reduce resistance to airflow. The AD cycle is then followed:

> Relaxed abdominal breathing to steady the breathing pattern.
>
> ↓
>
> Inhalation slowly through the nose to 1½ to twice tidal volume, slow enough for the breath not to be heard and using an abdominal breathing pattern if possible. Slow inspiration prevents secretions moving distally and encourages equal filling of all areas of lung.
>
> ↓
>
> End-inspiratory pause for 2–3 seconds with open glottis.
>
> ↓
>
> Exhalation similar to an active sigh, at maximum flow without collapsing the airways, and to a low enough volume (Fig 8.7) to locate the mucus, i.e. until the rattle of secretions is felt by the patient. Patients are advised to exhale through their nose or pursed lips unless this slows the flow, so that the extra resistance creates a form of PEP (p.235), especially if they are wheezy. The glottis should remain open, as indicated by a near-silent exhalation.

FIGURE 8.7 Cycles of autogenic drainage at increasing FRC as secretions move centrally. *IRV:* inspiratory reserve volume, *ERV:* expiratory reserve volume, *FRC:* functional residual capacity

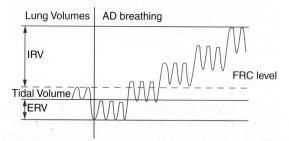

The location of secretions is identified by the patient exhaling until they can feel a rattle. The later the rattle, the more peripheral are secretions. This can also be palpated by the physiotherapist. When the secretions move mouthwards, i.e. the rattle is felt or palpated earlier on exhalation, breaths are taken at a higher FRC. Cycles at low FRC may need to be repeated several times before the rattle of secretions is felt. Cycles at higher FRC then move the mucus to the upper airways, from where they can be expectorated by a huff or gentle cough.

Patients at risk of bronchospasm can exhale 'as gently as when a receding wave ripples down the beach'. Exhaling against a tissue held at arm's length, or misting up spectacles, encourages maximum airflow and discourages noise in the throat which indicates upper airway closure. Cupping a hand over one ear accentuates the sound of airflow and enables the patient to keep it low.

Martins *et al* (2012) describe overpressure during exhalation: in side-lying, the patient is asked to breathe out to residual volume, keeping their throat open, while the physiotherapist compresses their abdomen to reduce lung volume further. This has only been studied in right side-lying, and in patients with stable COPD, but the outcome was increased clearance of secretions from the periphery of the dependent lung.

AD is best interspersed with relaxation, and positive expiratory pressure (p.235) may be incorporated.

POSTURAL DRAINAGE

Research into the traditional techniques of postural drainage (PD), percussion and vibrations often does not distinguish each component, but the combination appears to improve mucus transport (McCool & Rosen 2006), lung function and oxygenation (Andrews *et al* 2013). They rarely suit patients who are able to use more active techniques and can follow instructions, but for those who are not physically able and alert enough to use ACBT/AD, or the devices discussed later, these passive techniques may be suitable.

Effects

Using gravity to propel secretions mouthwards can be beneficial (Vliet 2005) but not if patients find it uncomfortable with acute disease or inconvenient with chronic disease. The movement of changing into a PD position may provide some of the benefit because expectoration can occur immediately after changing position. Some patients find this when gardening or cleaning the bath.

Technique

PD is usually combined with other techniques. For patients needing to clear individual lobes, 3–15 minutes may be spent in each position (AARC 1991). If a disease affects the whole lung, each lobe requires drainage, but a maximum of three positions per session keeps it tolerable. If bronchodilators are prescribed, these are best taken 15 minutes beforehand.

Patients are positioned with the area to be drained uppermost (App.F), bearing in mind that these positions may need modification for patient comfort or if lung architecture has been distorted by surgery, fibrosis, a large abscess or bullae. The most affected area is drained first to prevent infected secretions spilling into healthy lung. Patients on monitors should be checked for arrhythmias or desaturation before, during and after PD. The procedure is discontinued if the patient complains of headache, discomfort, dizziness, palpitations, breathlessness or fatigue.

Modifications include:
- alternate-side-lying only, the most commonly used positions for patients with general secretions
- sleeping in a modified postural drainage position, e.g. by using telephone directories to prop up the foot of the bed, so long as this does not cause coughing at night.

Indications

PD is used for people who find it preferable or more effective than other techniques. For patients with acute problems, modified positions are often required to accommodate dyspnoea. For people with chronic conditions, poor compliance is understandable and a week's trial should include motivating patients to find ways to fit the programme into their daily routine.

Contraindications to head-down PD

- cerebral oedema, e.g. recent stroke or acute brain injury

- trauma to the head or neck, including burns or recent surgery
- recent pneumonectomy or surgery to the eyes, spine, aorta, oesophagus or cardiac sphincter of the stomach
- epistaxis or haemoptysis
- risk of aspiration e.g. unprotected airway
- recent meal
- symptomatic hiatus hernia
- hypertension.

Precautions to head-down PD

- headache
- undrained pneumothorax or subcutaneous emphysema
- history of seizures (check with the neurologist)
- abdominal distension, including pregnancy or obesity
- acute spinal cord lesion
- bronchopleural fistula or empyema
- gastroesophageal reflux (Ch. 3)
- confusion
- breathlessness
- reduced cardiac reserve (Naylor & Chow 2005) e.g. pulmonary oedema, arrhythmias or cardiovascular instability.

MANUAL TECHNIQUES

Percussion or vibrations are usually performed in a postural drainage position. It is thought that they cause oscillations which increase ATP release and thereby hydrate mucus (Button & Boucher 2008), but research is hampered because of the inconsistency with which these techniques are performed (Jones *et al* 2005).

Manual techniques reinforce patient dependency but are suited to people who find them subjectively helpful. They may be useful for certain patients with chronic problems such as those with neurological disease, young children or those with learning disabilities. They may also suit patients who are too exhausted to use a more independent technique, e.g. if they have an exacerbation of disease.

Effects

When combined with PD, manual techniques can slow lung function decline in people with CF (Oermann *et al*

2000) and help clear secretions in those with COPD or bronchiectasis (Jones & Rowe 2000). Individual components have shown the following:

- percussion at 4 Hz increases upper airway mucociliary clearance (Ragavan *et al* 2010)
- vibrations shear secretions off the airway wall by increasing expiratory flow rates by an average 50% (McCarren *et al* 2006).

Self-percussion may be beneficial subjectively but can cause desaturation in patients with marginal reserve, and oximetry is advisable for the first session.

Technique

Percussion consists of rhythmic clapping on the chest throughout the respiratory cycle with a loose wrist and cupped hand, creating an energy wave that is transmitted to the airways. A sheet or pyjama top should cover the patient, but thick covering dampens transmission through the chest wall (Frownfelter & Dean 2006 p. 345), and correct cupping of the hand ensures that the procedure is comfortable. Indeed, when performed correctly it can soothe children and sometimes give relief to people who are acutely breathless. Patients choose whether they prefer a slow rhythmic single-handed or a rapid double-handed technique. Carers can use adult Palm Cups (Ch. 10).

Vibrations consist of a fine oscillation of the hands against the chest, down and inwards against the direction of the bucket handle act of breathing (Ch. 1), performed throughout exhalation after a deep inhalation. **Shaking** is a coarser movement in which the chest wall is rhythmically compressed. Both are less effective on a squashy mattress.

Vibrations, shaking and percussion should be interspersed with relaxed deep breathing to prevent airway closure, desaturation or bronchospasm.

Contraindications

- Osteoporosis
- Rib fracture, or potential rib fracture e.g. metastatic carcinoma
- Loss of skin integrity, e.g. surgery, burns or chest drains
- Recent epidural
- Lung contusion

- Recent pacemaker placement
- Recent or excessive haemoptysis, e.g. due to abscess or lung contusion.

Precautions

- Pain such as pleurisy or post-herpetic neuralgia
- Potential bleeding, e.g. platelet count <50,000
- Undrained pneumothorax or subcutaneous emphysema
- Active pulmonary TB
- Unstable angina or arrhythmias

Patients at risk of bronchospasm may need a break every 30 seconds for relaxed breathing, particularly with vibrations.

CLINICAL REASONING

Connors *et al* (1980) stated that 'postural drainage and chest percussion in patients without sputum production is not indicated'.

No chest clearance technique is indicated in patients without sputum production.

MECHANICAL AIDS

Positive expiratory pressure (PEP)

PEP is the application of positive pressure at the mouth during expiration. Breathing out against resistance is thought to stabilize airways, prevent airway closure, reduce gas trapping, improve ventilation (Johnston *et al* 2013) and force air through collateral channels so that it can get behind the mucus (Fig 8.8). PEP also helps counteract airway closure caused by floppy airways or coughing (Fig 8.9), helps stabilize airways that are sensitive to bronchospasm and can be more effective than postural drainage and manual techniques (Fink 2002b). People with COPD have found short term gain (Olsén & Westerdahl 2009), and for those with CF, improved lung

FIGURE 8.8 Ventilation ($\dot{V}$) finding its way through collateral channels to get behind a mucous plug (black oval)

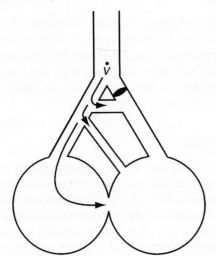

function and S_pO_2 have been identified (Darbee *et al* 2004).

Resistance to expiration is provided by a narrow orifice (Fig 8.10), the spring of a threshold resistor (Fig 8.11), a floating ball (Fig 8.12) or a blowing instrument such as a harmonica which is short on research but long on enjoyment.

Indications

PEP is mostly used by people with CF or bronchiectasis, and sometimes by those with COPD. It can be used by children as young as four. Patients with large quantities of mucus may need to add ACBT/AD.

FIGURE 8.9 (a) Forced exhalation compressing the airway. (b) Exhalation against positive pressure, stabilizing the airways and preventing collapse

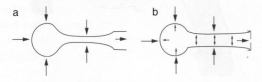

FIGURE 8.10 Mask PEP

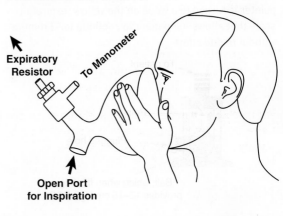

Expiratory Resistor

To Manometer

Open Port for Inspiration

Contraindications

Positive pressure techniques are inadvisable in the presence of:

- an undrained pneumothorax, which might lead to air being forced into the pleura
- haemoptysis, which might be exacerbated by the positive pressure
- raised intracranial pressure.

Technique

1 Patients take up their position of choice, but for those with advanced disease, sitting

FIGURE 8.11 TheraPEP Mouthpiece PEP

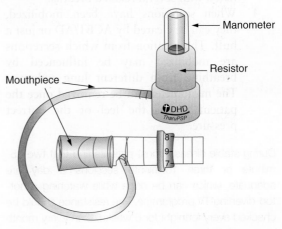

Manometer

Resistor

Mouthpiece

FIGURE 8.12 Mediflo PEP device, in which the pointer is turned to a value on the yellow 'expiration' scale that allows the patient to continue for 2 minute without undue effort

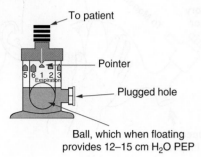

To patient

Pointer

5 6 1 2 3
Exspiration

Plugged hole

Ball, which when floating
provides 12–15 cm H₂O PEP

with their elbows resting on a table may protect the lungs from over-distension.

2   The resistance is chosen which the patient can use comfortably for 2 mins, usually 10–20 cmH₂O during mid-exhalation. The manometer is observed by the physiotherapist but not the patient at first, who might otherwise try to reach the target pressure by altering their breathing pattern.

3   After relaxing their breathing, the patient inhales slowly to slightly higher than tidal volume, holds their breath briefly at end-inspiration, then exhales actively but not fully or forcefully through the resistance. They should experience a comfortable effort, as if giving way to the resistance. Exhalation should last no more than 4 seconds. About 10 PEP breaths are alternated with several relaxed breaths.

4   When secretions have been mobilized, they can be cleared by ACBT/AD or just a huff. The location from which secretions are mobilized may be influenced by breathing from different lung volumes. The manometer can be removed once the patient knows the feel of the correct pressure.

During stable disease, most patients find that two 15-minute or three 10-minute sessions a day are adequate, which can be done while watching a not-too-diverting TV programme. The resistance should be checked every fortnight for 6 weeks, then every month

for 3 months. A mouthpiece may need a higher pressure (Larsson & Olsén 2006).

EzPAP

A hand-held device is available that amplifies a flow of air or oxygen approximately four times to create positive pressure throughout the breathing cycle. Research is limited but claims have been made that it can help clear secretions, increase lung volume (Elliott 2014) and improve oxygenation (Rieg et al 2012).

PEP tube

The thin tubing used for oxygen therapy can be cut to a length of about 30 cm, into which patients blow to create positive pressure (Fig 8.13). The technique is research-light but can be clinically reasoned to have a similar result to the PEP mask, albeit it more modestly, and patients can confirm whether or not it helps them. The positive pressure created by airflow resistance in the tube depends on the length of tubing and how hard patients blow, both of which they are usually able to judge and modify. The tube is cleaned in hot soapy water.

Oscillatory PEP

Oscillations can be added to further aid mucociliary clearance by means of ATP-mediated airway surface liquid secretion (Button & Boucher 2008). Patients breathe in to above tidal volume, then breathe out through the device hard enough to create the optimum oscillations. This may be less tiring than ACBT but is often most

FIGURE 8.13 PEP tube

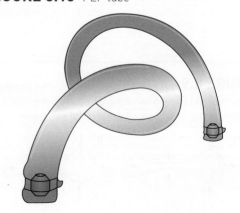

effective when used during the exhalation phase of ACBT/AD. They are suited to anyone who can blow bubbles. Contraindications and technique are as for PEP, with extra details below and in App.B. Cleaning instructions come in the package.

Bubble PEP

A cheap way of creating positive pressure and oscillations is by blowing out through water (Ch. 11).

Flutter

The Flutter (Fig 8.14a) resembles a short fat pipe and may assist people with bronchiectasis (Figueiredo *et al* 2012) or CF (Gondor 1999). By exhaling into the device, the patient creates a positive pressure of about 10 cmH$_2$O which varies with the angle at which it is held. Oscillations, created by a vibrating steel ball, are facilitated by slow breathing.

Patients inhale through their nose, then exhale through the mouthpiece as if using the PEP mask. They must keep their cheeks taut on exhalation and avoid blocking the holes on the device with their fingers.

The aim is for maximum oscillation, not maximum force. This is assessed subjectively by the patient and objectively by the physiotherapist palpating for vibrations over the chest. Mobilization of distal secretions is emphasized by tilting the Flutter slightly upwards, and for proximal secretions it is held more horizontal. The device is used for between 5 minutes (e.g. COPD) and 15 minutes (e.g. CF) at a session. The steel ball should

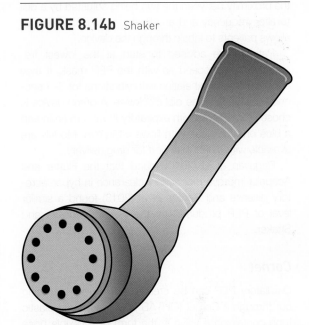

FIGURE 8.14b Shaker

be kept away from toddlers. The Flutter is available on prescription in the UK.

Shaker

The Shaker (Fig 8.14b) is similar to the Flutter but with a moveable mouthpiece (Santos *et al* 2013).

Acapella

The Acapella (Fig 8.14c) is popular because patients do not need to generate high flows and it can be used at any angle, being dependent on magnetic attraction rather than gravity. Exhaled gas causes oscillations by interaction of magnets and a counterbalanced lever,

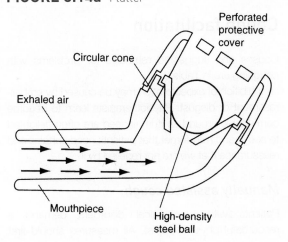

FIGURE 8.14a Flutter

Perforated protective cover

Circular cone

Exhaled air

Mouthpiece

High-density steel ball

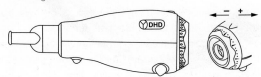

FIGURE 8.14c Acapella, with the frequency dial on the right

the proximity between the two being adjusted by a dial to alter frequency and amplitude. An inspiratory valve allows patients to inhale through the device.

Patients are advised to start at the lowest frequency, then proceed as with the PEP mask. If they cannot maintain exhalation with vibrations for 3–4 seconds, they adjust the dial clockwise. A green device is chosen for patients with expiratory flows >15 l/min and a blue one for those with flows <15 l/min. Models are available with a nebulizer port for drug delivery.

Ragavan *et al* (2010) found that the Flutter and Acapella improve mucociliary clearance in hypersecretory disease and Santos *et al* (2013) found a similar level of PEP produced by the Flutter, Acapella and Shaker.

Cornet

Oscillatory PEP can be created by actively breathing out through a Cornet (OHTAS 2009), a curved plastic tube containing a valve in the form of a flexible hose (Fig 8.14d). It can be used in any position and provides variable flow and pressure. There is limited research and it is fiddly to clean, but it suits some patients.

Machines

The following allow patients to be passive and sometimes take nebulized drugs at the same time.

High-frequency chest compressors

The 'Vest' delivers pulsatile compressions through an inflatable jacket round the torso, with adjustments for

frequency and pressure to create expiratory flow bias (p. 465) and 'mini-coughs' (Rand *et al* 2012). It can be started from age two, is convenient for families and popular with patients, who can use their social media at the same time. Compared to oscillatory PEP, which is particularly beneficial for excess secretions, the Vest appears suited to thick secretions (Ragavan *et al* 2010).

Intrapulmonary percussors

High gas flows at 60–400 cycles/minute send vibrations directly into the airway via a mouthpiece, mask or tracheal tube, along with nebulized saline or medication (Toussaint *et al* 2012). Intrapulmonary percussors may also recruit collapsed alveoli (Rand *et al* 2013).

High frequency oscillators

High frequency oscillation can be applied either directly to the airway or via the chest wall with the 'Hayek' oscillator (Hristara *et al* 2008). Chest wall oscillation has been found comfortable postoperatively for adults (Park 2012), but for some children it has caused discomfort and occasionally oxygen desaturation (Rand *et al* 2011).

Intermittent positive pressure breathing

Some weak or drowsy patients with sputum retention may respond to IPPB (Ch. 8), which can promote deep breaths and has the advantage of aerosol delivery. In-exsufflators (p.240) have a vibratory mode that delivers intrapulmonary percussion.

COUGH

Cough facilitation

Causes and suggested remedies for problems with coughing are in Table 8.2.

Inhibition of expectoration may be caused by embarrassment or disgust. Physiotherapists learn to become comfortable around sputum (indeed are often delighted to see it) and may forget that patients need curtains and reassurance that we are not repelled by it.

Manually assisted cough

Patients with neurological disorders demand a resourceful physiotherapist. All measures should first

---

FIGURE 8.14d Cornet

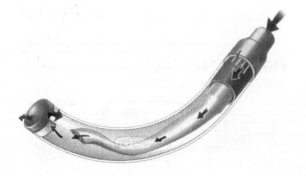

TABLE 8.2 Difficulties with coughing

Problem	Management
Pain following surgery	Pain relief and manual support (Ch. 16)
Thick secretions	Hydration Humidification
Dry mouth	Hydration Hot steamy drink Sips of water or juice Ice or semi-frozen pineapple or lemon juice Mouth care
Poor technique	Positioning upright (Ragavan *et al* 2010) Demonstration
Inhibition due to anxiety	Information (e.g. postoperative stitches, stress incontinence, fits of coughing)
Unstable airways	AD for bronchospasm, PEP for floppy airways
Upper airway obstruction e.g. tumour	Try different positions
Weakness	Manual or mechanical assistance (below)
Semiconsciousness	Abdominal co-contraction (Fig 6.7) Gentle skin pressure upwards over the trachea, just above the suprasternal notch
Last resort (1)	Blow out through straw into glass of water
Last resort (2)	Gentle stimulation at entrance to one or other outer ear canal (Irwin *et al* 1998) to stimulate Arnold's nerve response, but without using any instrument

be taken to bring the secretions proximally. Physical assistance is then given by helping the patient sit over the edge of the bed if possible. The abdomen is compressed manually, inwards and upwards, while either sitting beside (Fig 8.15) or kneeling behind the patient. Abdominal thrusts are co-ordinated with the patient making an expiratory effort and leaning forward, assisted by the physiotherapist. If the patient cannot sit up, it is done in supine.

Abdominal thrusts should be avoided or modified in patients with the following:

- unstable angina or arrhythmias
- rib fracture: if pain is controlled with a nerve block, manual assistance may be acceptable with modified hand positions
- high muscle tone the patient may require antispasmodic drugs
- spinal fracture

- gastroesophageal reflux (GOR)
- paralytic ileus or abdominal injury/surgery.

Some patients can assist themselves by sitting with a pillow pressed against their abdomen, then after a deep breath, bending forward while exhaling sharply.

Mechanically assisted cough

Mechanical insufflation-exsufflation (MIE) is provided by the CoughAssist (Fig 8.16) or Nippy Clearway (App. A). They apply gradual positive pressure to the upper airway, usually by a mask held by the physiotherapist or carer, then rapidly shift to negative pressure creating a high expiratory flow to simulate a cough.

It is best to start on manual mode and talk the patient through what to expect. Inspiratory and expiratory pressures may start equally at 10–20

FIGURE 8.15 Manually assisted cough

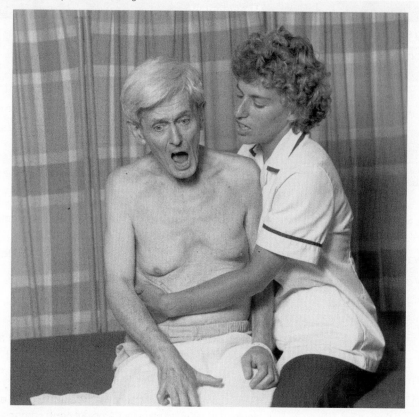

cmH$_2$O, and some patients like a pause between the two. The expiratory pressure can be gradually increased to 40–45 cmH$_2$O. By watching the breathing pattern, the exsufflation 'cough' can be switched on at the end of the patient's exhalation. Three to five cycles of in-exsufflation (with or without an abdominal thrust during exsufflation) are followed by about 30 seconds of rest, during which the patient is asked about timing and pressure, and the machine adjusted accordingly. The automatic mode can then be used.

Potential complications include abdominal distention, aggravation of GOR, discomfort, increased BP, and, rarely, haemoptysis or pneumothorax. Bradyarrhythmias can occur in people with high spinal cord injury. The risk of complications is reduced by adequate rest between applications and avoidance of hyperventilation.

Insufflation alone acts as a form of breath-stacking (p.111) and can facilitate a cough, but the full MIE cycle has been found more effective than a manually assisted cough (Jones *et al* 2012). MIE can also be used with a mouthpiece or tracheal tube. It is not suited to patients with floppy airways, as can occur with COPD or advanced CF.

MIE should be avoided in patients with:
- inadequate bulbar function
- undrained pneumothorax or subcutaneous emphysema
- bullous emphysema
- nausea
- chest pain of unknown origin
- severe acute asthma
- recent lung surgery
- raised intracranial pressure
- inability to communicate
- haemodynamic instability.

Both manual and mechanical assistance should be avoided after eating.

FIGURE 8.16 'CoughAssist' insufflator-exsufflator

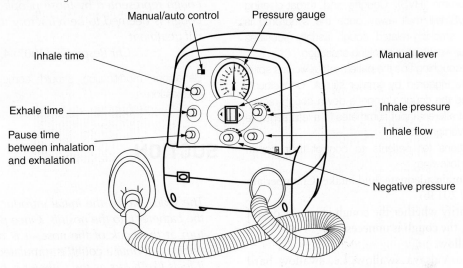

Cough control

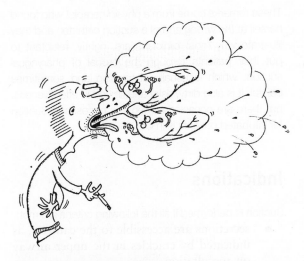

The cough is subject to more voluntary control than other respiratory reflexes such as sneezing and may need to be inhibited in the following situations:

- during ACBT/AD, before secretions are accessible
- after eye or cranial surgery, or if there is an aneurysm, raised intracranial pressure, surgical emphysema or recent pneumonectomy
- if the cough is dry and irritates the airways, or is unnecessary.

Unnecessary coughing may lead to stress incontinence (Ahmed *et al* 2013), which can be treated by pelvic floor exercises (Bø & Herbert 2013). It also disrupts sleep, work and social life, and suppression when appropriate has shown improved cough-related quality of life (Patel *et al* 2011).

Some patients inhibit their cough for social reasons. This is not advisable and can be avoided by ensuring patients know how to clear their chest effectively before a social event. Inappropriate cough suppression can lead to 'Lady Windermere syndrome' and bronchiectasis, caused by retention of secretions and inflammation of the long narrow dependent airways of the middle lobe and lingula, both served meagerly by collateral ventilation (Mori *et al* 2012).

The first step when dealing with a dry unproductive cough is to identify the cause (Ch. 2). A cough caused

KEY POINT

Unnecessary coughing can cause bronchospasm, paroxysm of coughing, desaturation or distress.

by asthma should disappear once inflammation is controlled, unless the actual cause is comorbid hyperventilation syndrome (HVS). Coughs and throat-clearing due to HVS will melt away once the syndrome is treated. A smoking-related cough usually subsides three to four weeks after smoking cessation.

Excess coughing tips the patient into a vicious spiral so that it is triggered by smaller stimuli. Consciously suppressing the cough dampens down cough receptors so that afferent input summates to a less sensitive threshold (Vertigan 2007).

Suggestions for patients to control their cough include the following:

- maintain adequate fluid intake (Chamberlain *et al* 2013b)
- identify whether the cough is wet or dry; if dry, the cough is unnecessary
- swallow
- try a Valsava swallow, i.e. swallow hard with neck flexion and while tightening the muscles in neck and shoulders
- take sips of water or cold grape juice
- take slow and/or shallow breaths
- breathe in through the nose, breathe out through pursed lips
- keep throat relaxed
- take repeated short sniffs
- use autogenic drainage techniques to control airflow
- suck non-medicated lozenges, ice pops or frozen seedless grapes
- chew gum
- inhale the steam from hot water poured over root ginger, then drink the warm solution (with honey, cinnamon and/or lemon)
- for a nocturnal cough, avoid supine.

Honey has been found moderately beneficial in children (Meremikwu *et al* 2012). Drugs to suppress a cough are in Ch. 5.

Occasionally a dry cough may be helpful and need not be suppressed, e.g. if a patient finds that one brief cough will settle it as if scratching an itch.

CLINICAL REASONING

Behaviour modification is appropriate for a subset of the total population with chronic cough represented by those people whose cough is deemed to be refractory to medical treatment.

Chr Respir Dis (2007) 4, 89–97

Behaviour modification should come before medication.

SUCTION

The worst part is the initial introduction of the catheter into the nostrils. Once past the turn at the back of the nose, it is not too unpleasant until a cough is stimulated; then it feels like hours as the catheter is brought back up. It felt as if I was choking.

Ludwig (1984)

These remarks come from a physiotherapist who found herself at the wrong end of a suction catheter, and they illustrate why most clinicians are, rightly, reluctant to put their patients through the ordeal of pharyngeal suction, which is usually distressing and sometimes painful. It is also dirty, risky and limited in effectiveness, but there are occasions when it is necessary. Suction for intubated patients is in Ch. 18.

Indications

Suction is performed if all the following criteria are met:

- secretions are accessible to the catheter, as indicated by crackles in the upper airway on auscultation
- secretions are detrimental to the patient
- the patient is unable to clear the secretions by other means.

Patients who are semiconscious, weak or neurologically impaired may require suction, but those who are fatigued rarely do because, unless fatigue is extreme enough for the patient to need ventilatory support, coughing is usually possible. Risks are increased in a combative patient, and those who need physical restraint for suction rarely need to undergo the procedure because they are usually strong enough to cough effectively, even though they choose not to. Suction against a patient's wish is unethical, illegal in the UK and acceptable only if the patient is deemed to lack capacity to give consent and their health will otherwise suffer significantly.

Catheters

Catheters have an end hole through which the mucus is suctioned and side eyes to relieve the vacuum if the end hole becomes blocked. The side eyes should not be too large (Fig 8.17c) or they will reduce suction efficiency, and their total size should be less than that of the end-hole so that they do not become suction channels. The ideal catheter is flexible, with a smooth rounded tip and small multiple countersunk side eyes.

Complications

Untoward effects of suction may be subclinical and include the following (AARC 2004):

1   The vacuum can cause atelectasis.
2   Hypoxia can result from atelectasis, suction of oxygen from the airways, enforced apnoea or increased oxygen demand.
3   Hypoxia, stress or irritation of the vagus nerve can cause hypertension or arrhythmias.
4   Vomiting may occur, in which case the patient should be helped to sit up, but suction continued to avoid aspiration.
5   Airway mucosa is exquisitely sensitive and is damaged by both passage of the catheter and pull from the vacuum (Kleiber *et al* 1988), exacerbated by poor technique.
6   Infective organisms find an easy target once the protective mucosa is damaged.
7   Laryngospasm is rare but may cause the catheter to become stuck and the patient unable to breathe, in which case the following steps should be taken:

   ● press the crash button and call for help
   ● ask the patient to sniff (Sandhu 2013)
   ● press hard into both postcondylar notches behind the earlobe (between

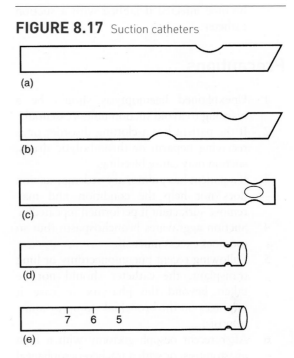

FIGURE 8.17 Suction catheters

(a)

(b)

(c)

(d)

(e)   7   6   5

the base of the skull, the mastoid process and the mandible) while displacing the mandible forward in a jaw thrust
   ● apply 100% oxygen (Cooper *et al* 2012).

CLINICAL REASONING

Pneumothorax has been described as a complication of suction, but it is difficult to find original controlled studies for this in adults, and it would require rather enthusiastic suction to poke a catheter through the airway wall, through a lung, then through the visceral pleura.

Contraindications

1   Stridor indicates a dangerously narrowed airway which could become obstructed if pharyngeal suction is attempted.
2   After basal skull fracture, nasopharyngeal suction is contraindicated in case there is cerebrospinal fluid leak, which could

become infected if jabbed with a suction catheter.

Precautions

1   Unexplained haemoptysis should be a warning to avoid suction unless essential.
2   If the patient has a clotting disorder or is receiving heparin or thrombolytic drugs, suction may cause bleeding.
3   If a patient has pulmonary oedema, suction does not help the condition and may remove surfactant if performed repeatedly.
4   Suction aggravates bronchospasm (but so too does excess mucus).
5   Following recent pneumonectomy or lung transplant, the catheter should not be taken beyond the pharynx in case it impinges on the bronchial stump or anastomosis.
6   After recent oesophagectomy with a high anastomosis, or with a tracheo-oesophageal fistula, the catheter may enter the oesophagus. Insertion should therefore not go beyond the pharynx, or a minitracheostomy can be requested.
7   Raised intracranial pressure is exacerbated with suction.

Technique

The patient should be talked through each step. The following are suggested:

1   Explain to the patient how it will feel, how long it will last and that they may ask for a pause at any time, a request that must be responded to. Obtain consent. Unconscious patients also need an explanation.
2   Check resuscitation status.
3   Choose a size 10 FG catheter, or occasionally size 12. Large sizes are more uncomfortable and increase the negative pressure (Palazzo & Soni 2013).
4   Ensure the patient is upright or side-lying in case of vomiting.
5   Pre-oxygenate for two minutes if this is not contraindicated. The oxygen mask should then be kept close to the patient's face throughout.
6   Ask the patient to take a few rapid breaths, if they can. There is no evidence that reducing P_aCO_2 prolongs tolerance to suction, but it enables patients to feel a little more in control. Reassure them that their oxygen is monitored.
7   Put on a visor, or mask and goggles.
8   Set the suction pressure to no more than -20 kPa (-150 mmHg) (Palazzo & Soni 2013). The pressure should be set with the machine turned on and the end of the suction tubing occluded.
9   Partially unpeel the catheter pack and attach to the suction tubing, while keeping the rest of the catheter in the pack, which can be tucked under the arm.
10 Put a sterile glove on the dominant hand. This hand must now not touch anything except the sterile catheter.
11 Remove the catheter from the pack and lubricate the tip with water-soluble jelly, while maintaining sterility of catheter and glove.
12 With the suction port open, slide the catheter gently into the nostril, directing it parallel to the floor of the nose. If resistance is felt at the back of the pharynx, rotate the catheter slowly between the fingers and ease very gently forwards.
13 To reduce the risk of entering the oesophagus, ask the patient to tilt their head back, stick out their tongue and cough. If coughing is not possible, slide the catheter down during inspiration, when the glottis is more open. If the patient swallows, the catheter has slipped into the oesophagus, in which case it should be slightly withdrawn, the head repositioned and the procedure continued. The catheter is usually in the airway if the patient coughs.
14 When resistance is felt, the catheter should be withdrawn slightly before applying vacuum pressure in order to limit trauma.
15 Block the catheter port with the non-dominant hand to apply suction, though not too suddenly, at the same time bringing up the catheter slowly and smoothly,

avoiding catheter rotation or sudden intermittent suction. Slow withdrawal reduces the need for a second attempt, but total apnoeic time should not exceed ten seconds and if the patient appears distressed, the catheter should be partially withdrawn until distress stops, then the vacuum removed, again not too suddenly, and oxygen applied with the catheter still *in situ*, until the patient is ready to continue.

Rotation is unnecessary and intermittent suction involving the sudden on/off application of vacuum pressure may damage mucosa (Day *et al* 2002) while reducing effectiveness because the flow can be reduced from 19 to 8.5 l/min (Brown 1983), making further suction passes more likely. Protection of mucosa is best maintained by continuous withdrawal, without stopping to change the position of the dominant hand on the catheter. If suction pressure rises unacceptably, the rocking thumb technique should be used, which is the smooth and partial removal of the non-dominant thumb from the control port of the catheter to reduce negative pressure gently.

PRACTICE TIP

Obtain an endotracheal tube and catheter. Insert the catheter, then withdraw it while rotating. Observe the tip to identify if the rotation transmits to the tip of the catheter.

If, during withdrawal, it becomes apparent that a second suction pass will be required, i.e. continuing crackles are heard, it is best to withdraw the catheter until the patient can breathe, then stop suction with the catheter *in situ*. The patient is then helped to sit forward and given oxygen, and once S_pO_2 has returned to normal and the patient has got their breath back, consent is obtained for a further suction pass. Keeping the same catheter *in situ* avoids repetition of the sometimes painful process of passing a new catheter through the bend in the throat, and clinical reasoning suggests that passing another catheter through the nose (whose job is to catch dirt) increases infection risk. If the catheter is removed and further suction is required, a fresh catheter must be used.

Afterwards, wind the catheter round the sterile glove, remove the glove inside out over the catheter and discard, rinse out suction tubing using tap water in a jug. Give the patient oxygen and comfort, check monitors and auscultate. Discard water in jug.

If the nasal route is uncomfortable, the other nostril can be tried or the oral route used. The catheter is inserted into a Guedel airway, which is a plastic tube shaped to conform to the palate with a flange to prevent it slipping into the throat (Fig. 8.18a). A size 4–6 airway is average, but it is best sized by holding it against the side of the face and measuring it from the corner of the mouth to the angle of the jaw below the ear.

After explanations and obtaining consent, the catheter is first inserted into the Guedel airway, then with the tip protruding just beyond the end of the airway, both airway and catheter are passed into the mouth (after removal of dentures), curve upwards to avoid pushing the tongue towards the throat. The patient is then advised to 'breathe it in'. It is rotated so that the curve is downwards, then passed gently into the throat. During insertion it should be pressed downwards onto the tongue so that it does not impinge on the soft palate and cause gagging. Introducing the airway is not painful but may be distressing, and the patient should be talked through the process and reassured that it will not stop them breathing (the clinician can demonstrate first with a separate airway passed into their own throat). Passage of the catheter then proceeds through the airway, as described above.

PRACTICE TIP

Hold your breath throughout the time the patient is unable to breathe.

Nasopharyngeal airway

A nasopharyngeal airway (Fig 8.18b) can be used for patients who need frequent suction, but insertion is painful and sinus infection is a risk. Size 6 mm is usually suited to women and 7 mm to men, or about the diameter of the patient's little finger. It is lubricated with aqueous or lignocaine gel before insertion, passed gently into the straightest (often the right) or largest nostril, then directed backwards along the floor of the nose parallel to the hard palate until the flange is flat with the nostril.

FIGURE 8.18 (a) oral Guedel airway and
(b) nasopharyngeal airway

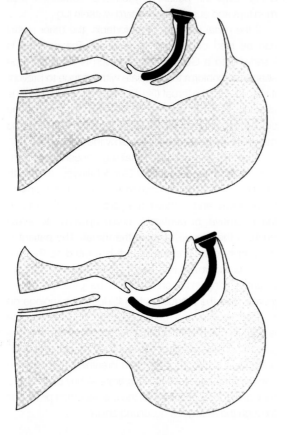

FIGURE 8.19 Minitracheostomy

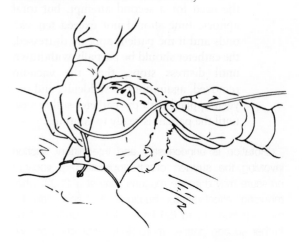

The size is correct if the airway can be moved slightly inside the nose. The tip rests behind the tongue just above the epiglottis. A safety pin across the top, outside the nostril, prevents it disappearing into the patient.

Suction can then proceed through the airway, which avoids the discomfort of passing a catheter each time through the bend at the back of the throat. The airway can be left in place for a maximum 24 hours, after which if necessary it can be cleaned and re-inserted. It should not be used in patients who have polyps, congenital deformities, old nose fractures, cerebrospinal fluid leak or bleeding from the nose or ear.

Minitracheostomy

A minitracheostomy (Fig 8.19) allows access for safe and comfortable suction. It is usually performed under local anaesthesia on the ward, and left in place for as many days as necessary. Suction with a size 10 catheter can then be performed through the aperture, with the patient breathing normally throughout. Some secretions are too thick for a minitracheostomy, although saline instillation may be helpful. A spigot protects the airway when the tube is not in use.

A minitracheostomy tube is uncuffed and preserves the function of the glottis so that natural humidification is maintained and the patient can cough, speak, eat and breathe spontaneously. It is often performed later than optimal, so the physiotherapist can act as instigator to ensure that it is used early enough to be effective, or obtain training in minitracheotomy themselves. Prophylactic placement during surgery is useful for patients at high risk of postoperative sputum retention (Beach *et al* 2013).

CLINICAL REASONING

Is the following statement logical (or kind)?

Indications for tracheal suction include … to assess endotracheal or tracheostomy tube patency.
Cardiopulmonary Physiotherapy, Oxford
(2002)

It is unclear why a patient should be put through this procedure in order to identify what could be ascertained by asking them to breathe or observing the ventilator screen.

Home suction

The carers of patients requiring domiciliary suction should be taught how to suction, or, better still, the patient can be taught to suction themselves. This is first assessed in hospital in case oxygen is required. The discharge summary should indicate individual modifications for the patient and their subjective and objective responses. Detailed guidelines are in AARC (1999a).

OUTCOMES FOR AIRWAY CLEARANCE

> *Lacking evidence that any technique is superior to another, patient preference is an important consideration.*
> Hess 2002

The following can be used to evaluate the effectiveness of techniques for clearing secretions:

- the patient's opinion
- ↓ crackles on auscultation or by sound analysis (Marques *et al* 2012)
- ↑ volume of sputum cleared
- ↑ S_pO_2, so long as other variables are excluded
- ↑ independence of patients to manage their own secretions.

Physiotherapists can evaluate their manual techniques through a bronchoscope, if their patient is to undergo this procedure. The effect can be impressive.

For patients with hypersecretory disease, functional outcome measures are in Ch. 3.

Using the literature to identify effective techniques is a minefield. Studies *in vitro*, or in people with normal lungs, bear limited relation to clinical practice. Studies that do not correct for cough alone are suspect because most techniques include coughing. Studies that do not follow up secretion clearance for several hours after treatment are of limited use. Studies that measure sputum volume or sputum weight do not compensate for saliva or swallowed secretions. Sputum volume is adequate for outcome measurement but is not valid for research.

Mucociliary clearance can be assessed by delivering a radioisotope as an inhaled aerosol. This is caught by the mucus and the subsequent decline in radioactivity measured (Bennett *et al* 2013). Cough should be excluded because this can affect the clearance rate.

For people with hypersecretory disease, research tracking the change in FEV_1 over time could indicate that clearing mucus from the larger airways is beneficial, on the assumption that stagnant secretions lead to damage that causes airflow obstruction. However, the procedure itself alters bronchial *status quo* by shearing secretions off the airway wall. The measurement of gas mixing efficiency may be more useful, based on the same assumption about secretions and airway damage (Robinson *et al* 2013).

DISCHARGE FROM PHYSIOTHERAPY

> *... I come home and I'm so weak I can't do the exercises.*
> Patient quoted by Lewis & Cramp 2010

Discharge planning should begin at the outset and involve all team members including the patient and family (DoH 2010b). Communication with relatives, the patient and primary care or continuing care teams are the basis of a smooth transition and can reduce readmission rates by 12%–75% (Harrison *et al* 2011). Follow up phone calls can also reduce readmissions and increase patient satisfaction (Naffe 2012). Copies of all letters should be sent to the patient.

CASE STUDY : MS

A 17 y.o. patient is admitted with an exacerbation of advanced cystic fibrosis

Social history

- MS lives with his parents and is about to start college.

Home management

- Brief morning session and longer evening session using ACBT, Flutter and postural drainage.
- Exercise mainly by biking to school; little exercise in holidays.
- Regular reviews with community physiotherapist.
- Frequent admissions.

Subjective assessment

- Bored.
- Not feeling ill.
- Not clearing phlegm.
- Not hungry or thirsty.

Objective assessment

- Hyperinflated chest.
- Thin.
- Top-up feeding by gastrostomy at night.
- Intravenous antibiotics.
- Clinically dehydrated.
- S_pO_2 95%
- Spiking temperature.
- Auscultation: widespread crackles.
- Frequent small non-productive coughs.
- Radiograph as Fig 8.20.

Questions

1 Analysis?
2 Problems?
3 Goals?
4 Plan?

FIGURE 8.20 MS

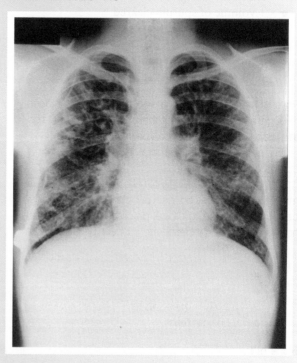

CLINICAL REASONING

Are the following statements problem-based and/or evidence-based?
  1   Deep breathing exercises have been proposed to assist the tachypnoeic patient.
  2   IPPB is claimed to be useful in delivering aerosolized bronchodilators.
  3   … available evidence suggests that postural drainage and controlled coughing or FET may
      be the most effective components.

IPPB: intermittent positive pressure breathing; FET: forced expiration technique (predecessor to ACBT)

Eur Resp J (1993) 3, 353–5

Response to Case Study

1   Analysis

  ● Radiograph shows widespread cystic shadowing.
  ● Lack of eating may indicate depression because MS's anorexia is not related to feeling ill, and although he is undoubtedly bored, his use of this term might also indicate depression because a 17 y.o. is unlikely to admit to this.
  ● Lack of fluid intake may be contributing to sputum retention.
  ● Frequent small non-productive coughs are ineffective and may cause fatigue or strain the pelvic floor.

2   Problems

  ● Depression → inactivity → sputum retention
                    → dehydration → sputum retention
                    → poor nutrition → immunocompromise → slow resolution of infection
  ● Ineffective cough → sputum retention
  ● Long term: lack of exercise in holidays

3   Goals

  ● ↓ depression
  ● Control cough
  ● Clear chest
  ● Long term – review chest clearance regime

4   Plan

  ● Liaise with team including community physiotherapist re. (a) management of depression including possible discussion on end-of-life care, (b) increasing fluid intake through IV.
  ● Re-educate cough: suppress ineffective coughs, cough only when secretions accessible.
  ● Check ACBT technique, suggest gym.
  ● If patient is tired or weak, discuss which passive techniques might suit him, e.g. postural drainage, manual techniques, intermittent positive pressure breathing (IPPB).
  ● Consider mask for biking to college.

None of the conventional techniques were effective until hydration took effect. However the patient enjoyed IPPB because he was shown how to administer it himself, then used it frequently to good effect. He was coaxed down to the gym, chose which equipment to use and was then able to use it whenever it was staffed. Both these techniques, chosen by himself, facilitated autonomy. He was discharged to the care of the community team.

Response to Clinical Reasoning

1   Tachypnoea indicates increased work of breathing, not loss of lung volume.
    If deep breathing exercises 'have been proposed', by whom?
    Deep breathing is counterproductive for breathless patients.
2   The words 'claimed to be' are unreferenced.
    IPPB is an expensive and inefficient way of delivering medication.
3   The 'available evidence' is unreferenced.

RECOMMENDED READING

Andersen T, Sandnes A, Hilland M (2013) Laryngeal response patterns to mechanical insufflation-exsufflation in healthy subjects. *Am J Phys Med Rehabil;* **92**(10): 920–9.

Bach JR (2013) A historical perspective on expiratory muscle aids and their impact on home care. *Am J Phys Med Rehabil;* **92**(10): 930–41

Bennett WD, Laube BL, Corcoran T et al (2013). Multisite comparison of mucociliary and cough clearance measures using standardized methods. *J Aerosol Med Pulm Drug Deliv;* **26**(3): 157–164

Brusasco C (2013) In vitro evaluation of heat and moisture exchangers designed for spontaneously breathing tracheostomized patients. *Respir Care;* **58**(11): 1878–85

Cross J, Elender J (2012) Findings from the MATREX study: a treatment protocol for the delivery of manual chest therapy in respiratory care. *Respir Care;* **57**(8): 1263–6

Iyer VN, Lim KG (2013) Chronic cough: an update. *Mayo Clin Proc;* **88**(10): 1115–26

Lai SK, Wang Y-Y, Wirtz D et al (2010) ''http://www.ncbi.nlm.nih.gov/pmc/articles/PMC2736374/?tool=pmcentrez'' Micro- and macrorheology of mucus. *Adv Drug Deliv Rev;* **61**(2): 86–100

Lv J, Wu J, Guo R et al (2013) Laboratory test of a visual sputum suctioning system. *Respir Care;* **58**(10): 1637–42

Munkholm M, Mortensen J (2013) Mucociliary clearance: pathophysiological aspects. *Clin Physiol Funct Imaging.* Sep 30

Nadel JA (2013) Mucous hypersecretion and relationship to cough. *Pulm Pharmacol Ther;* **26**(5): 510–3

Nikinmaa M (2013) Control of mucus secretion in airway inflammation. *Acta Physiologica;* **208**: 218–219

Rush EC (2013) Water: neglected, unappreciated and under researched. *Eur J Clin Nutr;* **67**: 492–495

Sears PR, Thompson K, Knowles MR et al (2013) Human airway ciliary dynamics. *Am J Physiol Lung Cell Mol Physiol;* **304**(3): L170–83

Yiallouros PK, Papadouri T, Karaoli C et al (2013) First outbreak of nosocomial Legionella infection in term neonates caused by a cold mist ultrasonic humidifier. *Clin Infect Dis;* **57**(1): 48–56

CHAPTER 9
Pulmonary rehabilitation

LEARNING OBJECTIVES

On completion of this chapter the reader should be able to:

- identify appropriate patients for a pulmonary rehabilitation programme and assess them as safe to participate

- deliver the physiotherapy components of the education sessions

- select suitable exercises and supervise training safely and effectively

- enable participants to integrate and maintain what they have learnt into their daily life

- evaluate outcomes of the programme.

INTRODUCTION

> *It's really been such a breakthrough in being able to mix with people and not being so afraid. All ... the new people that come, they're all in the same boat.*
>
> Patient quoted by Gysels & Higginson (2009)

Rehabilitation for people disabled by breathlessness is one of the most rewarding aspects of physiotherapy.

Irreversible disease does not mean irreversible loss of function, and multidisciplinary pulmonary rehabilitation (PR) is now enshrined in most national guidelines. People who have become entangled in a web of inactivity and helplessness are able to improve their independence and quality of life (QoL) through the following:

- understanding their disease, treatment options and coping strategies
- reducing symptoms
- improving exercise tolerance and activities of daily living (ADL)
- becoming less dependent on family and medical resources.

The need is greater now that patients are being discharged from hospital 'quicker and sicker', and post-exacerbation PR should begin within a month of discharge (BTS 2013), taking advantage of the 'teachable moment' when patients are most receptive.

Effects

> *Pulmonary rehabilitation is the only approach to chronic lung disease short of lung transplantation that improves the long-term outlook for these patients.*
>
> Tiep 1991

Participants report a sense of wellbeing from gaining control over symptoms, especially the fear of breathlessness. Benefits are independent of age, lung function or disability (Morgan 2009) and include the following:

- ↓ dyspnoea, ↑ exercise capacity, quadriceps strength, ADL ability and health status (BTS 2013)
- ↓ anxiety and depression (Bhandari *et al* 2013), sleep quality (Soler 2013)
- ↓ cardiovascular risk factors (Reis *et al* 2013)
- ↑ cognition (ACCP 2007)
- ↓ fatigue (Mikelsons 2008)
- ↑ well-being and empowerment (Pinto *et al* 2013)
- ↓ fear and panic (Williams & Bruton 2010)
- ↓ emergency and outpatient visits (Al Moamary 2012), ↓ need for bronchodilators (Behnke *et al* 2003), overall cost savings (ACCP 2007)
- double the quit rates for smokers (ACCP 2007)
- if inspiratory muscle training and ribcage mobilization are included: ↓ hyperinflation (Yoshimi *et al* 2012)
- ↑ QoL and independence, ↓ disability, exacerbations (Postolache & Cojocaru 2013) and hospital admissions (Fig 9.1).

Participants

> *No patient is 'too sick' or 'too well' to benefit from pulmonary rehabilitation.*
>
> Menier 1994

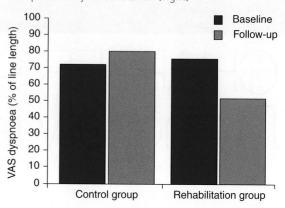

FIGURE 9.1a Increased shortness of breath on exertion without pulmonary rehabilitation (left) and with pulmonary rehabilitation (right)

For people with chronic obstructive pulmonary disease (COPD), PR is a fundamental treatment rather than an optional extra (BTS 2013). There is also value for people with bronchiectasis, asthma (with precautions to prevent exercise-induced exacerbation), interstitial lung disease (BTS 2013), scoliosis (Al Moamary 2012), cystic fibrosis (CF), neuromuscular disorders, lung cancer and pre- and post-surgery (Hodgkin *et al* 2009). Patients benefit if they have coexistent stable cardiovascular disease, chronic respiratory failure

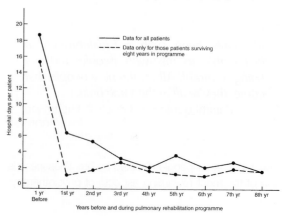

FIGURE 9.1b Reduced hospital admissions after initiation of pulmonary rehabilitation

(BTS 2013), are very elderly (Corhay *et al* 2012) or at the end stage of their condition (Ngaage 2004). Participants have described the benefit of being in a group of mixed severity and how this motivated them to persevere (Mein et al 2007). For people with interstitial lung disease, hypoxaemia rather than respiratory mechanics usually limits exercise (Markovitz & Cooper 2010) and close monitoring is required.

The programme usually includes eight to ten participants. Selection criteria are the following:

- shortness of breath (SOB) limiting activity
- medical management optimized
- adequate ability to hear or otherwise communicate
- motivation towards self-help and lifestyle change
- ability to attend the full programme, apart from exacerbations.

The set up

The options are:

- an outpatient programme in a physiotherapy gym
- an inpatient programme in a dedicated rehabilitation ward
- a community programme in a day or leisure centre, where the education component can be delivered in person or remotely (Stickland *et al* 2011)
- a home-based programme, facilitated by visits and/or online (Mosa *et al* 2012), the latter requiring much encouragement
- a seamless discharge programme after exacerbation, in- or outpatient based.

Pre-discharge wards are an ideal environment for PR, especially with frail elderly people who would otherwise remain in an acute medical ward, becoming deconditioned and prey to hospital infection.

Home-based programmes are becoming popular because, although they lack peer support, exercise and energy conservation can be adapted to an individual's environment, the family are easily involved and telehealth is becoming more sophisticated.

For group PR, the options are a rolling programme, with one or two new patients each week, which means that patients who miss an education session due to illness can make it up easily, or a cohort programme.

KEY POINT

Group programmes should incorporate precautions against the risk of cross-infection, especially when including people with CF or bronchiectasis.

Resources

The following are essential for group PR:

- oxygen
- oximeters and blood pressure monitors
- crash trolley and team members trained in life support
- accessible toilet.

The following are preferable:

- large warm room with easily-opened windows, cheerful atmosphere, wall space and non-slip floor, free from dust-collecting furniture
- treadmill, exercise bike, steps, trampoline, quoits, weights, stretchy bands and any available gym equipment
- comfortable chairs for family members, and comfortable upright chairs for participants
- name labels
- fans
- sputum pots and tissues
- high walking frame
- teaching aids
- demonstration inhalers
- handouts, exercise booklets, diaries, writing materials
- refreshments
- door-to-door transport, e.g. volunteer drivers, to avoid the stress and delays of public or ambulance transport.

Financial planning needs to take account of staffing, venue, equipment, stationery and administration time.

The team typically comprises a physiotherapist, occupational therapist, respiratory nurse, physician, dietician and clinical psychologist or social worker.

Structure and timing

Twice weekly supervised sessions are required, and 6–12 weeks are recommended (BTS 2013). The initial session involves assessment and goal setting, and provides the foundations for motivation. A group session prior to assessment has been shown to increase success by improving knowledge, reducing fear of failure or discomfort (Graves *et al* 2010) and correcting concerns about exercise (Fischer *et al* 2012). Other aids to motivation are avoiding early mornings, and participants having to travel in rush-hour or in the dark.

Each session is typically based on exercise, brief relaxation, a break for a drink and socializing, and an education component. A half-way review helps participants to take stock. Many of the components from Ch 7 are incorporated into the programme.

ASSESSMENT

Assessment incorporates the ICF domains:

1 respiratory impairment: ↓ lung function, e.g. FEV_1
2 activity limitation: the effect of this impairment, e.g. ↓ exercise capacity
3 participation restriction, e.g. anxiety.

There is much variation between degree of impairment and how much patients are restricted in their participation. Lung function tests are checked to confirm diagnosis but are not used as outcome measures.

Participants are assessed as in Ch. 2, with factors relating specifically to rehabilitation below.

Background information

The case notes are scrutinized to check that exercise training is safe. Contraindications include (AARC 2001):

● symptomatic angina or recent myocardial infarct
● uncontrolled arrhythmias or hypertension
● second or third degree heart block or other unstable heart condition
● deep vein thrombosis or recent embolism or other unstable vascular condition
● abdominal aortic aneurysm >5.5 cm (BTS 2013).

Relative contraindications include:

● resting systolic BP >200 mmHg or diastolic >110 mmHg
● disabling stroke or arthritis, if exercises cannot be adapted
● haemoptysis of unknown cause
● unstable asthma
● impaired cognition to the extent of being unable to follow instructions
● underweight, until nutrition supplementation is established (Slinde *et al* 2002)
● abdominal aortic aneurysm <5.5 cm (where surgery has been deemed inappropriate), indicating the need to avoid high intensity or resistive exercise (BTS 2013).

Liaison with the physician is suggested if P_aCO_2 is above 8 kPa (60 mmHg).

People with comorbid cardiovascular disease benefit (Ch. 12) and those with osteoporosis gain from impact exercise (Mazokopakis 2011). People with insulin-dependent diabetes require specific precautions (Ch. 3) and referral for treatment of other comorbidities may be required (BTS 2013).

The following drug history is relevant:

● drugs such as beta-blockers render the BP and pulse unreliable for monitoring purposes
● if prescribed and indicated, bronchodilators and anti-angina drugs should be taken before exercise
● steroids should be at the lowest effective dose to minimize muscle weakness.

Body mass index should be measured before and after rehabilitation, and education adjusted accordingly (Vestbo *et al* 2006).

Subjective measurements

Participants are often relieved to be asked if their SOB is frightening, because this may not have been acknowledged before. Breathlessness must be explained to participants so that they distinguish it from sensations such as chest tightness.

Questionnaires include the following:

For respiratory symptoms:

● Breathlessness, Cough and Sputum Scale (McCarroll et al 2013).

FIGURE 9.2 Modified Borg Scale

Modified Borg Scale		
0	Nothing at all	
0.5	Very, very slight (just noticeable)	
1	Very slight	
2	Slight	
3	Moderate	
4	Somewhat severe	Training zone
5	Severe	
6		
7	Very severe	
8		
9	Very, very severe (almost maximal)	
10	Maximal	

Specifically for breathlessness:

- Borg and MRC scales (Fig 9.2, Table 9.1), or, to identify how SOB affects function, multidimensional scales (Norweg *et al* 2011).

For PR and exercise:

- Self-Efficacy Scale (Vincent *et al* 2011) or Rating of Perceived Exertion (Ritchie 2012).

For education:

- LINQ scale (Jones & Haskell 2012)
- Inpatient Respiratory Rehabilitation Questionnaire (Pasqua *et al* 2012).

For anxiety and depression:

- Hospital Anxiety and Depression Scale (Norton 2013): a score above ten for either anxiety or depression should be reported.

For health-related QoL:

- SGRQ or CRQ (Jones & Price 2011)
- CAT questionnaire (Kon et al 2013).

Other scales are summarized by Crisafulli (2010) and Williams & Frei (2012). Scales are useful if they take account of participants stopping 'wanting' to do what they cannot do, and if they distinguish SOB and distress. Causes of distress include frustration, embarrassment, dependency, difficulty with conversation, reduced capacity for spontaneity, and the sensation of dyspnoea itself. It is also useful at this stage to ask patients how they see their illness working out, check their understanding of PR, address any concerns and explain the benefits of the programme (BTS 2013).

TABLE 9.1 Medical Research Council dyspnoea scale

1	Not troubled by breathlessness except on strenuous exercise
2	Short of breath when hurrying or walking up a slight hill
3	Walks slower than contemporaries on level ground because of breathlessness, or has to stop for breath when walking at own pace
4	Stops for breath after walking about 100 m or after a few minutes on level ground
5	Too breathless to leave the house, or breathless when dressing or undressing

Exercise tests

Assessment for exercise desaturation (Ch.5) is required (Dyer *et al* 2012), using an oximeter validated under exercise conditions. Participants are discouraged from becoming too focused on their oximeter and to maintain awareness of their subjective response to exercise.

Six Minute Walk Test (6MWT)

This easily-understood endurance test is reflective of ADL (Tomkinson & Bruton 2009). It is also used to confirm diagnosis of COPD, interstitial lung disease and heart failure, assist in pre-surgical evaluation (Pichurko 2012) and predict mortality (Golpe 2013). Participants are asked to walk for six minutes as fast as reasonably possible, along a corridor or around two cones, following standardized instructions:

1   You have six minutes to complete as many laps as you can.
2   You can stop or sit down as often as you like but these will be part of the six minutes.
3   Walk around each cone.
4   Say if you feel any pain, giddiness or other unexpected symptom.

The patient should be told when each two minutes has been completed. Encouragement is fine but must be standardized.

Participants should feel at the end that they have performed to their maximum capacity, but for those with severe disease, it is best that they walk as fast as they like rather than their maximum, in order to avoid excessive symptoms, tachycardia or oxygen desaturation without increasing the distance walked (Mattia *et al* 2004).

The data to record are the distance, symptoms, heart rate (HR) and SpO_2. Repeat tests should be performed at the same time in relation to bronchodilator drugs. Normal 6MWT is 800 m − (5 × age).

Incremental Shuttle Walk Test (ISWT)

This is more reproducible and less dependent on motivation than the 6MWT, being externally paced.

Participants are asked to walk around a 10 metre oval circuit with a cone at each end. The speed of walking is dictated by a taped bleep which increases in line with walking gradually rising from one to five mph. Instructions are standardized and no verbal encouragement is given. The physiotherapist walks alongside for the first minute to discourage the participant from exceeding the initial speed. Thereafter, if the cone is reached early, the patient waits for the beep before continuing. The test ends when the patient cannot complete the circuit before the beep. Some participants have trouble co-ordinating the cones with the beep, and a three minute shuttle walk test can be substituted (Sava *et al* 2012).

The minimal clinically important improvement is 54 m for the 6MWT (for people with COPD) and 47.5 m for the ISWT (BTS 2013). The 6MWT correlates with oxygen consumption ($\dot{V}O_2$), and the ISWT correlates with maximum oxygen consumption ($\dot{V}O_2max$) (Stroescu *et al* 2012). Both require a practise walk before the programme (but not afterwards), with a rest of 15 minutes between the practise walk and test walk (Hodgkin *et al* 2009 p.135/336).

Endurance shuttle test

This is thought to be more responsive than the incremental shuttle test (Eaton *et al* 2006). It uses the same 10 m shuttle course and is a paced walk at 85% of $\dot{V}O_2max$, as assessed by a prior ISWT. No practise walk is needed (Revill *et al* 2009) but the three walking tests required make this too exhausting for many patients.

Other tests

Simpler tests include the chair-stand test, which counts standing up and sitting down over 30 seconds (Cho *et al* 2012a), the stair-climbing test, which counts the steps climbed up and down in two minutes, and the 4-metre gait speed (Kon 2013).

Walking tests take little notice of upper limb work and do not assess ADL. Arm exercise capacity can be measured by arm ergometry (Janaudis *et al* 2012) or the unsupported-arm-lift test (Datta *et al* 2013).

Observation of the participant during exercise tests indicates tension and fatigue. SMART goals (Ch. 6), are re-assessed throughout the programme to assist motivation.

EDUCATION

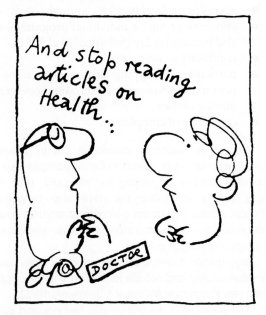

Mel Calman

Education underpins all other components of PR and facilitates adherence (ACCP 2007). It improves self-management (Mousing 2012) and provides a non-threatening atmosphere for discussion and mutual support, especially if a buddy system is in place in which 'expert' patients work alongside the team (Hancock & Cox 2008).

Hypoxia can impair memory, and retention of information is optimal if:

- the room is free of distractions
- the teaching plan is set out clearly
- the most important points are made first
- language is simple and jargon-free
- advice is specific rather than general
- information is reinforced regularly throughout the programme
- booklets and handouts are included.

The physiotherapist's job is to teach the management of breathlessness, the rationale of exercise training, chest clearance and, if included, inspiratory muscle training. The respiratory nurse or pharmacist covers drugs, inhalers, and the importance of pneumococcal and flu vaccinations (NICE 2012a). The occupational therapist discusses stress management, welfare benefits and relaxation. The dietician suggests six-meal-a-day menus, advises on healthy eating and explains which foods are constipating, hard to digest or gas-forming. A final session might include a question-and-answer discussion with the physician or all team members, and plans for the future.

The physiotherapist, nurse or physician explains the practicalities of oxygen therapy and discusses advance directives in relation to life-prolonging treatment. Less than 5% of patients are given the opportunity to discuss their options about life-prolonging treatment ahead of time (Curtis 2000), even though most value this (Burge *et al* 2013). Group discussion is often less threatening than individual discussion for delicate subjects such as death, sex and stress incontinence. However, about 10% of patients do not want to know about advance directives and 4% do not want to participate in end-of-life discussions (Heffner 2000) and patients from varied cultures will have different preferences. It is therefore useful to advise patients of the content of the next educational session so that they can absent themselves if they prefer. Curtis *et al* 2008 describe approaches to communicating prognosis to patients with life-limiting illnesses. Education topics are in App. C and Ch. 7.

> *Information does not equal education.*
> Tolomeo & Waldman 2013

KEY POINT

Pulmonary rehabilitation is not a course of treatment to make patients better, but more of a life plan.

Motivation

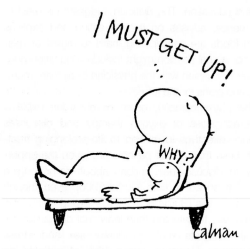

Mel Calman

> *The therapist-patient relationship can suc-*
> *ceed or fail depending on the care that the*
> *therapist takes in understanding the needs*
> *and circumstances of her patients.*
>
> Walker 1995

Motivation is the best predictor of success (Brannon *et al* 1998 p. 346). Patients may be used to the hierarchical hospital environment which can encourage the sick role and an assumption that experts know best. This is counterproductive in the rehabilitation process, where education is more than just feeding information into an empty vessel and pressing the right buttons.

Factors that increase motivation are:

- self-efficacy, i.e. patients having confidence in their autonomy (Davis 2007), including taking responsibility for their own management and setting goals (Krasny-Pacini *et al* 2013)
- realistic expectations
- clear advance information
- active participation, e.g. self-monitoring, encouragement to question and contribute ideas
- praise, warmth, humour, honesty and responsiveness from the rehabilitation team

- family involvement
- focus on health rather than disease
- early success, reinforced by progress charts
- access to medical notes if required
- choice of group or individual programmes and minimal delay (Sohanpal *et al* 2012)
- continuity of personnel
- participants swapping ideas, sharing transport to the sessions and exercising together outside classes
- certificate of completion.

Reduced motivation to exercise is due to advice that is inconvenient or difficult to follow, boredom (e.g. repetitive exercise or waiting for transport), fear of injury, not understanding the relationship between physical activity and health (Hartman *et al* 2013) and fatigue, which may be more common than anxiety or depression (Wong *et al* 2010).

Reassurance, if used blandly or indiscriminately, can increase anxiety and reduce motivation if it does not bring new information (Warwick & Salkovskis 1985).

Most participants are enthusiastic learners, and liberal use of teaching aids can explain the disease process in a way that is enjoyable. A large-print diary is useful to log daily exercise, symptoms, feelings, diet, drugs and side effects. The diary can record functional goals, the time to achieve them, and obligations of the patient and the PR team. Achievement of their first goal gives participants a motivating boost.

Memory aids include stickers at home on kettles and the fridge, and the use of dead time for exercises, e.g. TV advertisements or 'grey bar time' while waiting for the computer to process.

Most smokers want to stop (Talbot & Palmer 2013). Cessation advice should avoid telling participants that they should stop (they know this) but acknowledge how difficult it is, provide positive information and patient-friendly literature (App. B/C) and check that they know about local resources. Hospital admission provides an opportunity for behavioural interventions (Rigotti *et al* 2012). Other smoking cessation options are drugs (Ch. 5), exercise, mindfulness practice and falling in love (Xu *et al* 2012a).

> *There's nothing to giving up smoking. I've*
> *done it hundreds of times.*
>
> Mark Twain

Understanding reactions to the disease

Depression is the top-ranking cause of disability worldwide.

O'Neil *et al* (2013)

Participants can be advised that feelings are closely connected with breathing for all people including those with normal lungs, and that it is natural for breathless people to feel depressed and anxious, these being expressions of humanity, not weakness.

Anxiety is a frequent accompaniment to SOB and uncertainty. It is exacerbated by fears, e.g. that they might forget to breathe during sleep, or that death will be by suffocation, a common misconception that can contribute to panic attacks. Most respiratory patients, if they die from their disease, will do so after lapsing into a coma.

When depression and anxiety coexist, depression may not be recognized, and when it is, this is often accepted as a manifestation of the disease and not addressed, even though depressive symptoms of poor appetite, social isolation, low energy and insomnia can sabotage PR. Insomnia may be reduced by behavioural treatment (Williams *et al* 2013), yoga (Vidyashree *et al* 2013), Pilates (Aparecida 2012) or acupressure (Carotenuto 2013).

Care should be taken with language because the word 'psychological' may be interpreted as psychiatric, and the word 'disabled' is difficult for people who have not thought of themselves in this context. To use emotionally charged words without preparation is like using the word 'stump' to a new amputee without preparation.

Family relationships may be affected by lack of spontaneity because breathless people often cannot waste breath in expressing anxiety, anger, love or happiness. This emotional straightjacket can isolate partners from each other, sometimes worsened by guilt or the bitterness of dependence, and relationships may change during PR (Ashmore 2005). Denial may also complicate relationships, but some level of denial may be a necessary coping strategy.

Relationships with others may require a patient to explain about walking slowly or using oxygen, to ask that adequate time is allowed for speaking, and to find strategies to use if the legitimacy of an invisible condition is doubted.

It is natural for chronically disabled people to harbour resentment at the loss of their dreams. This may be projected onto their family or any of the PR team. Allowing patients to talk gives them an opportunity to understand this process. If there is no outlet, resentment turns inward and can augment depression. People who are depressed usually respond to a receptive ear. Time is always needed when working with troubled people, but this is time well invested by a member of the team with whom the participant feels comfortable.

Self-esteem and sexuality are closely linked, and loss of sexual expression reinforces low confidence. Education can clarify the benefit of building up exercise tolerance, and help discriminate between the effects of myth, illness and drugs on sexual activity. Myths perpetuated by society include the expectation that elderly people cannot have, do not want, or should not want sexual relations, and that disabled people are sexually neutered. The reality is that dyspnoea may limit the duration of kissing, and that during sex it may be useful to have a fan, oxygen and inhalers to hand. Alternative positions may be helpful (App. B). Libido can be affected by steroids, anticholinergics, antihypertensives, theophyllines, antidepressants, sedatives or alcohol, so a drug review may be helpful. Sometimes a partner may think that abstention is in the patient's interest, whereas the opposite may be the case.

Some physiotherapists are comfortable to listen to patients talking about feelings, but referral to other agencies may be required. The relevance of participants' feelings is shown by evidence that attitudes and beliefs bear more relation to exercise tolerance than ventilatory capacity (Morgan *et al* 1983).

Psychological dimensions carry a remarkable weight in the way patients ... face rehabilitation.

Lera 1997

EXERCISE TRAINING

You've gotta be joking ... I can't walk, I can't talk, how do you think I can do exercise?
Patient quoted by Gysels & Higginson (2009)

Patients are usually surprised and gratified that not only can they exercise, they can also build up exercise tolerance and improve their quality of life. This can occur whether exercise is limited by:

- breathlessness
- fear of breathlessness, or
- leg fatigue, which is common in people with COPD (Singer *et al* 2012).

These contribute to a vicious circle of SOB and deconditioning (Fig 9.3). An exercise programme enables patients to extricate themselves from this, but it must show tangible benefits and be designed so that it can be maintained unsupervised at home. Long term commitment is needed because de-training occurs faster than training.

Effects

> ### KEY POINT
>
> *Physical inactivity is the strongest predictor of all-cause mortality in patients with COPD.*
>
> Waschki *et al* 2011

The benefits of exercise for people with normal lungs are well known (Ch. 1). Extra benefits are found for people with respiratory disease:

- ↓ SOB (Gagliardi 2014), ↓ gas trapping (Vogiatzis & Zakynthinos 2013), a more efficient breathing pattern and lower minute volume (Collins *et al* 2001)
- ↑ exercise tolerance and ventricular function (Brønstad *et al* 2013)
- ↑ maximum oxygen uptake for people with asthma (Carson *et al* 2013)
- ↑ balance and QoL, ↓ falls, hypertension, high cholesterol and mortality (Kortianou 2010) potential to attenuate some elements of cachexia (Maddocks 2013)
- ↑ ADL ability, ↓ fatigue, anxiety and depression, ↑ endurance even when training at just 30% of maximum, with no correlation between degree of impairment and degree of improvement (Hodgkin *et al* 2009, p. 131/137/279)
- ↑ cognition due to increased blood flow and neurotransmitter release (Emery *et al* 2001)
- ↓ smoking (Ussher *et al* 2000)
- ↓ risk of chest infection (Karper & Boschen 1993)
- ↓ lung function decline (Garcia-Aymerich 2007).

Mechanism of training

Benefits occur by enhanced oxidative capacity, higher capillary density in muscle and lower ventilatory

---

FIGURE 9.3 Vicious circle that contributes to reduced exercise tolerance in breathless people

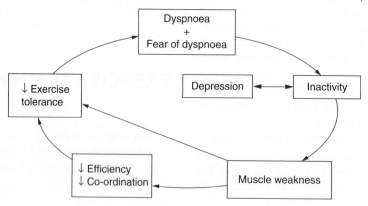

requirements for exercise (Ambrosino 2006). Half of patients with moderate to severe COPD cannot reach their anaerobic threshold (Thirapatarapong et al 2013) and their improved exercise tolerance is thought to be due to greater mechanical skill which reduces the oxygen cost of exercise, a more efficient ventilatory pattern and desensitization to dyspnoea (Cooper 2009).

Safety

Dyspnoea may prevent exercise from stressing the cardiovascular system, but contraindications are on p.254 and safeguards are below (AARC 2001):

- scrutiny of the notes following comprehensive medical screening
- treatment of comorbidities such as anaemia
- drug review, optimum nutrition and fluid intake
- steady exercise with no rushing at the start or finish
- discouragement of competition
- adequate rest, with placement of chairs at intervals
- emphasis on isotonic rather than isometric exercise, to reduce the risks of hypertension, impaired blood flow, and, in COPD, possible muscle damage (Rooyackers et al 2003)
- oximetry to ensure that SpO_2 stays above 90% (Langer et al 2009).

Exercise or exercise testing should be stopped if there is (AARC 2001):

- angina, cyanosis, pallor, cold clammy skin, unusual fatigue, confusion, headache, dizziness, nausea or palpitations
- BP rise to >250 mmHg systolic or >120 diastolic
- failure to raise systolic BP at least 20 mmHg above its resting level
- after the normal rise with exercise, a fall in systolic BP to below pre-exercise level or fall of >20 mmHg
- failure to increase HR
- arrhythmias.

Technique

Strength: capacity of muscle to generate force

Endurance: capacity of muscle to maintain a certain force over time

Even if a conventional training response is not anticipated, the three principles of training are followed:

- overload: intensity must be greater than the muscle's normal load
- specificity: only the specific activities practiced will show improvement.
- reversibility: cessation of training loses the benefit gained.

Endurance training, comprising low-resistance, high-repetition exercise such as walking, forestalls the onset of inefficient anaerobic metabolism and enhances the use of oxygen.

Strength training includes quadriceps exercises and may bring the added benefit of reducing knee pain (Chiu et al 2012), and arm weights which lead to reduced SOB during ADL, especially with unsupported arms (Romagnoli 2013).

Interval training (Brønstad et al 2013) more resembles a patient's ADL, alternating 15–60 second episodes of exercise with rest. This allows exercise to be sustained at an intensity which would otherwise be intolerable and prevents lactic acidosis, along with the extra SOB that this causes. Patients with severe disease can obtain a physiological training effect without ventilatory limitation, leading to a near tripling of the total exercise duration with lower metabolic and ventilatory responses (Kortianou 2010).

Preliminaries

You need to be taught to overcome the fear of exercise.
    Patient quoted by Lewis & Cramp 2010

Participants are reassured that exercise is not synonymous with pumping iron. Inpatients are best dressed in their day clothes, and all participants should have cleared their chests before exercising. Music can be used for pleasure but not as a metronome, and participants often bring their own favourites.

Warming up (Table 9.2) in a group allows participants to enjoy movement for its own sake and helps distract them from preoccupation with their SOB. Five

TABLE 9.2 A selection of warm up and stretching exercises

- Look up slowly, then look down slowly, keeping breathing steady
- Keeping shoulders still, turn head slowly to look over each shoulder
- Facing forward, bring each ear down towards each shoulder
- Roll shoulder girdle up, back, down and forwards, slowly and with a good stretch
- In sitting, raise alternate heels and toes
- With arms crossed and keeping hips facing forwards, turn to each side while breathing out and return to the front while breathing in. Feel the spine stretch. Repeat with hands on shoulders. If sitting, finish by pulling on the back of the chair to get an extra stretch
- In standing or sitting, with hands on hips, push chest forward and shoulders back while breathing in, then relax while breathing out.
- Lock hands, stretch arms forward at shoulder level while breathing out, feel the stretch between shoulder blades, then relax while breathing in
- Bend forwards, breathing out on going down and breathing in on coming up
- Hands on hips, tilt pelvis forwards on breathing in and back on breathing out. Feel stretch in lower back
- In standing, march on the spot, keeping breathing rhythmic
- Hold the back of a chair, stand up on tiptoes. Repeat without holding the chair if possible
- Stretch arm out sideways, then circle in progressively increasing circles, keeping breathing steady. Repeat with other arm
- Reach for the stars with right arm, stretch fingers, then bend to the left so that the arm goes up and over in order to side-flex the trunk. Repeat with other arm
- Hands on shoulders, circle elbows forwards and then backwards
- Sideways walking
- Raise an arm, then bend elbow and drop hand behind back so upper arm feels stretched, then bring hand back down and move it to small of the back. Repeat with other arm
- Breathing out, lunge forward so that the calf of the back leg feels a good stretch. Repeat with other side. Keep near something to hold on to
- Swimming action with arms, in time with breathing

minutes is usually sufficient for respiratory patients, and for those who are severely breathless, warm up may simply mean starting their exercise slowly. Participants are encouraged to maintain rhythmic quality of movement and avoid breath-holding.

Exercise prescription

Four components make up the exercise prescription: mode, intensity, duration and frequency.

The **mode** of exercise depends on the patient. Some prefer the stationary bike or treadmill because they feel in control, can use oxygen easily and have support for their arms. Others enjoy activities that can easily be continued at home such as walking and stair-climbing. Upper limb exercises reduce arm fatigue with ADL (Janaudis & Brooks 2012) and should include

strength and endurance components (McKeough *et al* 2012).

Exercises are best alternated between upper and lower limbs, and those which cause achey muscles and those which cause SOB. Patients are advised to exhale during the most effortful part of an exercise ('blow as you go') such as arm raising (Dolmage *et al* 2013). Balance exercises and fall prevention strategies should be included for people with COPD because of their impaired postural control (Roig *et al* 2012).

Instructions can be pinned to the walls, and participants record their scores and progress on their clipboard, with, if indicated from their assessment, their S_pO_2 or HR. They rest between each exercise until their breathing returns to normal. Table 9.3 provides examples of exercises. Each exercise is continued for between 15 seconds and 2 minutes.

TABLE 9.3 Circuit exercises

- **Biceps curls** – Sitting with elbows supported: lift and lower weight. Repeat with other arm.
- **Leg squats** – With back to wall, slide down the wall while breathing out, breathe in gently, then push back up while breathing out. Progress by increasing depth of squat.
- **Ball** – Throwing and catching in pairs, or bouncing on floor or wall, without breath-holding.
- **Quadriceps exercises** – In sitting, while breathing out, straighten one knee slowly until it is completely straight, hold for count of three while breathing steadily, lower leg slowly. Repeat with other leg. Graduate to weights.
- **Lift ups in sitting** – Push down with both hands and lift pelvis off seat, or just take some weight through arms, then let yourself down slowly.
- **Step ups** – Breathe out, step up with one foot. Breathe in, bring up other foot. Step down with one foot and then the other. Graduate to carrying 'shopping'.
- **Wall press-ups** – Stand with feet shoulder-width apart, put hands on wall, lean forward and bend elbows while breathing out, breathe in gently, then push back while breathing out. Graduate to increasing distance from wall.
- **High knee marching** – Holding back of chair with one hand, lift alternate knees high without breath-holding. Progress to high-knee walking.
- **Arm raise** – Sitting or standing, raise alternate arms above head, with or without weight.
- **Sit to stand** – Using a firm chair, breathe out on standing up, breathe in while standing, breathe out on sitting down. Repeat without using arms of chair. Graduate to holding a ball.
- **Equipment** – Static bike, hula-hoops, trampet, treadmill, gym ball, multigym
- **Pectoral stretch** (Fig 9.4) – Place elbows at shoulder height on either side of a doorway, then lean forward until a stretch (but no pain) is felt across the front of the upper chest. Alter position of elbows as required.

FIGURE 9.4 Pectoral stretch

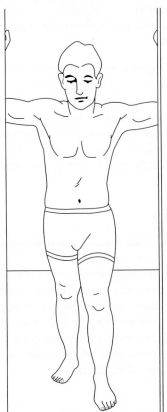

The **intensity** of exercise varies from a laissez-faire 'breathless but not speechless' approach to precise physiological monitoring. Moderate intensity is at 50% of $\dot{V}O_2max$, calculated from a walking test (Langer *et al* 2009), and higher intensity is at 70% (Zainuldin *et al* 2012). Self monitoring can be at 3–5 on the Borg scale (Jenkins *et al* 2011) or grades 2–4 on a Breathless scale (Table 9.4). Short exercise bouts, or sprightly patients, allow higher intensity.

For upper limb resistance training, patients with severe disease may fare best by working at <50% of maximum workload, measured by arm ergometry, because high-intensity exercise can lead to hyperinflation, reduced efficiency and shortened endurance time (Colucci *et al* 2011). For the lower limbs, Langer *et al* (2009) suggest working in 2–5 sets of 8–15 repetitions at 60–80% of 1RM.

The balance of **duration** and **frequency** depends on individual preference because the result is similar if total work is the same and one or both increase.

Supervised training sessions usually last for 30–60 minutes, but for home practice, respiratory patients are advised on up to 15 minutes two-three times a day or >20 minutes once a day (Watchie 2010 p. 304), with a

TABLE 9.4 Breathless scale

Rating 1	Comfortable breathing throughout
Rating 2	During exercise: deeper breathing After exercise: recovery 2–5 minutes Day after exercise: comfortable
Rating 3	During: harder breathing After: recovery 4–7 minutes Day after: comfortable
Rating 4	During: breathless but not speechless After: recovery 5–10 minutes Day after: not tired
Rating 5	During: breathless and speechless After: recovery >10 minutes Day after: tired

brief warm up and cool down, e.g. by slow walking. Patients need to exercise every day except on the days they come for PR, or if they feel ill.

People who tend to rush at their exercise, in an attempt to get it over quickly, may find that counting breaths with their steps helps them to pace themselves in the early stages, e.g.: *in/one out/one*, or *in/one out/one/two*. For others this disturbs their rhythm and distracts them from focusing on awareness of their breathing and level of effort. If a position or breathing technique (Ch. 7) has been found beneficial, individual patients may need reminding of this when getting their breath back.

Some participants find that breathing out against positive pressure during exercise eases their SOB by reducing exercise-induced hyperinflation (Monteiro *et al* 2012). For many this would be impractical, but for some it might enhance motivation. Other accompaniments include biofeedback, hydrotherapy (Jenkins *et al* 2011), non-invasive ventilation and for those unwilling to do active exercise, neuromuscular electrical stimulation (BTS 2013).

Progression

Progression is usually in weekly increments, either by frequency or duration (Hill *et al* 2012), or intensity (Stroescu *et al* 2012). Improvement usually continues for 4–6 months, and when a plateau is reached, moderate exercise should be maintained.

RESPIRATORY MUSCLE TRAINING

The concept that strengthening respiratory muscles would allow a patient to sustain increased exercise tolerance is an attractive one, but does it stand up to scrutiny?

Rationale

The following questions provide an overview of why some patients might benefit. These are followed by more precise evidence on the effects of respiratory muscle training.

Question 1

Respiratory disease can make inspiratory muscles either weaker or stronger than normal. How?

Weak muscles could be due to:

- systemic inflammation as in COPD or bronchiectasis
- poor nutrition (Singer 2012)
- inadequate oxygen delivery to the muscles
- steroid-induced weakness
- inactivity
- mechanical disadvantage, e.g. hyperinflation

Strong muscles could be due to working against the extra resistance of obstructed airways or stiff lungs.

Therefore, for weak inspiratory muscles, the cause should first be addressed when possible, after which respiratory muscle training may be beneficial. Strong inspiratory muscles are less responsive to training (Decramer 2009) and it is probably unnecessary to add a further load.

Question 2

Training can make the diaphragm either more or less susceptible to fatigue. How?

A diaphragm that becomes more susceptible to fatigue after training is thought to have reached maximum adaptability and is at risk of 'overuse atrophy' and muscle damage (Orozco-Levi *et al* 2001). A diaphragm that becomes less susceptible to fatigue after training, in an optimally-managed patient, is in a fit state to adapt to the training stimulus.

Effects

When used appropriately, inspiratory muscle training (IMT) in rested and nourished patients improves inspiratory muscle strength and endurance, but this is only relevant if it relieves SOB, improves exercise tolerance or enhances quality of life. The following outcomes have been reported:

- ↑ exercise capacity compared to exercise training alone (Markovitz & Cooper 2010)
- ↓ SOB in people with COPD (Petrovic *et al* 2012) including very severe COPD (Covey *et al* 2001)
- ↑ QoL (Mikelsons 2008) and ↓ fatigue (Hill *et al* 2007)
- ↓ days in hospital (Beckerman *et al* 2005)
- compensation for steroid-induced (Weiner 1995) or statin-induced (Chatham 2009) respiratory muscle weakness
- for ventilated patients, speedier weaning (Bissett *et al* 2012)
- for people with progressive neurological disease, possible slowing of the decline in respiratory muscle function (Cheah *et al* 2009)
- for people with normal lungs, ↑ VO$_2$max, probably as a result of blunted afferent sensations which reduce the discomfort of exercise at high ventilatory loads (Edwards 2013).

Specifically training the expiratory muscles has shown improved exercise performance in patients with COPD, and in other patients may improve cough and reduce SOB during exercise (Beckerman 2003). It can also strengthen the cough in people with multiple sclerosis (Ch. 3).

Indications and precautions

Most studies have investigated people with COPD (Yoshimi *et al* 2012), but benefits have been reported for people with CF (Enright *et al* 2004), asthma (Gomieiro 2011), restrictive lung disease (Chatham 2000), heart failure (Ch. 12) and those having surgery (Ch. 16). Patients likely to respond are those who:

- find breathing re-education difficult, in which case using the device might familiarize them to an altered breathing pattern, before progressing to self-regulation of breathing

- are fearful of exercise or unable to take up PR, in which case IMT can be used to desensitize them to breathlessness prior to venturing into exercise training
- are unable to participate fully in whole-body exercise training for other reasons (Simms *et al* 2011), e.g. prior to lung surgery (Benzo 2011) while awaiting transplantation (Janssen *et al* 2010), recovering from injury (Chatham 2000) or when activity is limited by arthritis, cancer (McConnell 2005), obesity (Edwards *et al* 2012), spinal cord injury (Russian 2011) or old age (Copestake & McConnell 1994).

A history of spontaneous pneumothorax is a relative contraindication (McConnell 2005).

Technique

A pressure-threshold device (Fig 9.5) incorporates a spring-loaded one-way valve which allows patients to exhale without resistance, but requires them to reach a pre-set load to inhale, set at a percentage of their maximum inspiratory pressure (MIP) (Ch. 2). In the UK the PowerBreathe (App. A) is available on prescription.

As with systemic training, exercise should be alternated with rest, and distressing levels of fatigue avoided. For strength training, the target is generally

---

FIGURE 9.5 Inspiratory muscle trainer (PowerBreathe)

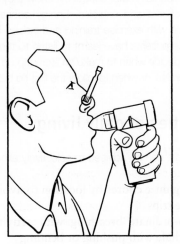

>30% of an individual's MIP (Myrrha *et al* 2013). If the aim is desensitization to breathlessness, resistance should be at a level that leaves the patient more breathless than normal but not speechless. If they are able, patients should work at different volumes to prevent muscle fatigue, but hyperinflation should be avoided. Oxygen can be delivered by nasal cannula if required.

Training should be at least daily (McConnell 2005) and preferably little and often, e.g. from about 5 minutes b.d. to about 15 minutes t.d.s. Interval training has produced the highest training loads and led to a greater sense of mastery (Hill *et al* 2006). Excessive overloading, as reported by patient discomfort, should be avoided in people with COPD (Puente-Maestu *et al* 2012).

When patients have mastered the art, IMT can be combined with watching TV or reading. It must be maintained once a plateau is reached (Weiner *et al* 2004), assisted by training diaries (App. C). For patients who find IMT boring, swimming has shown similar improvements in respiratory muscle strength (Santos *et al* 2012).

ENERGY CONSERVATION

> They tell you: 'Don't use a towel, use a towelling dressing gown', it's fantastic, it's such a simple thing.
> Patient quoted by Gysels & Higginson (2009)

Strategies to conserve energy tend to be used in the later stages of disease, but they are best taught early to give participants greater control over how they achieve a balance of rest and exercise. Energy conservation is compatible with exercise training and indeed is integral to it. Once patients have learnt to listen to their bodies, they can decide when to make an extra trip up the stairs as an exercise, or when to follow the first tip below.

Activities of daily living

Participants can be advised to selectively allocate their energy, e.g.:

- organize chores by location to avoid multiple trips
- co-ordinate breathing with activities, e.g. exhale with pushing or bending

- move smoothly, avoid extraneous movements or breath-holding
- prioritize activities, plan in advance, use pacing and work in stages
- notice where there is muscle tension and release it
- organize work space to reduce clutter and minimize reaching and bending
- keep heavy items on worktops; slide rather than lift them
- prepare large one-dish meals and freeze leftovers to use on breathless days
- soak washing up; drain dishes instead of towel-drying
- use a stool in the kitchen and bathroom; rest elbows on worktop or basin
- reduce bending by crossing one leg over the other to put on socks, trousers and shoes
- use pacing on stairs
- place chairs at strategic locations
- use pursed lips breathing for upper limb activities (Fig 9.6)
- use a rollator rather than a zimmer frame because the latter destabilizes the accessory muscles and requires twice the $\dot{V}O_2$ (Foley *et al* 1996), or use other energy-efficient walking aids (Fig 9.7).

FIGURE 9.6 Pursed lips breathing while doing unsupported upper limb activities

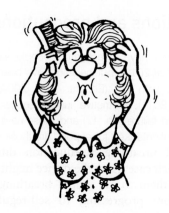

FIGURE 9.7 Rollator for efficient mobility (Vaes *et al* 2012)

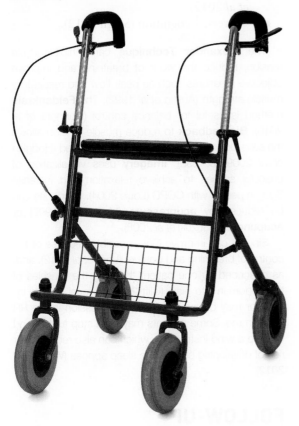

FIGURE 9.8 Energy conservation in the shower (Ries *et al* 2001)

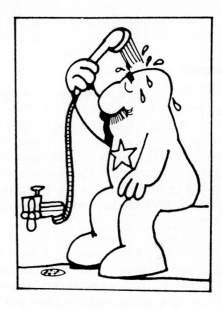

tried to counteract fatigue with prolonged rest, which tends to promote fatigue (Radbruch 2008).

Stress reduction

> *Voluntary control of respiration is perhaps the oldest stress-reduction technique known. It has been used for thousands of years to reduce anxiety and promote a generalized state of relaxation.*
>
> Everly 1989

Individuals vary:

- some may find it more important to use their energy to get to the shops than to be independent with dressing
- some prefer to sleep downstairs rather than suffer the 'stigma' of a stairlift
- some find sitting in a shower (Fig 9.8) easier than using a bath, while others find that water on their face upsets their breathing
- some are not happy to have their spouse bathe them.

Participants can share their own strategies such as using inconspicuous 'puffing stations' during shopping trips or leaning on shopping trolleys. Activity analysis with the occupational therapist helps break down their ADL and identify problem areas. Many patients have

Stress is physiologically detrimental (Ch. 1), and putting a tense person through a physical training programme without advice on stress management is silly. People with chronic lung disease suffer muscle tension from breathlessness and the body positions needed to ease their breathing. A continually active muscle such as the diaphragm is in particular need of relative relaxation by returning to its resting position after contraction, especially when it is being overused as in hyperinflation. Some patients have become accustomed to muscle tension as their default position and forget how it feels to be relaxed. Stress is reduced by education, occupational therapy and the measures below.

I was amazed how [relaxing my shoulders] had this calming effect ... it helps my lungs to expand.

Patient quoted by Wood et al (2013)

Relaxation

Relaxation (Payne 2010) should be taught early and re-inforced throughout, often in brief snippets. Daily practice is then needed until the sensation is appreciated and the skill mastered, whereupon a degree of relaxation is integrated into everyday life by identifying stressful situations and practicing in different positions. Even walking can be maintained in a way that does not waste energy. Spot checks during the day identify body tension.

Relaxation can be achieved in other ways, e.g. jigsaws or watching a lighted aquarium at night. Even looking at views of nature can reduce BP (Gladwell et al 2012). Activities such as circle dancing provide rhythmic exercise with a meditative effect and also emphasize trunk rotation, posture and balance. Patients who have spent their working lives with the forward head postures associated with computer work may require extra attention (Kang et al 2012).

The best way to still the mind is to move the body.

Roth 1990

Complementary therapies

Complementary therapies may help ease SOB and stress. It is useful to have some knowledge of effective local resources for participants who request this information.

Described as 'cosmic rehabilitation' (Gilbert 1999b), **yoga** incorporates breathing techniques, meditation and postures that consume minimal energy and induce the physiological effects of deep relaxation. It can increase adherence to exercise (Bryan 2012), reduce stress (Chong et al 2011), build bone mineral density (Fishman 2009) and reduce the distress of SOB in people with COPD (Donesky et al 2009). Meditation has shown the following benefits:

- ↑ exercise capacity compared to exercise training alone (Markovitz & Cooper 2010)

- ↓ depression and insomnia (Thompson 2009)
- ↓ respiratory rate, HR and BP (Melville et al 2012)
- ↓ stress, ↑ cognition (Singh 2012).

The **Alexander Technique** can inhibit muscle tension, reduce the work of breathing and improve objective measures such as peak flow and respiratory muscle strength (Austin et al 1992). The **Feldenkrais** method is useful for balance control (Connors et al 2010). **Biofeedback** to reduce muscle tension allows the sensation to be recognized and controlled (Hodgkin et al 2009, p. 230). **Imagery** uses visualization of peaceful scenes to achieve relaxation and increase S_pO_2 in people with COPD (Louie 2004). Dyspnoea can be reduced by **acupressure** (Maa et al 1997) or **acupuncture** (Suzuki et al 2008).

Singing can improve QoL, possibly because of the control of breathing and posture (Lord et al 2012), and, as described by one patient 'bringing the muscles of the abdomen into play' (Clift 2013). A local singing instructor may be available to take a session in the PR programme. Some patients may go a step further and take up a wind instrument, which can also reduce their risk of developing obstructive sleep apnoea (Ward et al 2012).

FOLLOW-UP

Wellbeing needs to be understood not as the end point, but as a precarious balance needing skilful maintenance and hard work.

Gysels & Higginson (2009)

A follow-up self-management programme has shown:

- a universally positive attitude towards exercise (Spencer 2013)
- maintenance of improved exercise tolerance (Soysa *et al* 2012)
- ↓ hospital admissions and SOB, ↑ QoL (Lomundal 2012).

Maintenance needs to be stressed at the start of PR because detraining occurs quicker than training. Some supervised training is best continued for a period after the initial programme, if possible, to prevent demotivation. Thereafter, follow-up in patients' homes, or by phone, newsletter or further training sessions, may be needed, three- and then six-monthly.

Motivation is helped by addressing depression (Heerema *et al* 2013) and by individuals choosing their own form of exercise, e.g. interactive exercise (Albores 2013), dance (Mejia-Downs 2011), T'ai Chi, which can reduce the distress of dyspnoea (Norweg & Collins 2013), hydrotherapy (Shead 2012), paced music (Ho *et al* 2012) or walking with pedometers (Houchen *et al* 2012). Patients may not realize how hard they are working if their exercise is enjoyable and distracting, e.g. bowling or Wii bowling.

Other motivators are a flexible routine (Effing 2012), home diary, metronome (Pomidori *et al* 2012), and either telehealth technology (Holland 2013) or home visits, which provide the opportunity to check for safety hazards and provide support for the family: a spouse may be stressed, neglect their own health, feel guilty or fearful of sleeping lest their partner die at night.

Urban patients are advised to choose the least polluted times and places for outdoor exercise. Those who walk by the sea usually find that they breathe easier when the tide is coming in than going out. For leisure centres, fitness instructors can be reassured that patients bringing oxygen are responsible for this, as with any other drug.

Half-an-hour of exercise five times a week is advised (BTS 2013). Once a week, participants should put themselves back on the same programme as on the final day of their training. If this is difficult, they have lost fitness and will need to increase their maintenance exercise. If training is interrupted by illness, their programme is restarted at a lower level. Attending a further PR programme may be considered if resources allow (BTS 2013).

The mutual support that develops between participants during PR may become one of its most enduring assets, and patients often prefer ongoing exercise with their peers, sometimes in a structured environment, without the embarrassment of a public setting (Hogg *et al* 2012). This support can be built into self-help groups using Breathe Easy (App. B) or peer outreach when patients are visited by volunteers with lung disease. Social outings together are particularly supportive for people who do not like to be seen in public with their oxygen.

OUTCOMES

Evaluation of rehabilitation should be embedded from the start and can include the following:

- number of participants completing the programme
- daily activity, e.g. by using an accelerometer (Gorzelniak et al 2012) and home exercise diaries
- return to hobbies or job
- smoking cessation
- weight ↑ or ↓ as appropriate
- patient satisfaction (BTS 2013)
- wellbeing of carers
- sustained improvement in exercise tolerance
- ↓ GP visits or admissions to hospital (Fig 9.9).

The scales and exercise tests on p.255–6 can be used for outcomes. Measures to identify behaviour change are the Obstacles to Exercise Survey and the

FIGURE 9.9 Number of days spent in hospital before and after pulmonary rehabilitation

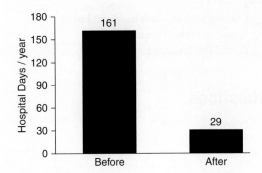

Self-efficacy to Exercise Scale (Artistico *et al* 2013). Follow up benefit can be measured by the Nijmegen Clinical Screening Instrument, a short online questionnaire which includes an automated monitoring system (Vercoulen 2012) or the use of activity monitors and video clips (Lareau 2006) which demonstrate flexibility, posture and gait.

It is hoped that an abiding legacy of the programme is the friendship and courage that participants give each other. For those labouring under the double burden of disease and ageing, the outcome should be a more optimistic attitude towards a life that can be both active and fulfilling.

> *I'm thankful that I have one leg,*
> *to limp is no disgrace.*
> *Although I can't be number one*
> *I still can run the race.*
>   Hart quoted by deLateur (1997)

CASE STUDY: Mr EH

Identify the problems of this 66 y.o. man with COPD from Medellin who was referred as an outpatient after disappointment following rejection for transplantation. Then implement a treatment plan.

Background
- **Social history:** lives with wife, first floor flat with lift.
- **Drugs:** bronchodilators, steroids, diuretics.
- **History of present complaint:** Recent admission for exacerbation, discharged with home oxygen, making slow recovery.

Subjective
- Can't do much since leaving hospital. Able to look after self. Unable to walk any useful distance. Don't go out. Unable to help in house or with shopping. Poor sleep since hospital. Not hungry. Don't use oxygen much. No phlegm.

Objective
- Leaning forward with hands on knees.
- Speaking in short sentences.
- Pursed lips breathing.

Questions
1 Analysis?
2 Problems?

CLINICAL REASONING

Do we need to read further than the title of the following article?
Preoperative pulmonary rehabilitation versus chest physical therapy in patients undergoing lung cancer resection: a pilot randomized controlled trial.

Arch Phys Med Rehabil (2013), 94, 1, 53-58

Response to Case Study

1 Analysis
   - Loss of confidence and exercise tolerance since discharge.
   - Lack of sleep and appetite may relate to depression, possibly triggered by rejection for transplantation and contributing to vicious circle of inactivity.

2 Problems
   - Breathlessness.
   - Inefficient breathing pattern.
   - ↓ exercise tolerance.
   - Possible depression.
   - Misuse of oxygen.

3 Goals
   - Short term: daily walk to bandstand.
   - Medium term: return to pre-admission function including steps up to front door.
   - Long term: lifelong exercise programme.

4 Plan
   - Obtain further information from patient on fluids, nutrition, assessment for oxygen therapy and limitations to exercise tolerance (e.g. anxiety, SOB, deconditioning).
   - Identify cause of poor sleep, discuss possible depression, liaise with multidisciplinary team.
   - If oxygen is indicated, educate Mr H on its use. Check knowledge of medication. Provide information on pulmonary rehabilitation.
   - If patient declines PR, refer to dietician for nutritional advice, educate on SOB and exercise, initiate written daily exercise programme, follow up in a week to maintain motivation, then monthly, then six-monthly reviews.

Response to Clinical Reasoning

Pulmonary rehabilitation and 'chest physical therapy' (chest clearance) are for different problems.

RECOMMENDED READING

Afolabi G, Stevens R, Turner M *et al* (2013) Development of a pulmonary rehabilitation service for people with COPD. *J Cardiopulm Rehab Prev;* **33**(5): 323–7

Apps LD, Mitchell KE, Harrison SL *et al* (2013) The development and pilot testing of the Self-management programme of activity, coping and education for COPD. *Int J Chron Obstruct Pulmon Dis;* **8**: 317–27.

Beekman E (2013) Course length of 30 metres versus 10 metres has a significant influence on six-minute walk distance in patients with COPD. *J Physiother;* **59**(3): 169–176

Castro AA, Porto EF, Iamonti VC (2013) Oxygen and ventilatory output during several activities of daily living performed by COPD patients stratified according to disease severity. *PLoS One;* **8**(11): e79727

Dassios T (2013) Aerobic exercise and respiratory muscle strength in patients with cystic fibrosis. *Respir Med;* **107**(5): 684–90

Garvey C (2013) Pulmonary rehabilitation exercise prescription in COPD. *J Cardiopulm Rehab Prev;* **33**(5): 314–22

Gillespie P, O'Shea E, Casey D *et al* (2013) The cost-effectiveness of a structured education pulmonary rehabilitation programme for chronic obstructive pulmonary disease in primary care. *BMJ Open;* **3**(11): e003479

Gupta SS, Sawane MV (2012) A comparative study of the effects of yoga and swimming on pulmonary functions in sedentary subjects. *Int J Yoga;* **5**(2): 128–33

Harrison SL (2013) Physical activity monitoring: addressing the difficulties of accurately detecting slow walking speeds. *Heart Lung;* **42**(4): 361–364

Heerema-Poelman A, Stuive I, Wempe JB (2013) Adherence to a maintenance exercise program 1 year after pulmonary rehabilitation. *J Cardiopulm Rehabil Prev;* **33**(6): 419–26

Holland AE, Wadell K, Spruit MA (2013) How to adapt the pulmonary rehabilitation programme to patients with chronic respiratory disease other than COPD. *Eur Respir Rev;* **22**(130): 577–86

Jörres RA, Nowak D, Ochmann U (2012) Long-term efficacy of pulmonary rehabilitation: a state-of-the-art review. *J Cardiopulm Rehab Prev;* **32**(3): 117–126

Kovelis D, Zabatiero J, Furlanetto J (2012) Short-term effects of using pedometers to increase daily physical activity in smokers. *Respir Care;* **57**(7): 1089–97

Lan C-C (2013) Benefits of pulmonary rehabilitation in patients with COPD and normal exercise capacity. *Respir Care;* **58**(9): 1482–8

Markovitz GH, Cooper CB (2010) Mechanisms of exercise limitation and pulmonary rehabilitation for patients with pulmonary fibrosis/restrictive lung disease. *Chr Respir Dis;* **7**(1): 47–60

Moy ML, Weston NA, Wilson EJ *et al* (2013) A pilot study of an Internet walking program and pedometer in COPD. *Respir Med;* **106**(9): 1342–50

Osthoff AR (2013) Association between peripheral muscle strength and daily physical activity in patients with COPD. *J Cardiopulm Rehab Prev;* **33**(6): 351–9

Reid WD, Yamabayashi C, Goodridge D *et al* (2012) Exercise prescription for hospitalized people with COPD and comorbidities. *Int J Chron Obstruct Pulmon Dis;* **7**: 297–320

Shirreffs SM (2007) Milk as an effective post-exercise rehydration drink. *Br J Nutr;* **98**(1): 173–80

Spruit MA, Singh SJ (2013) Maintenance programs after pulmonary rehabilitation. *Chest;* **144**(4): 1091–3

Spruit MA, Singh SJ, Garvey C *et al* (2013) An official ATS/ERS statement: key concepts and advances in pulmonary rehabilitation. *Am J Respir Crit Care Med;* **188**(8): e13–e64

Suler Y, Dinescu LI (2013) Safety considerations during cardiac and pulmonary rehabilitation program. *Phys Med Rehabil Clin N Am;* **23**(2): 433–40

Wardini R, Dajczman E, Yang N *et al* (2013) Using a virtual game system to innovate pulmonary rehabilitation: safety, adherence and enjoyment in severe COPD. *Can Respir J;* **20**(5): 357–61

Zhang C (2013) Development and validation of a COPD self-management scale. *Respir Care;* **58**(11)

PART III PHYSIOTHERAPY FOR SPECIFIC GROUPS OF PEOPLE

PART III
PHYSIOTHERAPY FOR SPECIFIC GROUPS OF PEOPLE

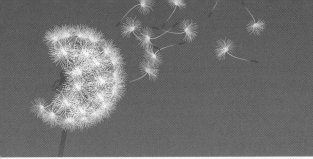

CHAPTER 10
Physiotherapy for Infants

LEARNING OBJECTIVES

On completion of this chapter the reader should be able to:

- describe the anatomical and physiological differences between adults and infants

- discuss the common medical and surgical conditions of infants

- understand the principles of care for infants on a neonatal ICU

- identify the main physiotherapy problems in relation to neonatal conditions, and describe their management.

INTRODUCTION

Central to a baby's universe is his or her mother, and physical separation is recognized by the baby from birth (Nagasawa *et al* 2012), leading to possible neural dysfunction in later life (Wieck *et al* 2013). Babies need to hear and feel their mother, and parents need to be involved in the care and comfort of their baby. Handling by health staff can destabilize preterm infants, but stroking and gentle handling have shown beneficial effects (Harrison 1996) while handling by the mother can reduce stress and oxygen consumption (Ludington 1990).

Premature infants are those born before 37 weeks' gestation. Neonates are preterm or term infants from birth to the age of 28 days of postnatal life. Infants are children under one year old.

Anatomical and physiological considerations

Infants are not small adults. Changes are more abrupt than in adults because of their different cardiorespiratory functioning:

1   The respiratory rate (RR) of infants and children has an extensive range that is more responsive to disease and emotion than in adults. Irregular breathing and occasional periods of apnoea may occur, which if frequent and combined with prematurity are the 'perfect storm' of tissue injury (Di Fiore 2013).

2   Work of breathing (WOB) is two to three times that of adults (Hoffman 1995).

Physiological reasons are immature inter-costal muscles, cartilaginous and horizontal ribs, under-compliant lungs and an over-compliant ribcage that is easily sucked in (Robinson 2012), leaving the diaphragm to do most of the work (Button 2005).

3 Anatomical reasons for increased WOB include narrow airways so that broncho-spasm, oedema or secretions lead to a disproportionate increase in airway resistance. Peripherally, the narrow airways leave infants and young children prone to obstructive diseases such as bronchiolitis. Proximally, the relatively large tonsils, adenoids and tongue contribute to upper airway obstruction.

4 Babies are preferential nose breathers and the mouth is normally reserved for ingestion, exploration and communication (Trabalon & Schaal 2012). Nasal secretions or a nasogastric tube can significantly increase the WOB (Schechter 2007) and may leave the mouth as the sole passage for breathing.

5 A tendency to atelectasis is caused by lack of collateral ventilation until age two to three, and a functional residual capacity (FRC) that is sometimes below closing volume due to the compliant ribcage and immature respiratory control (Primhak & Kingshott 2012).

6 In side-lying, the compliant ribcage increases the difficulty of expanding the dependent lung, leading to inspired air preferentially ventilating the uppermost lung regions, reversing the ventilation gradient that occurs in healthy adults (Ch. 1). However, this is variable (Frerichs et al 2003) and it is best to rely on the S_pO_2 when positioning an infant.

7 Response to heavy workloads is an increased rate rather than depth of breathing.

8 Hypoxaemia tends to cause bradycardia rather than tachycardia, leading to reduced cardiac output (Barrington 2011).

9 Blood pressure (BP) regulation is unrefined (Gao & Raj 2010).

10 Preterm infants are at extra risk of atelectasis because the surfactant system does not mature until 35 weeks' gestation.

Prematurity

The emergence of the baby into the outside world is perhaps the most cataclysmic event of his or her life.
West (2012) p.155

The full-term neonate is biological work in progress, but premature babies have the added shock of being displaced foetuses and experiencing heightened responses to stimuli (Honda 2013). Prematurity leaves them with limited defence mechanisms and sometimes without the basic capacity for respiration or temperature control. Of infants born at <32 weeks gestational age or weighing <1500 g, approximately 10% have motor deficits and up to 60% have cognitive disabilities (Selip et al 2012). The sequelae for the lowest birth weight preterms appear to be lifelong (Saigal et al 2000), particularly cardiorespiratory morbidity (Nanduri 2013) including asthma in later life (Wilmott 2014).

Prematurity is increasing in prevalence (Heaman et al 2013). The lower the gestational age, the more keenly sensitive are preterms to their environment, including their mother's pain during labour (Thistlewood 1988). The more premature the baby, the more beneficial is skin-to-skin contact (Mörelius et al 2012).

Care of the family

I longed as I have never longed for anything so badly, to hold her... to whisper that I was here, that it was all right ... Feeling her minute pink fingers holding so hard to mine, I was hit sideways and bowled over by the purest, tenderest, most passionately committed love I have ever felt ...
I couldn't bear to not be able to help her myself ... I wanted to pick her up and hold her to my breast, even if it meant that she died in a few minutes. That would be better

> *than having her suffer the pain, fear, noise, bewilderment . . .*
>
> *Every time I touched her, she relaxed and the monitors showed it, her heart rate set- tled, her limbs were calmer, her eyes searched less frantically about . . .*
>
> *I had never held her to me and I ached to do so, she seemed so alone in there amongst all the wires and drips and tubes and monitors.*
>
> Hill (1989)

Parents need to be involved in all aspects of care in order to reduce the helplessness that is one of the greatest stresses for parents (Matricardi *et al* 2013) and to help avoid the 'medicalization of parenting'. Parental presence during invasive procedures is rec- ommended, and, with support, during resuscitation, if acceptable to the parent (Curley *et al* 2013). Parents require confidence in their own competence and acknowledgement that they are the experts on their children. Unrestricted visiting should include grandpar- ents and siblings. Siblings require involvement because they may feel a variety of responses including jealousy, anxiety, isolation and guilt. If their brother or sister is disabled, they are likely to suffer bullying at school.

MEDICAL CONDITIONS

Meconium aspiration syndrome

Infants who suffer distress in utero or asphyxia during labour or Caesarian section (Swarnam *et al* 2012), may pass meconium (faecal material) before birth, then gasp and suck it into their mouth. Meconium aspiration occurs when this is inhaled into the lungs. Meconium aspiration syndrome is when this sets up a chemical pneumonitis, causing alveolar inflammation, surfactant depletion and epithelial injury. This leads to hypoxae- mia, poor lung compliance and sometimes pneumo- thorax. Airflow obstruction causes hyperinflation if incomplete, and atelectasis if complete.

Supplemental oxygen is required, and, although oro- pharyngeal suction compromises a normal baby at birth (Graves & Haley 2013), suction of the mouth and nose is needed if sticky meconium needs removal. A non- vigorous infant requires continuous positive airway pres-

sure (CPAP) or mechanical ventilation (MV) (Maayan- Metzger *et al* 2013), sometimes with high pressures to ventilate the stiff lungs. Inhaled surfactant may be required (AARC 2013b) or extracorporeal membrane oxygenation (ECMO) (Swarnam 2012) to allow the lungs to recover with less risk of barotrauma. Most infants survive without complications (Dargaville 2012).

If caught early, physiotherapy can clear the fresh meconium by intensive postural drainage, percussion, vibrations, saline instillation and suction. This is contin- ued until secretions are free from the dark colour of meconium. Bronchoalveolar lavage (BAL) may be used to clear the debris (Hahn *et al* 2013).

Persistent pulmonary hypertension of the new-born

In utero, a high pulmonary vascular resistance shunts blood away from the lungs through the ductus arterio- sus. After birth, the pulmonary circulation dilates within a few breaths, enabling oxygen to enter the bloodstream so that the placental circulation becomes redundant. If the pulmonary circulation does not dilate, the pressure in the lungs remains high and the ductus arteriosus stays open, shunting blood away from the lungs through the patent foramen ovale and ductus arteriosus, leading to profound and unremitting hypoxaemia.

Risk factors are birth asphyxia, an obese or diabetic mother and some medications (Delaney & Cornfield 2012). Signs are cyanosis, tachypnoea, respiratory dis- tress, hypoxaemia and tachycardia. Medical manage- ment is aimed at improving oxygenation, reducing pulmonary vasoconstriction and optimizing circulation, sometimes with ECMO (Rocha *et al* 2012).

Intraventricular haemorrhage

Prematurity may cause bleeding into the cerebral ven- tricles due to swings in BP or arterial blood gases. Pre- cipitating factors are pain (Mainous & Looney 2007), intubation without sedation (Wren 1989) and MV (Aly 2012). Physiotherapy is contraindicated, including suc- tion unless essential.

Pulmonary haemorrhage

Pulmonary haemorrhage is an acute, often cata- strophic event in which bleeding may involve more than a third of the lungs, sometimes spreading to other areas (Zahr 2012). Causes are prematurity, birth asphyxia, bleeding disorders, toxaemia of pregnancy, breech birth, hypothermia, infection, respiratory distress syndrome or interventions such as surfactant inhalation or ECMO. Management includes immediate suction, oxygen and MV with high airway pressures to inhibit the bleed. Physiotherapy is contraindicated.

Respiratory distress syndrome

Respiratory distress syndrome (RDS), also known as hyaline membrane disease, may occur in premature infants, especially if delivered by Caesarean section, and is the commonest cause of death in the preterm infant (Smart & Princivalle 2012). Lack of surfactant leads to patchy atelectasis, stiff lungs and increased WOB. Alveoli inflate with difficulty and collapse between respiratory efforts.

Signs of respiratory distress develop in the first hours of life. Reduced breath sounds are heard on auscultation, along with diffuse fine crackles. The chest x-ray shows hyperinflation, mottling and air bronchograms. Respiratory distress may persist for 24–48 hours, followed by improvement over several days as surfactant is produced, or protracted disease.

Prevention is by prophylactic instillation of artificial surfactant on delivery of preterm babies, administered in different positions to ensure even distribution (Rojas-Reyes 2012).

Management is by regulation of temperature, fluid and nutrition, and respiratory support using oxygen, CPAP, non-invasive ventilation or MV (Ramanathan 2012). Both oxygen and MV come with their own complications: oxidative stress predisposes to chronic lung disease of prematurity (Chakraborty 2010), high pressure ventilation in surfactant-deficient alveoli can lead to atelectrauma, and high tidal volumes can cause barotrauma.

Physiotherapy is limited to advice on positioning in the early stages. Periods in alternate side-lying assist secretion mobilization and postural orientation, with the head of the incubator raised to minimize reflux. Prone improves oxygenation (Gillies *et al* 2012). Intubation irritates the airways and may stimulate excess secretions, which need to be cleared in the recovery phase when the infant is stable, usually with suction and occasionally with percussion. Monitoring should be continuous because deterioration can be sudden.

Chronic lung disease of prematurity (CLD)

With prematurity comes the risk of a continuum of lung injury, progressing from RDS, pulmonary interstitial emphysema (PIE) (Ch. 17), oxygen toxicity and then CLD, also known as bronchopulmonary dysplasia. The process is exacerbated by the interaction of immature lungs with high volume MV, but the risk is reduced with bubble nasal CPAP, early surfactant treatment and rapid extubation (Friedman *et al* 2013).

Inflammation is the core process, interfering with surfactant production and leading to scarring, disordered lung growth, stiff lungs and pulmonary hypertension (Del Cerro *et al* 2014). Signs are persistent respiratory distress and high oxygen requirements. X-ray changes vary from 'grey' lungs to widespread cystic areas interspersed with collapse (Agrons 2005).

Support is by lung protective ventilation using minimal volumes. Treatment is by steroids (Cheong 2013), targeted S_pO_2, caffeine, vitamin A and optimum nutrition (Tropea 2012).

The damaged lungs are prone to recurrent infection and atelectasis, for which physiotherapy is usually indicated, preceded by bronchodilators if required. This includes alternate side-lying with the head elevated, percussion, vibrations and suction. Manual hyperinflation may be required if atelectasis is present in an intubated baby. Treatment should be modified or discontinued if the child becomes wheezy or develops pulmonary hypertension.

After long hospitalization, parents need comprehensive preparation for discharge so that they build up confidence and do not feel that they have 'borrowed' their baby to take home. Domiciliary oxygen or non-invasive ventilation may be required, and sometimes advice on physiotherapy. The lungs repair as they grow, but survivors may enter adulthood with suboptimal lung function (Marlow 2014) and low exercise tolerance (Tsopanoglou *et al* 2014).

Bronchiolitis

Acute viral bronchiolitis is the most common disorder and the leading cause of respiratory failure in infants under 2 years old, with respiratory syncytial virus (RSV) being the main culprit (Postiaux *et al* 2013). Infants born prematurely or those with conditions such as congenital heart disease or immunodeficiency may develop severe disease. Respiratory syncytial virus (RSV) is responsible for 80% of cases (Anil *et al* 2010).

The infection depletes the mucous layer water content, damages epithelial architecture and impairs mucociliary clearance. Sputum retention and mucosal oedema lead to airway obstruction and hyperinflation. Signs are excess oral secretions, wheeze, fine crackles, nasal congestion and breathlessness. Air trapping may prevent sternal recession, unlike croup or pneumonia. Admission to hospital is required if the infant is too breathless to feed or manage a cough, or has a RR >50/min (SIGN 2006).

Treatment is by maintenance of the head-up position, environmental temperature regulation, hydration, assisted feeding, minimal handling, and oxygenation by humidified oxygen therapy, high-flow nasal cannulae (Da Dalt *et al* 2013) or CPAP (Essouri *et al* 2014). If associated with recurrent apnoea or exhaustion, non-invasive or invasive ventilation may be required. Antibiotics are only effective if there are bacterial complications (Postiaux *et al* 2013).

Nebulised hypertonic saline reduces oedema by osmotic action on the submucosa (Postiaux *et al* 2013). Normal saline nebulized half-hourly has shown swift improvement in mild disease (Anil *et al* 2010). The acute illness subsides in approximately a week, with recovery over two to three weeks, but over 50% of infants experience recurrent cough and wheeze (Midulla *et al* 2012).

Physiotherapy is not recommended in the acute stage because of the risk of desaturation, wheeze or vomiting (Roqué *et al* 2012). If sputum retention is a problem, however, an experienced physiotherapist can sometimes coax the secretions mouthwards using judicious percussion and vibrations in alternate side-lying, while monitoring closely.

There is no evidence that nasopharyngeal suction is required for spontaneously breathing infants, apart from maintaining patent nostrils to aid nose breathing (Mallory 2003). Deep suctioning has been associated with longer hospital stay (Mussman 2013).

Tracheobronchomalacia

Repeated upper airway infections or prolonged intubation can lead to softened airway cartilages, causing a cough, harsh wheeze, chest recession and sputum retention (Tan *et al* 2012), especially with increased workload such as crying, feeding, pain or discomfort. Often the first sign is inability to wean from MV. Protracted ventilatory support and tracheostomy may be needed until the infant grows and the airway enlarges. If physiotherapy is required, positive pressure in the airway must be maintained to minimize airway collapse, unless a stent has been inserted.

SURGICAL CONDITIONS

Congenital heart disease (CHD)

CHD is the most common congenital condition in infants, but it may be missed after birth and routine oximetry has been advised (Ewer 2014). Classification is according to whether the baby is blue or not (Table 10.1), cyanosis indicating that 30–40% of the blood supply is shunted from the right to left heart without passing through the lungs. Other features are compression atelectasis from an enlarged heart

TABLE 10.1 Non cyanotic and cyanotic congenital heart disease

Acyanotic defects	Cyanotic defects
Ventricular septal defect (VSD)	Fallots tetralogy
Atrial septal defect (ASD)	Transposition of the great arteries (TGA)
Patent ductus arteriosus (PDA)	Tricuspid atresia
Aortic stenosis	Total anomalous pulmonary venous drainage
Pulmonary stenosis	Truncus arteriosus (may be acyanotic)
Coarctation of the aorta	Pulmonary atresia with VSD
Atrioventricular septal defect	Pulmonary atresia with intact ventricular septum
Aorto-pulmonary window	Hypoplastic left heart syndrome
Partial anomalous pulmonary venous drainage	Ebstein's anomaly of the tricuspid valve

(Healy *et al* 2012), pulmonary oedema and, later, exercise intolerance. Over 90% of patients survive to adulthood (Zomer 2013), but neurodevelopmental problems become apparent by school age in up to half the children (Raheem 2012).

Some defects require surgery immediately. Staged surgery may be needed throughout life, including transplantation (Stewart & Mayer 2014). Trauma from surgical repair may include:

- damage to the recurrent laryngeal nerve, leading to a weak cough, hoarse voice, difficulty weaning from MV and vocal cord palsy (Sachdeva *et al* 2007)
- damage to the phrenic nerve, causing unilateral diaphragmatic palsy (Sanchez de Toledo *et al* 2010), which may require surgery to take tucks in the diaphragm (plication).

Physiotherapy precautions are the following:

1 The target saturation should be ascertained before treatment.
2 Robust analgesia is required (see below) e.g. neuraxial drugs added to local anaesthesia around the nerves of the central nervous system, which has shown improved outcomes (Walker 2012).
3 Newly diagnosed infants with TGA are on a drug called dinoprostone (Prostin) to maintain a patent ductus arteriosus. The antagonist to this drug is oxygen, so medical staff should be consulted before F_iO_2 is increased as this may cause the duct to close.
4 Pulmonary vasoconstriction can cause right to left shunt and hypoxaemia (Moudgil 2005). Supplemental oxygen may be required, but it can upset the balance between pulmonary and systemic blood flow (AARC 2002b). Pre/postoperative S_pO_2 levels will be specified for each child.
5 Infants can desaturate spectacularly and without warning if they become stressed.

Congenital diaphragmatic hernia

In around 1:3,000 births the diaphragm fails to fuse properly during foetal development and the abdominal contents push up into the thorax (Mesdag *et al* 2014), inhibiting lung development and leading to pulmonary hypertension and lung hypoplasia. Antenatal diagnosis by ultrasound improves the likelihood of safe delivery and timely surgery. Physiotherapy depends on cardiovascular stability.

Necrotizing enterocolitis

This condition is characterized by bowel necrosis and multisystem failure, affecting 5% of preterms who weigh <1500 g and 10% of those under 1000 g, with mortality rates of 25% if the condition is severe enough for surgery (Patel & Shah 2012). It typically becomes evident in the second to third week of life, causing abdominal distension, bloody stools and air in the bowel wall. Prevention is by probiotics (Fernández-Carrocera 2013), treatment is by antibiotics, and supportive care includes bowel rest by parenteral nutrition, gastric decompression and control of fluids, electrolytes and BP. If the abdomen is sufficiently distended to require MV, physiotherapy consists of assessment to ascertain if respiratory care is needed, and involvement in the team management of positioning, usually avoiding prone and supine. Bowel perforation requires resection of the dead bowel and/or formation of a colostomy.

NEONATAL INTENSIVE CARE

A neonatal intensive care unit (NICU) provides the technology and skill to care for sick infants or those born prematurely. It is not an ideal environment, with its bright lights, noise that can be ten times above recommended levels (Marik 2013), frequent disturbances and resistant bacteria (Inglis *et al* 2008). The infant's neurological system is vulnerable to injury, sensory bombardment and the deprivation of normal stimuli and maternal skin contact (Symington & Pinelli 2009). Bonding between child and mother is hindered by the barrier of the incubator and the mother's fear of touching equipment. NICU 'graduates' run an above-average risk of educational disability (Odd *et al* 2012), and follow-up clinics are advised (Ralser *et al* 2012).

Stress management

The brain undergoes a dramatic sequence of maturation in the third trimester of pregnancy and the first

FIGURE 10.1 Kangaroo care, skin on skin is a baby's ideal ecological niche

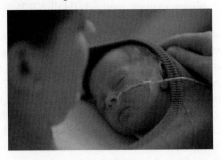

months of postnatal life. Untimely exposure to some environmental influences, especially in preterms, can affect brain function throughout life (Arichi *et al* 2012).

> ### KEY POINT
>
> A stressed parent means a stressed baby.

Parents benefit from help to cuddle their child when attached to awesome equipment, and advice on baby massage, which can improve growth in preterms, alleviate motor problems, enhance immune function and reduce stress for parent and infant (Matricardi *et al* 2013).

Skin-to-skin and chest-to-chest contact ('kangaroo care') with a parent (Fig 10.1) is associated with decreased stress for the baby and parent, reduced infection risk, hypothermia and mortality, and greater paternal involvement after discharge. Benefit is greatest when started straight after birth and continued for as much time as possible (Blomqvist *et al* 2013). Being close to the mother brings the added advantage of her familiar heartbeat, smell and voice (Welch 2012).

Noise and light

The auditory, visual and central nervous systems are the last to mature, and for premature babies these stages occur in the incubator. Exposure to noise can lead to disrupted breathing (Fig 10.2), physiological instability (Hassanein 2013), hearing impairment, sleep disturbance and delayed emotional development (Wachman & Lahav 2011). Noise and light are also obstacles to parental presence (Heinemann 2013). Simple remedies are ear muffs, soft-close bins, dimmed lights when not needed, avoiding putting equipment on the incubator, quiet conversation and most importantly, education for the NICU team (Milette 2010).

Sleep

Babies require 16 hours of sleep a day, evenly distributed in 2–4 hour periods (Primhak & Kingshott 2012). Maintenance of this pattern promotes brain development (Tarullo *et al* 2012). This is aided by skin contact (Flacking 2012) and 'I am sleeping till … pm' signs above the cot.

FIGURE 10.2 The effect of noise on the breathing pattern of a premature infant

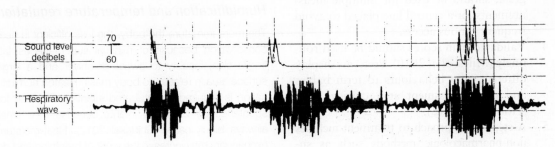

Pain

> *Painful procedures in the NICU are common, undertreated and lead to adverse consequences.*
>
> Hall 2012

Physiological effects of pain are:

- ↑ BP, RR, heart rate (HR), intracranial pressure and P_aCO_2
- ↓ S_pO_2, vagal tone, peripheral and cerebral blood flow
- in preterms, apnoea of prematurity (Karen *et al* 2013).

Pain can lead to long-term neurological, social and cognitive outcomes (Honda 2013) including altered pain processing extending into adulthood (Low 2012). Greater harm is caused to preterm infants (Marlow 2014), for whom it can be life-threatening (Cong *et al* 2012).

Behavioural responses diminish when acute pain abates, but physiological responses may continue, risking intraventricular haemorrhage in the short term (Cong *et al* 2012) and changed brain circuitry in the long term (Low & Fitzgerald 2012).

Preterm infants are subjected to 10–16 invasive procedures per day, leading to detrimental outcomes in all major organ systems (Cong *et al* 2012).

Suggestions to reduce pain are below.

1. Kangaroo care modulates the stress regulation system involved in pain and should be used whenever possible during stressful procedures (Campbell-Yeo *et al* 2013).
2. Breastfeeding (Gabriel 2013) and expressed breast milk (Ou-Yang *et al* 2013) has analgesic properties.
3. One blood sample, following topical analgesia, should be used for multiple measurements, or a central line placed to avoid frequent venous access.
4. Validated pain scores should be used routinely (Milesi *et al* 2010). Preterms display different pain behaviours to term babies and need assessment at a cortical level (Holsti *et al* 2012).
5. A stepwise approach to treatment includes non-pharmacologic methods such as su-

crose, non-nutritive sucking to stimulate mechanoreceptors (Gibbins 2002), swaddling and massage therapy, progressing to pharmacologic methods (Hall 2012).

Sucrose influences endogenous opioid medication and when sucked is activated through taste receptors on the tip of the tongue. Despite it being known as an effective analgesic for heel lances (Gibbins 2002), it is strange that it is not used more widely, despite being proved beneficial in 145 trials (each trial requiring a control group of infants who received no analgesia) (Harrison 2012). Heel lances are more painful than venepuncture (Shrestha 2012) and behavioural sensitivity to heel pain persists for at least a year after repeated lances.

Some health staff do not realize that pain is experienced before birth. Noxious information is transmitted to the preterm infant cortex from 35 weeks (Honda 2013) and anatomic connections for nociception are in place half-way through pregnancy. The foetus mounts sizeable stress responses, so analgesia has been recommended for intrauterine procedures (Bellieni 2013) or late termination (Fisk *et al* 2001). Even during the first trimester of pregnancy, invasive procedures can lead to impaired lung function after birth (Greenough *et al* 1997). Memories are acquired in the third trimester (Anand *et al* 2001), and as the child grows up, long-lasting effects have been identified on biological, psychological (Erni *et al* 2012) and neurological (Diz-Chaves *et al* 2013) systems.

Support systems

Preterms should have blood samples from an umbilical artery catheter withdrawn slowly to protect the brain from hypoxia (Schulz *et al* 2003).

Humidification and temperature regulation

The more immature the baby, the less efficient is heat conservation because of minimal subcutaneous fat, fragile skin, inability to sweat or shiver and a large surface area in relation to body mass. Heated humidification is required for intubated infants, and often for spontaneously breathing infants because their small airways block easily (Chidekel 2012). Heat-moisture exchangers may increase the work of breathing and do not prevent loss of body heat. During physiotherapy, the head, in particular, must be protected from heat loss.

Oxygen therapy

Antioxidant systems to counteract toxic oxygen-free radicals do not develop until late in the third trimester (Walsh *et al* 2009) and the developing brain, eyes and lungs of premature infants can be damaged by high, low or fluctuating oxygen levels. Excessive or oscillating oxygen pressures can disrupt the development of the delicate retinal capillaries, leading to a form of blindness called retinopathy of prematurity (Fleck 2013), but fine tuning is required because oxygen restriction (Fig 10.3) may increase mortality (Vaucher *et al* 2012), especially in extremely preterm infants, whose oxygen saturation must not drop below 90% (Stenson *et al* 2013).

Non intubated infants do not tolerate oxygen masks, and supplemental oxygen is by soft-pronged nasal cannulae or humidified perspex head box. Disadvantages of the box include a variable F_iO_2, the need for a minimum 7 l/min flow to prevent accumulation

of CO_2, bacterial contamination and harmful noise levels (Walsh *et al* 2009). High-flow nasal cannulae (Ch. 5) provide a more reliable F_iO_2 and a degree of CPAP. Algorithms help to maintain a steady F_iO_2 (Walsh *et al* 2009). Entrainment devices are available for low-resource countries (Coghill *et al* 2011).

Continuous positive airway pressure (CPAP)

The low FRC of infants requires them to avoid exhaling too far, using eccentric diaphragmatic activity and glottic closure during exhalation. CPAP fulfils this function when the baby is unable to do so, raising both FRC and tidal volume (Miedema *et al* 2013).

The extra pressure is provided by heated and humidified flow from either a neonatal ventilator, high flow nasal cannulae (Petty 2013) or a bubble system (Youngquist *et al* 2013) (Fig 10.4). If no gas source is available, bubble CPAP can be provided cheaply using consumer-grade pumps, tubing, and regulators expensively (Fig 10.4) or cheaply (Brown *et al* 2013a). The

FIGURE 10.3 Estimate of survival to hospital discharge or one year of life with different levels of inspired oxygen

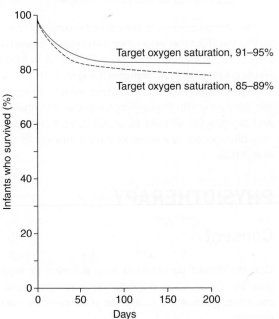

FIGURE 10.4 Bubble CPAP. Pressure is generated at 3–10 cmH₂O, controlled by the amount of water in the CPAP generator on the left

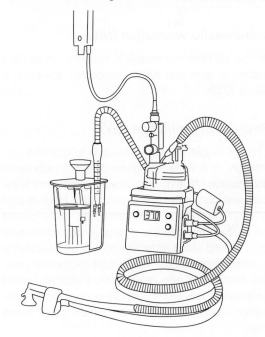

pressure can be delivered through an endotracheal tube (ETT), nasal mask or nasal prongs.

Feeding

Term babies can co-ordinate breathing and sucking, but this is compromised in preterms, who may aspirate while feeding (Trabalon & Schaal 2012) or drop their S_pO_2 (Sakalidis *et al* 2012). Breastfeeding minimizes the risk, but if this is not possible, a bottle nipple is available which feels like a normal breast and vents to air when the child sucks (Jenik *et al* 2012). Otherwise the F_iO_2 can be increased during feeds.

Infants who become breathless with oral feeds are usually fed by nasogastric tube, sometimes via a pump to reduce intermittent loads on the diaphragm. Severely compromised babies require intravenous feeds.

Drugs

The influence of developmental changes on the pharmacokinetics and pharmacodynamics of drugs varies widely (Tayman *et al* 2011). Analgesia is usually required before physiotherapy, but infant and monitors should be observed for post-analgesia respiratory depression, which can happen suddenly.

Drugs can be delivered direct to the lung by inhalation (Steinhorn 2012) or instillation (Jeng *et al* 2012). As with adults, paralyzing drugs are used as little as possible (Da Silva *et al* 2010).

Non-invasive ventilation (NIV)

NIV can be used successfully in neonates, infants and children in term and preterm neonates (Bancalari & Claure 2013).

Mechanical ventilation (MV)

If neither oxygen nor CPAP are able to maintain oxygenation, or if ventilatory failure does not respond to NIV, invasive MV is needed. The subglottic area is the narrowest part of the airway and young children tend to move their heads more than adults, so to protect the mucous membranes, a nasal endotracheal tube (ETT) is used which either has no cuff or, if ventilation is compromised by the leak, a high-volume low-pressure microcuff (Weiss *et al* 2009). Elaborate fixation systems are required to prevent such a heavy contraption becoming disconnected from such a tiny nose.

Intubation without anaesthesia is almost always fatal in injured adults (Lockey 2001) and babies should be anaesthetized for this procedure (Barois & Tourneux 2013) to prevent systemic and pulmonary hypertension, bradycardia, intracranial hypertension and hypoxia (Barrington 2011). Accidental intubation of the right main bronchus and beyond the right upper bronchus leads to right upper lobe collapse more often than with adults.

Pressure control ventilation is used in order to avoid high peak airway pressures and to compensate for the leak of the cuffless tracheal tube. Infants intubated but not ventilated should receive CPAP rather than oxygen via T-piece (AARC 2002a) in order to substitute for their lost physiologic PEEP (p.8).

Complications are similar to those in adults, with barotrauma being more likely because the compliant ribcage and low lung collagen afford little protection against overdistension:

1 Pulmonary interstitial emphysema (PIE) is identified radiologically as lucent streaks radiating from the hila, representing air in the interstitium. Unlike air bronchograms, the streaks do not branch or taper. Extension of PIE to the periphery can lead to pneumothorax.

2 Pneumothorax is suspected if there is rapid deterioration without obvious cause. Chest drainage in a female infant requires careful placement to avoid long term breast damage (Rainer & Gardetto 2003).

The stress response is reduced if the ventilator is set so that the infant can trigger their own breaths (Brown & DiBlasi 2011). Ventilator-induced lung injury is reduced by using lung protective strategies (Feng *et al* 2013).

MV requires continuous analgesic infusion to maintain synchrony with the ventilator, improve oxygenation and stabilize BP (Ancora *et al* 2012). Prolonged MV may be reduced by inspiratory muscle training (Smith *et al* 2013).

PHYSIOTHERAPY

Consent

Consent should be obtained from a parent or legal guardian (Table 10.2), but if this is unavailable, treatment may be given if it is deemed in the patient's best interests.

TABLE 10.2 Parental responsibility in the UK

Child's mother	Responsible unless the child is adopted, placed for adoption or under a placement order.
Child's father	Responsible if married to the mother or has legal responsibility by: • joint birth registration with the mother • parental responsibility agreement with the mother • parental responsibility order made by the court
Social services/court	Responsible if parental responsibility is removed. May be temporary or permanent.

Assessment

The main role of the physiotherapist is to judge if intervention is required. Treatment itself may be carried out by the physiotherapist, neonatal nurse or in part by the parent. The approach is to assess, identify problems and balance up the benefits and risks of treatment. Scrutiny of the notes is complemented by reports from nursing and medical staff, including acceptable limits for S_pO_2 and other vital signs.

History

Medical and birth history provide the first indications of precautions to be taken, e.g.:

1   Gastroesophageal reflux (GOR) is common and requires the infant to maintain the head up position to minimize aspiration (Jung 2012a).
2   Neurological insults such as intraventricular haemorrhage or encephalopathy may present with altered tone, abnormal postures, aspiration or difficulty clearing secretions. The head-down position is banned in these infants.
3   A recent history of self-limiting bradycardia or periods of apnoea suggests that suction might be indicated, but discussion with the nurse is required to identify other possible causes.

Subjective

Close attention to information from the parent or guardian provides a wealth of information, e.g.:

1   Handling: infants may desaturate or stop breathing if disturbed.
2   Feeding regime: assessment can take place at any time but treatment should be given at least an hour after a feed to minimize the risk of vomiting.
3   Pain: an infant behaves differently from an older child. Signs include inconsolable crying, clenched fists, withdrawal, increased extensor tone and irritability, but it should not reach this extreme. Subjective report from the carer is complemented by pain scales, e.g. Fig 10.5.

Objective

The chart identifies trends in age-related normal values (Table 10.3), as well as ventilator parameters, fluid balance and oxygenation related to F_iO_2. Preterm infants have a left-shifted dissociation curve because of foetal haemoglobin, and desaturation may reflect a lower P_aO_2 than in an adult. The chart also documents weight gain or loss, mode and frequency of feeds, response to handling and suction, results of the last suction, and whether the baby has rested since the last intervention. Much reliance is placed on objective information because of the limitations of clinical and subjective assessment.

Before touching the infant, signs can be listened for and observed. The ear picks up stridor, wheeze, grunting and the coarse crackles of upper airway secretions. Observation identifies alterations in colour, e.g. skin pallor, flushing or cyanosis. Cyanosis is a late sign of deterioration. Observed signs of respiratory distress are in Fig 10.6 and Table 10.4. If much of the

FIGURE 10.5 Pain scale for babies from 32 weeks gestational age

	0	1	2
Crying	No cry or cry which is not high pitched	High pitched cry but consolable	High pitched cry and inconsolable

Characteristic cry of pain is high pitched

	0	1	2
Requires O_2 to maintain $SpO_2 > 95$	No	Requiring $O_2 < 30\%$	Requiring $O_2 > 30\%$

Consider other reasons for desaturation, e.g. pneumothorax, oversedation

	0	1	2
Vital signs	HR and BP +/- 10% baseline	10–20% increase in HR or BP	>20% increase in HR or BP

Take BP last as this may wake the infant causing difficulty with other assessments

	0	1	2
Expression	Neutral	Grimace	Grimace/grunt

Grimace characterized by brow bulge, eyes shut, deepening naso-labial furrow, open mouth

	0	1	2
Sleeplessness	No	Wakes frequently	Constantly awake

Based on infant's state during the hour preceding assessment

respiratory excursion is occurring abdominally, respiratory distress is severe.

Physical assessment must avoid noise, sudden movement and cold hands.

Auscultation, with a warmed stethoscope, identifies atelectasis or secretions. Sounds are often referred through such a diminutive chest: upper lobe collapse can sometimes only be detected posteriorly and the crackles of secretions are difficult to localize. In ventilated infants, the slight hiss of the intentional air leak can be heard by ear or stethoscope.

Atelectasis or consolidation show on x-ray, the middle and upper lobes being especially inclined to collapse. A large thymus may look similar to right upper lobe consolidation, and atelectasis of the left lower lobe may be missed on a portable x-ray if it is hidden by the heart. Air bronchograms projected against the heart shadow may not be significant but are pathological when seen peripherally.

Monitoring

Non-invasive monitoring is available for arterial blood gases (Ganesan et al 2002), and end tidal CO_2 (Tingay et al 2013). For S_pO_2, the oximeter probe site must be changed four-hourly to prevent pressure

TABLE 10.3 Normal values for infants

	Premature infant	Infant
RR	40–60	30–40
S_pO_2	92–95%	93–98%
P_aO_2	8–10.6 kPa (60–80 mmHg)	10–13 kPa (75–100 mmHg)
P_aCO_2	5–6 kPa (37–45 mmHg)	5–6 kPa (37–45 mmHg)
HR	120–200	100–150
BP	50/25–60/30	70/40–80/50

Note: *RR:* respiratory rate, *HR:* heart rate, *BP:* blood pressure

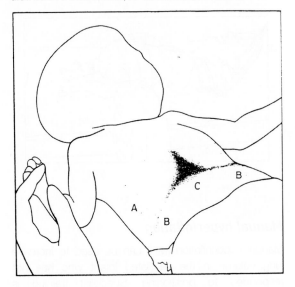

FIGURE 10.6 Recessions indicating respiratory distress. *A:* intercostal, *B:* subcostal, *C:* substernal

sores. Conscious level can be assessed with bispectral monitoring (Sammartino *et al* 2010).

KEY POINT

The maxim that routine treatment is taboo is never more apt than with infants.

Indications for treatment

Physiotherapy is indicated if there is evidence of atelectasis or excess secretions which cannot be cleared by humidification and suction. Increased work of breathing (WOB) may be responsive to physiotherapy unless it is due to a pathological process. Poor gas exchange is responsive if is caused by the above. Treatment may also be indicated after extubation if airway irritation has created secretions that the infant does not cough and swallow spontaneously.

Precautions

Hand washing and universal precautions are required even more strictly than with adults because of the immature defence mechanisms of infants. Staff with any infection should not enter the NICU.

Treatment is contraindicated if the infant is hypothermic, has suffered a pulmonary or intraventricular haemorrhage or had surfactant treatment in the last six hours. Other contraindications are cardiovascular instability (unless this is due to hypoxia), or fresh blood-stained secretions (unless there are significant problems with mucous plugging). Manual hyperinflation is contraindicated if there is PIE or other barotrauma, and any physiotherapy is contraindicated in infants with an undrained pneumothorax.

If treatment is necessary within an hour of feeding, the gastric contents can be aspirated by syringe through the nasogastric tube and replaced afterwards. If the infant is receiving phototherapy for jaundice, it can be suspended temporarily for treatment.

Treatment should only take place after the patient has been stabilized medically. Observation and monitoring

TABLE 10.4 Signs of respiratory distress in an infant

- ↑ RR
- If severe: ↓ RR, or apnoea
- Chest recessions
- Tracheal tug
- Head bobbing, representing unfixed accessory muscle contraction
- Nasal flare
- Grunting (equivalent to pursed lip breathing in adults)
- Unstable HR
- Inability to suckle

are required more frequently during treatment than with adults. Large swings in BP, in particular, risk causing brain injury (Marlow 2014).

Desaturation episodes may be precipitated by suction or caused by secretions, breath holding, pulmonary hypertension or upper airway obstruction. The infant's head falling into flexion can obstruct the airway and may cause stridor. Following extubation, subglottic oedema may develop immediately or over 24 hours.

After treatment, the cot sides must be raised or incubator ports closed.

PRACTICE TIP

Physiotherapy sessions should be structured into the daily plan so that infants can receive prolonged rest and adequate sleep.

Methods to increase lung volume

Positioning

The lungs are not happy to remain in the same position for prolonged periods, and infants should have their position changed as regularly as their condition and response to handling allows.

Raising the head of the incubator lessens the risk of GOR (Button 2005) and in spontaneously breathing infants reduces the load on the diaphragm.

Side-lying allows greater diaphragmatic excursion than supine, with trunk and limbs supported in a flexed position to optimize neurodevelopment. If there is a pneumothorax or unilateral PIE, side-lying with the affected lung dependent may assist absorption of the gas, with close monitoring of SpO$_2$.

The prone position (Fig 10.7) stabilizes the breathing pattern, HR and S$_p$O$_2$ (Maynard et al 2000), but spontaneously breathing infants must be monitored because of the risk of sudden infant death syndrome (Kinney & Thach 2012). Extended time in prone may lead to a flattened frog position because of hypotonia, which can be avoided by raising the pelvis on a roll (Vaivre-Douret et al 2004).

The effects of repositioning should be closely monitored, especially in preterms. For ventilated babies, traction on the ETT must be avoided, and the leak around the ETT re-assessed in the new position.

FIGURE 10.7 Prone positioning of an infant on CPAP with nasal prongs

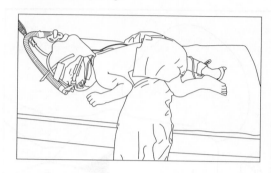

Manual hyperinflation

Manual hyperinflation (MH) can be used to increase lung volume in the ventilated infant who has not responded to positioning. Specialist training is required, particularly for MH of younger infants, because of the risk of barotrauma (Morrow et al 2008). Precautions to MH are similar to adults, with three additions:

- hyperinflation conditions such as meconium aspiration and bronchiolitis
- extreme prematurity (<28 weeks gestation) due to the increased risk of pneumothorax
- infants whose RR is over 40/min because it is difficult to achieve an effective hyperinflation at such a high rate; extra sedation and muscle relaxants may be helpful.

A 500 ml reservoir bag is used for infants and children under two years old. These bags have an open tail which is squeezed between finger and thumb to regulate the pressure more sensitively than a valve (Fig 10.8). The following technique is suggested:

1   A manometer is incorporated into the circuit, and a pop-off valve that opens above 40 ± 5 cmH$_2$O (Oliveira et al 2011), which is especially important because pressure varies with flow (Oliveira et al 2013b).

2   Each hyperinflation should be interposed with 2–3 tidal breaths and the chest should rise just slightly more than during MV.

FIGURE 10.8 Hand position for manual hyperinflation

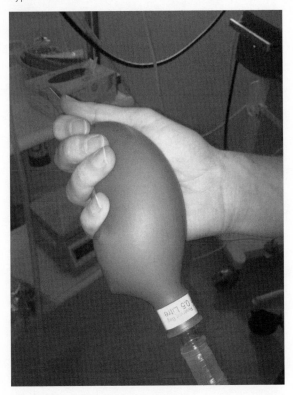

3 Some positive pressure should be maintained at the end of expiration to maintain PEEP and prevent derecruitment.
4 The monitors must be kept under observation, any significant drop in BP indicating a need to return the infant to MV and advise nursing or medical staff.

Methods to reduce the work of breathing

Excess WOB can be for respiratory, neurological or postural reasons. An unstable breathing pattern may be caused by excess WOB or by hunger, pain or stress (Schwartzstein 2010). Once distress has been minimized, repositioning may reduce the WOB. Non-invasive ventilation for infants who become exhausted, hypercapnic and acidotic has been used in the youngest age groups so long as apnoeas and technical problems are overcome (Abadesso 2012).

Methods to clear secretions

Postural drainage

Preterm infants, or term infants who tolerate handling poorly, should have their position changed minimally. Other babies can be posturally drained in alternate side-lying or prone, preferably on a parent's lap. The head-down position is inadvisable because it facilitates GOR and splints the diaphragm.

Percussion and vibrations

Manual techniques are fruitful because of the compliant ribcage of infants, who may also find them soothing. Vibrations with the finger tips can be applied on every second or third exhalation. Percussion can be performed with a soft-rimmed face mask or a 'Palm Cup' (Fig 10.9) directly on the skin, taking care to stay within the surface markings of the little lungs.

Precautions are similar to adults, with the following additions:
1 The head must be supported throughout because of the risk of causing a form of brain damage similar to 'shaken baby syndrome' (Hassam & Williams 2003).
2 Manual techniques should be avoided in premature infants or others at risk of rickets (Nehra *et al* 2013).

FIGURE 10.9 'Palm cups' made for percussion on babies and young children (Henleys)

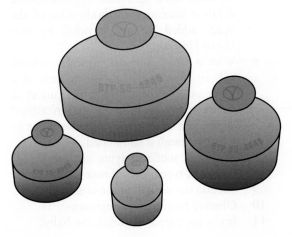

3   Monitoring must be maintained throughout because responses can be unpredictable.

4   Hefty chest vibrations may increase air-flow resistance (Schechter 2007).

Suction

For **non-intubated infants**, positioning and manual techniques may mobilize secretions so that they are swallowed. If not, suction may be necessary, but with minimal distress because it is associated with the physiological responses that accompany other painful interventions (Ivars *et al* 2012) and crying increases transpulmonary pressure swings and the risk of lung damage (Walsh *et al* 2011). Nasopharyngeal airways (Ch. 8) should not be used in infants routinely because the reduced airway lumen increases WOB. Oral airways should not be used unless the infant is unconscious or does not have airway protective mechanisms. The precautions and techniques described in Ch. 8 are modified by the following:

1   Have the baby in side-lying, wrapped up comfortably but firmly, and with a second person supporting the infant behaviourally (Cone *et al* 2013).

2   For preterm infants, pre-oxygenate by no more than 10% above baseline (Walsh *et al* 2011).

3   Set the vacuum pressure to 8–10 kPa (60–80 mmHg) (GOSH 2013).

4   Use a catheter that is no more than half the diameter of the smallest nostril, usually size 5–6 FG.

5   Measure the depth of suction from the tip of the nose, to the tragus of the ear, and then to the base of the neck (Fig 10.10). If the child has a significant kyphoscoliosis, depth is measured on both sides of the head, added up and divided by two (Alder Hey 2009).

6   With a small amount of water-soluble jelly or the child's nasal secretions as a lubricant on the catheter tip, insert it gently into the nose to the measured depth, but no further than the point at which a cough is stimulated.

7   Withdraw while applying suction.

8   Reassess, repeat only if necessary.

9   Suction the nostril on the other side.

10 Observe monitors throughout.

11 Invite the parent to cuddle the baby.

FIGURE 10.10 Measurement for nasopharyngeal suction in an infant

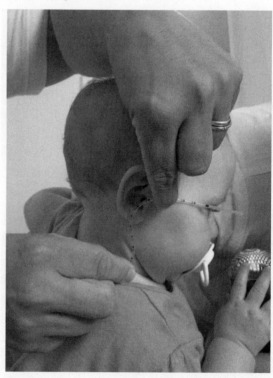

FIGURE 10.11 Hypertension in an infant during suction

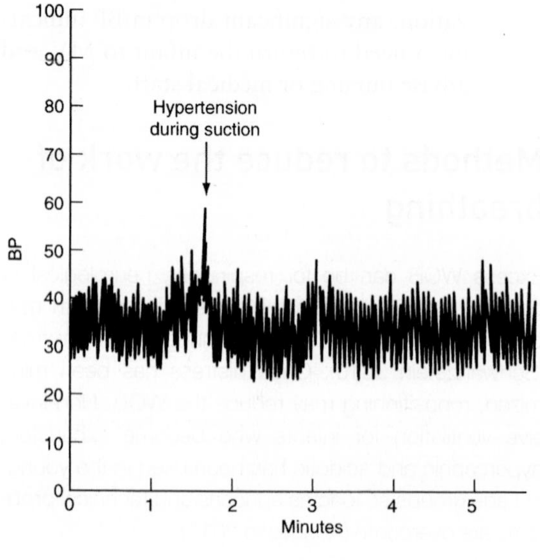

For **ventilated infants**, secretions may be present even if not heard on auscultation or felt on palpation. Liaison with the nurse is helpful, but for babies without hypersecretory disease, suction every 6–12 hours is adequate if no indication for more frequent suction is apparent (Walsh 2011).

Complications include hypoxaemia, bradycardia, tachycardia, atelectasis, infection, arrhythmias (Cone et al 2013) and abrupt peaks in BP (Fig 10.11), but these are less likely if step 4, below, is followed. For preterms, closed suction brings less complications than open suction (Pirr et al 2013). Suction should be avoided if there is low cardiac output or shock (pallor or cyanosis, sweating or decreased peripheral temperature).

Modifications to technique are the following.

1   Extra sedation may blunt the stress response, so long as the infant is not at risk of hypotension.

2   Preoxygenation is by increasing ventilator F_iO_2 to 10–20% above baseline (Walsh et al 2011), or by using MH, with monitoring by oximetry.

3   If there is difficulty passing the catheter, sterile saline may be used as a lubricant.

4   The catheter should not advance more than 1 cm beyond the end of the ETT. Its length can be checked against the length of an equivalent-sized ETT, which is usually taped to the outside of the incubator for emergencies, or a graduated catheter can be used (Ritson 2000).

5   The catheter diameter should be less than half the diameter of the airway (Walsh 2011):

   - 5 FG for ETT size 2.5 mm
   - 6 FG for ETT size 3.0 mm
   - 7 FG for ETT size 3.5 mm
   - 8 FG for ETT size 4.0 mm.

a) For postoperative infants, ensure that someone supports the wound.

b) After disconnection from the ventilator (for open suction), the catheter is inserted to the premeasured depth. If resistance is felt, it is withdrawn 0.5 cm before suction is applied. Suction should be kept to five seconds if possible, or a maximum ten seconds.

c) After reconnection to the ventilator, the mouth and nostrils usually need suction.

d) When S_pO_2 has stabilized, F_iO_2 is titrated slowly to the target S_pO_2. If values do not return to baseline, or the infant is unsettled, further suction may be indicated.

If the infant does not respond as expected, or does not settle, liaison with nursing or medical staff is required. The nurse will know if bradycardia caused by stress might be reversed by physical input such as gently rubbing the sternum.

If sputum retention continues despite efficient humidification and the above techniques, saline instillation may be required, preferably with a low-sodium solution to reduce infection risk (Walsh et al 2011). Suggested boluses are 0.5 ml for preterm infants and 1–3 ml for term babies, but this varies with the stability and tolerance of the infant (Ridling et al 2003).

Therapeutic bronchoalveolar lavage (BAL)

For persistent atelectasis caused by mucous plugging, BAL has been found effective in 84% of ventilated infants who have not responded to conventional physiotherapy (Morrow et al 2006).

Two suggestions for blind BAL have been described, both under close monitoring:

1   For open suction, Downs (1989) describes the following with babies at low risk of hypoxaemia:

   - inject saline into an unconnected sterile catheter, still partly in its package, until the catheter is filled; keep the syringe connected
   - disconnect the ventilator and insert the filled catheter into the ETT
   - instil saline directly to the distal end of the tracheal tube, using the syringe
   - withdraw saline, along with any mucus, using the syringe
   - disconnect catheter from the syringe, connect to the suction circuit, then apply suction and withdraw
   - re-oxygenate and monitor.

2   Prasad (2008) describes the following:

   - preoxygenate and sedate
   - position the baby with the affected side downwards

- instil saline, 2–5 ml for infants and 10–15 ml for older children
- manually ventilate with tidal volume breaths
- reposition with affected side uppermost
- apply manual techniques and MH
- suction
- monitor.

Either can be repeated if necessary.

Precautions include raised intracranial pressure, haemodynamic instability, pulmonary hypertension and coagulation disorders. The catheter remains in the airway for longer than conventional suction, and complications include hypoxaemia or cardiovascular instability, which may require escalation of respiratory of haemodynamic support.

Exercise and rehabilitation

Passive movements are normally unnecessary, but for very low birth-weight babies, daily gentle exercise can improve weight and bone mineralization (Moyer-Mileur 2000). Monitors should be observed throughout. Referral to specialist colleagues is required for infants needing developmental input, including rehabilitation for ventilator-dependent infants with chronic respiratory insufficiency (Dumas et al 2013).

CASE STUDY

Holly is a 1 week old neonate, born at 38 weeks gestation, after which she aspirated her feed. She was sedated, intubated and ventilated, using pressure support ventilation with F_iO_2 of 0.75, and showing the following:

- S_pO_2 94%
- pH 7.23, P_aO_2 9.3 kPa (70 mmHg), P_aCO_2 10.2 kPa (77 mmHg), HCO_3^- 22
- auscultation: ↓ breath sounds L side and R upper zone, crackles throughout
- X-ray shows bilateral upper lobe collapse (App.D)
- suction → thick creamy secretions.

Questions

1   Analyze the arterial blood gases.
2   Overall analysis?
3   Problems?
4   Goal?
5   Plan?

CLINICAL REASONING

Consider the following:

Unless it can be shown that the foetus has a conscious appreciation of pain ... the responses to noxious stimulation must still essentially be reflex.

Do foetuses feel pain? *BMJ* (1996), 313, 795–9

Response to Case Study

1 Blood gases

- Uncompensated respiratory acidosis, borderline oxygenation with high F_iO_2.

2 Analysis

- X-ray and secretions suggest mucous plugging.

3 Problems

- Loss of volume both lungs and retained secretions.

4 Goal

- Reinflate upper lobes and clear secretions.

5 Plan

1. Care with positioning throughout because of the high ETT on X-ray.
2. Instil saline to right lung, monitor.
3. Turn to left side-lying.
4. MH, vibrations and suction, monitor.
5. Re-assess.
6. Instil saline to left lung, monitor.
7. Turn to right side-lying.
8. MH, vibrations and suction, monitor.
9. Re-assess.
10. Plan for improvement.
11. Plan for deterioration.

Response to Clinical Reasoning

The assumption is not evidence-based. A foetus cannot be asked if it consciously appreciates pain. There is no reasoning behind the statement that his or her responses 'must' be reflex. Perhaps a foetus should be given the benefit of the doubt.

(Brugger 2012)

RECOMMENDED READING

Allegaert K (2014) Neonatal clinical pharmacology. *Paediatr Anaesth*; **24**(1): 30–8

Byrne E, Campbell SK (2013) Physical therapy observation and assessment in the neonatal intensive care unit. *Phys Occ Ther Ped*; **33**(1): 39–74

Cerritelli F (2013) Effect of osteopathic manipulative treatment on length of stay in a population of preterm infants. *BMC Pediatr*; **13**: 65

Gold JI, Nelson LP (2012) Palliative care in a neonatal intensive care unit. *J Crit Care*; **27**(1): 95–6

Gupta P (2014) Caring for a teen with congenital heart disease. *Pediatr Clin North Am*; **61**(1): 207–28

Meena N (2013) Impact of early physiotherapy intervention on neuro-development in preterm low birth weight infants during the first six months of life. *Indian J Phys Med Rehabil*; **24**(1): 3–8

Neumann RP (2014) The neonatal lung – physiology and ventilation. *Paediatr Anaesth*; **24**(1): 10–21

Hooper SB et al (2013) Evaluating manual inflations and breathing during mask ventilation in preterm infants at birth. *J Pediatrics*; **162**(3): 457–63

Vutskits L (2014) Cerebral blood flow in the neonate. *Paediatr Anaesth*; **24**(1): 22–9

Walker SM (2014) Neonatal pain. *Pediatr Anesth*; **24**: 39–48

Zareen Z, Hawkes CP, Krickan ER et al (2013) In vitro comparison of neonatal suction catheters using simulated 'pea soup' meconium. *Arch Dis Child Fetal Neonatal Ed*; **98**(3): F241–3

CHAPTER 11
Physiotherapy for children

LEARNING OBJECTIVES

On completion of this chapter the reader should be able to:

- describe the anatomical and physiological differences between adults and children

- discuss the common medical and surgical conditions of children

- understand the principles of care for children on a paediatric ICU

- identify the main physiotherapy problems and describe their management

- develop an insight into palliative care in children.

INTRODUCTION

> We should look at the care of children with a child's eyes, in a child's manner.
> Collins 1999

Adult patients can say to themselves: 'I understand that I'm not in hospital for the rest of my life and that the nasty things they are doing to me are for my own good'. Young children do not have these resources of reasoning and may be overwhelmed by bewilderment, uncertainty about the behaviour expected of them and sometimes feelings that they are abandoned or being punished.

Despite progress in humanizing children's experience in hospital, long term emotional disturbance can still occur. Children need to be listened to, believed and given some control over what is done to them. Teenagers in particular need autonomy because they often feel that they have outgrown the paternalistic environment of a paediatric unit. It is not surprising that children in hospital can exhibit different behaviours than those that are normal for them.

Children appreciate having the same physiotherapist throughout their stay. They need their own toys and belongings, and all but the sickest are best dressed in their day clothes.

A child is defined as aged from one year to adolescence. Adolescence is between 10 and 19 years.

Differences between children and adults

There are the following differences:

1 By two years old, the bucket handle action of the ribs has developed and the ribcage and lungs become equally compliant.

2 By age two to three, collateral ventilation is established but the lungs are still vulnerable to atelectasis.

3 By three years old, when more time is spent upright, the ribs are oblique rather than horizontal.

4 Children are physically resilient, with bones and wounds healing quickly, but emotionally they are only resilient if they have a background of emotional security and are encouraged to express what they are thinking and feeling.

Children over age 10 are considered adults anatomically and physiologically, but they are not psychologically and emotionally mature for many years. At any age they may show an exaggeration of the behaviour patterns that they normally use to cope with stress, and social maturation may be delayed by potentiation of the sick role from professionals and families. From age three, they should be involved in treatment planning with health staff and their parents.

The move from paediatric to adult care needs to be managed sensitively, with attendance at the transition clinic by age 14. For inpatients, the provision of an adolescent unit means that teenagers do not have to sit in a ward full of toys or be surrounded by elderly patients with advanced pathology (Srivastava 2012). Teenagers also appreciate having some control of which visitors they receive.

CARDIORESPIRATORY CONDITIONS

Modifications from Chapter 3 are below.

Cystic fibrosis

For chest clearance, regular physical exercise is suited to children and can slow the decline in airflow obstruction (Almajed & Lands 2012). When combined with forced expiratory manoeuvres, it may be an acceptable substitute for the active cycle of breathing (ACBT) in children with mild disease (Reix *et al* 2012).

Children should normally avoid the head-down tip because of the likelihood of reflux (Ch. 3). Withers (2012) makes the following observations for adolescents:

- From their early teens, patients should have some private time with their clinician.
- Some problems such as delayed puberty are more visible and unwelcome at this age.
- The full significance of a life-limiting condition becomes apparent to the patient, and screening for depression should be routine.
- The need for independence is hampered by on going dependence on the health system, and some dependence on their family may continue if employment is limited.
- Adherence may be improved by 'motivational interviewing' (Duff & Latchford 2013).

Irons *et al* (2013) identify singing as a beneficial change from the gruelling daily ritual, and recommend the children and youth version of the ICF as an outcome measure.

Asthma

> *Cough as a symptom of asthma has been so drummed into us, that there is a real danger that every cough of any duration is treated as asthma.*
>
> Bush (2002)

A misdiagnosis of asthma is often made from self-limiting infections or persistent cough (Craven & Everard 2013). However, asthma is still the most common chronic disease of children in developed countries, and its incidence is rising (Hansen et al 2013). Below are paediatric aspects of prevention, education and medication.

Prevention is best started before conception by ensuring that intended mothers understand the association of asthma with prenatal factors (Ch. 3). Exacerbations may be triggered by allergens, tobacco smoke (Rubin & Pohanka 2012) or occasionally drinks such as Coca Cola (Bush 2002).

Most children outgrow their asthma, and it is thought to be more than coincidence that this is the time when they outgrow their fears (Gillespie 1989). Education is therefore the key, e.g.:

- colourful diaries and stickers, available from asthma organizations or manufacturers (App. B)
- inhaler practise, preferably in front of a group to improve confidence at school
- for children over six years, practise in electronic monitoring of peak flow (BTS 2012a)
- healthy eating, especially fresh fruit (Varraso 2012)
- hard, enjoyable, controlled physical activity because many children with asthma are de-conditioned and associate exercise with anxiety.
- cough control because of an above-average incidence of incontinence (Soyer 2013).

During adolescence, depression, anxiety or panic attacks may increase and complicate symptoms (McCauley et al 2007). Management may be facilitated by:

- screening for early identification of those at risk
- allowing expression of feelings and worries
- part of the clinic appointment being without a parent
- identification of hyperventilation syndrome.

Teenagers with asthma should be referred to the adult services to avoid them disappearing into a void (Srivastava 2012).

Nedocromil (Ch. 5) inhibits histamine release and is an unfashionable drug, partly because its patent is out of time, but it is effective in 70% of children, in which case steroids can often be avoided (Korhonen et al 1999).

However, asthma may require steroids if it is persistent (Vichyanond et al 2012) or acute (Redman & Powell 2013), and for those aged 5 or older with a severe exacerbation this should be within an hour of presentation (NICE 2013a). CPAP may be required for oxygenation and bronchodilation (Gomes 2013). Immunotherapy may be effective in children (Vichyanond et al 2012).

Fatalities are rare in children but have shown a link with obesity and low income (Rubin & Pohanka 2012).

Chest infections

The risk of infant chest infection is reduced by breast feeding (Ghimire 2012), increased by prematurity (Drysdale 2011) and doubled by passive smoking (Sconce 2013). Young children react more severely to respiratory infection than adults because of their narrow airways. Lower respiratory tract infection with the respiratory syncytial virus is a leading cause of hospitalization for severe bronchiolitis and pneumonia, the risk being increased by chronic lung disease of prematurity or congenital heart disease (Szabo et al 2013).

Children with flu-like symptoms should not be given aspirin because it can cause Reye syndrome.

Croup

Croup is acute obstructive inflammation of the upper airway, usually caused by viral infection. It occurs mainly from ages six months to six years, with children born prematurely being most at risk. Clinical features include a harsh barking cough, hoarseness, painful breathing and sometimes stridor, which is a rasping sound on inspiration indicating upper airway obstruction. It is usually benign and self-limiting, requiring just encouragement of fluids. Severe disease with stridor requires hospitalization, steroids, sometimes nebulized adrenaline (Daniel 2012) and occasionally intubation.

Epiglottitis

Epiglottitis is a less common but more vicious form of upper airway obstruction, caused by fulminant infection of the soft tissues around the entrance to the larynx. Tachypnoea is evident, along with a severe sore throat so that swallowing saliva is difficult and drooling occurs. The child usually sits bolt upright or in a tripod position with neck extended and arms providing support for the accessory muscles. Prompt antibiotics and steroids are required.

With both croup and epiglottitis, physiotherapy is contraindicated in the acute phase because of the risk of increasing obstruction, but if the airway is protected with an endotracheal tube (ETT) and sputum retention is evident, chest clearance may be indicated. Table 11.1 identifies the differences between the two conditions.

Pneumonia

The clinical course of pneumonia is more acute than in adults, with chest recession and a respiratory rate (RR) sometimes reaching 50 bpm. Diagnosis is by x-ray or ultrasound (Don *et al* 2013) and oral antibiotics are usually effective (Bradley *et al* 2011).

Physiotherapy may include positioning to improve gas exchange, and airway clearance is sometimes needed in the later stages if the child is unable to clear airway debris.

Pertussis (whooping cough)

Whooping cough is a lower respiratory tract bacterial infection caused by bordetella pertussis and is one of the most contagious bacterial infections in children. Immunization has reduced the incidence, and deaths are rare, but a recent resurgence has been linked to parental mistrust of vaccines (Glanz 2009).

Signs are coughing spasms which terminate in a 'whoop' as air is gasped into the lungs, accompanied in younger children by vomiting and apnoea. The disease can be lengthy (hence the nickname '100-day cough') and coughing severe, leading to fatigue in the short term and sometimes airway damage and bronchiectasis in later life. Physiotherapy is only required if there is sputum retention, and treatment must avoid any stimulus which irritates the sensitive airways and sets off more coughing.

Inhaled foreign body

Children are notorious for inserting objects into their noses and mouths, from where the object may find its way into the airway. Physiotherapy is contraindicated until removal of the object.

Hypertension

Hypertension in children has tradionally been secondary to kidney disease, but obesity, sedentary life styles and faulty diets have led to increased prevalence of primary hypertension. Older children may present with symptoms related to end organ abnormalities involving the heart, eye and brain, and prompt recognition is needed to prevent further damage (Anyaegbu 2014).

Hyperventilation syndrome

Hyperventilation syndrome is commonly missed and may incorporate vocal cord dysfunction, fear of suffocation, throat clearing or habit cough (Grüber *et al* 2012). It occurs in about 18% of children, or 55% of those with asthma (Gridina *et al* 2013). Treatment is similar to adults (Ch. 13).

TABLE 11.1 Upper airway obstruction

	Croup	Epiglottitis
Age	6 months to 3 years	2–6 years
Aetiology	Viral	Bacterial
Onset	Days	Hours
Temperature	<38.5	>38.5
Cough	Barking	Minimal
Stridor	Only if severe	Yes
Voice	Hoarse	Weak
Can drink?	Yes	No
Child active?	Yes	No

CONDITIONS WITH CARDIORESPIRATORY COMPLICATIONS

Gastroesophageal reflux (GOR) disease

Episodes of GOR are common in infancy and childhood. This is not considered pathological unless frequent enough to cause gastrointestinal or respiratory symptoms (Schechter 2007). It is thought to occur in up to 80% of asthmatic children, with half symptomatic (Blake 2013). Signs include regurgitation or vomiting after meals, failure to gain weight, unwillingness to eat, eating small amounts and choking, or wheezing after food. General treatment is by feeding little and often with thickened feeds, and an antacid (Horvath et al 2008).

Physiotherapy must be avoided after eating. If postural drainage is required, opinions are conflicted. Some observers have described the head-down tilt as safe (Doumit et al 2012) but others have claimed the opposite (Schechter 2007). Clinical reasoning suggests that in the absence of convincing evidence, head-down postural drainage is inadvisable if symptoms are present. Prone and left-side-lying give some protection (Ewer et al 1999). However, children vary in the position at which reflux occurs, and symptoms should be monitored closely.

Neuromuscular conditions

Children with neurological disease may have respiratory muscle insufficiency, low lung volumes, impaired cough, swallowing dysfunction, GOR, chronic aspiration, recurrent chest infections or sleep disordered breathing (BTS 2012c). In children and adolescents, vital capacity of <1.1 litres or peak cough flow <160 l/minute denotes a risk of chest infection serious enough to require hospital admission (Bush 2007).

For children with **cerebral palsy**, side-lying and supported sitting may be the most effective positions for reducing respiratory rate and effort, while supine is least tolerated (Littleton et al 2011).

For children with **spinal muscular atrophy** or **Duchenne muscular dystrophy**, regular assessment of pulmonary function when awake and asleep enables early recognition of deterioration and the instigation of non-invasive ventilation (NIV) when required, for which humidification is needed (BTS 2012c). Respiratory failure is the primary cause of death and NIV has improved both quality and longevity of life (Katz et al 2013). Respiratory function may be enhanced by positioning, and the most comfortable position may be upright or high side-lying. For chest clearance, augmented cough techniques may be needed if peak cough flow is <270 l/min (BTS 2012c). Mechanical in-exsufflation (Ch. 8) shortens the time taken for airway clearance (Chatwin & Simonds 2009), usually with the child supported in their wheelchair, and can reduce the risk of respiratory failure (Goncalves et al 2012).

Trauma

Trauma is the main cause of childhood morbidity and mortality worldwide (Ivashkov 2012). Brain injury is responsible for >85% of the deaths (Cullen 2012), leaving survivors with a 10–50% incidence of behavioural and psychiatric problems, which may get worse over time (Linda & Jianghong 2013). Child survivors of trauma also show surprisingly high rates of post-traumatic stress disorder, at 69% in the short term (Herbert 2005) and 27% in the long term (Holbrook et al 2005). Parental distress is a contributing factor, underlying the importance of care for the family. Children tend to mistake flashbacks for reality and to keep their feelings to themselves so as not to upset their parents.

SURGERY

Preoperative care

Parents have not always explained an operation to the child. Without explanation, the boundary between reality and fantasy may be blurred, e.g. being 'put to sleep' can have fearful connotations if this has happened to a family pet. Children have been known to mistake a bone marrow test for a 'bow-and-arrow test' and a dye injection for a 'die injection'. Young age and preoperative anxiety increase postoperative pain (Pagé 2012) and the 60% of children who are anxious before surgery are in particular need of preoperative information (Vaezzadeh et al 2011).

Explanations can be helped by pictures, visits, discussions with children who have had the same operation and rehearsal of procedures such as trying the anaesthetic mask (Fortier 2011). Physical sensations and their reasons should be explained, and a play specialist enrolled when possible. Truth is essential, otherwise co-operation is lost. For cardiac patients, preoperative advice on breathing and mobility can lead to more rapid recovery (Carmini et al 2000). Parents require highly detailed explanations.

Children must not be excessively starved, and should be allowed oral fluids two hours preoperatively to reduce the risks of dehydration, nausea, hypoglycaemia and hypotension (Friesen et al 2002).

Parental presence at induction of anaesthesia reduces postoperative agitation (Zand et al 2011). Children are more accepting of the face mask if their choice of flavoured lip balm is smeared inside before induction (Walpole 2003).

Postoperative care

To improve co-operation with physiotherapy, multimodal analgesia should be used, including regional analgesia (Russell et al 2013), and patient-controlled analgesia (Rai 2013). Children are more prone than adults to vomiting, which needs to be treated (Bassanezi 2013).

Tachycardia may be due to pain, anxiety or fluid deficit. Bradycardia may be caused by hypoxia or medication. Oxygen saturation must not be allowed to drop below 93%. Post-extubation laryngospasm is a greater risk than in adults, and is three times higher in infants than in older children, with stridor being a risk if the endotracheal tube has been tight (Pawar 2012).

Children like to be touched as little as possible after surgery. Manual techniques to the chest are usually counterproductive and are not effective in preventing atelectasis (Schechter 2007). However, if required, preoperative and postoperative chest clearance, with adequate analgesia and including early mobility, can reduce complications (Felcar et al 2008). Following lung surgery, positive expiratory pressure can assist sputum clearance and mobilization can improve lung expansion (Kaminsk 2013). Following heart surgery, atelectasis due to mucous plugging may respond to mucolytic drugs (Ozturk 2013). If coughing is necessary, children prefer to splint the incision themselves by leaning forward with their arms crossed and using a clean teddy bear or rolled up towel. Multidisciplinary management is emphasized by Bacha & Kalfa (2014), the goal being to 'treat more while hurting less'.

PAEDIATRIC INTENSIVE CARE UNIT (PICU)

The PICU is a high technology, high stress environment. Children waking up in the PICU are subject to extra fears if explanations are not full and clear. Restraints should not be used unless children are in danger, e.g. pulling out lines and tubes, and sedation requires specific paediatric protocols (Deeter et al 2011). The physiotherapist should be watchful after the sedative propofol, which can cause tachycardia in young children (Dewhirst et al 2013), and dexmedetomidine, which can cause bradycardia and hypotension (Kim et al 2014).

Pain management

The young and the elderly have the most to fear from pain because they are the most defenseless against it.

Fine (2001)

Children at risk of inadequate pain assessment and treatment are those who are critically ill, pre-verbal (Brahmbhatt 2012) or neurologically impaired (Parkinson et al 2013). Children who are cognitively impaired are thought to be more sensitive to pain if they have been subject to prior pain experiences in the NICU (Baeyer et al 2013), which can sensitize pain pathways and damage central nervous system development (Walker 2014). Guidelines are often not adhered to (Ozawa & Yokoo 2013), and the consequences could bring prosecution if applied to animals.

The causes of poor pain management in children include the following:

1   Children's subjective complaints may not be taken seriously.
2   Distinguishing pain from agitation is challenging in young children, and some do not express pain in terms that are easily understood by adults. Absence of crying does not always mean absence of pain.
3   Inexperienced doctors may underprescribe analgesia due to fear of side effects. They can be reassured that adequate analgesia is safe in the youngest children (Misra et al 2008) and from age three months, ventilatory depression from morphine or fentanyl

is no greater than that seen in adults with similar plasma concentrations (Ivashkov 2012). Meticulous prescription is required (Taylor 2013).

4   Children may not report pain if they think they are to receive the dreaded needle, especially if extra pain is caused by the accompanying sympathetic vasoconstriction (Anderson 2013).

5   Children are easily held down by force.

Parents' opinions must be actively sought because they tend to assume that everything to minimize pain is done automatically. Older children can be asked directly about their pain, which gives an indication of any associated fear. Children over three can use colour intensity scores, charts with body outlines or face scales using six (Fig 11.1) or three (Baeyer *et al* 2013) faces. Those aged over seven can use an adult visual analogue scale. Most children benefit from a combination of self-report and at least one other measure (Brahmbhatt 2012). Assessment tools are also available for prelingual and non-verbal children (Voepel-Lewis 2002).

Physiological measures such as changes in RR, heart rate, BP and S_pO_2 are not specific to pain, not sustained with continued pain and only occur with extreme pain, as evident by a trebling of serum cortisol levels (Paix & Peterson 2012). Apparent sleeping after a painful procedure may be 'dissociative shock' rather than an indication that all is well.

Multimodal analgesia includes local anaesthetic infiltration, patient-controlled analgesia (Liu *et al* 2013a), nasal (Regan *et al* 2012), or sublingual preparations (Neri *et al* 2013), virtual reality games (Das *et al* 2005) and Entonox (Hjortholm *et al* 2013). If a needle is required, children need local anaesthetic cream (Schreiber *et al* 2013). Having a measure of control over the process is essential (Brown *et al* 2012).

Respiratory drugs

For non-ventilated children, whether in or outside the PICU, inhalers are required that are adapted to a child's lack of co-ordination, short inspiratory time, reduced ability to breath-hold and low inspiratory flow rate. The following are suitable but must be reviewed regularly (BTS 2011):

1   A face mask is required until the child can use a spacer mouthpiece. If a mask is frightening, it can be used to gently stroke the child's cheek beforehand. Crying means that most of the aerosol does not reach the lower airways (Amirav & Newhouse 2012).

2   Some large-volume spacers need to be tipped downwards during inhalation to allow the valve to open.

3   From birth to age five, a metered dose inhaler (MDI) and spacer are preferred.

4   If any of the above are ineffective, a nebulizer can be used.

5   Children aged three years or older can use a dry powder inhaler, or inhaler with spacer.

6   A child aged ten years upwards can manage an MDI.

If symptoms do not respond as expected, poor inhaler technique or lack of adherence may be the cause.

Nebulizers can be tried on a teddy first, or may be used with some supervised children when asleep.

FIGURE 11.1 Faces pain scale, for children aged three years and over. Point to each face, using the words to describe the pain, then record the number

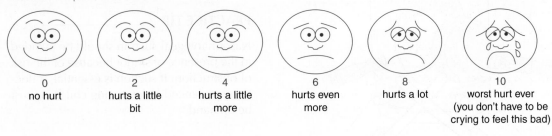

0	2	4	6	8	10
no hurt	hurts a little bit	hurts a little more	hurts even more	hurts a lot	worst hurt ever (you don't have to be crying to feel this bad)

In countries where spacers are not available, a 500 ml plastic bottle can be substituted. Comprehensive instructions (App. B) and regular checks are needed to ensure reliable technique.

Continuous positive airway pressure and non-invasive ventilation

For spontaneously breathing children, continuous positive airway pressure (CPAP) or non-invasive ventilation can be used if adequate oxygenation or ventilation cannot otherwise be maintained (Platt 2014). Administration can be by face mask, nasal prongs or a hood (Fig 11.2).

In the absence of chronic lung pathology, a starting pressure of 5 cmH$_2$O is used for CPAP, then gradually increased until grunting stops or oxygenation is optimum, so long as the child does not start to exhale forcefully, indicating excess work of breathing. Pressures above 10 cmH$_2$O bring a risk of gastric distension and diaphragmatic splinting, so if the child has a nasogastric tube, it should be left on free drainage to enable escape of trapped gas. Accurate monitoring of pressure using a separate manometer is required to minimize the risk of pneumothorax.

For non-invasive ventilation, inspiratory pressures of 8–12 cmH$_2$O are set initially, then gradually adjusted to a level that overcomes the work of breathing, as observed by a stable breathing pattern. Expiratory pressures start at 3–5 cmH$_2$O and are adjusted to

achieve upper airway patency at end-expiration, as reflected by improved S_pO_2 (Baird 2012).

> **PRACTICE TIP**
>
> Children at risk of vomiting should not use a hood or full face mask without a nasogastric tube, in case of aspiration.

Mechanical ventilation (MV)

Intubation and MV can cause haemodynamic deterioration in children (Jones 2012) and inotropic support (Ch. 17) may be needed to stabilize BP. This acts as a warning that if physiotherapy is indicated, the response to each intervention should be monitored before proceeding to the next step. A nasal ETT and pressure control ventilation are commonly used (Jauncey-Cooke et al 2010). Falling tidal volumes may be due to retained secretions or bronchospasm.

Intubation means that the child cannot grunt when in respiratory distress, and loss of positive end-expiratory pressure (PEEP) may result in derecruitment and hypoxia. If manual hyperinflation is indicated, PEEP should be maintained (Boriosi et al 2012).

Extubation

Upper airway obstruction is the commonest cause of extubation failure (Ivashkov 2012), and children who have been ventilated for several days, or have increased risk of post extubation stridor (e.g. Down's syndrome or cerebral palsy) may need steroids beforehand to minimize airway swelling (Lukkassen & Markhorst 2006). Stridor can be managed by heated humidified oxygen, nebulized adrenaline and sometimes heliox (Martinón-Torres 2012).

FIGURE 11.2 Hood for CPAP or NIV

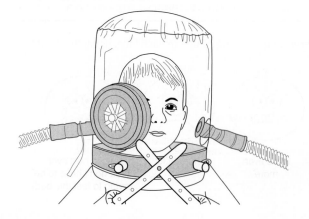

> **PRACTICE TIP**
>
> Nasopharyngeal suction should be avoided in the presence of stridor because of the risk of obstruction. If suction is essential, a doctor experienced in intubating children must be on hand.

Tracheostomy

Tracheostomy is only performed on the PICU if a child requires long term airway management. Fenestrated tubes are rarely used for small children due to the risks of obstruction with granulation tissue and misdirection of suction catheters.

For preverbal children, delayed communication can be prevented by speech-language therapy (Jiang & Morrison 2003). To assist communication, an uncuffed tube can be occluded with a gloved hand on expiration if the child is attempting to talk, laugh or cry. This must only be done if there is sufficient leak to move air past the vocal cords to allow the child to breathe out. Occlusion must be brief and explained to the child beforehand. Toddlers learn to drop their chin to occlude the tube when wanting to talk.

Decannulation is usually preceded by downsizing to a tube that is small enough to let the child breathe around the tube but wide enough to allow suction if required. The smaller the child, the more likely are problems related to airway resistance created by a smaller tube, unexpected anatomical problems or a mucous plug. Close monitoring is required, particularly at night.

The families of children going home with a tracheostomy will need training in suction, feeding, bathing, tracheostomy care and resuscitation. Unlike adults, children requiring an on-going tracheostomy need humidification rather than a heat-moisture exchanger (McNamara et al 2014).

PHYSIOTHERAPY

Parents should be welcomed during assessment and treatment. If this causes the child to express anxiety more noisily than when unaccompanied, this is healthier than withdrawal. Children must not be discouraged from crying, nor told to be brave. If they are 'difficult', it is usually because they are frightened (Weaver & Battrick 2007). For an anxious child, it is advisable to avoid touch until a degree of trust has been established.

Babies can be given rattles and toys to watch during treatment. Older children need clear, honest and simple explanations, assisted by demonstrations on a teddy or doll. Hand puppets can give instructions in funny voices, sometimes hiding under clothes. The puppet can fall down with a squeal of joy if good breaths are done, or sulk if not so good. If the child's favourite toy, TV programme, food or game is documented, these can be used to engage their interest.

Story-telling can enable the child to look forward to the rest of the story in the next session.

Children must be reassured that the procedure can be stopped, sometimes temporarily, at any time. Reluctance can often be overcome by giving the child a choice, e.g. whether to keep the TV on or off, to have incentive spirometry or a walk outside, or have parents present or not. Requests to stop treatment should almost always be respected, though this can usually be overcome by cajoling, distraction, joking and enlisting the help of a parent or play specialist.

Consent

Children should not simply be deemed competent if they agree and incompetent if they disagree. People aged over 16 are able to consent to treatment unless they lack capacity (p.414). A child under 16 may consent to treatment if they fully comprehend what is involved. If they refuse treatment it can be overridden by an adult with parental responsibility (see Table 10.2), from whom consent must be obtained (Lynch 2010). The early teenage years are a useful time for patients to be informed that confidentiality between them and their clinician can only be broken if they or someone else might be harmed.

Emergency treatment can be given without consent if this is required to prevent serious deterioration. Treatment may also be provided in the absence of a guardian if that treatment is deemed in the patient's best interests, so long as this is not used as an excuse to avoid seeking consent.

Assessment

Assessment can be on a parent's lap, with a description of what is being examined and why. Wound drains and intravenous lines can inhibit children from moving and they should be reassured that all lines and drains will be supported throughout. If the child is nil-by-mouth they can be distressed and not understand why they are not allowed to drink.

The notes and charts indicate any variation in normal values (Table 11.2).

Subjective

Both the parent and child's views are required. Asking the child to draw a picture may indicate the effect of the illness on them, or some suggested questions are in Box 11.1.

TABLE 11.2 Normal values for children

Parameter	Values
RR	16–30
S_pO_2	93–98%
P_aO_2	10–13.2 kPa (75–100 mmHg)
P_aCO_2	5–6 kPa (35–45 mmHg)
HR	60–100
BP	90/55–110/65

BOX 11.1

Questions to ask a child, which can be modified for other conditions

1 What do you think asthma is?
2 How did you learn that you had asthma?
3 What do you think can be done to help it go away?
4 How do you feel when you have an attack?
5 Why do you think you got asthma?
6 How do you feel about asthma?

Fatigue may manifest as a change in sleep-wake times, continuous lack of interest or concentration difficulties (Radbruch 2008). Breathlessness can be measured with picture scales (Tulloch et al 2012).

A cough may caused by GOR, foreign body aspiration, hyperventilation syndrome or passive smoking. It can disrupt sleep and schooling, and disturb other family members.

Objective

PRACTICE TIP

Children in respiratory distress assume a position that promotes airway patency and they should be allowed to maintain this position, especially if stridor is present.

BOX 11.2

Signs of respiratory distress

As with Table 10.4:

● unstable RR or apnoea, unstable HR, tracheal tug, nasal flare or grunting
● apical breathing pattern
● see-saw breathing (abdominal paradox)
● increased accessory muscle use ± tripod position
● lethargy.

RR: respiratory rate, *HR*: heart rate

Observation indicates if respiratory distress is present (Box 11.2).

Before auscultation, children can be given the opportunity to see and feel the stethoscope, and use it to listen to themselves or a doll. The diaphragm or bell should be warmed before use.

Deteriorating gas exchange may be indicated by pallor, sweating, restlessness, agitation, glazed eyes and, in ventilated children, fighting the ventilator. Cyanosis or reduced consciousness may indicate severe hypoxia.

Precautions

The assessment, in particular questioning the nurse and parents, indicate if the child is unstable and should be touched minimally.

All forms of physiotherapy except education, and sometimes positioning, are contraindicated if there is:

● an undrained pneumothorax
● airway compromise not caused by secretions.

Most forms of physiotherapy should be avoided if there is cardiac instability or blood-stained secretions. Ventilated children requiring inhaled nitric oxide (Ch. 17) and who are stable enough for manual hyperinflation should have the gas continued throughout in order to prevent swings in pulmonary artery pressure.

Reassessment is necessary throughout treatment as deterioration can occur rapidly. Desaturation episodes may be caused by secretions, breath holding, distress or suction.

Some modifications of the techniques described in Part 1 and Chapter 10 are discussed below.

Methods to increase lung volume

Positioning is fundamental to both respiratory and developmental physiotherapy. For respiratory care, alternate high side-lying and supported upright sitting are usually effective and well tolerated. When positioning for gas exchange, the distribution of ventilation is opposite to that in healthy young adults (Ch. 1), but gas exchange varies and oximetry is the best guide.

Breathing exercises can be done by children aged >2 years if taught imaginatively, or a paediatric incentive spirometer can be motivating. The use of blowing games utilizes the deep breath that is taken before blowing out, e.g. paper mobiles, bubble-blowing, blowing a tissue or, better still, messy paint blowing. Abdominal breathing can be taught by placing a toy on the abdomen, 'like a boat on the sea'. Crying upsets the flow rate without increasing volume (Fig 11.3) and should be avoided, particularly in children with stridor.

For intubated children, **manual hyperinflation** uses an open tail 500 ml bag for those aged <2 years or a 1 litre valved bag above 2 years. The usual precautions apply (Ch. 18).

Methods to reduce work of breathing

Breathlessness is caused by increased work of breathing, deconditioning, anxiety, metabolic acidosis or decreased power due to muscle weakness or structural abnormalities. As with adults, it may be relieved by positioning, a fan or non-invasive ventilation. Pharmacology is based on opioids (Robinson 2012).

Methods to clear secretions

Children have more viscous secretions and relatively more mucus-secreting glands than adults. They benefit from airway clearance according to their condition (Table 11.3).

FIGURE 11.3 Breathing patterns of (a) a two y.o. child at rest and (b) a 20-month-old child while crying (left half) and sobbing (right half)

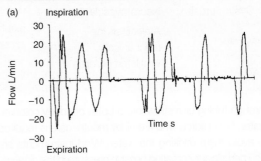

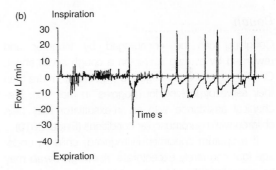

To aid motivation, the choice of airway clearance technique is best chosen by the child when possible.

Mucociliary clearance

Postural drainage can be enjoyable over a bean bag, or wedges and frames can be used for the longer term, with the usual precautions in case of GOR (p.299). For infants, who spend much time in supine, the sitting position helps drain the apical segments of the upper lobes, with particular attention to the right upper lobe. **Manual techniques** are modified according to the child's age and comfort.

The **active cycle of breathing** and **autogenic drainage** can be done by children from ages four to five, but they are usually unable to put the components together consistently until aged six to seven. Huffing can be facilitated by misting up a mirror, using a peak flow mouthpiece to blow cotton wool or ping-pong balls, or using the story of the big bad wolf who 'huffed and puffed and blew the house down'. For younger children, the physiotherapist can apply passive autogenic drainage.

Positive expiratory pressure can be modified by using 'bubble PEP' (Fig 11.4), when the child blows out

TABLE 11.3 Evidence of benefit from airway clearance with some conditions

Proven benefit	Probable benefit	Possible benefit	Minimal or no benefit/counterproductive
Cystic fibrosis	Neuromuscular disease Atelectasis in mechanically ventilated children	Prevention of post extubation atelectasis in neonates	Acute asthma Bronchiolitis Respiratory distress syndrome Respiratory failure without atelectasis

through tubing or a straw into a bottle of soapy coloured water. For children who are nil by mouth, care is required to avoid them drinking the water. Wind instruments are also beneficial for creating positive pressure in the airways.

Cough

Coughing can be encouraged by laughter and rewarded by earning a star on a cough score sheet. Children can be encouraged to expectorate more than their saliva by looking for 'froggies' in their spit. Mechanical assistance with an in-exsufflator may help children with neuromuscular conditions (Finder 2010).

If a sputum specimen is required, children under age four can rarely expectorate. A **cough swab** may be successful, in which the child coughs and secretions are collected from the back of the throat by a swab, then sent to microbiology in a sterile container. If a specimen of **nasopharyngeal aspirate** is requested in order to obtain epithelial cells for diagnostic pur-

poses, nasal suction should be performed into the post-nasal space, to a depth that has been measured from nose to ear (Fig 11.5). However, contamination by oral flora limits success, and even secretions from intubated children usually carry bacteria from the upper airway (Blaschke et al 2011). **Nasal swabs** are as sensitive as nasopharyngeal aspirate for the detection of major respiratory viruses except respiratory syncytial virus (Blaschke et al 2011).

> ### PRACTICE TIP
>
> Nasopharyngeal suction is unnecessary if the child is coughing effectively, even if secretions are swallowed.

Suction

Variations from the procedure in Ch. 10 are the following:

- If regular suction is anticipated in an older child, a nasopharyngeal airway can be inserted to minimize trauma.
- Depth of insertion of the suction catheter is measured from the tip of the nose to the tragus of the ear and then to the base of the neck, with the head facing forwards (Fig 11.6). If the child has a significant kyphoscoliosis, depth is measured on both sides of the head, then the measurements added up and divided by two.
- There is little research on the pressure at which damage occurs, but pressures of 13.3–16 kPa (100–120 mmHg) have been advised (AARC 2004).

Non-bronchoscopic bronchoalveolar lavage (BAL)

For diagnostic BAL, large aliquots of normal saline (1 ml/kg body weight) are administered deep into the airways to sample fluid from the lower respiratory tract

---

FIGURE 11.4 Bubble PEP, particularly popular with children if water sprays over the physiotherapist

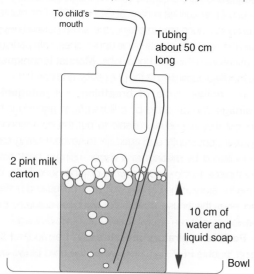

To child's mouth

Tubing about 50 cm long

2 pint milk carton

10 cm of water and liquid soap

Bowl

FIGURE 11.5 Measurement for nasopharyngeal suction

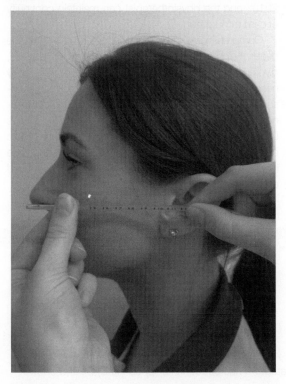

FIGURE 11.6 Measurement for nasopharyngeal aspirate

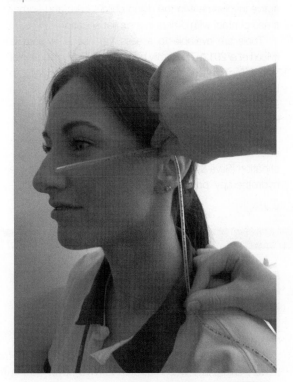

in order to identify pathological organisms. This technique picks up less contamination than using specimens from the upper respiratory tract. Therapeutic BAL (Ch. 8) is used to reverse atelectasis caused by mucous plugging (Morrow *et al* 2006).

Exercise

Physical activity may open up the lung or assist airway clearance. Games can become increasingly energetic as the child progresses, building up to wheelbarrow races. Paediatric rehabilitation programmes for asthma and cystic fibrosis can reduce symptoms and enhance self-management (Jung *et al* 2012b), and early mobilization in the PICU is advised (Choong *et al* 2013).

A valid discharge planning tool has been developed (Ellerton *et al* 2011).

PALLIATIVE CARE

Children have a right to grieve. They have the capacity to do so, and begin to develop an understanding of

death from two to three years old (Slaughter & Griffiths 2007). They may be prevented from grieving because of a natural desire by others to protect them from suffering. Children understand more than they can articulate and it is thought that they usually know that they are going to die (Tamburro *et al* 2011). Evasion can leave them with a sense of bewilderment, betrayal and fantasies that are more frightening than reality.

Communication with dying children should be based on honesty. If death is compared to sleep, for example, they may develop an unhealthy fear of bedtime. Many children are able to take decisions about whether to have active or supportive therapy (Tamburro *et al* 2011). As well as experiencing their own responses to dying, children have the burden of their parents' grief. Parents, grandparents, brothers and sisters may carry the added burden of being avoided by friends.

Siblings may be as upset as their (Sandler 2013) parents but with less opportunity to express this and sometimes the functional loss of their parents (Gillance 1997). They may worry about their own vulnerability or feel confused by a mixture of what they have been told, overheard, observed or imagined.

They should not be fed 'Susie-is-going-away-on-a-long-trip' euphemisms or they may wait for her return. They need information, open family communication, active involvement in the dying child's care and sometimes contact with others in a similar situation.

Tools are available to assess the needs of parents (Meert et al 2012). The family benefit from timely palliation of symptoms, continuity of personnel, the opportunity to bathe and hold their child, clear explanations and written summaries of options before making any decisions, including the timing of withdrawal of life support if necessary.

Physiotherapy focuses on symptom control, e.g. abdominal breathing and abdominal massage for constipation (Silva & Motta 2013), and children can use the hydrotherapy pool with oxygen cannulae, tracheost-

omies and ventilators, with appropriate management. Withdrawal of intensive care support sometimes enables the child to transfer to a hospice (Gupta & Harrop 2013), and the physiotherapist can maintain continuity of care throughout.

Comprehensive family support before and after the death helps reduce the high incidence of distress, divorce and sibling neglect that may ensue. The family need respect for the child's body, and sometimes keepsakes, such as locks of hair, attendance of staff at the funeral and follow-up phone calls (Brooten et al 2013). It is unhelpful to tell parents that they will get over their child's death and is rarely true. Parents can sometimes find ease in reflecting that it may have been better to have loved and lost a child than not to have had the child at all.

CASE STUDY : MK

Four year old Mark has cerebral palsy. He was admitted with a severe chest infection, then developed respiratory failure and was ventilated for two days. Now extubated, he has suddenly dropped his S_pO_2 and shows the following signs:

- RR 40, F_iO2 0.6, S_pO_2 88%
- ABGs: pH 7.10, P_aCO_2 13.2 kPa (100 mmHg), P_aO_2 7.9 kPa (60 mmHg) HCO_3^- 29
- Auscultation: ↓ breath sounds and crackles on the left
- ↓ expansion left chest
- See-saw breathing pattern
- Secretions thick and yellow.

Questions

1 Analyze the ABGs
2 Analyze the X-ray (right)
3 Overall analysis?
4 Problems?
5 Goal?
6 Plan?

ABGs: arterial blood gases, *RR*: respiratory rate

FIGURE 11.7 Chest X-ray of MK

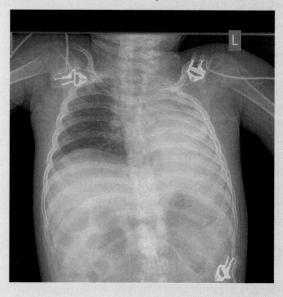

CLINICAL REASONING

... these patients vigorously object to having an arterial puncture done even if they are relatively sick. Because of this, more than one person is usually required to obtain the sample.

(Deming 1995 p. 213)

Response to Case Study

1 **ABGs**
   - Severe partially compensated respiratory acidosis. Poor oxygenation with high F_iO_2.

2 **X-ray**
   - Left lung collapse with mediastinal shift to left.

3 **Analysis**
   - Acute left lung collapse, probably due to mucous plugging.
   - Poor respiratory function, borderline for CPAP/NIV or intubation and ventilation.

4 **Problems**
   - Loss of volume left lung.
   - Retained secretions.

5 **Goal**
   - Left lung re-inflated within two treatments.

6 **Plan**
   - Preoxygenate patient, monitor.
   - Administer nebulized saline or hypertonic saline.
   - Position patient into right side-lying, monitor.
   - Percussion and vibrations, monitor.
   - Cough stimulation.
   - If unsuccessful, consider cough augmentation with in-exsufflator.
   - If unsuccessful, consider nasopharyngeal suction, monitor.
   - Re-assess.
   - Plan for improvement.
   - Plan for deterioration, including the need for mechanical assistance.
   CPAP: continuous positive airway pressure, *NIV:* non-invasive ventilation

Response to Clinical Reasoning

This demonstrates the low priority given to children's pain by some medical textbooks and shows little awareness of the ethical, legal and humane implications of forcibly holding down a child in order to impose a procedure that causes significant pain.

RECOMMENDED READING

Alzouebi M, Roberts I (2005) Paediatric chest radiographs. *Student BMJ;* **13**: 309–52

Barkman C (2013) Clowning as a supportive measure in paediatrics. *BMC Pediatr;* **13**: 166

Berlinski A (2013) Nebulized albuterol delivery in a model of spontaneously breathing children with tracheostomy. *Respir Care;* **58**(12): 2076–86

Boschee ED, Cave DA, Garros D *et al* (2014) Indications and outcomes in children receiving renal replacement therapy in pediatric intensive care. *J Crit Care;* **29**(1): 37–42

Brooten D, Youngblut JM, Seagrave L *et al* (2013) Parent's perceptions of health care providers actions around child ICU death. *Am J Hospice Palliat Med;* **30**(1): 40–49

Carnevale FA, Gaudreault J (2013) The experience of critically ill children. *Dynamics;* **24**(1): 19–27

Carroll CL, Sala KA (2013) Pediatric status asthmaticus. *Crit Care Clinics;* **29**(2): 153–66

Chikata Y, Sumida C, Oto J (2012) Humidification performance of heat and moisture exchangers for pediatric use. *Crit Care Res Pract;* 439267

Clark L (2011) Pain management in the pediatric population. *Crit Care Nurs Clin N Am;* **23**(2): 291–301

Cooley WC (2013) Adolescent health care transition in transition. *JAMA Pediatr;* **167**(10): 897–9

Crook J (2013) The agreement of fingertip and sternum capillary refill time in children. *Arch Dis Child;* **98**(4): 265–8

Davies FCW (2013) A patient survey for emergency care designed by children, for children. *Arch Dis Child;* **98**(4): 98–247

Davis GA, Purcell LK (2014) The evaluation and management of acute concussion differs in young children. *Br J Sports Med;* **48**(2): 98–101

Dumas HM, Fragala-Pinkham MA, Rosen EL *et al* (2013) Cardiorespiratory response during physical therapist intervention for infants and young children with chronic respiratory insufficiency. *Pediatr Phys Ther;* **25**(2): 178–85

Duyndam A, Ista E, Houmes RJ (2011) Invasive ventilation modes in children. *Crit Care;* **15**(1): R24

Giessen L (2012) Nocturnal oxygen saturation in children with stable cystic fibrosis. *Pediatr Pulmonol;* **47**(11): 1123–30

Gilmer MJ, Foster TL, Bell CJ *et al* (2013) Parental perceptions of care of children at end of life. *Am J Hospice Palliat Med;* **30**(1): 5358

Grüber C, Lehmann C, Weiss C *et al* (2012) Somatoform respiratory disorders in children and adolescents. *Ped Pulmonol;* **47**: 199–205

Hawcutt DB (2013) Review: paediatric pharmacogenomics. *Arch Dis Child;* **98**(3): 232–7

Kheir JN (2013) Comparison of 2 lung recruitment strategies in children with acute lung injury. *Respir Care;* **58**(8): 1280–90

Kwok S-Y (2013) Resting heart rate in children and adolescents: association with blood pressure, exercise and obesity. *Arch Dis Child;* **98**(4): 287–91

Lanza FC, Wandalsen G, Dela Bianca AC *et al* (2011) Prolonged slow expiration technique in infants: effects on tidal volume, peak expiratory flow, and expiratory reserve volume. *Respir Care;* **56**(12): 1930–5

Mantzouranis E (2014) Childhood asthma: recent developments and update. *Curr Opin Pulm Med;* **20**(1): 8–16

Mata AF, Sarnaik AA (2013) Bronchoscopy with N-acetylcysteine lavage in severe respiratory failure from pertussis infection. *Pediatrics;* **132**(5): e1418–23

Meucci M, Curry CD, Baldari C *et al* (2013) Effect of play-based summer break exercise on cardiovascular function in adolescents. *Acta Paediat;* **102**(1): e24–e28.

NICE Guideline (2013) Sedation in children and young people (CG112)

Packel L, Sood M, Gormley M *et al* (2013) A pilot study exploring the role of physical therapists and transition in care of pediatric patients with cystic fibrosis to the adult setting. *Cardiopulm Phys Ther J;* **24**(1): 24–30

Payne D (2013) Meeting the needs of young people in hospital. *Arch Dis Child;* **98**(12): 930–932

Shields MD, Bush A, Everard ML (2008) Recommendations for the assessment and management of cough in children. *Thorax;* **63**: 1–15

Tovar JA, Vazquez JJ (2013) Management of chest trauma in children. *Paediatr Respir Rev;* **14**(2): 86–91

Ullman A, Long D, Horn D *et al* (2013) The kids safe checklist for pediatric intensive care units. *Am J Crit Care;* **22**(1): 61–9

Vincent E, Faustino S, Hirshberg EL *et al* (2012) Hypoglycemia in critically ill children. *J Diabetes Sci Technol;* **6**(1): 48–57

Walter JK (2013) How to have effective advanced care planning discussions with adolescents and young adults with cancer. *JAMA Pediatr;* **167**(5): 489–490

Watts R, Vyas H (2013) An overview of respiratory problems in children with Down's syndrome. *Arch Dis Child;* **98**(10): 812–817

Werkman MS, Hulzebos EH, Helders PJ *et al* (2014) Estimating peak oxygen uptake in adolescents with cystic fibrosis. *Arch Dis Child;* **99**(1): 21–5

White CC (2013) Bronchodilator delivery during simulated pediatric noninvasive ventilation. *Respir Care;* **58**(9): 1459–66

CHAPTER 12
Physiotherapy for people with cardiovascular disorders

LEARNING OBJECTIVES

On completion of this chapter the reader should be able to:

- understand the physiotherapist's role in the management of patients with heart failure, coronary heart disease and peripheral arterial disease

- outline the importance of patient education in reducing risk and improving adherence

- describe the principles of exercise therapy for patients with cardiovascular disorders

- identify a range of outcome measures suitable for this group of patients.

INTRODUCTION

It has been estimated that if everyone walked briskly at 3–4 mph on most days, about 30% of deaths from cardiovascular disease would be prevented.
WCPT (2009)

Physiotherapists treat problems of movement and function. Cardiovascular (CV) disorders cause symptoms such as chest pain, breathlessness and fatigue, which affect the ability to move and provoke a fear of moving, leading to a spiralling decline in function and quality of life.

Physiotherapy includes education, exercise and relaxation. Exercise helps prevent cardiovascular disease and reduce some of its complications once it has occurred (Yoshikawa *et al* 2013). Education is provided by all team members and includes motivation to sometimes change the habits of a lifetime. Patients may not remember advice, not understand it or not know how to follow it (Myers & Abraham 2005). They may feel too ill, too well, too tired or too busy. Knowledge alone is not enough, and clinicians need to maximize patients' understanding (Box 12.1) and ensure autonomy (Teixeira et al 2012).

Treatment follows the usual physiotherapy approach of assessment, setting patient-centred goals, following through a plan and assessing outcome.

PROBLEMS ASSOCIATED WITH HEART FAILURE (HF)

> *I can't breathe even if I did exercise.*
> Patient quoted by Rodriguez et al 2008

Pulmonary oedema associated with HF increases the work of breathing, especially during exercise (Cross et al 2012). Exercise capacity is also limited by fatigue and muscle weakness, augmented by 'heart failure myopathy' and dyspnoea caused by increased ventilatory response to exercise (Witte & Clark 2008).

HF can progress over decades (Liu 2014), and patients should be under the care of a specialist team, which enables them to improve their quality of life, reduce hospitalization and extend life (OHTAC 2009).

Management of patients with acute disease

Breathlessness from pulmonary oedema may be relieved in acutely unwell patients by a hand-held fan (Wong 2013) and upright positioning to displace the fluid downwards, with support of the feet to prevent the inexorable slide down the bed. Poor gas exchange may require continuous positive airway pressure (CPAP), which has the added bonus of improving the neural control of heart rate (HR) in patients who have comorbid COPD (Reis et al 2010). As soon as the patient is willing, mobilization should follow, after a check for anaemia which has a prevalence of 10–56% (Piña 2013) but is missed by most cardiologists (Doehner et al 2013).

BOX 12.1

Tips for improving adherence

- Ask the patient what they want to know rather than tell them what you think they should know.
- Give the most important information first.
- Be specific: 'Walk for 30 minutes every day' is better than 'Do as much walking as you can'.
- Link self-treatment to an event or location ('whenever you make a cup of tea . . .' is more effective than 'three times a day').
- Tell them what you are going to tell them, then tell them, then tell them what you have told them.
- Write it down or use easy to read material.
- Use clear sentences and repeat key information.
- Recruit family members to help with remembering.
- Tailor advice to the individual.
- Promote self-efficacy with motivation and encouragement.
- Ask patients to repeat what they have been told, to check understanding of key points.
- Encourage questions.

Rehabilitation that is maintained after discharge improves survival (Catanzaro *et al* 2012).

Education

> *If I knew I was going to live this long, I would have taken better care of myself.*
> Patient quoted by Menezes *et al* (2012)

Patients often feel overwhelmed when they first receive their diagnosis (Rodriguez *et al* 2008). Education should therefore start with an explanation that the alarming term 'heart failure' simply means that the heart isn't pumping as hard as it should and is different from a heart attack or cardiac arrest. Advice (Table 12.1) can be aided by strategies to maintain cognitive functioning (Alosco *et al* 2013).

Sodium restriction may be prescribed, but patients are advised against low salt substitutes due to their high potassium content (SIGN 2007). When discussing advance care planning, many patients prefer to enhance their quality of life rather than prolong survival (Dev *et al* 2012).

The benefits and side effects of medication are explained so that patients can make informed decisions. For example, they may prefer to take their diuretics at a time to minimize frequency (Hwang *et al* 2013).

Patient-directed goals, along with provision of blood pressure (BP) machines, weight scales, pedometers, DVDs and booklets, can improve autonomy, lower BP and reduce admissions (Shively *et al* 2013). Consideration should be taken of barriers to adherence such as unappetising diets or depressed mood. Nearly half of patients have clinically significant depression, which may be helped by cognitive therapy (Dekker 2011), support for the spouse (Chung 2009) and cardiac rehabilitation. The phone can assist in providing education (Piamjariyakul *et al* 2013).

TABLE 12.1 Topics for patient education

Topic	Patient skills and self-care
What is heart failure?	• Background, causes and symptoms
How do I manage it?	• Daily weight • If increased dyspnoea or oedema or sudden weight gain of >2 kg in 3 days, diuretic dose to be increased and/or health team alerted
What do the drugs do?	• Indications, doses, effects and side effects
What about drinking and eating?	• Healthy eating and correct weight • Fluid restriction of 1.5–2 l/day if significant symptoms (weight-based fluid restriction may cause less thirst) • Restriction of hypotonic fluids if hyponatraemia is a problem
Can I smoke?	• Smoking and illicit drugs to be avoided
How does exercise help?	• Benefits explained • Flexibility to suit the patient • Activities of daily living
Can I have sex?	• Normal sexual activity is fine if the condition is stable and undue symptoms are not provoked
Do I need a flu jab?	• Vaccinations protect against influenza and pneumococcal disease
What about how I feel?	• Social support and treatment options for depression and cognitive dysfunction
What's my future?	• End of life choices

Motivation to exercise is assisted by education that dyspnoea on exercise is not harmful (Witte & Clark 2008).

Exercise

Exercise training can relieve symptoms, increase exercise capacity, reduce hospitalization (Piepoli 2013), improve peripheral vascular and skeletal muscle function (Arena et al 2013), improve quality of life and reduce mortality (Fernhall 2013). With appropriate prescription (Box 12.2), improvements in health status occur early and persist over time (Flynn et al 2009).

Most cardiac rehabilitation programmes exclude patients with a primary diagnosis of HF (Dalal 2012), and these patients form a different population to those who have been through a sudden event such as myocardial infarct or heart surgery. A dedicated HF rehabilitation programme is preferable, but patients can successfully join a pulmonary rehabilitation programme because people with COPD and HF have a similar background of slowly progressive disease, and the disorders often coexist (Evans 2011).

Interval training allows higher-intensity training levels, improves quality of life (Chrysohoou 2013) and may reduce arrhythmias (Guiraud et al 2013). Dancing can bring functional and cardiovascular benefits similar to formal exercise training and brings greater motivation (Kaltsatou et al 2014). Patients with implanted devices to restore synchronized contraction between right and left ventricles require specific precautions (Haennel 2012).

PRACTICE TIP

Warm-up and cool-down before and after exercise counteract the risks of ischaemia, post exercise hypotension and arrhythmias.

Inspiratory muscle weakness impairs exercise tolerance (Ribeiro et al 2012) and the inclusion of inspiratory

BOX 12.2

Exercise prescription for patients with heart failure

● Incorporate aerobic and resistance exercise.
● Start with frequent 5–10 minute activities for de-conditioned or compromised patients.
● For interval approach: work for 1–6 minutes and rest for 1–2 minutes.
● Consider ratios of work:rest at 1:2 or 1:1, sitting:standing at 1:1 or 1:3 and strength:endurance at 1:1 or 2:1.
● Intensity for aerobic exercise: 55–80% HRR or use RPE.
● Intensity for strength and endurance exercise: 50–70% of 1RM for lower body, 40–70% for upper body.
● Include low to moderate intensity large muscle group work e.g. walking, stationary cycling, muscle groups for ADL.
● Emphasize posture and core strength.
● Include breathlessness management and recovery strategies.
● Promote energy conservation and pacing.

HRR: heart rate reserve, *RPE*: rating of perceived exertion

muscle training can improve functional capacity and reduce dyspnoea, according to a systematic review (Lin *et al* 2012) and a meta-analysis (Plentz *et al* 2012). Functional electrical stimulation can improve exercise capacity, quality of life and endothelial function (Karavidas 2013).

A home-based programme can reduce hospital admissions (Harris 2013), and telephone reinforcement can increase survival (Hoekstra *et al* 2013).

PROBLEMS ASSOCIATED WITH CORONARY HEART DISEASE (CHD)

For patients with acute problems related to CHD, the physiotherapist becomes involved when they are admitted with myocardial infarction or for heart surgery. Once the patient has stabilized, they are best managed through a multidisciplinary cardiac rehabilitation programme.

CARDIAC REHABILITATION

> *Despite the evidence supporting its cardio-protective properties, physical activity is not taken seriously as a prescription. Health services rely on medication without considering the long-term consequences.*
> Stamatakis & Weiler (2010)

Following hospitalization for heart disease or heart surgery, disability rates of 45–75% have been identified (Dolansky *et al* 2011). Cardiac rehabilitation (CR) addresses the causes of this, including exercise intolerance, comorbidities and anxiety.

CR involves education, exercise and relaxation, supervised by a multidisciplinary team. Participation rates are low at 20–30%, due to patient and health system factors (Grace *et al* 2012) and a gender bias towards men (Beckstead *et al* 2014). Older patients show higher adherence (Azad 2012), and have demonstrated greater improvements in function, quality of life (QoL) (Lavie 2000) and depression (Fig 12.1) but older people are underrepresented, possibly because of low expectations and inadequate referrals (Menezes *et al*

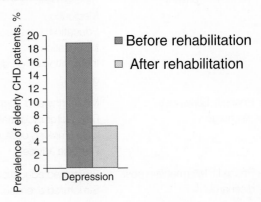

FIGURE 12.1 Prevalence of depression in elderly heart disease patients before and after cardiac rehabilitation

2012). Attendance can be maximized by sending phone reminders, arranging parking or volunteer drivers, and considering home-based programmes for lower risk patients, which are cheaper and can be as effective (Brual *et al* 2012).

CR shows the following benefits:
- ↑ endothelial function (Cornelissen 2014)
- ↑ heart rate recovery, reflecting vagal reactivation and improved mortality (Beckie *et al* 2014)
- ↓ morbidity and mortality (Beckstead *et al* 2014).
- ↓ myocardial reinfarction, anxiety, depression, re-admission, ↑ QoL, exercise capacity and return to work (ACPICR 2012).

In Europe rehabilitation is separated into four phases (Table 12.2), while the US combines phases II and III.

Structure

In-patient phase

In phase I, the patient's physical ability is compromised by the effects of heart disease or surgery, and sometimes by bed rest. Automatic referral for CR is advised (Leger *et al* 2013). Once vital signs are stable, the aim of physiotherapy is to maintain suitable levels of activity

TABLE 12.2 Cardiac rehabilitation phases.

Timing	Content	Staff
Phase I: In-patient	Assessment. Medication. Education: lifestyle and medication Mobilization. Information on cardiac support groups.	Hospital-based nurses, physiotherapist, doctors, dietician, pharmacist, psychologist, occupational therapist (OT).
Phase II: Early post-discharge	Monitoring and support. Risk factor modification, e.g. weight loss, smoking cessation, relaxation. Exercise advice.	Community specialist team.
Phase III: Intermediate post discharge	Structured education. Structured exercise.	Specialist nurse, physiotherapist, OT, pharmacist, dietician, clinical psychologist.
Phase IV: Maintenance	Long term follow-up. Local support groups.	Community specialist team.

(App. C), with exercise intensity governed by heart rate (HR) or perceived exertion (Table 12.3).

Early post discharge phase

Most post-discharge morbidity and mortality has been attributed to failure to adhere to the new medication regime (Bernal *et al* 2012), which underlines the importance of monitoring and support in this Phase II. Education is usually provided by specialist nurses and involves a combination of home visits, telephone monitoring and clinic appointments.

In this transition stage physiotherapists can advise patients to build up their activity gradually to around 20–30 minutes of walking each day, including power walking (Kim *et al* 2012a), depending on previous fitness levels. Dolansky *et al* (2011) describe how education and a family-focused low-intensity exercise programme can improve exercise tolerance and motivation to attend Phase III.

Intermediate post discharge phase

The structured part of the programme occurs in Phase III. When started from one week after discharge, it can reduce readmissions (Haykowsky *et al* 2011). Patients

need to be screened, including an exercise ECG (stress test) to detect ischaemic changes on graded

TABLE 12.3 Rate of perceived exertion

	Intensity	Breathing equivalent
6	No exertion	
7		Can sing full songs
8	Extremely light	
9	Very light	Can sing partial verses
10		
11	Light	Can talk in full sentences
12		
13	Somewhat hard	Can talk in short sentences
14		
15	Hard	Breathing hard
16		
17	Very hard	
18		
19	Extremely hard	
20	Maximal	

exercise (Stickland *et al* 2012). Patients with a variety of CV disorders can be included (Box 12.3) irrespective of age or clinical status, but a change in condition requires re-assessment.

Programmes are usually group-based and last 6–12 weeks, comprising one to three sessions a week of education and supervised exercise, with partners and carers present when possible. Patients may prefer individual sessions, sometimes at home, or use of a self-help heart manual (NHS Lothian 2011).

Long-term maintenance

Phase IV is indefinite, the goal being to encourage life-long adherence to the healthy habits established during earlier phases. An exercise regime maintains the benefits of the programme (Freyssin *et al* 2012), and is advised as working to 50–70% of maximal predicted HR on most days (Golbidi & Laher 2012) or 150 mins/week (Pinto *et al* 2011).

Education

Education aims to build confidence and facilitate autonomy. It should include the principles in Box 12.1 and most of the topics in Table 12.1, plus:

- pathology and symptoms
- other risk factors such as hypertension
- occupational and vocational factors
- pharmaceutical and surgical options
- basic life support
- living with uncertainty, advance care planning and end of life decisions (BACPR 2012).

Discussion on other therapies is also advised because the majority of patients use dietary supplements or complementary therapies (Prasad *et al* 2013). Stress management has a direct bearing on QoL (Arena 2012), and treatment options for depression should be included because CV disease and depression influence QoL in an additive fashion, with QoL

BOX 12.3

Patients suitable for cardiac rehabilitation

Coronary heart disease

- stable angina
- myocardial infarction
- revascularization by angioplasty or coronary artery bypass graft

Other types of heart surgery

- pre and post heart transplant
- heart valve repair/replacement

Other heart conditions

- stable heart failure
- following implantation of cardiac defibrillator or resynchronization device
- adults with congenital heart disease

Vascular conditions

- peripheral vascular disease
- transient ischaemic attack

outcomes being as important as survival outcomes (O'Neil et al 2013).

> The availability of [healthy] foods and better access to recreational and sporting facilities may have a greater impact … than health professional advice.
>
> Ebrahim et al (2011)

Exercise

Exercise training is well-established for improving QoL and survival in patients with CV disease (Piepoli 2013). As well as improved arterial compliance, both artery diameter and arteriolar density are increased. This increase does not occur with pathological myocardial hypertrophy (e.g. from hypertension or aortic stenosis) when capillary rarefaction occurs (Laughlin et al 2012).

Patients need to build up their exercise tolerance slowly because, although sustained physical training reduces platelet reactivity, acute activity brings an increased risk of atherosclerotic plaque rupture during and immediately after physical exercise, especially in those who have been sedentary (Kumar et al 2012).

Assessment

Participants should bring their anti-angina drugs with them for all sessions. Those with diabetes need to bring their glucose tablets. Drinking water must be available throughout, but energy drinks are not recommended because of the risk of adverse cardiac events (Goldfarb 2014).

The six-minute and shuttle walk tests (Ch. 9) relate to maximum oxygen consumption ($\dot{V}O_2$max) (Mandic 2013), or the 2-minute-walk test can be used for debilitated patients (Casillas et al 2013). Symptom-limited exercise testing can be performed safely and effectively in patients with implanted cardioverter defibrillators, but, as always, strategies must be place in case of ventricular arrhythmias (Flo et al 2012).

Intensity monitoring can be by:
- $\dot{V}O_2$max derived from an exercise test.
- 'System-limited' peak oxygen consumption, which is the highest oxygen consumption reached during an exercise period and

is considered a valid index of $\dot{V}O_2$max (Mezzani et al 2013).
- The measures in Table 12.4.

The history and assessment identifies any contraindication to exercise training (Box 12.4) and patients are then stratified as low, moderate or high risk (App. C) for exercise prescription and level of supervision.

BP should be taken with the cuff as near heart level as possible. BP and HR are required before each exercise session as well as in the formal assessment.

If HR is irregular or >100 or unusually low for the patient, especially if associated with dizziness, palpitations, chest discomfort, dyspnoea, nausea or sweating, the patient should sit or lie down in a semi-recumbent position. If it does not resolve, exercise is contraindicated and the doctor should be called.

Exercise can usually be modified for patients with arthritic conditions, but on days when joint pain is increased by exercise, the patient can take their own decision on whether to continue, with or without analgesia, so long as the pain is not prolonged and they are fully informed about joint protection. They may prefer non-weight-bearing maintenance exercise such as swimming.

The assessment provides an opportunity to offer literature or advice on clinics for smoking cessation, without which the benefits of CR are limited (Mlakar 2013), dietetics or erectile dysfunction. A minimum of two staff members is required at all times, with a staff to patient ratio of 1:5 for moderate risk patients.

Procedure

Patients on anti-coagulation drugs should avoid high-impact activity or contact sports in case of bruising or bleeding, and those on diuretics should avoid prolonged exercise in hot weather in case of reduced potassium and fluid volume. Patients must not exercise after a large meal or in extremes of heat or cold. For post-sternotomy patients, the mode of exercise should not cause a shearing stress on the sternum before union at 8–12 weeks. Warm up and cool down periods of exercise are required for all patients.

A progressive training effect can be achieved by increasing the frequency, intensity and/or duration of exercise (Table 12.4), to include both endurance and resistance training (Uhlemann et al 2012).

TABLE 12.4 Exercise prescription

Requirement	Frequency	Intensity	Time in minutes per day	Type of exercise
Health benefit	Every day – incorporate into daily routine	RPE 11–13 e.g. brisk walking	30 min. (can be done in bouts of 10–15 min.)	Structured exercise or lifestyle activities e.g. walking, stairs, washing car, cleaning windows, gardening, cycling
Cardiovascular fitness	2–3 times per week	Initially 40–60% $\dot{V}O_2$max progressing to 70% i.e.: • 40–60% HRR, progressing to 70%, or • 12–14 RPE, progressing to 15	45–60 min. continuous: • 15 min. warm up • 20–30 min. workout • 10 min. cool down	Aerobic activity, starting with interval then progressing to continuous
Muscle strength and endurance	2–3 times per week	• Upper body 30–40% 1 RM • Lower body 50–60% 1 RM	1 set of 10–15 repetitions	8–10 different muscle groups
Deconditioned patient with functional capacity < 3 METS	Every day – incorporate into daily routine	RPE 12, 40% HRR, 60% HR max or lower intensity for very low functioning patients.	5–10 min. bouts (gradual increase to accumulated 30 min. per day)	Activities to improve function, strength, endurance, posture, balance and co-ordination e.g. walking, low step-ups, sit to stand, seated activities.

1RM: one repetition maximum, *HRR*: heart rate reserve, *Max HR*: available from a stress/exercise test, or calculated as 220 minus age; *RPE*: rating of perceived exertion

BOX 12.4

Factors which preclude a patient from joining or continuing the exercise component of cardiac rehabilitation

- unstable angina
- resting systolic BP >200 mmHg or diastolic BP >110 mmHg
- exercise-induced hypotension or orthostatic BP drop of >20 mmHg with symptoms
- critical aortic stenosis (valve area <1 cm^2)
- acute illness or fever
- uncontrolled arrhythmias
- acute pericarditis or myocarditis
- uncompensated congestive cardiac failure
- 3rd degree atrioventricular block (without pacemaker)
- thrombophlebitis or recent embolism
- resting ST segment displacement >2 mm, indicating ischaemia
- uncontrolled diabetes
- high or low potassium levels
- severe rejection following cardiac transplantation
- severe orthopaedic or arthritic condition that would prohibit exercise or exacerbate the orthopaedic/arthritic problem.

The physiotherapist learns to identify the characteristics of each patient's angina and the feel of their pulse. If HR is used for monitoring, participants take their pulse during exercise to ensure that it is within their prescribed target range, and after the cool-down period to check that it has returned to the pre-exercise rate. Excessive HR is inadvisable because a short diastole prevents the blood from nourishing cardiac muscle (Böhm & Reil 2013).

Beta-blockers and calcium channel blockers dampen the heart's response to exercise, and patients on these drugs should monitor their RPE rather than HR. The RPE is valid for monitoring and prescribing exercise intensity (Scherr 2013) and is explained to patients as the inner feeling of exertion, not leg ache or breathlessness. Self-monitoring encourages exercise maintenance in Phase IV (Izawa et al 2005).

A check ECG should be requested if the pulse behaves abnormally, if exercise tolerance declines over two or three sessions, or if a patient feels that their heart is not 'right'. Patients often detect that something is amiss before it becomes obvious, and reports of 'impending doom' need to be taken seriously (Chhabra & Spodick 2013). Referral for drug review is required if angina occurs, side effects increase or exercise tolerance is reduced by pulmonary oedema.

If a patient says they do not feel well or feels unusually tired, they should sit down and have their BP, HR and respiratory rate taken. If a patient gets angina during exercise, the following steps should be taken:

- the patient sits down and takes their glyceryl trinitrate, 1–2 sprays or 1–2 tablets, under the tongue, if prescribed, unless the patient is hypotensive or feels dizzy
- they wait five minutes for relief of symptoms
- two further doses may be taken at five minute intervals

- if symptoms are relieved, they should rest for a further five minutes, then re-join the class at a lower intensity; if they wish to leave they must be fully recovered beforehand
- if symptoms are unrelieved after 15 minutes of repeated medication, the doctor should be called.

If there is an irregular pulse which takes more than a minute to recover, the patient should lie down. Myocardial infarction is suspected if the pain is more severe than normal or the patient is grey, short of breath and sweaty, in which case assistance is summoned.

When one participant feels unwell and is being cared for, spare staff should attend to the other participants.

Relaxation

Relaxation improves haemodynamic variables beyond that promoted by CR alone (Neves *et al* 2009), and 5–10 minutes' practice should be slotted into each session so that patients understand how it can be fitted into their daily life. Relaxation also helps combat the fatigue that is commonly cited as a barrier to exercise (Barnason *et al* 2008). T'ai Chi promotes relaxation and

shows beneficial effects on BP, $\dot{V}O_2$max and QoL (Ng *et al* 2012).

Follow up

Patients have described on-going support as imperative to help them maintain lifestyle changes and navigate a new way of life (Pryor 2014), e.g. community programmes run by fitness instructors (Adsett *et al* 2013).

PROBLEMS ASSOCIATED WITH PERIPHERAL ARTERIAL DISEASE (PAD)

Intermittent claudication (Ch. 4) limits exercise tolerance and impairs quality of life (Fig 12.2). Goals negotiated with the patient may include increasing distance walked or time spent walking, walking to a location which is meaningful to the patient or managing a specific activity.

Education

The aims of education are to help the patient modify risk factors associated with atherosclerosis, explain

---

FIGURE 12.2 Functional consequences of PAD

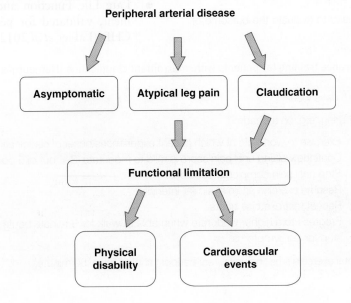

how exercise helps their condition and advise on foot care.

Exercise

Exercise training can improve walking ability more than stent revascularization (Murphy *et al* 2012). Muscle oxidative capacity is enhanced, functional performance and quality of life improved (Monteiro *et al* 2013) and cardiovascular risk reduced (McDermott *et al* 2009).

Treadmill walking is suitable for many patients, but for those who are elderly, frail or at risk of falling, the circulation can be improved by lower limb exercises in sitting (Castro-Sánchez 2013) or devices to facilitate plantarflexion (Tebbut *et al* 2011). Interval training is recommended, and some success is possible without eliciting leg pain (Lefebvre 2013).

Exercise testing may reveal signs and symptoms of hitherto occult coronary heart disease, which should be reported. As exercise tolerance improves, these symptoms may become a limiting factor. Cardiac rehabilitation can be adapted for patients with PAD but patients classified at the severest level (Ch. 4) should not join the exercise sessions. Exercise prescription is suggested in Table 12.5.

For simple cramps at night, patients may find it helpful to do three 30-second calf stretches during the day, lowering alternate heels from the edge of a step (Daniell & Pentrack 2013).

OUTCOMES

The following can be used to evaluate the outcome of cardiac rehabilitation.

Exercise capacity

- Accelerometer (Pinto *et al* 2011).
- Six minute walk test (Bellet *et al* 2012) or tests which correlate with this such as the Timed Up and Go Test (Adams *et al* 2013).
- Incremental shuttle walk test (Shoemaker *et al* 2013).
- Chester Step Test (Sykes & Roberts 2004).
- Treadmill or cycle ergometer tests (Lauer 2008).
- Treadmill walking ability and questionnaires (Mays *et al* 2011).
- Measure Yourself Medical Outcome Profile (Salisbury *et al* 2009).

Quality of life

- Minnesota Living with Heart Failure questionnaire (Naveiro-Rilo *et al* 2012).
- Hospital Anxiety and Depression Scale (Eng *et al* 2011).
- SF36 and SF12 (Mays *et al* 2011).
- Heart QoL Questionnaire (Oldridge *et al* 2014).
- EQ–5D and QLMI questionnaires (Dyer *et al* 2010).
- Dartmouth COOP Domain (Eaton *et al* 2005).
- Cardiovascular Limitations and Symptoms Profile (Lewin *et al* 2002).
- Late Life Function and Disability Instrument, validated for people >age 60 with CHD (LaPier *et al* 2012).

TABLE 12.5 Endurance training for patients with intermittent claudication (Hamburg & Balady 2011)

Frequency	3–5 days/week
Modality	Walking, e.g. on a treadmill
Intensity	• Exercise to work rate at which patient experiences onset of claudication. • Continue walking until pain score is mild to moderate (3–4 out of 5 points). • Stop until pain completely subsides. • Resume exercise again at similar intensity. • Repeat rest/exercise bouts. • Progress to a higher work rate when able to walk for 8 minute bouts without needing to stop for leg symptoms.
Duration	Total exercise time (including rest periods) should equal 50 minutes.

CASE STUDY : MR BG

Identify the problems of this patient awaiting discharge following inguinal hernia repair.

Background
- COPD
- Smoker

Nurse report
- Possible chest infection

Subjective
- Feeling unwell
- Breathless, especially when lying flat
- Coughing up white secretions

Objective
- Pale
- Apyrexial
- Bilateral basal crackles and wheeze on auscultation
- Swollen ankles
- S_pO_2 94%
- Radiology as Fig 12.3

Questions
1. Analysis?
2. Problems?
3. Goals?
4. Plan?

FIGURE 12.3 Enlarged heart and hilar flare indicative of pulmonary oedema

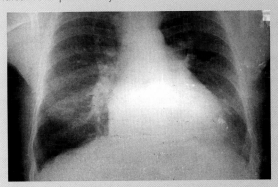

CLINICAL REASONING

Cardiac rehabilitation including exercise, group discussion, breath focus, meditation, mindfulness, visualization and cognitive restructuring was found to reduce BP, blood lipids and BMI, and to improve psychological measures and exercise response. The conclusion was that a mind/body CR programme reduced medical and psychological risks.

J Cardiopulm Rehabil Prev, 29, 230–8

Response to Case Study

1 **Analysis**

- X-ray suggests pulmonary oedema.
- Absence of green sputum or pyrexia suggests there is no chest infection.
- Sudden onset suggests MI rather than HF.
- Need to liaise with medical team for further investigations.

Note 1: beta-agonist bronchodilators may induce tachycardia.

Note 2: airway clearance techniques are not effective for pulmonary oedema.

2 **Problems**

- Increased WOB, due to pulmonary oedema.

3 **Goals**

- Reduce WOB.
- Rehabilitate to home environment.

4 **Plan**

- Once patient is stabilized and on appropriate medication, advise on upright positioning and progressive mobility.
- Multidisciplinary rehabilitation, preferably HF rehabilitation, otherwise pulmonary or cardiac.

HF: heart failure, *MI:* myocardial infarct, *WOB:* work of breathing

Response to Clinical Reasoning

Multiple components mean that no conclusion can be drawn about any one modality. The lack of a control group means that improvements cannot definitely be attributed to the intervention.

RECOMMENDED READING

Chiari S (2013) Dynamic pulmonary hyperinflation occurs without expiratory flow limitation in chronic heart failure during exercise. *Resp Physiol Neurobiol;* **189**(1): 34–41

Delise P (2013) Long-term effect of continuing sports activity in competitive athletes with frequent ventricular premature complexes and apparently normal heart. *Am J Cardiol;* **112**(9): 1396–1402

ESH/ESC (2013) Guidelines for the management of arterial hypertension. *Eur Heart J;* **34**(28): 2159–219

Gąsiorowski A, Dutkiewicz J (2013) Comprehensive rehabilitation in chronic heart failure. *Ann Agric Environ Med;* **20**(3): 606–12

Hamm LF, Jones AM, McBride PE *et al* (2012) Aerobic exercise intensity assessment and prescription in cardiac rehabilitation. *J Cardiopulm Rehab Prev;* **32**(6): 327–50.

Han HR, Song HJ, Nguyen T *et al* (2014) Measuring self-care in patients with hypertension. *J Cardiovasc Nurs;* **29**(1): 55–67

Haykowsky MJ (2013) Meta-analysis of aerobic interval training on exercise capacity and systolic function in patients with heart failure and reduced ejection fractions. *Am J Cardiol;* **111**(10): 1466–9

Johnson FL (2014) Pathophysiology and etiology of heart failure. *Cardiol Clinics;* **32**(1): 9–19

Karapolat H, Engin C, Eroglu M *et al* (2013) Efficacy of the cardiac rehabilitation program in patients with end-stage heart failure, heart transplant patients, and left ventricular assist device recipients. *Transplant Proc;* **45**(9): 3381–5

Lopez-Jimenez F, Kramer VC, Masters B *et al* (2012) Recommendations for managing patients with diabetes mellitus in cardiopulmonary rehabilitation. *J Cardiopulm Rehab Prev;* **32**(2): 101–12

Orr JL, Williamson P, Anderson W *et al* (2013) Cardiopulmonary exercise testing. *Anaesthesia;* **68**: 497–501

Patarroyo-Aponte M (2014) Evaluation of patients with heart failure. *Cardiol Clinics;* **32**(1): 47–62

Scalvini S (2013) Home-based versus in-hospital cardiac rehabilitation after cardiac surgery. *Phys Ther*; **93**(8): 1073–83

Shoemaker MJ (2013) Clinically meaningful change estimates for the six-minute walk test and daily activity in individuals with chronic heart failure. *Cardiopulm Phys Ther J*; **24**(2): 21–29

South F, Upton D, Upton P (2013) The impact of Ramadan on lifestyle behaviours and implications for cardiac rehabilitation. *Internat J Rehabil Res;* **20**(7): 328–34

White A, Broder J, Campo TM (2012) Acute aortic emergencies. *Adv Emerg Nurs J*; **34**(3): 216–29

CHAPTER 13
Physiotherapy for people with hyperventilation syndrome

LEARNING OBJECTIVES

On completion of this chapter the reader should be able to:

- appreciate the relationships between the origin, triggers, pathophysiology and consequences of hyperventilation syndrome

- recognize symptoms of the disorder and ensure that all team members are aware of the syndrome and its presentation

- plan a flexible management regime related to the patient's needs

- ensure that the patient is able to maintain improvement

- evaluate the outcomes of treatment.

INTRODUCTION

Respiration is situated strategically at the interface of mind and body.
Wilhelm *et al* (2001)

Hyperventilation is breathing in excess of metabolic needs. Acute hyperventilation is an adaptive response preparing for fight or flight. Chronic hyperventilation may be linked to stress, disorders associated with shortness of breath or both. It occurs in all age ranges (Munemoto et al 2013) and has been found in 9.5% of adults (Jones et al 2013a) and 20% of children and teenagers, or twice this if they also had asthma (Gridina 2013). It is associated with some alarming effects, often intermittently, which deplete the body's stress-coping mechanisms.

Chronic hyperventilation may be termed 'dysfunctional breathing', or more specifically 'hyperventilation syndrome' (HVS). Attempts to understand the condition have led to other labels such as irritable heart, autonomic imbalance, cardiovascular neurosis, effort syndrome, neurocirculatory asthenia, soldiers' heart, factor X syndrome and, as a last resort, fat folder syndrome. Links with cardiology and warfare (Magarian 1982) relate to its symptomatology and its association with stress (Munemoto *et al* 2013). The condition was first identified during the American Civil War and again in the 20th century World Wars, when many thousands of young soldiers were invalided out with 'heart disease'. Symptoms that mimic heart disease led to both Florence Nightingale and Charles Darwin being diagnosed with cardiac problems at an early age, but both lived long lives and their ill-health has since been ascribed to HVS (Timmons & Ley 1994).

Widespread failure to identify the syndrome is because:

- there is cursory coverage in medical texts
- physiological adaptation has taken place so that not all patients are conspicuously breathless
- it occupies the boundary between body and mind, a no-mans-land in Western medicine
- symptoms are non-specific and variable
- there is no unequivocal diagnostic test.

If HVS is not identified, patients trek from clinic to clinic, accruing ever fatter case files, being labelled as neurotic and submitting to invasive investigations and sometimes years of debilitating medication. Without treatment, the condition persists or worsens in 75% of people, through intertwining vicious circles (Fig 13.1). The majority of children with HVS appear to go undiagnosed (Joorabchi 1997), and Enzer *et al* (1967) found that 86% were misdiagnosed with epilepsy, seizures and panic disorders. HVS is eminently treatable, however, with symptoms being abolished in 75% of patients (Timmons & Ley 1994, p. 113). Relaxation and breathing re-training appear to be more effective than

---

FIGURE 13.1   Interrelation of some of the factors which cause and exacerbate hyperventilation syndrome

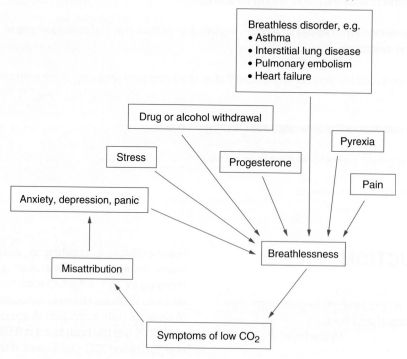

psychological methods or drugs (Kraft 1984), and sedatives such as diazepam are inadvisable (Munemoto *et al* 2013).

Much of this chapter is based on physiological reasoning and the author's patients, due to limited coverage in the health literature.

CAUSES, TRIGGERS AND EFFECTS

> *The thread of the breath is woven throughout the tapestry of a person's life experience.*
> Harris 1996

Some religious sects and individuals deliberately hyperventilate in order to attain trance-like states of consciousness (Perera 1988). Some of these effects are similar to the symptoms of HVS, but they do not incorporate the anxiety and lack of control that accompany unintentional and chronic hyperventilation. The overlap between cause, effect, pathophysiology and clinical features reinforces the difficulty in identifying HVS, even though physiologically the syndrome is simply an abnormality of respiratory control (Chenuel 2008).

A person's respiratory drive varies two- to four-fold under normal circumstances, but this can be modulated by life events (Strohl *et al* 1998). HVS may originate from bereavement, a traumatic birth (Brennan 2011), adverse life experiences (Bakal 2013) especially if crying out is prevented, or incidents around fear and breathing, including seemingly minor events such as a ducking in the school swimming pool or a forcefully applied anaesthetic mask. The common outcome is a hyperventilatory respiratory drive (Jack *et al* 2004). Breathing occupies a central role in translating psychological changes into somatic symptoms (Gilbert 1999a), and body memory is thought to be held particularly in the breathing pattern (Harris 1996). Other causes are chronic pain (Glynn 1981), withdrawal from opiates (Brashear 1983) or alcohol (Roelofs 1985), and hypermobility syndrome affecting thoracic joints (Innocenti & Troup 2008).

Whether or not an original cause is identified, there is usually a trigger, often stress-related, which the patient may identify as setting off an acute episode. This may be as simple as prolonged conversation, or a recognized stressor such as viral illness or surgery (Moon *et al* 2011).

The trigger sets off an overly sensitive 'suffocation alarm' which may have become sensitized by the original cause. This can lead to disproportionate dyspnoea, fear of asphyxia and a cascade of panic symptoms. One patient described how she constantly listened for her next breath and did not like travelling in cars because she could not hear it (Paulley 1990).

P_aCO_2 tends to be kept low by chronic hyperventilation in order to avoid triggering the alarm (Meuret *et al* 2012), but hyperventilation-induced alkalosis can itself increase serum lactate and set off a panic attack (Ridder *et al* 2010).

Cause and effect then become interchangeable. The question that continues to tease researchers is whether hyperventilation or anxiety comes first, but in practice they augment each other. Either way, the syndrome is associated with:

- conditions which cause over breathing and may reprogramme the respiratory centres, e.g. asthma, heart failure, pain, interstitial lung disease, long term low grade fever or acidosis caused by liver cirrhosis (Karetzky 1967)
- other conditions such as chronic fatigue syndrome (Ocon 2013), hypertension, sleep disorders, Raynaud's disease, migraine, agoraphobia and vocal cord dysfunction, the latter mimicking or coexisting with asthma and being set off by autonomic imbalance (Ayres & Gabbott 2002)
- exercise deconditioning due to avoidance of activities that cause dyspnoea, as also occurs with asthma (Troosters 1999)
- spinal and pelvic instability (Chaitow 2007) or poor balance (David *et al* 2012)
- the premenstrual week because progesterone is a respiratory stimulant (Moon *et al* 2011)
- chemical sensitivities, food allergy, irritable bowel syndrome (Kanaan *et al* 2007) or high caffeine intake (Wemmie 2011)
- emotional factors such as fear, suppressed anger, depression, orgasm or laughter
- occupations which entail deep breathing or prolonged speaking such as singing, call centre work, teaching or playing a wind instrument (Widmer *et al* 1997)
- restrictive clothes, leading in Victorian times to corseted women collapsing with

the 'vapours', and a century later the alternative name for HVS of 'designer jeans syndrome'

- in children, family discord or anxieties, sometimes leading to fainting in school assembly or possibly 'mass psychogenic illness' (Jones *et al* 2000).

There is overlap between hyperventilation, panic attacks and agoraphobia (Wemmie 2011), the latter being found in 60% of people with HVS, while HVS has been found in 60% of people with agoraphobia (Garssen 1983). These respond to breathing retraining (Meuret *et al* 2012).

Although hyperventilation is a recognized stress response, it is not known why some people respond to stress with chronic hyperventilation while others develop different somatization disorders. Somatization has been considered one of medicine's blind spots and may be the body's way of expressing distress via autonomic dysregulation without conscious appreciation (Dreher 1996).

Personality plays a part because people who respond to stress in this way tend to suppress their emotions and are often conscientious, sensitive, perfectionist and enthusiastic. It is these qualities, along with the high motivation that accompanies their relief at finding constructive help, which makes people with HVS a delight to treat.

PATHOPHYSIOLOGY

Body and mind can live in two different worlds ... this odd mismatch can create a morass of symptoms and no end of distress.
                                                                    Gilbert 1999a

Over breathing washes out the body's CO_2 stores, leading to high and sometimes unstable pH in blood and cerebrospinal fluid. Alkalosis leads to:

- ↓ hydrogen ions in intracellular fluid, shifting extracellular potassium ions into the cells to maintain the balance of intracellular ions → hypokalaemia → upset ECG.
- ↓ calcium ions in plasma → excitable sensory and motor neurons → stiffness, spasms, tetany and in severe cases seizures (Weiss 2009).
- ↓ cerebral blood flow (Pearson 2007), leading to headaches (Moon *et al* 2011).

- autonomic instability of other blood vessels (Fig 13.2c) causing widespread symptoms
- Oxygen dissociation curve shifted to the left → less oxygen released to the tissues, which reinforces the cerebral hypoxia caused by unstable blood vessels.
- ↓ phosphate levels → fatigue, disorientation, paraesthesia and muscle cramps (Widmer *et al* 1997).
- ↓ magnesium → further muscle spasm, fatigue, headache and ECG upset.

An increased drive to breathe re-sets the respiratory centres in order to maintain normal pH, obliging the patient to continue low-grade hyperventilation despite a persistently low P_aCO_2.

FIGURE 13.2 Hyperventilation causing (a) respiratory alkalosis, (b) hypocapnia, (c) vasoconstriction

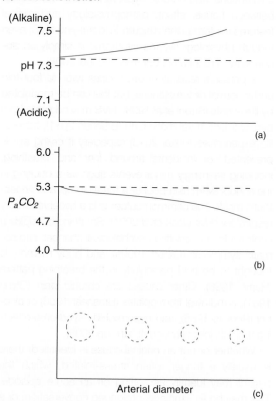

CLINICAL FEATURES

Breathing is the very essence of life. When this function is under threat it is impossible not to feel frightened.

Syrett & Taylor 2003

Once pH reaches 7.5, symptoms emerge in some people, and at 7.6 they are universal (Gilbert 1999a). When compensation has returned pH to normal, albeit with some instability, a low P_aCO_2 may be maintained with occasional deep breaths or sighs, which can be imperceptible subjectively (Moynihan 2001) and only noticeable by an attentive clinician. Patients whose minute volume is not labile and has stabilized at a higher level may not complain of dyspnoea.

Added to the symptoms outlined previously are those described below:

1   Cerebral vasoconstriction can cause nausea, dizziness, blackouts, fainting (David 2003), fear of falling (Clague 2000), visual disturbance and sometimes a dissociated state of unreality that feels like the person is floating outside their body.

2   Coronary vasoconstriction, compounded by decreased oxygen yield to the tissues, may cause angina (Magarian 1982) or atypical chest pain. Up to 90% of noncardiac chest pain is thought to be associated with HVS (DeGuire *et al* 1992) but a misdiagnosis of heart disease may occur (Kannivelu 2013). Unlike heart pathology, however, the ST segment may be depressed and T wave flattened (Moon *et al* 2011), and changes may disappear with exercise (Missri & Alexander 1978).

3   Musculoskeletal imbalance may be caused by overuse and tension in the accessory respiratory muscles or dysfunctional postures, especially with tasks involving sustained concentration such as computer work (CliftonSmith & Rowley 2011).

4   Despite chronic pain sometimes being a cause or trigger (Kvåle *et al* 2002), one of the effects of neuronal excitability on large nerve fibres is to dampen down pain. Hyperventilation is sometimes used as a

coping strategy for pain, and HVS can be one of the outcomes for survivors of torture (Hough 1992).

5   Misdiagnosis of asthma is common (Hagman *et al* 2011) because HVS and asthma augment each other's symptoms and hypocapnia can cause bronchoconstriction (Lehrer *et al* 2008) or chest discomfort on exercise (Hammo 1999). Gardner (2004) found that 80% of patients with acute hyperventilation had evidence of asthma, and half of these were undiagnosed. Thomas *et al* (2001) found that a third of women and a fifth of men diagnosed with asthma had HVS. So-called 'steroid resistant asthma' may be HVS (Thomas 2003). People with HVS may associate breathing with a need to concentrate, while those with asthma may describe a sense of effort (Anon 2012).

Alkalosis and paraesthesia may lead to further misdiagnoses, one study finding that 86% of patients referred with carpal tunnel syndrome had HVS (Aslam *et al* 2012).

The dyspnoea of HVS is distinctive. It is disproportionate, fluctuating, poorly correlated with exercise, greater with inspiration than expiration and exacerbated with crowds, conversation and social situations. It is sometimes described as air hunger, heaviness on the chest or a smothering feeling. Negative trials of nitroglycerin or bronchodilators help to eliminate a diagnosis of heart disease or asthma, and a normal peak flow reading when breathless can be reassuring.

Exercise may relieve symptoms due to metabolism catching up with breathing, but sometimes loss of fine tuning means that breathing may not adjust to activity and symptoms may worsen or become chaotic (Fig 13.3). Even though fatigue is a common symptom, some patients choose to work out because it provides the opportunity to take deep breaths. Activities which heighten arousal without an accompanying increase in activity, e.g. driving, can worsen symptoms.

Breathing usually stabilizes at night when it is driven by the metabolic system (Slutsky & Phillipson 1994), but patients with unstable blood sugar, e.g. after a late carbohydrate-laden meal, sometimes complain of feeling dreadful on waking, when their blood sugar has plummeted.

Signs and symptoms are summarized in Table 13.1.

FIGURE 13.3 Ventilatory response to graded exercise in a patient with HVS before (top 2 lines) and two weeks after (bottom 2 lines) education on the disorder. The coloured area represents the range in normal subjects

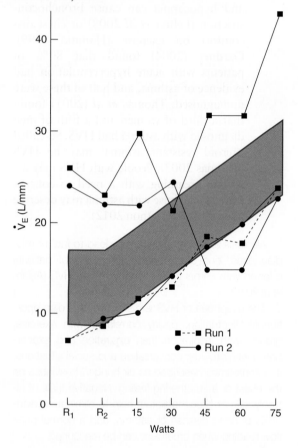

ASSESSMENT

Hyperventilation is the great mimic

Lum 1981

People with HVS may have received a selection of diagnoses from peripheral neuropathy or neurosis to myocardial infarction or multiple sclerosis. Some have been dismissed as malingerers or told that it is all in their mind. Others have been told that it is 'only hyperventilation', somehow disqualifying further consideration. The first priority therefore is to ensure that patients feel welcome and know that their problem is taken seriously. They need space, time, privacy and an attentive ear.

The case notes should be scrutinized for conditions that cause breathlessness and for concomitant or alternative diagnoses. Low haemoglobin, for example, means that breathing retraining can exacerbate the dyspnoea of anaemia. If patients are on β-blockers, these can either exacerbate HVS by causing bronchospasm, or ameliorate autonomic symptoms and help break the vicious circle of sympathetic stimulation and hyperventilation. Beta$_2$-agonists given for asthma can provoke palpitations and agitation (Criner & Isaac 1995). If patients are being weaned off sedatives, relaxation will be difficult unless treatment coincides with the peak effect of the drug.

KEY POINT

Whether the patient has been medically screened or not, an open mind must be maintained because some symptoms may indicate serious disease.

Subjective

Feelings of flying apart, absolute terror, falling down through the world, spinning through the universe . . .

Patient quoted by Bradley, 2012

SCENARIO

A young woman was referred in some distress following bilateral carpal tunnel release.

Surgery had been performed due to tingling and numbness in both hands, but these symptoms were related to undiagnosed HVS and her paraesthesia was unrelieved. Postoperatively she developed reflex sympathetic dystrophy and the resulting hyperaesthesia led her to cool her hands by blowing on them. This exacerbated her HVS.

Parasthaesia and other HVS symptoms resolved after physiotherapy but her reflex sympathetic dystrophy remained.

TABLE 13.1 Clinical features associated with hyperventilation syndrome

System	Manifestation
Neurological & vascular	Tingling or numbness of extremities or around mouth
	Cold extremities
	Tremor or tetany, especially in extremities
	Chest, shoulder or arm pain
	Headache, dizziness, migraine, blurred vision
	Weakness
	Poor memory and concentration
	Hypersensitivity to lights and sounds
	Palpitations
	Faintness or a spaced out feeling
Emotional	Depersonalized feelings of unreality
	Depression
	Suppression of emotion
	Anxiety ± heightened vigilance
	Panic attacks ± fear of going mad or dying
	Phobias (especially claustrophobia & agoraphobia)
	Mood swings
Gastrointestinal	Gastroesophageal reflux
	Difficulty swallowing
	Dry mouth
	Nausea
	Indigestion
	Flatus and belching
	Irritable bowel
	Food intolerance
Musculoskeletal	Tense and/or fatigued neck & shoulder muscles
	Tense posture
	Myalgia, stiffness, cramps
	Weakness
General	Air hunger
	Fatigue
	Insomnia
	Hypoglycaemia
	Blurred body image

Feelings vary from anxiety to a fear of impending madness or dying (Timmons & Ley 1994, p. 142). There may be fear of flying, of being trapped in a lift or feeling unable to escape from a crowded supermarket. Patients may complain of an inability to take a satisfying breath, or may in fact be unaware of any breathing abnormality. If symptoms worsen while they are on the waiting list, this may be because a common response to a diagnosis of a breathing disorder is to practice deep breathing exercises.

It is useful to identify factors that precede symptoms and the patient's interpretation of them. Patients are often puzzled as to why symptoms affecting so many parts of the body can be caused by a breathing disorder, and may not report 'irrelevant' symptoms. Specific questions about symptoms that are likely to be caused by HVS help elicit these, and also facilitate acceptance of the diagnosis.

Questions on lifestyle may reveal a hyperactive trait and a pattern of rushing to meet deadlines. Many patients are high achievers, and a majority tend to perform tasks quickly, impatiently, often several simultaneously and with a tendency to think ahead, whereas only 20% of normal subjects show these characteristics (van Dixhoorn 1986). Other common factors are a general sensitivity and hyperresponsiveness (Garssen 1980), as shown in the patient's breathing, emotions, and sometimes allergy to food or medication.

Patients should say all they want at this stage because it reduces their need to talk during treatment, which upsets their breathing pattern.

Objective

People who chronically hyperventilate may have a labile breathing pattern, e.g.:

- sighs, yawns, sniffs, throat-clearing or a dry cough
- shallow, fast, apical and/or irregular breaths
- excessive thoracic movement, sometimes with abdominal paradox (Ch. 2)
- breath-holding
- cogwheel breathing, as if the patient dare not let the air out
- prolonged inspiration and curtailed expiration, as if the patient wants to hold on to their precious air.

Dyspnoea and hyperventilation are not synonymous and changes may not be obvious. The breathing

required to maintain hypocapnia is less than that required to induce it, and resting CO_2 levels may be halved with only a 10% increase in minute ventilation (Gardner 2004).

Other signs are a stiff posture and gait, lack of co-ordination between talking and breathing, rapid speech as if the patient is trying to cram several sentences into one, excessive hand movements or other indication of tension, and strategies to sneak in more air such as chest heaving before speaking. Belching may be caused by air swallowing, and cold hands by vasoconstriction. If chest wall tenderness is present, palpation can reassure patients that it is not cardiac pain. Patients are further reassured if thoracic mobilizations ameliorate this tenderness (Innocenti & Troup 2008).

Questionnaires

Suspicions of HVS are raised when there is an unusual mix of clinical features which include some of the above. The Nijmegen questionnaire (Table 13.2) is then used, which demonstrates a sensitivity of up to 91% and specificity up to 95% (Vansteenkiste et al 1991). The normal score is 5–11 out of 64, but for those with HVS it may be above 23 (Courtney et al 2011).

Tests

The following are not validated but may aid acceptance of the diagnosis.

1   A short breath-hold time is suggestive of HVS. People with normal control of their breathing can often hold their breath for 60 seconds at end-inspiration, while those with HVS can reportedly manage only 20 seconds (Courtney et al 2011).

2   People with HVS have an exaggerated increase in ventilation when changing from supine to standing (Stewart et al 2006).

3   A provocation test entails the patient taking 20 consecutive deep breaths or breathing rapidly for 3 minutes (Warburton & Jack 2006). This may bring on familiar symptoms in people with HVS, not just the dizziness which is a normal response to acute hyperventilation. If capnography

TABLE 13.2 Nijmegen questionnaire Tick the relevant box and add up the score

	0	1	2	3	4
Chest pain	☐	☐	☐	☐	☐
Feeling tense	☐	☐	☐	☐	☐
Blurred vision	☐	☐	☐	☐	☐
Dizzy spells	☐	☐	☐	☐	☐
Feeling confused	☐	☐	☐	☐	☐
Faster or deeper breathing	☐	☐	☐	☐	☐
Short of breath	☐	☐	☐	☐	☐
Tight feelings in chest	☐	☐	☐	☐	☐
Bloated feeling in stomach	☐	☐	☐	☐	☐
Tingling fingers	☐	☐	☐	☐	☐
Unable to breathe deeply	☐	☐	☐	☐	☐
Stiff fingers or arms	☐	☐	☐	☐	☐
Tight feelings around mouth	☐	☐	☐	☐	☐
Cold hands or feet	☐	☐	☐	☐	☐
Palpitations	☐	☐	☐	☐	☐
Feelings of anxiety	☐	☐	☐	☐	☐

is available, the CO_2 takes longer than normal to return to baseline (Fig 13.4). The provocation test can be distressing for patients, but may reassure them of the validity of their symptoms and show that they have some control, but it is neither sensitive nor specific (Malmberg *et al* 2000). Vasospasm may be caused by the test and a crash trolley should be on hand. Cerebral vascular disease, epilepsy, sickle cell disease (Brashear 1983) and coronary heart disease are contraindications.

4 A low P_aCO_2 is not itself diagnostic because the syndrome is intermittent, but HVS is suspected if resting CO_2 is low or erratic, if a low CO_2 is sustained during an exercise test (Warburton & Jack 2006), or voluntary over breathing reduces it to <4 kPa (30 cmH$_2$O). Capnography may also be used to provide feedback for patients and outcome measures for physiotherapists (Fig 13.5).

EDUCATION

The main sustaining factor with hyperventilation is misattribution of symptoms to a sinister cause (Singh 2001) and clinical reasoning therefore dictates that education comes first. If a waiting list precludes prompt treatment, education can begin in advance. Sending a handout (App. B) or information about a patient-friendly book such as that by Bradley (2012) will do much of the physiotherapist's work, and sending a Nijmegen questionnaire to be filled out saves time and gives the patient some 'aha' moments as they identify familiar symptoms.

At the first appointment, expectations are checked and goals agreed e.g. in the short term to cope with panic attacks, and in the long term to integrate a normal breathing pattern into everyday life, as identified by elimination of symptoms. The mechanism of HVS can be explained using the vicious circle on the handout, and this information itself normally reduces anxiety. Patients are reassured that HVS does not cause harm, nor does it indicate physical damage. It is a response to stress or other triggers, not a psychiatric illness.

FIGURE 13.4 Capnography measurement of end-tidal CO_2 measured at baseline and for 15 minutes after provocation

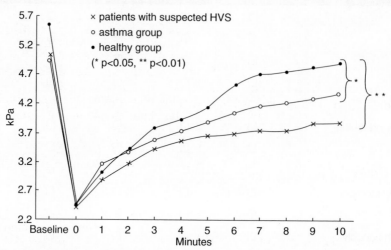

When patients understand that their symptoms stem from chemical changes in the blood, they may feel exonerated from the stigma of not having had their complaints validated by a 'proper' diagnosis.

FIGURE 13.5 End-tidal CO_2 trace (%) before and after physiotherapy

HV: voluntary hyperventilation

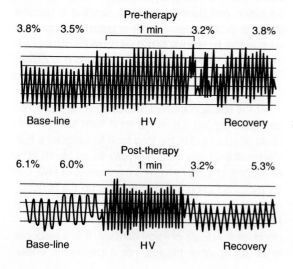

The following advice may be helpful:

1 Physiotherapy will not eliminate the original cause nor remove precipitating factors, but triggers should be identifiable.
2 Commitment is required, in the early stages when learning to control the breathing, and later when incorporating practice into everyday life.
3 It is useful, and sometimes essential, to integrate a small but fundamental shift in attitude and lifestyle that allows time for relaxation and reflection.
4 A nice deep breath does not help relaxation.
5 Re-learning a new lower level of breathing involves experiencing the discomfort of air hunger, but after practice the respiratory centres become re-tuned to registering and regulating a more normal breathing pattern.

To anticipate the feelings experienced with breathing retraining, 'bad breathlessness' can be explained as the patient's familiar and distressing sensation of uncontrolled air hunger, while 'good breathlessness' is a similar physical feeling but without distress because this can now be consciously initiated and controlled as part of the treatment. Although 'good', this breathlessness is not comfortable, and patients appreciate acknowledgment of this.

Patients are advised that physical symptoms may occasionally become worse during or after the first session. This may be due to a paradoxical but transient increase in minute ventilation if the respiratory centres interpret the effects of the breathing re-education as a form of smothering.

Education enables patients to step out of their vicious circle and begin to take control of their breathing. Fig 13.3 shows the ventilatory response to graded exercise before and after gaining insight into the nature of the condition.

BREATHING RETRAINING

According to psychoanalyst Wilhelm Reich, changing a person's breathing pattern is tantamount to emotional surgery (Gilbert 1999b), which may relate to the blocking of emotions caused by tension in chest wall and postural muscles (Kvåle *et al* 2002). The safe environment of a physiotherapy department is unlikely to excavate the depth of emotion that emanates from the analyst's couch, but feelings may surface, and if this brings tears, a proffered box of tissues lets patients know that this is acceptable.

A quiet room is required with an open window or fan. The patient is positioned in any relaxed position, e.g. half-lying with a pillow under their knees and head supported.

Awareness of breathing

Patients learn the feel of their breathing, using some (but not all!) of the following:

1   Rest one hand on your upper chest and one on your abdomen to distinguish chest and abdominal breathing.
2   Experiment with slight alterations in the depth and rate of breathing, to distinguish the two.
3   Try alternate nose and mouth breathing to feel the difference.
4   Feel the passage of the breath as it passes through your nose, down your windpipe and into your lungs, then visualize the air gently returning along the same route.

5   Feel cool air on the in-breath and warm air on the out-breath.
6   To help keep the throat relaxed, imagine breathing in gently through the eyes (Brennan 2011).
7   Try a pause between the out-breath and the in-breath.
8   Check for tension in the rest of your body.

The patient will need to be observed closely throughout the above to ensure that minute volume does not creep up.

Nose breathing

Man should no more breathe through his mouth than take food through his nose.
Clifton-Smith 2004

A habit of breathing in and out through the nose should be established during the session, after explanation, with on going role modelling from the physiotherapist. This may be combined with localized relaxation by the patient keeping their jaw loose and lips together. Reminders may be needed throughout the session.

PRACTICE TIP

Patients can use their time watching TV to remind themselves to nose-breathe.

Relaxation

Breathing cannot be re-educated in a tense person, and most patients need to learn relaxation. Some people find that the thought of being 'obliged' to relax causes tension itself and may prefer to do their relaxation after the breathing practice.

In the West, tense people sometimes find relaxation an alien concept, and it may be easier after a brief neck massage, during which it is helpful for patients to focus on the experience and not feel that they have to talk or 'do' anything. Localized heat can also be helpful prior to relaxation, usually to the shoulders and neck, or to the back with the patient prone. Lying prone may facilitate relaxation, possibly because this is a less vulnerable position than supine.

Focusing on the breath itself helps relaxation, especially if patients are encouraged to gently 'breathe in the good air' and 'breathe out the tension', as if freeing the breath. Control of breathing is central to many methods of relaxation because focusing on breathing forms a mini-meditation and helps link mind and body (Gilbert 1999d). Physiotherapists should ensure that they themselves are relaxed.

A highly developed sense of success and failure is often present with HVS patients, and the relaxation session is an opportunity to remind them that there is no right or wrong way to relax.

Throughout treatment, a relaxed state can be maintained by bringing the patient's awareness to areas of tension, including the jaw and throat.

Abdominal breathing

To settle the breathing pattern, the physiotherapist encourages regular and gentle speed, depth and synchrony, using a rhythmic voice. If the patient is able, breathing abdominally (Ch. 7) is a useful way of settling the breathing because it reduces the abnormal proprioceptive input of upper chest breathing (Bruton et al 2011) and may reduce chest pain (Gilbert 1999c), so long as patients do not increase their depth of breathing. Abdominal breathing may be facilitated with the hands behind the head or back, while maintaining relaxation and slow gentle breaths. Occasionally abdominal breathing is easier after reducing the minute volume rather than before.

Reducing the minute volume

A combination of education, relaxation and settling the breathing into an abdominal pattern may be sufficient (Pinney et al 1987), but patients with established HVS sometimes require further intervention to reduce minute volume. Patients can be asked simply to 'breathe less', but very gently in order to avoid tension and exacerbation of abnormal breathing patterns. Some patients need an explanation that this means reducing the rate or depth of breathing, or both, but thinking too hard about an automatic process may be counterproductive. If the patient understands that the aim is to achieve the slight discomfort of 'air hunger', they can often achieve this independently without too much control by the physiotherapist. Meuret et al (2008) found that reducing the depth of breathing contributes more to raising the P_aCO_2 than reducing the rate.

'Low and slow' is the key. Some patients need only a pause at end-exhalation, so long as this does not go further than air hunger and cause tension. If patients tense up, they should focus on returning to smooth, gentle, steady breathing.

To help patients maintain their rhythm, it is best not to ask for verbal feedback during the practice, although they can nod or shake in answer to quiet questions.

Observation of the breathing pattern indicates if tension develops, suggesting that the patient has reduced their minute volume too much and needs a reminder not to allow more air hunger than is just uncomfortable. They are then advised to gently get their breath back.

The physiotherapist watches the patient closely and may need to give selective advice on rate or depth of breathing, or a suggestion to pause at the end of the out-breath. The patient may have developed manoeuvres to slip in a covert deep breath such as a subtle change in position, breathing pattern or body movement, or preceding speech with a sharp intake of breath. The physiotherapist and patient can compete as to who notices these first! However, much of the time is in silence as the patient focuses on their breath and achieving air hunger, with occasional verbal nudges from the physiotherapist.

In the first session, when the patient feels the air hunger, they are congratulated and advised to start getting their breath back by allowing themselves slightly deeper and/or slightly faster breathing, without gasping. When they are able to tolerate the air hunger, they are asked if they can experience it for a few moments so that their respiratory centres can begin experiencing normal breathing as normal. The patient gradually learns the right balance for themselves of 'slight discomfort but no tension'. It is similar to the 'slight breathlessness' taught to respiratory patients when desensitizing them to dyspnoea (Ch.7). The periods of air hunger can then be gradually extended.

If this is too nebulous for the patient, more structured support can be given by pacing the patient's breathing to the physiotherapist's voice. The patient is asked to breathe in time with the physiotherapist's words, the rate of which is slightly slower than the patient's rate. Counting or pacing may be used e.g.:

- 'In-and-out, in-and-out …'
- 'In-and-out-two-three, in-and-out-two-three …'
- 'In-and-relax-out, in-and-relax-out …'
- 'In-and-let-it-out, in-and-let-it-out …'

Words and timing should be flexible to suit the patient, but instructions need to be repeated rhythmically, and the patient observed to ensure that slower breathing is not counteracted by deeper breathing. Some patients find that counting brings a sense of security in the early stages, the words acting as a 'breathing pacemaker'. Progression is aimed at independent control without the physiotherapist's voice.

If patients feel an irresistible need for air, they can take a conscious and controlled deeper breath, then get back gently into rhythm, sometimes with a preliminary breath-hold as compensation (but not if this causes tension). The concept of control is important for people who hyperventilate because they have felt out of control of their most fundamental physiological need. Advice can be given at intervals if necessary:

1 Keep it smooth/shallow/slow.
2 Swallow if you need to suppress a deep breath.
3 Keep the rhythm going, you don't need to hold your breath.
4 Maintain relaxation, avoid trying too hard.
5 Don't fight your breath, befriend it.
6 Be assured that you are in control and can stop at any time.

By establishing a lower more normal minute volume, it is thought that the normalized P_aCO_2 resets the air hunger threshold, reducing the sensitivity to bodily sensations and/or desensitizing the suffocation alarm system (Meuret et al 2008). The Buteyko technique (p.90) is also based on the principle of reducing the minute volume.

Variations

A process as individual as breathing needs a flexible approach. Suggested variations are the following:

1 Physiotherapists may use themselves or a mirror to demonstrate the patient's breathing pattern and different options.
2 Patients can slow down by 'breathing in' to areas of muscle tension, then 'breathing out' the tension.
3 They can visualize inhalation as if going up a hill and exhalation as if coming down the other side.
4 Feeling less cold in their nose reminds patients that they have succeeded in 'breathing less'.
5 Some patients slow down if the physiotherapist moves physically away and asks them to 'breathe from where I am'.
6 Humming may slow the breath.
7 The simple yoga technique described on p.211 suits the most hardened workaholic because it is so brief.
8 Neurophysiological facilitation (p.186) may be beneficial.
9 Capnography can be used as biofeedback (Meuret et al 2012).

Musculoskeletal input includes:
- in prone: thoracic mobilizations
- in supine: pectoral stretches
- in side-lying: intercostal stretch, holding the upper elbow so that the shoulder is abducted and applying gentle pressure on the mid to lower ribs.

By the nature of the syndrome, it is essential that patients are not hurried, and an undisturbed hour should be set aside for the first session, and if possible for subsequent sessions.

MANAGEMENT OF PANIC ATTACKS

Panic attacks occur in 50% of people with HVS (Cowley 1987). Once patients understand that these episodes are not themselves harmful, they can start gaining control over them. Breathing retraining itself may block an attack (Pappa 1993).

Coping strategies include identifying trigger factors, talking through the process, using an internal dialogue to acknowledge the fear but act as a reminder that panic attacks are not damaging, behavioural strategies such as rehearsals or distraction, and a choice of the techniques used to manage breathlessness (Ch. 7) or paroxysms of coughing (Ch. 8). People with claustrophobia may benefit from neurolinguistic programming (Sturt et al 2012). Breathing into a paper bag to retain CO_2 is no longer recommended because there have been occasional episodes of post-hyperventilation apnoea (Munemoto et al 2013) but breathing into cupped hands may be beneficial.

Self-management plans which focus on regular symptom monitoring may be less helpful for people with panic tendencies because preoccupation with bodily sensations can be reinforced (Dowson 2010). Drugs for panic disorders are sometimes associated with addictive properties, but relaxation or cognitive behavioural therapy may be helpful (NICE 2011c).

PROGRESSION AND INTEGRATION

> The centrality of breathing in human emotion, health and consciousness is obvious from references to it in intellectual domains as wide ranging as literature, philosophy, religion and physiology.
>
> Wilhelm et al (2001)

As control is established, abdominal breathing and reducing the minute volume is repeated in sitting, standing, walking and activities that might cause breath-holding such as bending, stair-climbing or eating. Patients are also encouraged to practice selectively relaxing parts of their body during their activities.

Particular attention is required during speech. If prolonged talking brings on symptoms, slowing down speech may be practiced by reading aloud, starting with poetry in order to use the natural pauses, then reading stories to children. Tips for maintaining control during speech are to:

- check shoulder relaxation and the breathing pattern
- take small breaths and inhale through the nose between sentences instead of gulping through the mouth
- add mental commas (Bradley 2012).

Pacing functional activities is often beneficial, though difficult for people with a hyperactive tendency. Exercise is encouraged that is steady, rhythmic and enjoyable, with the patient avoiding either anticipatory hyperventilation or obsessive over-achieving.

Posture and breathing can be affected by tense abdominal muscles, which may compress the abdomen on inspiration. Allowing outward abdominal movement needs to be balanced with patients feeling comfortable with their appearance. Tight clothes and belts should be avoided when possible.

Patients can be given recordings of advice and relaxation, sometimes including the physiotherapy session, because of the forgetfulness that sometimes accompanies HVS (Ocon 2013). If counting is used, this can be taped at fast, medium and slow speeds. If commercial relaxation tapes are used, patients are reminded to ignore instructions to breathe deeply.

Patients can also be given recordings of pacing tones with a rise in pitch to indicate inhalation and a fall for exhalation. They are advised to match their breathing to these tones for ten minutes a day, preferably abdominally, followed by five minutes without auditory guidance to help the transfer to daily life. The tones are set at gradually slower rates each week (Jeter et al 2012).

It is worth motivating patients to work hard during the first crucial week. Practice in breathing retraining should take place little and often, after brief relaxation and with the phone silenced. At first this could be around three times a day for 15 minutes, or minisessions of 3 minutes every hour. This is reduced for the second week, with times flexible to suit the individual. However, patients who tend to become preoccupied with a daily programme should not be burdened with excessive homework. Flexibility is particularly necessary for parents with young families, who find a tight routine impossible. One patient found that sitting beside her child as he fell asleep enabled her to slow her own breathing by pacing it to his breathing as it slowed and steadied.

Patients should maintain a steady blood sugar by ensuring that they have breakfast (including protein which is slow to metabolize), not going without a snack for more than three to four hours, and avoiding sugar binges which may lead to reactive hypoglycaemia. This should be emphasized for patients who are too busy to eat during the day and eat heavily at night, which can produce nocturnal or early morning symptoms. Meals should be slow (if possible) and enjoyable, avoiding excessive caffeine because of its respiratory stimulant and vasoconstrictive effects (Tal 2013). If patients must smoke, deep inhalations are to be avoided.

Spot checks throughout the day can be assisted by memory aids and use of opportunities such as red traffic lights, sitting on the bus, coffee breaks, and 'grey bar time' (p.258). Laptops can have beeps programmed at set intervals to act as reminders. Gradually the practice sessions can be less defined as the correct minute volume becomes automatic.

Vocal cord dysfunction may require speech language therapy, and the occupational therapist provides activity analysis and pacing. If patients ask for advice on complementary therapies, many techniques are helpful for relaxation, so long as they exclude deep breathing. Acupuncture may be beneficial by reducing anxiety levels and symptom severity (Gibson et al 2007). Hypnotherapy is unwise for people who suffer episodes of depersonalization.

Much encouragement is needed to help patients integrate their new breathing pattern and approach to life into the distractions of everyday living, but the obsessional tendencies of some patients means that adherence is usually high (Williams 2001). If progress is slow, attention can be given to identifying individual fears and precipitating factors. Reassessment of the abnormally high demands to which patients often subject themselves may be fruitful.

Physiotherapy is needed weekly until self-management is stabilized, usually after a few sessions, then sometimes monthly for adjustment and encouragement, followed by advice that patients can ask for a review session if required. Once learned and reinforced, the new breathing pattern can be maintained automatically because there has been no physical damage, as there is with respiratory disease. Self-awareness and stress management however must last a lifetime. Patients are advised that hyperventilation may return at stressful times, but they will recognize it and should be able to control it.

If patients do not improve after several sessions, and it becomes apparent that they are not practicing at home, or if they exhibit a 'yes but …' tendency, it is possible that they subliminally 'need' their hyperventilation to block out memories, in the same way that some patients with chronic pain express their emotional distress on a physical level (Bruera 1997). This is not a conscious process and makes the disorder no more tolerable, but if this is the case, physiotherapy is unhelpful and may just 'feed' the somatization, so referral is required.

OUTCOMES

Reduced symptoms are the most relevant outcome for the patient. Objective outcomes include a reduced RR, stable breathing pattern and shorter breath-holding time. Nijmegen score and capnography should also be normalized.

The following outcomes have been documented:

- ↓ depression, ↓ Nijmegen scores in people who also have asthma (Holloway & West 2007)
- doubling of breath-holding times (Maskell et al 1999)
- ↓ symptoms, ↓ RR (Bastow 2000)
- improvements in capnography, anxiety, depression and other symptoms (Tweeddale et al 1994)
- ↓ anxiety and improved breathing pattern (Han et al 1996)
- ↓ panic attacks (David 1985)
- ↓ Nijmegen scores, anxiety and depression in all patients audited after just two treatment sessions and a phone call (Williams 2001)
- ↑ quality of life, ↓ physical symptoms (Hagman et al 2011), ↓ emergency room visits (Fig 13.6).

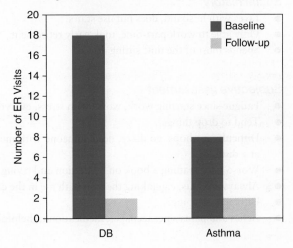

FIGURE 13.6 Reduction in emergency room (ER) visits over one year in people with dysfunctional breathing (DB) and asthma after physiotherapy

Discharge letters to both GP and consultant help raise awareness of the syndrome and show them the effectiveness of treatment.

> *To be wholly alive is to breathe freely, move freely and to feel fully.*
>
> Lowen (1991)

CASE STUDY : Ms SJ

Identify the problems of this 70 y.o. woman from Ankara with a 48-year history of fatigue and non-specific symptoms.

Background

Relevant medical history
- Investigated for multiple sclerosis: NAD (nothing abnormal discovered).
- Some depressive symptoms, labelled as 'abnormal illness'.
- Migraine with certain foods.
- Barium swallow: NAD, awaiting endoscopy.
- Many other investigations but NAD.

History of present complaint
- Since age 22: overwhelming chronic fatigue.
- 4–5 years: dysphagia.
- Two weeks: ↑ breathlessness.

Social history
- Lives with husband, does not use stairs.
- Only able to work part-time, took early retirement.
- Spends most of the time sitting down.

Subjective assessment
- Fatigue since starting work, worse with stress, everything is a great effort, feels like battery going down.
- Tend to drop things.
- Difficulty in shops, go dizzy, need someone with me in case I fall, use a stick to help balance and keep people at a distance.
- Worse since reading a book on relaxation and trying deep breathing exercises.
- Always anxious, e.g. taking the iron with me in the car when I go out to ensure I've not left it on.
- Difficulty sleeping.
- Aches and pains since teenager, medication unhelpful.

- It's like I can feel all my muscles.
- Nothing but reflexology has helped.
- Fed up with hospitals.

Objective assessment
- Nervous posture including excess hand movements.
- Breathing pattern normal in sitting, tense and rapid in lying.
- Sighing before speaking.
- Nijmegen score 28.

Questions

1 Analysis?
2 Patient's problems?
3 Goals?
4 Plan?
5 Outcomes?

CLINICAL REASONING

Does this statement accurately reflect the reference to which it refers?

'... *voluntary diaphragmatic movements ... improve the ventilation of their lower lung zones' (ref 10).*
Chest, 97, 1110–14, 1990
From ref. 10 – 'lower lung zone ventilation ... improved ... during voluntary deep breathing ...'.

Response to Case Study

1   Analysis
- Long term poor quality of life.
- Patient using excess energy to maintain breathing pattern and avoid falling.
- Original cause not explored because patient focused on improving quality of life.
- Symptoms and questionnaire suggest hyperventilation syndrome.

2   Problems
- Fatigue.
- Anxiety.
- Poor sleep.
- Poor exercise tolerance.

3   Goals

- Shop independently and without anxiety.
- Visit friends.

4   Plan

- Educate on interrelation of symptoms, breathing, anxiety and quality of life
- Relaxation and control of breathing
- Pacing and energy conservation
- Stairs
- ↑ Exercise tolerance

5   Outcomes: sequence

1   No change in symptoms, but 'husband says less huffing and puffing',
2   No change in symptoms, but 'I'm a little more in control of my breathing'.
3   Able to control nightly chest pain with shallow breathing.
4   Improved symptoms.
5   Improved function including stairs.
6   Visiting friends and distant family (without taking the iron!).
7   On discharge – some fatigue still present but not preventing activities, Nijmegen score 12.
8   Christmas card nine months later indicated that improvement was maintained.

Response to Clinical Reasoning

Deep breathing is not the same as diaphragmatic breathing.

RECOMMENDED READING

Decuyper M, De Bolle M, Boone E *et al* (2012) The relevance of personality assessment in patients with hyperventilation symptoms. *Health Psychol*; **31**(3): 316–22

Freire R, Perna G, Nardi AE (2010) Panic disorder respiratory subtype: psychopathology, laboratory challenge tests, and response to treatment. *Harv Rev Psychiatry*; **18**: 220–9

Han J, Zhu Y, Li S (2008) The language of medically unexplained dyspnea. *Chest*; **133**(4): 961–8

Kox M, Stoffels M, Smeekens SP *et al* (2012) The influence of concentration/meditation on autonomic nervous system activity and the innate immune response. *Psychosom Med*; **74**: 489–94

Lung FW, Lee TH, Huang MF (2012) Parental bonding in males with adjustment disorder and hyperventilation syndrome. *BMC Psychiatry*; **12**: 56

Munemoto T, Masuda A, Nagai N *et al* (2013) Prolonged post-hyperventilation apnea in two young adults with hyperventilation syndrome. *BioPsychoSocial Med*; **7**: 9

Nishino T, Ishikawa T, Nozaki-Taguchi N *et al* (2012) Lung/chest expansion contributes to generation of pleasantness associated with dyspnoea relief. *Resp Physiol Neurobiol*; **184**(1): 27–34

Sardinha A, Freire RC, Zin WA *et al* (2009) Respiratory manifestations of panic disorder: causes, consequences and therapeutic implications. *J Bras Pneumol*; **35**(7): 698–708

CHAPTER 14
Physiotherapy for elderly people with cardiorespiratory disease

LEARNING OBJECTIVES

On completion of this chapter the reader should be able to:

- differentiate changes with ageing that are inevitable and those which are modifiable

- identify suitable strategies for communicating with patients who are confused or have dementia, while optimizing autonomy

- plan the management of elderly people with cardiorespiratory disease, including liaison with the multidisciplinary team.

INTRODUCTION

The bulk of health care in the 21st century relates to older people, and increasingly frail older people.

Silver Book (2012)

Age is the dominant risk factor for cardiovascular disease (Chantler 2012), and some of the resulting morbidity can be ameliorated by rehabilitation. For older people admitted to hospital, this helps reduce the dependency and anxiety to which they are susceptible in this environment. Rehabilitation also helps maintain dignity, which elderly people associate with self-respect, autonomy and inclusion in decision-making (Woolhead 2004), and which will become ever more relevant as the older population is projected to double by 2030 (Kortebein 2009).

NORMAL EFFECTS OF AGEING

The normal age-related decline in lung function starts from around age 25 (DoH 2010), after which it is all downhill (Fig 14.1). Changes relevant to physiotherapy include the following:

- ↓ exercise tolerance by approximately 10% per decade (Strait 2013)
- ↑ energy cost of walking, leaving reduced reserves for other activities (Wert *et al* 2013)
- postural hypotension, particularly before and after meals (Abdel-Rahman 2012), ↓ balance (Reuter 2012), and coordination (Latash & Johnston 2012)
- ↑ systolic blood pressure (BP) due to vascular stiffness, while maintaining diastolic BP so that pulse pressure widens (Steppan *et al* 2011)
- ↓ ability to match oxygen delivery to consumption, especially in the transition from rest to exercise (Behnke & Delp 2010)
- ↓ elasticity of lung tissue and chest wall, ↓ diffusion of respiratory gases, ↓ ventilatory response to hypoxaemia and hypercapnia (Dyer 2012)
- narrowing of small airways, ↑ dead space, ventilation/perfusion ($\dot{V}_A/\dot{Q}$) mismatch and ↑ closing volume, which reaches FRC (see Fig 1.19) at average ages 44 in supine and 65 in sitting (Olsén 2005)
- ↓ respiratory muscle and cough strength, slower mucociliary clearance (Lowery 2013)
- ↓ perception of dyspnoea (Ebihara *et al* 2012) which may delay patients seeking assistance or taking suitable medication
- ↑ perception of pain (Cowan 2003) but ↑ stoicism (Abdulla *et al* 2013)

FIGURE 14.1 Effects of ageing on the cardiorespiratory system. *CVS*: cardiovascular system, $\dot{V}_A/\dot{Q}$: ventilation/perfusion, DO_2: oxygen delivery to the tissues

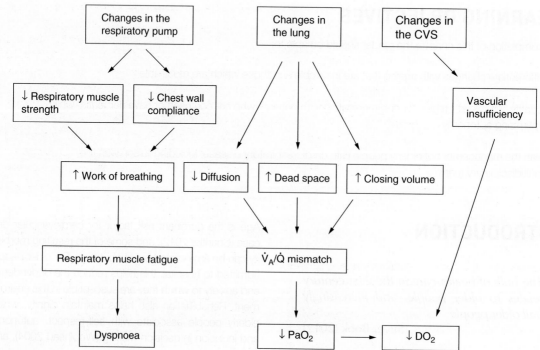

- cognitive impairment, associated with reduced independence on discharge from hospital (Law *et al* 2012)
- ↓ immunity (Layé 2013) and taste (Toffanello *et al* 2013), also dysphagia (Khan *et al* 2014) and gastroesophageal reflux (Soumekh *et al* 2014), leading to increased risk of pneumonia (Ebihara 2012)
- altered absorption, distribution and metabolism of drugs (Sera 2012)
- ↓ muscle mass (Fig 14.1) at 1–2% per year after age 50.

PREVENTABLE EFFECTS OF AGEING

The majority of patients admitted acutely to hospital are frail, elderly and cognitively impaired (McMurdo & Witham 2013). **Confusion** is increased by sleep fragmentation, lack of hearing aid or glasses, or relocation stress due to hospitalization. 'Hospital-acquired **delirium**' can be set off by surgery (Griffiths *et al* 2014), polypharmacy (Cudennec *et al* 2013) or insensitive handling, and leads to cognitive deterioration at twice the rate in the year after discharge compared with those who do not develop delirium, sometimes because of the continuation of psychotropic drugs (Bell 2013). Delirium may develop into post-traumatic stress disorder (Cunningham 2013) and Collier (2012) considers it an emergency. Preventing delirium on admission is cost effective (Akunne 2012), e.g. by orientation, by avoiding dehydration, constipation, pain or sleep disturbance, by the patient having access to clocks with large numbers, meals at central locations rather than in bed, and using toilets rather than bedpans. All team members, including the family, can be involved in preventive strategies (Martinez *et al* 2012).

Delirium predisposes to **dementia** (NICE 2010d), but only half of demented patients are diagnosed (Russ *et al* 2012) and a label of confusion or delirium should not be accepted without investigation by a specialist. Whittamore (2014) found that, of acute elderly patients admitted to hospital, 27% had delirium, 41% had dementia and 19% had both. Dementia is less likely in people of

African ancestry (Schlesinger 2013) but more likely in people with respiratory disease (Pivi 2012). Confusion differs from dementia in its acute course and reversibility.

Dementia is associated with dysphagia and **aspiration** (Sura *et al* 2012). Energetic oral hygiene reduces the incidence of aspiration pneumonia (Ortega *et al* 2014). A bidirectional relationship between pneumonia and cognition explains how a single episode of infection may lose a person their functional independence (Shah *et al* 2013).

Adverse drug events are more likely, along with both over- and under-prescription of medication. For example, underprescription of drugs for bone health (Conroy *et al* 2010) risks osteoporosis, and over-prescription of psychotropic drugs increases falls and cognitive decline (Cammen 2014).

Depression can accelerate the ageing process (Garcia-Rizo 2013) and hinder rehabilitation (Vieira *et al* 2014). It is common in later life, particularly in people who are institutionalized (Katona 2004) or suffer bereavement, isolation or functional impairment (Weyerer *et al* 2013). It leads to worse outcomes in hospitalized patients (Dennis 2012), increased risk of readmission, relocation and death (Büla 2001) and predisposes to dementia. Dementia impairs the diagnosis of depression, but depression is treatable within dementia (Katona 2004) and these must be distinguished because some antidepressants aggravate delirium (Meagher 2001). Studies have found that 94% of junior hospital doctors miss diagnosing depression in older people, and GPs treat only 10% of their depressed elderly patients (Katona 2004). Depression should always be considered in the presence of comments such as 'she's forgetful, she's beginning to dement'.

Sleep disturbance is common and impairs functional autonomy (Valenza 2013). It is associated with institutionalization, cognitive impairment and depression (Anderson *et al* 2014) but can be improved by exercise (Dzierzewski *et al* 2013).

Postural hypotension is a drop in systolic BP of 20 mmHg or more on moving from sitting or lying to standing, and in older people is usually due to vascular insufficiency (Moore & Lyons 2003). It is worsened by dehydration. **Dehydration** is common because ageing kidneys are less able to reabsorb water and electrolytes, and the thirst mechanism is blunted (Arai *et al* 2013). Nazarko (2000) found that the main cause of hyponatraemia in elders was the use of diuretics. Reduced mobility may inhibit fluid intake while increasing anxiety about incontinence. **Urinary incontinence** affects 15–50% of older women and is associated with functional decline (Omli *et al* 2013) and risk of falls (Hunter 2013). An assumption that incontinence is inevitable may lead to mopping up taking precedence over preventive action such as maintenance of mobility and ensuring access to the toilet.

Constipation may be due to dehydration, medication, change of diet, dementia, immobility, lack of privacy or feeling hurried when on the commode. As well as addressing the cause, it can be ameliorated by exercise (Costilla 2014).

Breathlessness affects 25–37% of adults aged over 70 (Parshall *et al* 2012) which may be why respiratory disease is often overlooked (Patterson *et al* 1999), especially as many patients do not report the symptom (Luce 1996). Reversible components of dyspnoea may not be treated even if a diagnosis is made (Sherman *et al* 1992).

Aerobic capacity declines with age (Buchman *et al* 2014) but can be attenuated by exercise, even in very elderly people (Krist *et al* 2013) and those with dementia (Garuffi 2013). One study found that gardening was the most significant predictor to mobility among all the health characteristics and social factors studied (Lêng *et al* 2013).

Poor mobility may be exacerbated by treatable conditions such as anaemia, painful feet, fear of exercise or lack of vitamin D which is common in elderly people and predisposes to depression (Lapid 2013). Vertebral fractures have been found in 51% of elderly patients (Jagt-Willems 2012). The risk of **osteoporosis** increases with age, diseases such as COPD and its medication, immobility and, for housebound people who have difficulty with food preparation, a diet deficient in musculoskeletal nutrients (Sharkey 2013). The role of the physiotherapist is to adapt impact exercises to the patient's lifestyle, to refer to a dietician if required, and sometimes to the GP because of widespread under-diagnosis, especially in men (Frost *et al* 2012).

Contractures are frequent in institutionalized elders (Müller 2013), where formal exercise is often absent. Families can be enrolled, with the help of exercise diaries, to ensure the basics of mobility.

Aches and pains are pathological and to be investigated, not accepted as part of ageing.

SPECIFIC NEEDS OF OLDER PEOPLE

> *Dignity refers to self respect and being valued by others.*
> *Autonomy refers to control of decision making.*
>
> BMJ (2001)

Patients may accept unnecessary symptoms with comments such as 'what can I expect at my age?' They should, however, be encouraged to ask for symptoms to be investigated, rather than acquiesce to the ageist attitudes that are common in the health system (Kydd & Wild 2013), e.g.:

- Stone *et al* (2012) found that fewer elderly people admitted with an exacerbation of COPD were seen by a respiratory specialist, even though they had greater comorbidity and higher mortality than younger people, and they were more likely to receive a 'do-not-resuscitate' order irrespective of comorbidities.
- Curtains were less likely to be pulled round older patients left exposed than around younger patients (Turnock & Kelleher 2001).

Respiratory health for elderly people was found by Hubbard *et al* (2009) to be best maintained by a personally-tailored programme of little-and-often exercise, recommended at 150 mins of moderate intensity or 75 mins of vigorous intensity, in bouts of at least 10 min duration (Taylor 2014). Other benefits of exercise are:

- ↑ cognition (Forte 2013), balance and functional ability (Chou 2012)
- ↓ agitation (Alessi 1999), length of stay (Fisher *et al* 2010) and urinary incontinence (Vinsnes *et al* 2012)
- ↓ age-related inflammation, ↑ muscle strength, balance and bone mineral density (Marques *et al* 2013)
- ↓ depression (Pereira *et al* 2013)
- ↓ morbidity and mortality (Ikezoe *et al* 2013).

Dance improves balance (Balingit *et al* 2013), video dance stimulates cognition (Jovancevic 2012) and people with dementia have responded well to Salsa dancing (Abreu & Hartley 2013). Other patients can improve their balance with Wii (Bieryla & Dold 2013).

Exercise programmes should include balance, co-ordination and fall prevention (Franklin 2013).

Risk of falls is increased by:

- dyspnoea, pain, ↓ confidence, ↓ balance, poor footwear, environmental hazards or postural hypotension (NICE 2004)
- respiratory and swallowing problems (Higashijima 2010), the most common swallowing disorder being associated with deconditioning during acute illness (Berner 2009)
- polypharmacy, urinary frequency, sensory impairment, ↓ cognition, depression, antidepressants or dizziness (Deandrea *et al* 2013)
- malnutrition (Neyens *et al* 2013)
- weakness, especially of the quadriceps (Regterschot *et al* 2014)
- anxiety, which can upset postural control and trigger a vicious circle of inactivity and reduced fitness (Yardley 2004).

Exercise is the main preventive intervention to reduce falls (Karlsson *et al* 2013), especially endurance training (Nam *et al* 2013). Coloured wristbands or named labels on walking frames are useful to identify how far a patient can walk and the assistance required, e.g. red for two staff, yellow for one and green for the patient being independently mobile.

2012) and meditation, which can improve sleep, mood and memory in people with dementia and their carers (Innes *et al* 2012).

Autonomy is central to rehabilitation. This can be facilitated by respecting patients' senior status, experience and wishes. This means, for example, ensuring privacy when required (Logan 2012) and allowing patients to return to bed when they request rather than enforcing unhappy hours slumped in hospital chairs. Discomfort reduces the depth of breathing, and the zeal with which patients are hauled out of bed for lengthy periods can lead to 'chairsores' becoming more prevalent than bedsores (Mulley 1993).

Another limitation to rehabilitation is untreated pain (Triggle 2013), which has been identified in 50% of people with dementia (Achterberg *et al* 2013) and 40–80% of nursing home residents, causing anxiety, social isolation, depression, and impaired posture, sleep, appetite and memory (Cowen 2003). Methods are available for assessing pain in people who are very old (Abdulla *et al* 2013), have had surgery (Falzone 2013) or have dementia (Ersek *et al* 2011), the latter tending to express their pain by agitation and aggression (Ahn 2013). People who have difficulty articulating their pain may also be handicapped by ageism (White 2014 and Fig 14.2).

Other problems which hinder rehabilitation are:

- Memory loss; most physiotherapy advice and exercise programmes should be written down and explained to the family.

KEY POINT

The elderly population represents a perfect population to benefit from exercise training.
Menezes *et al* (2012)

Exercise that is not aimed at conditioning includes:
- T'ai Chi, which improves strength, flexibility (Manson *et al* 2013), balance, sleep and cognition (Nguyen 2012), and helps reduce falls (Reyes 2013) and depression (Chi 2013).
- Yoga, which can improve patients' mental state and sleep quality (Alexander *et al* 2013).

Non-active stress reduction strategies include hand massage (Remington 2002), reflexology (Simonnet

FIGURE 14.2 Percentage of health staff who would expend maximum time and energy on patients' pain

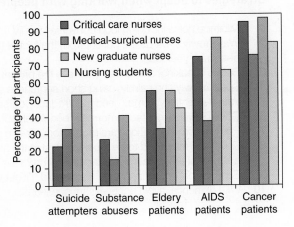

- Malnutrition, which can reach 40–50% in older adults living in care homes (Chau 2004), exacerbated by illness or depression.

Rehabilitation is facilitated by maintaining orientation, including:

- ensuring that patients know that they are heard (Ward & Cowley 2012)
- providing information consistently (Dahlen *et al* 2012)
- avoiding the use of first names uninvited, because for older generations this may be seen as a sign of disrespect rather than friendliness
- encouraging patients to bring to hospital their personal possessions and photos
- involving patients in goal-setting, which may reduce dependency (Parsons *et al* 2012)
- encouraging patients to wear their own clothes when possible
- ensuring communication between all parties, including the family, when patients are transferred to and from acute care (Lane *et al* 2013).

Some suggestions to assist communication are in Box 14.1.

KEY POINT

Use psychology before drugs.

Sharpe & Hanning 1999

A demented person's ability to feel emotions remains intact even as aphasia sets in, and it is thought that most patients are aware of, and feel distressed by, their limitations (Zimmermann 1998). Personal care may also cause distress, which can be ameliorated by keeping the patient covered, using the right water temperature, patting rather than rubbing dry and talking quietly; this approach was found to reduce crying out and the need for drugs (Adams *et al* 2012) but it is perplexing that we need research to tell us this.

Patients need their inhaler technique individually checked (Taffet 2013), and specific requirements include the following:

1   On surgical wards, postoperative cognitive decline is more likely in elderly people (Fineberg 2013), and communication and

BOX 14.1

Strategies to adopt when working with people who are confused or demented

1   Minimize noise including loud conversation, TV, radio and bleeps.
2   Walk slowly towards the patient from the foot of the bed, with eye contact and without the lighting obscuring your face.
3   Before speaking, check that you have the patient's attention.
4   Speak slowly and calmly, using short sentences and avoiding two questions in one sentence.
5   With dementia, you may need to introduce yourself each time you speak.
6   Gentle physical contact is normally beneficial, but not if the patient withdraws.
7   Positive communications are more productive, e.g. 'rest in the chair' rather than 'don't get up yet'.
8   Questions may need to be repeated, first in the same way and then in a different way, e.g. 'are you in pain?' a couple of times, then 'does anything hurt?'.
9   Echo the patient's input, e.g. 'you're cold, I'll get you a blanket'.
10 With dementia, avoid unnecessary questions.

orientation are a priority, especially following emergency surgery (Stoneham *et al* 2014). A general anaesthetic brings a 35% increased risk of dementia (Karran 2013), especially if this is followed by a chest infection (Terrando *et al* 2011).

2   On medical wards, early rehabilitation reduces length of stay and the likelihood of discharge to a nursing home (Kosse *et al* 2013).

3   In the ICU, most patients are elderly (Vasilevskis *et al* 2010) and they benefit from early mobilization (Josaleen 2013).

4   In residential and nursing homes, the majority of residents have been found to take unsuitable medications (Lima *et al* 2013). Patients also tend to have inadequate end-of-life care (Hanson *et al* 2008), particularly those with dementia, which is a terminal disorder and requires advance care planning (Steen *et al* 2013). Physiotherapists can take the initiative in referring patients to the palliative team when required.

OUTCOMES

> It is an error of youth to think that with age comes a readiness to accept the consequences of ageing and to tolerate its attendant illnesses.
>
> Gems (2011b)

Exercise capacity in elders can be measured by a sit-to-stand test (Bohannon 2011), shuttle test (Dyer *et al* 2002) or shortened walking tests of 10 m (Fritz 2013) or 3 m (Worsfold & Simpson 2001). Valid instruments include those for quality of life (Makai 2013, Wu *et al* 2013), physical activity (White *et al* 2012b), activities of daily living (Huiszoon 2014) and seven screening tools for functional ability (Beaton & Grimmer 2013). A robust model for breathless older people is the above combined with the modified Medical Research Council dyspnoea scale (DePew *et al* 2013).

For patients with dementia, multidimensional outcomes include the Comprehensive Geriatric Assessment (Bernabei 2010) and for exercise the six-minute walk test is valid, as are the Figure-of-Eight walk test, the 'TUG' test, the 'FICSIT' balance test and the Chair Rise Test (Blankevoort *et al* 2012).

Discharge requires multidisciplinary management and often a home visit.

> All unnecessary (and perhaps even some indicated) medications must be discontinued before discharge, thereby adhering to the tenets of geriatric pharmacology by prescribing as few drugs as possible.
>
> Green & Maurer (2013)

CASE STUDY : Mr MM

Analyze the problems of this 82 y.o. patient from Brighton who has COPD and was visited at home after a fall.

Social history

● Ex-professional singer.
● Lives with daughter and adolescent grandchildren. Tends 'to hibernate in my room to avoid them'.

Subjective assessment

- Recent pneumonia, continuous fatigue since then.
- Don't use stairs or go into garden. Can't go out. Just want to sit down all the time.
- Saw GP for swollen ankles, told to restrict fluid intake.
- Given oxygen by GP. Seem to get headaches when use oxygen.
- Not breathless at rest but main reason for limited activity is SOB, with some limitation due to fatigue, anxiety, loss of confidence after fall and avoidance of grandchildren.
- On questioning about falls, Mr M is unable to identify preceding dizziness or other cause.

Objective assessment

- No other signs of CO_2 retention such as flapping tremor or warm hands.
- S_pO_2 95% on room air.
- Patient leaning forwards and clutching arms of chair.
- Rapid shallow rhythmic breathing pattern.
- Auscultation: BS reduced but present and R=L. No AS.
- No obvious environmental falls hazard.
- No standby antibiotics or steroids.

SOB: shortness of breath, *BS*: breath sounds, *R*: right, *L*: left, *AS*: added sounds.

Questions

1 Analysis?
2 Problems?
3 Plan?
4 Progression?

CLINICAL REASONING

Comment on the logic of the following statement in a study evaluating exercise performance:

'[We] examined ... leg muscle training, inspiratory muscle training and postural drainage ... the largest effect occurring with leg muscle training.'

Austr J Physiother (1992) 38, 189–93

Response to Case Study

1 **Analysis**
   - Mr M has not returned to normal function since pneumonia.
   - He is unsure about when to take oxygen and has not been assessed for this. Headache may relate to CO_2 retention.
   - Multiple reasons for reduced exercise tolerance: physical, emotional and social.

- Fall may have been related to fatigue, weakness and/or loss of confidence.
- Requires overall management plan.

2 Problems

- Falls risk
- Inaccurate oxygen prescription
- Fatigue
- Breathlessness
- Anxiety and probable loss of confidence
- Exercise intolerance

3 Plan

- Explanation about oxygen and leaflet provided.
- Explanation of COPD and leaflet provided.
- Explanation of possible heart failure (HF). Advice on ankle exercises and leg elevation when resting. Patient agrees on referral to community HF team.
- Explanation about breathlessness; more relaxed forward lean sitting advised.
- Discussion on possible causes of fatigue: post-viral, loss of fitness.
- Discussion on possible triggers for pneumonia, stress contributing.
- Advice on building up immune system.
- SOB management strategies. Leaflet on SOB and exercise.
- Explanation on quadriceps exercises and leaflet.
- Stretchy bands and leaflet.
- Walk into garden, with pacing. Patient chooses to exercise at 'breathless but not speechless' level.
- Bottom three steps on stairs.
- Discussion on lifestyle and building in graded exercise. Walking aid declined.
- Discussion on pulmonary rehabilitation programme. Mr M prefers home exercise.
- Discussion on singing and breathing. Mr M to contact the singing teacher associated with pulmonary rehabilitation programme.
- Advice on when to take antibiotics or steroids, when to call community respiratory service, GP or ambulance.
- Continuous oximetry throughout session, including exercise: no desaturation. Advised to avoid oxygen until assessment.
- Patient agrees on referral to falls clinic and oxygen clinic.
- Email to GP: information on referrals, request for advice on HF diagnosis, request for standby antibiotics and steroids, information on discontinuation of oxygen and advice requested.

4 Progression

- Personalized exercise diary.
- Check headaches.
- Check breathing pattern, re-educate if this has not normalized.
- Follow up communication with GP, liaise with falls clinic.
- Build up exercise tolerance, including full flight of stairs and going out with friends.

Response to Clinical Reasoning

Not surprising. Training is specific. Exercise performance would not be expected to improve with postural drainage. Exercise performance may or may not improve with inspiratory muscle training, depending on the factors causing inspiratory muscle weakness.

RECOMMENDED READING

Albertson T (2013) The pharmacological approach to the elderly COPD patient. *Drugs Aging*; **30**(7): 467–77

Brauer S (2013) Falls in older people. *J Physiother*; **59**(3): 213

Choi M-H, Kim H-J, Kim J-H (2013) Correlation between cognitive ability measured by response time of 1-back task and changes of SpO_2 by supplying three different levels of oxygen in the elderly. *Geriatr Gerontol Internat*; **13**: 384–387

Denker MG, Cohen DL (2013) What is an appropriate blood pressure goal for the elderly? *Clin Intervent Aging*; **8**: 1505–1517

Egerton T (2013) Self-reported aging-related fatigue: a concept description and its relevance to physical therapist practice. *Phys Ther*; **93**(10): 1403–13

Falzone E, Hoffmann C, Keita H (2013) Postoperative analgesia in elderly patients. *Drugs Aging*; **30**(2): 81–90

Gobo S (2014) Effects of exercise on dual-task ability and balance in older adults. *Arch Geront Geriatr*; **58**(2): 177–187

Higashijima M (2013) Relationship between swallowing dysfunction and decreased respiratory function in dementia patients. *J Phys Ther Science*; **25**(8): 941–2

Hirosaki M, Ohira T, Kajiura M (2013) Effects of a laughter and exercise program on physiological and psychological health among community-dwelling elderly in Japan. *Geriatr Gerontol Internat*; **13**(1): 152–60

Inglés M, Gambini J, Villaplana L (2013) Potential role of physiotherapists in polymedication of the elderly. *Geriatr Gerontol Internat*; **13**: 1086–7

Kelaiditi E, van Kan GA, Cesari M (2014) Frailty: role of nutrition and exercise. *Curr Opin Clin Nutr Metab Care*; **17**(1): 32–9

Kirk-Sanchez NJ, McGough EL (2014) Physical exercise and cognitive performance in the elderly. *Clin Intervent Aging*; **9**: 51–6

Liu W, Cheon J, Thomas SA (2014) Interventions on mealtime difficulties in older adults with dementia. *Int J Nurs Stud*; **51**(1): 14–27

Maidan I (2014) Introducing a new definition of a near fall. *Gait Posture*; **39**(1): 645–7

McDonald VM (2013) Managing older patients with coexistent asthma and COPD. *Drugs Aging*; **30**(1): 1–17

NICE Clinical Practice Guideline (2010): Delirium

Pop-Vicas A (2013) Over-distension of the airways by mechanical ventilation in the elderly. *Crit Care*; **17**: 165

Puente KP (2014) Study of the factors influencing the preparation of advance directives. *Arch Geront Geriatr*; **58**(1): 20–24

Taffet GE (2013) Considerations for managing chronic obstructive pulmonary disease in the elderly. *Clin Intervent Aging*; **9**: 23–30

Rastogi R, Meek BD (2013) Management of chronic pain in elderly, frail patients. *Clin Intervent Aging*; **8**: 37–46

Torke AM, Sachs GA, Helft PR (2012) Timing of Do-Not-Resuscitate orders for hospitalized older adults who require a surrogate decision-maker. *J Am Geriatr Soc*, **59**(7): 1326–31

CHAPTER 15
Palliative respiratory physiotherapy

LEARNING OBJECTIVES

On completion of this chapter the reader should be able to:

- recognize, as part of the team, when the goals of management shift from cure of disease to control of symptoms

- ensure that the patient's wishes drive these goals

- use clinical reasoning to identify physiotherapy strategies to suit these goals

- develop empathetic communication skills, including adaptation to different cultures.

INTRODUCTION

It begins with an easy voice saying,
just a routine examination;
as October sunlight pierces the heavy velvet curtains.
Later it is the friends who write but do not visit . . .
it is doctors who no longer stop by your bed
. . .

it is terror every minute of conscious night and day
to a background of pop music.

Wilkes (1983)

Physiotherapists are suited to working with people who are dying, who often have similar needs to those who are disabled (Purtilo 1976). End-stage disease is not a time to withdraw physiotherapy because there is much that can be done to ease the passage towards a good death.

Palliative care focuses on patient-determined quality of life (QoL) and involves a multidisciplinary team including the patient and family. Symptom control, psychosocial and sometimes spiritual care are required, which may need to be prolonged.

In developed countries, most people die slowly, and usually in old age. Heart failure (Gadoud 2013) and COPD (Sorenson 2013) are terminal diseases, and the trend is towards early initiation of palliative care (Yoong et al 2013), starting from diagnosis (Fig 15.1). When initiated early, palliative care improves QoL and prolongs survival (Temel et al 2010).

Palliative care rehabilitation concentrates on the functional consequences of end-stage disease (Low et al 2012). This has been studied mostly in cancer patients who find that rehabilitation reduces anxiety, increases satisfaction and feelings of control, and may enable them to be discharged home (Fu 2012).

REACTIONS OF PATIENTS

> *Accepting loss of control and loss of movement is not something I want to come to terms with.*
> Patient quoted by Soundy *et al* (2012)

When informed that they are dying, most patients feel overwhelmed and experience a variety of reactions. Disbelief and then fear usually predominate at first, though not primarily fear of death itself (Murray-Parkes 1998). Patients may be frightened of symptoms and the dying process, of isolation, of being a burden or of the unknown.

With 21% of global cancer deaths caused by smoking (Rom 2013), guilt may be an extra burden. Anger is also an ever-ready emotion that may arise from feelings

FIGURE 15.1 Top: traditional model of care with a clear transition point. Bottom: model of care with palliation starting from diagnosis

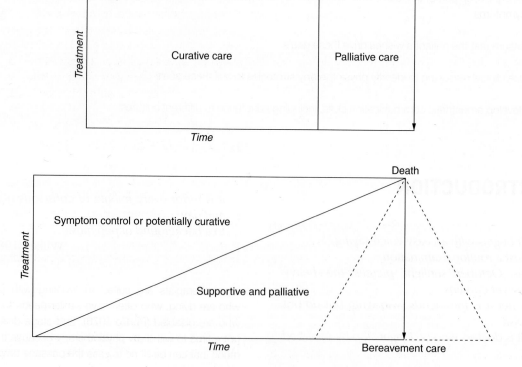

of helplessness or act as a defense against the experience of grief (Philip *et al* 2007). Grief can develop into depression, which amplifies pain, distresses relatives and erodes the patient's ability to do the emotional work of separating and saying goodbye (Block 2000). Patients should be allowed to express sorrow, anger, guilt, unusual humour or any other feeling, for which they do not need to apologize. As one patient said, 'I laugh because I don't want to cry' (Soundy *et al* 2012).

Many patients deny reality in order to avoid the pain of grief or fear, acting and talking as if they expect to get better. Denial may be a necessary cushion and is a defence mechanism to be respected. When and if patients are ready to confront the truth, they may sink into a dark place that can paradoxically be a creative process by which they begin to take responsibility for the way they respond to change. Then they may accept their loss and allow fear to dissolve.

These reactions are not stages that occur with defined boundaries, but may weave in and out of a patient's awareness, so that a moment of anger may open into acceptance, followed by the mind curling back into the darkness of fear. Time is needed, and patients with cardiorespiratory disease often have time. With support, time can be used wisely.

The media's focus on 'fighting' at the end of life does not support patients who prefer to seek peace and comfort in their last weeks. They and their family may feel stigmatized if they 'lose the battle'.

REACTIONS OF RELATIVES

When someone you love dies, you pay for the sin of outliving them with a thousand piercing regrets.

Simone de Beauvoir 1966

Family and friends can feel a kaleidoscope of emotions before and after a patient dies, e.g. remorse, relief, impotence at being unable to help, and similar reactions to those of the patient. 'Anticipatory grief' can be more difficult than after death and is especially common when the dying person has dementia (Johansson *et al* 2013).

Patient and family may try to 'protect' each other from reality, occasionally with the collusion of health staff. Just when they need each other the most, they may be separated by a conspiracy of silence. Patients and relatives usually need the opportunity to share the truth with each other.

A third of older spouses experience bereavement complicated by difficulties beyond those associated with 'normal' grief (Acierno 2012). Risk factors include:

- prior ambiguous or dependent relationship with the dying person
- families from a culture who are unable to follow their own customs
- relatives who have learning disabilities or dementia.

People with learning disabilities may manifest grief as behaviour change or self harm (Duffin 2000). If a bereaved person has dementia, they may repeatedly forget, feeling shock each time they are told. Complicated grief may lead to post-traumatic stress disorder, especially after a death in the intensive care unit (ICU) (Sanderson *et al* 2013).

Children benefit from open communication and need the opportunity to be close to their dying relative. They know their own limitations and may simply want to pop in and out of the sick room. Children often fantasize that they are to blame for the death of a parent or sibling, or they may feel that they must not distress the family and so avoid talking about it.

Assistance for families includes involving them in decisions when patients are unable do this themselves, helping them to provide physical comforts for their loved one, advice on support groups (Henriksson *et al* 2013) a communication diary (McEvoy 2012), and telephone contact after the death (Darbyshire *et al* 2013).

REACTIONS OF STAFF

To be ethically engaged is to be … mindful of their needs, values and goals, attuned to their illness experiences, and emotionally open to their suffering.

Jensen & Greenfield (2012)

Once a patient's condition is known to preclude recovery, this is sometimes interpreted as a failure by health staff and has been described as an 'institutional liability' (Risse & Balboni 2013). Reactions may include avoidance, heroic measures to prolong life, unsuitable bonhomie, the use of drugs to suppress patients' expression of emotion, inaccurate optimism (Billings 2000) or inappropriate reassurance. Reassurance has been criticized as 'social bromide' aimed at making staff feel better rather than the patient (Fareed 1996).

Health staff working with people at the end of life require support themselves. They need access to their own feelings because expression of feelings by staff, when appropriate, has been found therapeutic for patients, who can find professional detachment unhelpful and occasionally offensive (Fallowfield 1993).

WHERE TO DIE?

The end of a life in the critical care environment can become one of the most powerfully uncomfortable and inhumane experiences that any human will endure.

Angood (2003)

Most patients prefer to die at home, but the majority die in hospital (Gomes et al 2013). For those who have to die in the ICU, this usually follows a decision to withdraw or withhold treatment (Ranse et al 2012), in which case alarms and electronic monitoring should be disconnected, and if a tracheal tube is to be removed, plans need to be made in case of secretions or gasping.

Symptoms tend to be poorly managed in hospitals (Pinzón 2012) and care homes (Brooke 2012), and in these environments patients need to be under the care of a palliative team (Kao et al 2014). Hospice-at-home services are well established, including physiotherapy input (Cobbe et al 2013), and both home and hospice enable patients to achieve a similar QoL (Leppert 2012). People with heart failure can be managed at home even if they require inotropic infusions (Taitel et al 2012).

Palliative care services tend to be accessed late (Akashi 2012), especially for patients with end-stage respiratory disease, who have symptoms of similar severity to cancer but with a less predictable prognosis (Chadwick 2012). Information on advance care planning should be provided early and systematically, ideally in an outpatient setting such as during pulmonary rehabilitation. This should include options for different levels of support, bearing in mind that patients' wishes are often not those of their family or their doctor (Cook et al 2003). If the choice is for home care,

information should include preparation for untoward or frightening events.

COMMUNICATING WITH DYING PEOPLE

His yellow eyes watched us being taught at the bedside of each patient and when we came to his bed we all walked directly past him to the patient on his other side. Not a word was said. Not a greeting. Not even a nod ... Dismay turned to guilt with the thought that I, too, had no idea how to approach or comfort a dying patient.

Carmichael (medical student) 1981

It is not easy to find the right words to say to people who are facing death. The key is to listen. Patients find relief if they feel that it is acceptable to talk, and the astute listener can pick up indirect questions. Patients may drop hints that they would like to talk by mentioning other people who have died, joking about their future or asking how long before they get better. We can indicate a willingness to listen by sitting down, maintaining eye contact (in Western cultures) and asking non-threatening questions such as 'how do you feel in yourself?'

If a patient has just received a distressing prognosis, they are unlikely to focus on their physiotherapy, but they may need some space to ask questions that they did not ask when receiving the information. As one patient said 'The second the doctor told me I had cancer, the rest of the conversation was over; I don't remember anything' (Burt 2000). It is useful to ask how they understand what they have heard, and be guided by their response. Clarity of words is required, e.g. patients may understand the word 'severe' more clearly than the word 'advanced', or they may assume that the word 'cancer' equates to an inevitable or distressing death.

During and after talking, patients need time to process their thoughts, and silence can be used constructively. It is not helpful to rationalize patients out of their feelings, tell them what to do, or say that we know how they feel (we don't). It is however helpful to provide information that reduces anxiety and increases the ability to cope, and discussion itself helps to divest death of its power. Fear of the unknown is usually a heavier burden than the truth, and patients who are left in ignorance tend to feel a loss of control that shackles their coping strategies. This is illustrated in a study finding that patients who knew their cancer to be incurable experienced less fatigue, anxiety and physical symptoms than those unaware of their disease status (Lee et al 2013d) and another in which patients who were given specific information were less anxious and had improved QoL (Nakajima et al 2013). As described by Dewar (1995), 'bearing the agony of knowing one has a life-threatening condition is not as problematic as not being given adequate information'. Handover at the bedside rather than at the nurses' station aids communication (Ferri 2012).

We might also find it useful to ponder our own reactions: 'Am I feeling uncomfortable? Am I helping or hindering her flow of thought? Am I responding to his needs or mine?'

The majority of patients want to be told their diagnosis and feel that they should decide who else is told (Buckman 1996). Most people with COPD also desire end-of-life discussions, yet most often these conversations do not occur, leading to discordant care (Reinke et al 2013).

When patients ask questions about their prognosis, however indirect, it is unethical to avoid giving information and keeps patients in a subordinate position. This may be due to a false assumption that distress equals harm, or uncertainty about who should take the initiative. Physiotherapists have as much right and responsibility to inform patients as other health staff (Sim 1986) but it is acceptable for physiotherapists to refer difficult communications to other appropriate staff, ensuring that patient's questions are then addressed and that issues of power about who 'owns' the truth do not hinder this.

To reveal the diagnosis to the family without the patient's knowledge creates tension and mistrust, and is unethical. Other family requests, e.g. to suction a patient, should be respected and discussed, but should not take precedence over the rights of the patient. Some cultures favour family-based decisions rather than individual-based decisions and patients can be asked about the family's role in the decision-making process.

Reaction to bad news is varied and sometimes irrational, including regression to child-like behaviour, relief, despair at the loss of fulfillment, or projection of hostility. Patients should be left with some realistic hope, even if directed towards a minor achievement. And it is always worth casting a backward glance when leaving the bedside, because it is sometimes necessary to return and pick up the pieces.

> In 1672 a French physician considered the idea of telling the truth to patients, but concluded that it would not catch on.
> Buckman (1996)

MANAGEMENT OF SYMPTOMS

> All I want to know is that there will be someone there to hold my hand when I need it. I am afraid. Death may be routine to you, but it is new to me ... I've never died before.
> Patient quoted by Gallagher & Trenchar (1986)

This message from a dying student nurse advises her colleagues on how they can best help her towards a good death. Management of symptoms is consistently found to be the prime requirement of patients, especially control of breathing, bladder and bowels. As soon as it is known that patients are in need of care rather than cure, the emphasis is on allowing them a choice in both the method and timing of their treatment.

Physiotherapy is provided according to individual needs, including rehabilitation to maximize independence (Hanks 2010, p.1503). For people with cancer, exercise can improve sleep, body image and QoL, and reduce anxiety, fatigue and pain (Mishra et al 2012). In people with end-stage COPD, pulmonary rehabilitation improves exercise tolerance (Ngaage 2004) and a home-based walking programme can improve QoL (Lowe et al 2013). Supplemental oxygen, if indicated, maintains cerebral oxygenation (Fig 15.2). Autonomic dysfunction may be present in advanced cancer (Stone 2012), indicating a need to check for postural hypotension before mobilization.

Symptoms may respond to complementary techniques practiced by physiotherapists, e.g. reflexology or acupuncture for dyspnoea (Wyatt 2012, Towler *et al* 2013), massage for pain (Mitcienson 2014), and relaxation or manual modalities for mood disturbance (Ben-Arye *et al* 2012).

Breathlessness

> *Ms A avoided any activity that made her aware of her breathing because she believed that being breathless would make her cancer spread.*
>
> Bailey (1995)

Shortness of breath (SOB) engenders fear in patients (Johnson 2013) and helplessness and anxiety in their carers (Malik *et al* 2013), but is often undertreated at the end of life (Sangeeta 2013). It is experienced by 74% of people dying from non-cancer causes, 65% of those dying from general cancer (Burt *et al* 2010) and 90% of those dying from lung cancer or COPD (Sorenson 2000b). With cancer, SOB indicates a short prognosis (Booth *et al* 2008), but with COPD it

is slowly-progressive (Fig 15.3), allowing patients to develop some of their own coping strategies. The sensation may signal to patients the beginning of a loss of control, and in end-stage disease the symbolism of not getting enough breath is an ever present reminder of approaching death.

Dyspnoea may be caused by cachexia, a tumour, lung fibrosis due to disease or radiotherapy, or a coexisting condition. Treatable causes of SOB should be identified, e.g. pleural effusion, ascites, obstruction or compression of the lung, anxiety or anaemia. Anxiety is strongly correlated with SOB, especially for patients with cancer (Bruera *et al* 1999) because of unfounded fears of dying from suffocation (Mahler *et al* 2010). Disentangling this concept is aided by desensitization (p.205). The physical management of SOB is discussed in Ch. 7, and a physiotherapy-led breathless management programme has shown improved functional capacity and coping strategies (Wood *et al* 2013). Other measures are described below.

Opioids are the drug of choice (Lehto *et al* 2013), sometimes with added sedatives (Allcroft *et al* 2013) or antidepressants (Booth 2013). Fear of the side effect of respiratory depression is largely unfounded at the end

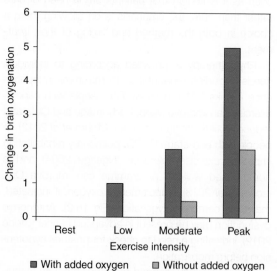

FIGURE 15.2 Increase in oxygen saturation in the brains of patients with end-stage lung disease during exercise, with and without added oxygen

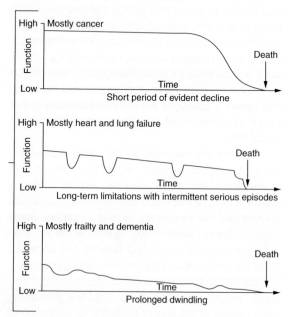

FIGURE 15.3 The effect of dyspnoea on function with different conditions over time

of life (Kamal 2012) if the dose is carefully titrated (Ahmedzai *et al* 2012, p.27). It is delivered subcutaneously if the patient cannot swallow. Nebulized morphine may be beneficial (Sorenson 2000b), and the reassuring presence of a nebulizer may reduce respiratory panic. Oxycodone helps some patients (Kawabata 2013) and steroids may relieve SOB associated with diffuse lung malignancy.

Non-invasive ventilation may palliate SOB (2013), sometimes with high-flow oxygen (Hui *et al* 2013). Other forms of oxygen are rarely beneficial objectively for normoxaemic patients (Campbell 2013) and set up a barrier between patient and family, but carry a strong placebo effect, as described by one observer: 'I realized that she was finding comfort receiving the oxygen, as she curled herself around the tube in an almost foetal position' (Scanlon 2003). If it is prescribed for this purpose, the patient needs to be informed that this is probably its mode of bringing relief, and a fan should be tried first (Kamal 2012).

Fatigue

> *I was too tired to think.*
>   Patient quoted by Eustace (2002)

Fatigue is under-recognized, under-assessed and under-treated (Radbruch 2008), with more importance being ascribed to it by patients than by health staff (Fig 15.4). It occurs in 70–100% of patients (Robinson & English 2010), can be aggravated by steroids (Matsuo & Yomiya 2013) and may not be relieved by rest (Brown 1999). Pharmacological management includes methylpheni-

date, which also helps depression (Kerr 2012). The exhaustion of cachexia can be eased by organ-specific nutrition (Zadák 2013) and sometimes non-steroidal anti-inflammatory drugs (Reid *et al* 2013). Physical management is by energy conservation (Yun *et al* 2012) and paced multimodal exercise (Kassab 2013).

Weakness

Weakness and the resulting lack of function are high on the 'unbearable suffering' spectrum (Ruijs *et al* 2012). Causes include immobility, cachexia or some drugs, in particular steroids which may be essential to treat raised intracranial pressure or spinal cord compression (Lo 2013). For cancer patients, the quadriceps are the most severely affected muscles (Brown 1999), indicating the need for little-and-often strengthening exercises. Other exercises are best related to an individual's activities of daily living, with always an awareness of potential osteoporosis from radiotherapy, chemotherapy or bony secondaries.

Cough

In the last year of life, 57% of patients complain of coughing (Leach 2010). When persistent, it can precipitate vomiting, chest or abdominal pain, rib fracture, syncope, insomnia or exhaustion. If pulmonary oedema, infection or bronchospasm contribute, they can be dealt with pharmacologically. For other coughs, linctus temporarily soothes the throat, and codeine and the opioids may suppress the central nervous system contribution to the cough (Yorke *et al* 2012). Nebulized local anaesthetics can relieve

---

FIGURE 15.4 Proportion of patients and oncologists reporting on whether fatigue or pain most affects daily life

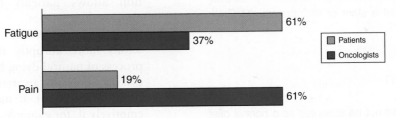

an intractable cough (Truesdale 2013), but eating and drinking are banned for an hour afterwards. Physical management depends on whether the cough is productive or not (Ch. 8).

Difficulty swallowing

Dysphagia, often due to weak mouth or throat muscles, may cause silent aspiration, in which ingested material ends up in the lungs without signs of swallowing difficulty or coughing. This may be first identified by the physiotherapist, who can then make a speech-language referral.

Dehydration and thirst

Some patients escape the symptoms associated with dehydration such as headache, nausea and cramps, but 36% of patients are reported to experience thirst (Arai 2013). In the UK it is illegal to withhold food or fluids before coma ensues (Dimond 2009 p.71), and Cohen (2012) found that patients who can communicate their wishes prefer to be hydrated because it improves their comfort, reduces pain and nourishes their body and mind. Artificial hydration has to be carefully balanced (Nakajima 2013) and the best option is often physical assistance using a spoon or feeding cup, with advice to the patient on when to swallow. This usually requires the time and patience of a relative. If the patient does not accept this, the relative can be reassured that a drink is probably not needed at that time.

A coated tongue or dry mouth can be relieved by the measures in Table 8.2, by semifrozen gin and tonic or unsweetened pineapple chunks (Regnard 1997).

Stridor

Treatment of stridor is by upright positioning, steroids, Heliox, insertion of a stent or radiotherapy (McGrath et al 2011).

Depression

Depression should not be accepted as a normal grief response. It is accompanied by symptoms such as fatigue, guilt and thoughts of suicide, yet is often undetected and poorly managed in palliative care settings (Mellor et al 2013). The majority of patients who express a wish to hasten their death are depressed, which may be due to feelings of helplessness or being a burden on their family (Billings 2000).

Several measuring tools are available (Johns et al 2013) but for physiotherapists a 'two question screening tool' identifies depression by first asking the simple question 'are you depressed?' followed by 'have you experienced loss of interest in things or activities that you would normally enjoy?' (Payne 2007).

A palliative team is usually able to offer medication, counselling or both, or the patient may prefer to talk to friends. Psychotherapy can be helpful for patients expected to live for more than six months, and a 'life review' can be helpful for those expecting to die earlier (Stagg & Lazenby 2012). The life review records patients as they reflect on their lives, then this is transcribed and given to the patient to share with whom they like. Benefits include affirmation of the patient's life, resolution of conflicts, comfort for the family, and help with closure for both patient and family (Csikai 2013).

Anxiety

Anxiety can be underestimated by both patient and physiotherapist (Taylor 2007). Information is always the first approach. Also helpful are music therapy (Black 2012), mindfulness meditation, which can also reduce depression (Halifax 2011) and Reiki, which can also ease pain (Marcus et al 2013).

Palliative sedation (Vayne-Bossert 2013) can be provided at three levels:

1 'Conscious sedation' is a patient-controlled state achieved after initial relief of symptoms, when sedatives are reduced to a level in which communication allows patients to continue to express their wishes.

2 'Deep sedation' renders patients unconscious more abruptly than during the process of natural dying but does not necessarily prevent awareness or distress (Rady et al 2013). It may be used preemptively if, for example, ventilatory support is to be removed (Berger 2012) and

its effects can be monitored by observational scales (Brinkkemper 2013).

3   'Respite sedation' is used for 24–48 hours and then reduced for re-assessment (Mazzotta 2012).

The use of sedation for existential suffering is more controversial, and addressing the root cause may be preferable, followed by strategies such as spiritual support, friendship or psychotherapy (Taylor & McCann 2005).

For both depression and anxiety, the physiotherapist's contribution is to maximize independence, if and as required by the patient, and to lend an ear.

Discomfort

Regular turning and positioning to suit the individual eases the discomfort of immobility. Some patients like to be propped up with their head well supported, while others like to be curled up on their side with generous quantities of pillows. The skin needs meticulous attention. Simple brief exercises are usually helpful, sometimes demonstrated to the relatives.

Immobility

The physiotherapist works with the family and staff to assist the patient with mobility, balance and transfers, and often to reduce the fear of falling. This may lessen anxiety, decrease injuries and restore dignity. Other reported outcomes are improved emotional functioning and reduced fatigue for people with cancer, and reduced depression and pain for those with spinal cord compression (Turner et al 2013).

Pain

No one should die while experiencing pain, for it obliterates all composure and the quiet business of the commendation of the soul.

Sewell 2012

Pain is a malevolent adversary of dying patients, but under-treatment is common, especially for those in hospital (Yao 2013). Assessment is available for people of all nationalities (Huang et al 2012) and those with special needs (Ch. 16). Acute and chronic pain may co-exist (Merlin et al 2013).

Fear that opioids will hasten death contributes to their underuse (Fromme et al 2008). Prescribers can be reassured that physical dependence is not the same as addiction (Hanks et al 2010 p. 691), that there is no upper limit (Silvestri 2000), that one patient who takes regular analgesics may need 100 times more than another, and that addiction when using opioids for pain relief occurs in less than 1% of patients (McCaffery 2001).

Co-prescription of laxatives and anti-emetics is needed, but tolerance to the side effect of sedation usually develops. Delirium can occur if opioids are used simply for anxiety, and a multidimensional approach that includes rotation of drugs and psychosocial support can reduce both intractable pain and delirium (Mori et al 2012).

The synthetic opioid fentanyl can be delivered transmucosally or transdermally (Bradley 2013). Intravenous lignocaine can be used for transient severe pain (Kintzel 2012) or intractable hiccups (Kaneishi 2013).

Micco et al (2009) caution against 'knee-jerk symptom relief that can dull or remove whatever subjective experience someone may have'. However, pain contributes to hopelessness (Sachs et al 2013) and patients should be able to make an informed choice about their pain relief.

Other pain-relieving strategies include TENS (Robinson & English 2010), massage (López et al 2012), pain meditations (Levine 1988) and reflexology (Hodgson & Lafferty 2012).

You can choose to sit in a corner and say 'I cannot do anything', or you can just get on with it and say, 'Well, I don't get any less pain from doing something'.

Patient quoted by Cour & Hansen (2012)

Nausea

Nausea is usually more difficult to control than vomiting, but haloperidol can reduce nausea, vomiting and delirium without the need for it to be processed through a fully functioning kidney or liver (Prommer 2012).

Insomnia

Sleep fragmentation may predispose to delirium in advanced illness (Kerr et al 2013). Any symptoms or environmental factors that disturb sleep need to be addressed. The patient can then choose from a variety of measures (pp.208/411), or, specifically for end-stage disease, acupressure (Tsay 2003), relaxation or cognitive-behavioural therapy, the latter being more sustainable than medication (Dambrosio 2013). Drugs include trazodone, which can sometimes also control nightmares (Tanimukai et al 2013), and there is now a tentative re-emergence of thalidomide, which also helps appetite (Davis et al 2012).'

Secretions and the death rattle

Half of patients develop secretions in their throat at the end of life if they are too weak to expectorate or swallow (Heisler 2013). Once the patient is unconscious, audible secretions are usually called a death rattle, heralding death within an average 16 hours (Bickel & Arnold 2008). The term 'lung congestion' is kinder for the patient and relatives. Campbell et al (2013) report that the secretions do not cause respiratory distress, and relatives can be reassured that the noise is a common occurrence at this stage.

The sound may ease with repositioning. Secretion formation can be prevented by hyoscine patches or syringe pump at the first indication of moist breath sounds, or by oral, subcutaneous, sublingual, transdermal, ophthalmic or parenteral atropine (Protus et al 2013). Once present, secretions can be dried up by low doses of a tricyclic antidepressant, beta-blockers, or for patients who are able, dark grape juice or sugar-free citrus lozenges (Voltz 2004). Chest clearance by percussion is unhelpful and

---

PRACTICE TIP

Suction is not indicated, even if the patient is unable to express distress, because it may cause distress which the patient cannot articulate, and its effect is transient.

---

unsafe because of the risk of fracture from boney secondaries.

Terminal restlessness

Delirium affects a patient's ability to communicate, their decision-making capacity, functional ability and quality of life (Hosie 2013). In the last few days of life it is called terminal restlessness and may be more related to anguish and spiritual pain, occurring in up to 85% of patients and complicating bereavement for the family. Risk factors are unfinished business, positional pain, physical restraint, SOB, dehydration, urine retention, constipation (Mazzarino 2010), sensory loss, pain, anxiety, fear, toxic levels of narcotics (Papadimos et al 2011) or the withdrawal of nicotine or alcohol, these last being avoidable by substitution (Ch.17).

Even for patients who are unconscious, quiet familiar music, a hearing aid if required and the presence of chosen family members are thought to be beneficial. Bright lights and strong environmental stimuli should be avoided. Medication may be helpful (Irwin et al 2013).

Deathbed visions of deceased family or friends are a more peaceful accompaniment to dying (Estle 2013). Near-death experiences occur in 10% to 18% of patients, and tend to bring feelings of serenity (Lawrence & Repede 2013).

ON DYING WELL

> Hope does not lie in a way out, but in a way through.
>
> Robert Frost

When patients are free from fears, they are more able to live their remaining life to the full. Conscious dying is possible when a balance of minimum symptoms without undue sedation has been achieved, so that patients are not trapped between perpetual pain and perpetual somnolence, and are able to take decisions on how much they may or may not like to experience the process. Dying is an event that not all cultures, nor all individuals, want to be sedated out of experiencing. Indeed, some patients find that life in the face of death allows for a more intense existence and awareness of the present (Cour & Hansen 2012), or as described by one author 'Dying had quickened his own livingness' (Brennan 2013).

There is no 'right' way to die, but death can be a positive achievement when patients are not consumed by anxiety about symptoms and have stopped fighting for life. Through the many little deaths of dying, they have plumbed the depths of their being, but fear has dissolved, there is peace without defeatism and they are free to look for some meaning in the experience. Open communication, on the patient's terms, is thought to contribute to acceptance of dying and the quality of the dying process (Lokker et al 2012).

Working with dying people is demanding and requires us to be emotionally healthy. It means sharing anguish, absorbing misdirected anger and providing comfort and dignity for people who are totally dependent. It includes emotional involvement, wherein lies its challenge and reward.

OUTCOMES

That's the trouble with death, all the loose ends.

Rousseau (2013)

Multiple-symptom evaluation is recommended to assess the effects of treatment (Lowery et al 2014). The Good Death Scale and Palliative Outcome Scale are examples (Cheng 2013, Saleem et al 2013). Specifically for advanced cancer are the Cancer Dyspnea Scale (Uronis 2012), Edmonton Functional Assessment Tool (Cobbe et al 2013) and Advanced Cancer Patients' Distress Scale (Fischbeck et al 2013). For patients unable to self-report, a behavioural test assesses respiratory distress (Campbell et al 2010). Carer burden is assessed using the Zarit Burden Inventory (Bausewein 2012).

CASE STUDY: Ms IU

You are called in to see a 69 y.o. woman with an exacerbation of COPD. There was no non-invasive ventilation service in the hospital at the time.

Social history
- Lives alone and independently.
- Supportive son lives in nearby town.

Subjective
- Can't breathe
- Dry mouth

Objective
- Medical notes state that a decision has been made not to ventilate the patient.
- P_aO_2 9.5 kPa (71.4 mmHg), P_aCO_2 11.3 kPa (85 mmHg), pH 7.21, HCO_3 32, BE 1.4
- S_pO_2 85% and fluctuating
- On 24% dry oxygen
- Temperature 36°C
- On infusion of salbutamol and doxapram (respiratory stimulant).

- Propped up in bed
- Rapid shallow breathing
- Body shaking continuously
- Difficulty speaking
- Appears fearful

Questions

1   Is the goal of medical treatment palliative or curative?
2   Give three possible reasons for Ms IU's shaking.
3   Problems?
4   What teamwork is needed?
5   Plan?

CLINICAL REASONING

Could the following signs and symptoms indicate anything else?
'Signs and symptoms which indicate a need for suctioning include: patient restlessness or anxiety, diaphoresis, increased blood pressure and heart rate.'

Acc Emerg Nurs (1997) 5, 92–8

Diaphoresis: sweating.

Response to Case Study

1   **Goal**
    - There appear to be conflicting goals. With this level of respiratory acidosis, Ms IU will die without supported ventilation, indicating that the goal is palliative. However, doxapram is a distressing drug, does not palliate symptoms and is normally aimed at keeping patients alive.

2   **Reason**
    - Fear, hypercapnia, doxapram

3   **Problems**
    - Anxiety
    - Dyspnoea and fatigue
    - Dry mouth
    - Hypoxaemia
    - Hypercapnia and acidosis

4   **Teamwork**
    - Liaise with referring doctor to revisit decision not to ventilate (declined).
    - Liaise with nurse to contact son.

5   Plan

- Fear: the patient was unable to speak, so she was reassured that her son was being contacted and that she would not be left alone and that her needs would be attended to; she was also told that one of the drugs in her drip was likely to be causing her shakes.
- Dyspnoea: fan, gentle back rubbing, positioning sitting over the edge of the bed, feet on the floor and leaning forward over a pillow on a table, with manual support.
- Dry mouth: mouth care, sips of water offered, mask changed to nasal cannulae; humidification was not attempted because the patient could not be left and the nurse was unable to fetch the equipment (it was 3 am and only one nurse was on duty).
- Hypoxaemia: F_iO_2 titrated using oximetry.
- Hypercapnia and acidosis: intermittent positive pressure breathing attempted but the patient was too weak to trigger the machine.

The patient died quietly two hours later.

Response to Clinical Reasoning

There are many possible causes of restlessness, anxiety, sweating and disturbed vital signs. If not identified and remedied, these could be increased by suctioning.

RECOMMENDED READING

Association of Chartered Physiotherapists in Oncology and Palliative Care (1993) *Guidelines for Good Practice*. Chartered Society of Physiotherapy, London

Bajwah S, Higginson IJ, Ross, Joy R *et al* (2013) The palliative care needs for fibrotic interstitial lung disease. *Palliat Med;* **27**(9): 877

Barawid EL (2013) Rehabilitation modalities in palliative care. *Crit Rev Phys Rehab Med*, **25**(1–2): 77–100

Baxter SK, Baird WO, Thompson S *et al* (2013) Use of non-invasive ventilation at end of life. *Palliat Med;* **27**(9): 878

Billings JA (2012) Humane terminal extubation reconsidered: the role for preemptive analgesia and sedation. *Crit Care Med*; **40**(2): 625–30

Brown-Saltzman K, Upadhya D, Larner L *et al* (2010) An intervention to improve respiratory therapists' comfort with end-of-life care. *Respir Care*; **55**(7): 858–65

Carson K, McIlfatrick S (2013) More than physical function? Exploring physiotherapists' experiences in delivering rehabilitation to patients requiring palliative care in the community. *J Palliat Care*; **29**(1): 36–44

Davis C, Guyer C (2013) Integrated care pathways for dying patients – myths, misunderstandings and realities in clinical practice. *Eur J Palliat Care*; **20**(1): 112–119

Department of Health (2007) Gold Standards Framework (GSF) for Palliative Care

Horton R, Rocker G, Dale A *et al* (2013) Implementing a palliative care trial in advanced COPD. *J Palliat Med*; **16**(11): 67–73

Hayle C (2013) Understanding the experience of patients with chronic obstructive pulmonary disease who access specialist palliative care. *Palliat Med;* **27**(9): 861–8

Kehl KA, Kowalkowski JA (2013) A systematic review of the prevalence of signs of impending death and symptoms in the last 2 weeks of life. *Am J Hospice Palliat Med;* **30**(6): 601–16

Killick S (2013) Managing the conflicting wishes of a woman on ventilatory support and her family. *Eur J Palliat Care*; **20**(4): 172–173

Mols A (2013) Palliative surgery in cancer patients. *Eur J Palliat Care*; **20**(1): 9–13

Morgan DD, White KM (2012) Occupational therapy interventions for breathlessness at the end of life. *Curr Opin Support Palliat Care*; **6**(2): 138–43

Nelson JE, Hope AA (2012) Integration of palliative care in chronic critical illness. *Respir Care*; **57**(6): 1004–13

NICE Guideline (2013) Opioids in palliative care (CG140)

Nogler AF (2014) Hoping for the best, preparing for the worst: strategies to promote honesty and prevent medical futility at end-of-life. *Dimens Crit Care Nurs*; **33**(1): 22–7

Payne C, Wiffen PJ, Martin S (2012) Interventions for fatigue and weight loss in adults with advanced progressive illness. *Cochrane Systematic Rev*, **1**: CD008427

Peereboom K, Coyle N (2012) Facilitating goals-of-care discussions for patients with life-limiting disease. *J Hospice Palliat Nurs*; **14**(4): 251–8

Primus CP, Flett AS, Cheung CC *et al* (2013) Palliative care provision in an advanced heart failure clinic: patients' experiences. *Eur J Palliat Care*; **20**(3): 127–129

Read S (2013) Palliative care for people with intellectual disabilities. *Palliat Med*; **27**(1): 3–4

Simon ST, Bausewein C, Schildmann E *et al* (2013) Episodic breathlessness in patients with advanced disease. *J Pain Symptom Management*; **45**(3): 561–78

Twomey S, Dowling M (2013) Management of death rattle at end of life. *Br J Nurs.*; **13;22**(2): 81–5

CHAPTER 16
Physiotherapy for people undergoing surgery

LEARNING OBJECTIVES

On completion of this chapter the reader should be able to:

- understand the complications of different types of surgery

- recognize the role of the physiotherapist in preventing and managing these complications

- describe the rehabilitation required before and after a variety of operations

- discuss the management of a patient with a tracheostomy.

INTRODUCTION

Physiotherapists working on a surgical ward need acumen in order to identify patients who need treatment, and empathy for the individual because what is routine for the clinician is a unique event for the patient. Patients anticipate surgery with their own mixture of hope and dread.

Open surgery with full-sized incisions (Fig 16.1) is becoming less common as more organs are accessible to video-assisted keyhole techniques. This minimally-invasive surgery involves the insertion of fibre optic endoscopes through small stab incisions, so that the operative field can be viewed by the team on a monitor (Spinoglio 2014). Surgery is also possible at the bed-side or in the intensive care unit (ICU) under local anaesthesia.

Respiratory complications are the leading cause of prolonged hospital stay, morbidity, and mortality (Branson 2013), and the need for physiotherapy has increased because of rapid rehabilitation, early discharges and the extra time required for sicker and older patients who can now be operated on. Less physiotherapy is required to deal with complications related to pain and bed rest.

FIGURE 16.1 Incisions for open surgery

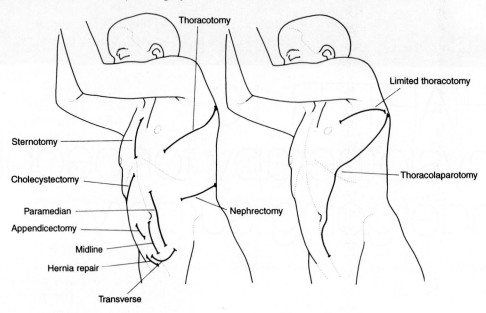

CARDIORESPIRATORY COMPLICATIONS OF SURGERY

Atelectasis

Functional residual capacity is reduced by up to one litre on lying down and a further half litre on induction of anaesthesia (Licker *et al* 2007). This predisposes to atelectasis (Fig 16.2) (Hedenstierna 2012) in dependent lung regions, lasting on average 24 hours after laparoscopy and 2 days after major surgery (Duggan 2005). Atelectasis becomes problematic in 0–5% of patients following lower abdominal surgery, 19–59% after thoracic surgery (Agostini & Singh 2009) and up to 88% after upper abdominal surgery (Dias 2008). Causes are the following:

1   Pain has a direct effect (Urell *et al* 2012), dull at rest and sharp on movement. After abdominal or chest surgery, guarding spasm of the trunk muscles and inhibition of breathing brings tidal volume down into the closing volume range (Ch. 1).

2   Prolonged recumbency reduces ventilation to the lung bases and causes pooling of intrathoracic blood to these regions, thus upsetting ventilation/perfusion matching.

3   Drowsiness and immobility obliterate the normal oscillations in tidal volume.

4   Abdominal surgery disrupts the diaphragm (Smith *et al* 2010).

5   Pleural effusion is a common, though usually minor, reaction to perioperative fluid overload.

6   Atelectasis creates a restrictive defect, reducing lung compliance and depleting surfactant (Davis 2012a). Greater efforts are needed to inflate the poorly-compliant collapsed alveoli (see Fig 1.5) than to prevent this occurring.

KEY POINT

Prevention is better than cure, and should begin preoperatively.

FIGURE 16.2 Interrelation of factors affecting lung function (*FRC:* functional residual capacity)

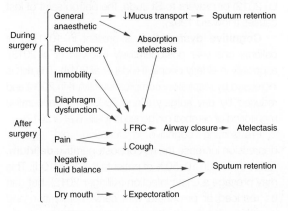

FIGURE 16.3 Oximetry readings showing damaging episodes of desaturation on the third postoperative night after major surgery

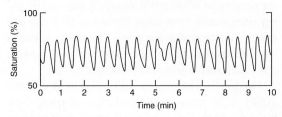

Hypoxaemia

Hypoxaemia is caused by the shunting of blood through airless lung and inhibition of hypoxic vasoconstriction (Ch. 1) by volatile anaesthetic agents (Davison & Cottle 2010). This can slow wound healing, destabilize the cardiovascular system and cause infection by encouraging bacterial translocation from the gut through the hypoxic gut lining and into the circulation (Strachan & Noble 2001).

When present briefly, hypoxaemia is related to the anaesthetic, and low risk patients only need brief postoperative oxygen therapy. When present for several days it is related to the surgery and postoperative factors, with supplemental oxygen being required for at least 72 hours following major surgery (Singh 2011). Night time is particularly precarious, high risk patients being hypoxaemic for 2–4 nights after surgery (Kehlet & Wilmore 2002) because they are catching up on their oxygen-hungry rapid-eye-movement sleep (Ch. 1) which has been obliterated by sleep disturbance and medication. Patients who have had major surgery, or those with respiratory or cardiovascular disease, should be monitored for nocturnal oxygen desaturation (Fig 16.3) to prevent premature cessation of oxygen therapy.

Chest infection

A slight pyrexia following surgery is a normal reaction to tissue trauma, but fever beyond 48 hours suggests infection, often of the wound or lungs. Intubation overrides upper airway defence mechanisms, and for longer operations the anaesthetic gases dry the airway and impair ciliary action, predisposing to chest infection. Signs usually emerge some days after surgery, e.g. crackles on auscultation, purulent bronchial secretions, malaise, fever and sometimes rapid breathing. The risk of pneumonia is reduced by a multidisciplinary 'pneumonia bundle' of education, incentive spirometry, for selective patients, oral care and mobility (Wren *et al* 2010).

Haemodynamic instability

Atrial fibrillation is a common complication in elderly people and is the most frequent complication after cardiovascular surgery. It tends to develop on the second postoperative day and predisposes to cardiovascular complications (Omae & Kanmura 2012).

Pre- and postoperative fluid restriction can cause electrolyte disturbance which may develop into unrecognized hypovolaemia and arrhythmias (Chelazzi 2011). Fluid overload also brings complications (Ch. 17). The risk is reduced with pre-emptive 'goal-directed therapy' to optimize haemodynamics by monitoring and manipulating fluid and drug therapy (Haas 2012). Postural hypotension may be a sign of unrecognized hypovolaemia and is a reminder to avoid sudden standing or position change.

OTHER COMPLICATIONS

Pain is a major risk factor for atelectasis and other complications (Ch. 16). **Anxiety** and **stress** increase the perception of pain, splint the diaphragm, compromize immunity and promote infection (Solowiej *et al* 2009). Psychological and physiological stress inhibit healing (Gouin 2012) and promote metastases in cancer patients (Neeman 2013). Anxiety is reduced by giving preoperative information (Sjoling *et al* 2003) and granting postoperative autonomy. The stress response can be modified by preoperative nutritional support and postoperative analgesia (Patel *et al* 2012).

Fatigue is related to pain (Rubin & Hotopf 2002). It is more prolonged than expected by most patients. Frequent short walks may need to be negotiated postoperatively rather than infrequent long ones.

Some drugs contribute to the 'big little problem' of postoperative **nausea**, which can be more distressing than pain, occurs in one third of patients and predisposes to pulmonary complications (Rawlinson *et al* 2012). Risk factors are anxiety, pain, abdominal or breast surgery and inadequate preoperative fluids. Nausea inhibits deep breathing and can lead to dehydration, electrolyte imbalance, wound dehiscence (opening of the incision) and bleeding (Gan 2006). It can be relieved by:

- hydration, pain relief and medication (Kovac 2013)
- preoperative relaxation (Seers *et al* 2008)
- acupressure (White 2012) or acupuncture (Grube 2009).

Depression may occur, especially if surgery affects body image, e.g. colostomy, head and neck surgery or mastectomy. An understanding ear or referral to a self-help group (App B) may prevent a natural sense of loss degenerating into long-term depression.

Urine retention, flatulence or **constipation** impair excursion of the diaphragm. Flatulence can be relieved by gentle bed exercises (Dainese 2004), e.g. pelvic tilting and knee rolling in crook-lying.

Wound infection, suspected if there is fever, swelling, redness or increasing pain, complicates 2-5% of operations (Mestral 2013) but is reduced if high FiO_2 is delivered during surgery (Hovaguimian 2013). Infection increases the risk of **dehiscence,** especially if the patient smokes, is malnourished, obese, immunocompromised, on long-term steroids or receiving radiotherapy (Singh *et al* 2011). Wound, chest or otherinfection may lead to **sepsis** (Moore & Moore 2013).

Incessant **hiccups**, due to irritation of the diaphragm, cause sharp pain at the wound site. Suggested remedies are drugs, sugar, breath-holding to raise P_aCO_2, pulling on the tongue, pressing on the eyeball, eating peanut butter, rectal massage (Chang & Lu 2012) or prayers to St Jude, the patron saint of lost causes (Howard 1992).

Cognitive dysfunction is present in 10–17% of patients one year postoperatively (Stewart *et al* 2013), especially in elderly people (Riedel *et al* 2014). The risk is increased by respiratory complications (Murkin 2006) and reduced by day surgery (Cane 2003) or intraoperative monitoring of cerebral oxygenation (Ballard *et al* 2012).

Pre-existing cognitive dysfunction, old age or depression increase the risk of postoperative **delirium**, which occurs in 10–50% of patients (NICE 2010d). This may presage a chest infection (Killinger 2012), but can be reduced or prevented with early mobilization and nutrition, a familiar clock and calendar, glasses or hearing aid, and ensuring a good night's sleep (Rudolph *et al* 2011). If sedation is required, dexmedetomidine is recommended (Zhang 2013).

Peripheral nerve injuries may become apparent 48 hours postoperatively, most commonly of the ulnar nerve, brachial plexus or spinal cord. They are caused by compression, stretch ischaemia or direct nerve trauma on the table (Lalkhen & Bhatia 2012).

Postoperative **haemorrhage**, due to surgical complications or deficient clotting, is suspected if there is:

- obvious bleeding
- rapid filling of drainage bottles
- signs of hypovolaemic shock (Ch. 19).

Deep vein thrombosis (DVT) complicates up to a quarter of operations (Dar *et al* 2012). Causes are calf compression on the table, immobility, fluid loss, manipulation of blood vessels and surgical stress which upsets clotting (Nimmo 2004). It can be clinically silent or cause signs and symptoms (Ch. 4). It may break free and cause **pulmonary embolism** by lodging in the pulmonary vascular bed, reportedly leading to 10% of hospital deaths (Dar *et al* 2012). Patients at risk are those who:

- are undergoing lengthy surgery, neurosurgery, or surgery which pulls on blood vessels such as knee, hip or pelvic surgery
- are elderly, obese, or have malignant, neurological, vascular or blood disorders
- have a history of DVT.

Awareness during anaesthesia is a feared but rare complication occurring in an average 0.15% of 1 in

15,000 patients and sometimes leading to post traumatic stress disorder (Avidan 2013). Risks are day surgery, when anaesthesia is minimized, and trauma surgery (Ghoneim 2000), but this can be reduced by brain monitoring (Pandit *et al* 2013).

PREOPERATIVE MANAGEMENT

> *The single most important preoperative intervention is to educate patients on manoeuvres to increase lung volumes.*
> Zarmsky 2001

Physiotherapy

Is physiotherapy necessary before surgery? Education on positioning, mobilization and, if necessary, chest clearance can reduce postoperative complications, increase S_pO_2 and improve mobility (Olsén *et al* 1997). Impaired physical capacity is associated with postoperative pulmonary complications (Soares 2013) and preoperative exercise has shown the following postoperative benefits:

- Improved exercise tolerance and functional independence (Soares 2013).
- Improved outcomes after major abdominal surgery (Dronkers et al 2013).
- Reduced complications after cardiac (Valkenet *et al* 2011), abdominal or thoracic surgery (Olsén & Anzén 2012).

Information is especially important for patients expecting to wake up in the ICU, where they will feel relieved at the sight of a familiar face (Scott 2004). Patients anticipating mechanical ventilation (MV) should be warned of their inability to speak. They need information on the experience of MV and suction, the fact that they may hear before being able to respond, and reassurance that there will be a nurse watching over them. Visits to the ICU by the patient and family are often helpful, and should be supplemented by written material (Scott 2004).

Accurate information relieves anxiety (Scott 2004) and anxious patients should be seen early if possible because worry at impending surgery inhibits receptivity (Cupples 1991). Some patients find it beneficial to have relatives present to help absorb the information. At the end of the discussion, it is useful to check patients' understanding (Scott *et al* 2003). If a patient is not admitted early enough to be seen, preoperative physiotherapy can take place in the pre-assessment clinic, or by phone (Carli *et al* 2010), or a hand out (App. B) can be sent.

Teamwork

Preoperative information includes advice for smokers to stop, preferably months previously (Wolfenden 2005). They are more likely to do so if they hear messages specific to surgery, e.g. that smoking increases wound infections (Gravante *et al* 2007). Some patients also benefit from the opportunity to discuss advance care planning (Redmann *et al* 2012).

The tradition of prolonged preoperative fluid and food restriction is now known to increase postoperative nausea, vomiting, pain (Maharaj 2005), dehydration, stomach acidity (Mackenzie *et al* 2010) and risk of aspiration (Stuart 2013). Patients should not fast for longer than six hours (Stuart 2013), and clear oral fluids two hours before surgery help maintain fluid and electrolyte balance and improve patient comfort (Itou *et al* 2012).

The 'enhanced recovery programme' incorporates interventions to minimize the stress response to surgery, including early mobility (Fig 16.4). It can halve 30-day morbidity and reduce length of hospital stay (Adamina *et al* 2013). Pre-emptive analgesia is included because less analgesia is required to prevent pain than to abolish it after it has started, noxious impulses gaining entry into the central nervous system and 'winding up' the response to subsequent afferent inputs (Ng & Vickers 2013). Attention to nutrition is included because it can reduce complications two- to threefold (Leach *et al* 2013). A leafy view through a window is not included but can speed recovery (Ulrich 1984).

PAIN MANAGEMENT

> *[There is] an enormous amount of unnecessary pain ... It seems almost as if many members of the medical profession view 'curing' and 'caring' as mutually exclusive.*
> Lowenstein (2000)

FIGURE 16.4 Components of the enhanced recovery programme. *CHO:* carbohydrate, *NG:* nasogastric

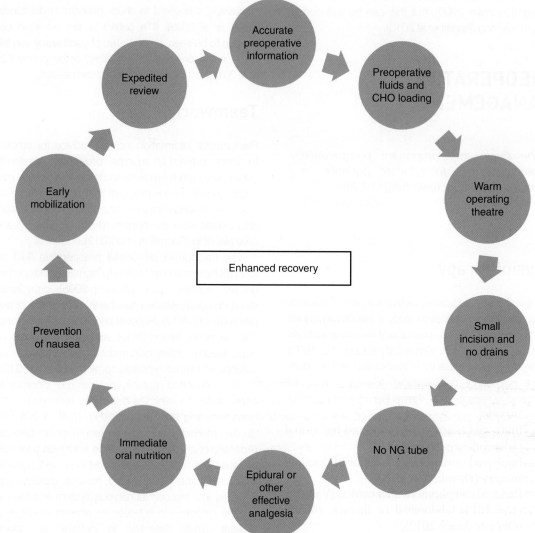

Inadequate pain relief has a direct bearing on post-operative complications (Patel 2012) including long-term pain and poor quality of life (Moore *et al* 2013). Unnecessary postoperative pain still occurs in up to 67% of patients in the UK (Wood 2010a).

The concept of pain includes both the sensation and the individual's reaction to the sensation, and there is wide variation in patients' perception of pain, as well as unpredictable responses to analgesics (Chapman *et al* 2012). However, it is not unusual to hear patients dismissed as having a 'low pain threshold' or accused of exaggerating their complaints (McCaffery *et al* 2005).

Other reasons for unnecessary pain are:
- ignorance of the difference between the use and abuse of opioids, some staff thinking that a request for pain relief indicates drug dependence (McCaffrey *et al* 2005)
- misunderstanding the difference between opioid euphoria and respiratory depression, or fear that opioids adversely affect

pain assessment despite evidence to the contrary (Ranji *et al* 2006)

- 'opiophobia', reinforced by British GP Harold Shipman using diamorphine to murder his patients in the 1990s
- patients' low expectations of pain relief and anxiety about side effects (Sutcliffe 1993)
- inexperience, staff shortage and poor pain assessment (Moore *et al* 2013).

Empathy for another's pain requires activation of the anterior insular and cingulate cortices (Gu *et al* 2012) and it is to be hoped that these precious parts of the brain in clinicians are not desensitized by exposure to poor practice in the health system.

Effects of pain

PRACTICE TIP

Next time you are in the dentist's chair and you see the needle advancing, try to take a deep breath.

Pain has the following effects:
- ↓ deep breathing and coughing (Figs 16.5/6)
- ↓ cardiorespiratory function, mobility and sleep, ↑ delirium (Reimer-Kent 2003)

FIGURE 16.5 The effect of pain on atelectasis

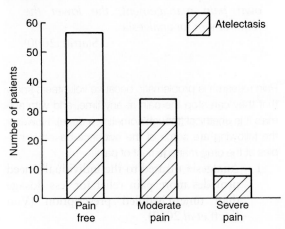

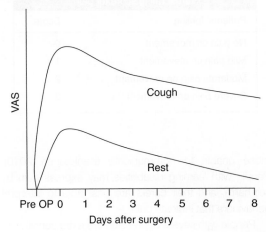

FIGURE 16.6 Postoperative pain with cough (top) and at rest (bottom) measured by visual analogue scale (VAS)

- ↑ sympathetic tone, inflammatory response, coagulation cascade and oxygen consumption (Piriyapatsom *et al* 2013)
- delayed hospital discharge (Kim *et al* 2013)
- ↓ opportunity for day surgery (Berg *et al* 2013).

The intensity of postoperative pain is a predictor of long-term pain, and one chronic pain clinic has reported an increase in patients whose pain originated postoperatively (Cho *et al* 2012b).

Assessment

*With rare exceptions, pain **is** as the patient describes it.*

Azzam & Alam (2013)

Pain should be assessed like any other vital sign, including at rest and on movement (Fig 16.7). Pain assessment is also a right for people with special needs, not just those who can complain in a way that is easy to understand. Verbal numerical rating scales are simple and give consistent results, and assessment tools are available for patients with confusional states or intellectual impairment (Macintyre *et al* 2010) and

FIGURE 16.7 Pain scale that can be used before physiotherapy

Verbal rating score for pain	
Patients' feeling	Score
No pain on movement	0
Mild pain on movement	1
Moderate pain on movement	2
Severe pain on movement	3

those unable to communicate (Kankkunen 2010). People with learning disabilities may express pain by self-harm, and their carers are best able to interpret behaviours that indicate pain.

People with severe depression are extra sensitive to pain because of the accumulating effect of emotional and physical pain (Savitz et al 2012). Elderly people are less likely to report pain and are at particular risk of under-treatment (Wood 2008) while the majority of patients with dementia have been found to suffer severe postoperative pain (Morrison & Siu 2000).

Objective signs are pallor, sweating, shallow breathing, breath-holding and increased pulse, BP and respiratory rate, but these indicate severe pain and can also reflect other conditions. Extreme pain causes nausea, vomiting and reduced pulse and BP.

Pain assessment for infants, children and older people are in Chapters 10, 11 and 14.

Reduction in the perception of pain

There are many things that make pain worse, such as the spirit in which it is inflicted. You are indeed acutely vulnerable to the attitude of people surrounding you.

         Patient quoted by Donald (1977)

Factors such as anxiety, depression and coping skills can affect the perception of pain more than the pathology or procedure itself (Davis 2012b). The effect of 'anticipatory anxiety' on pain (Lin et al 2013) is a reminder of the need for accurate information in terms the patient

understands (Hjortholm et al 2013). Relaxation techniques can reduce both pain and anxiety (Rejeh et al 2013) (Ch. 9).

Handling patients in pain

The sense of anticipation is honed, to hysteria almost, and one quickly learns to be thoroughly suspicious of the well-meant: 'this won't hurt'.

         Patient quoted by Brooks (1990)

There are few rewards greater than relief on the face of a patient whose pain we have eased, and handling and positioning can be as important in relieving acute pain as drugs (Sutcliffe 1993). Some suggestions are in Box 16.1.

For rolling into side-lying, patients are asked to bend their knees, shift away from the direction in which they are to roll, hold onto the bed rail on the side towards which they are to roll, push with their knees and roll in one piece. They are encouraged to push with their legs rather than pull with their arms, so that abdominal muscle work is inhibited. After laparotomy, any manoeuvre that entails abdominal muscle work, e.g. eccentric contraction when lying back against the pillows, is eased by facilitating active back extension and reciprocal abdominal relaxation.

During activity, patients need reassurance in words and actions that they will be heard and responded to. 'Tell me if it hurts and I'll stop', is music to their ears.

Medication

The more patients feel in control of their own pain management, the lower the requirement for analgesia.

         Starritt (2000)

Pain research is problematic because volunteers know that they can stop the pain at any time, and with animals it is unethical (though sometimes done). However the following are some of the evidence-based principles of the drug management of pain:

1   Analgesia titrated to the individual's need provides more pain relief for less dosage than time-scheduled prescription (Von Korff et al 2012).

BOX 16.1

Tips for handling patients in pain

- Proactive analgesia is required (Kim & Kang 2013), given automatically before physiotherapy instead of first checking to see if treatment causes pain, i.e. after the horse has bolted.
- Unnecessary handling should be avoided.
- Patients must be assured that they are in control, and allowed to move themselves at their own pace when possible.
- Patients should be informed of how and when each movement will take place. Words to avoid are 'just relax', which signals to any seasoned patient that they are about to be hurt, or 'sorry' after an unexpected movement instead of clear explanations before the movement. The 'wince-sorry' scenario is familiar to those who have witnessed patients being routinely hurt and then routinely apologized to.

2   Morphine remains the favourite opioid analgesic, with a half-life of several hours. Side effects include elimination of spontaneous sighs (Bell 2013), nausea, constipation, abdominal distension, and, in hypovolaemic patients, hypotension. Respiratory depression is recognized by a respiratory rate that drops below 8 bpm, which is reversible by the opiate antagonist naloxone (Boland et al 2013). Fentanyl and alfentanil are useful for physiotherapy because of their quick onset.

3   Multimodal analgesia combines drugs and delivery systems in order to influence different physiological processes, e.g. intraoperative wound irrigation with local anaesthetic, regional (epidural or nerve block) anaesthesia (Gasanova et al 2013), central-acting analgesics like paracetamol, peripheral-acting non-steroidal anti-inflammatories, and drugs for neuropathic pain.

4   Drugs are best co-ordinated by an acute pain team (Usichenko et al 2013).

The **intravenous** (IV) route works immediately and can be delivered continuously or in boluses. Fentanyl should be injected slowly to reduce the side effect of coughing (Hung et al 2010).

Patient-controlled analgesia (PCA) delivers a pre-set dose of drug when the patient presses a button. This encourages mobility, requires less drug to achieve the same pain control, minimizes respiratory depression and can include anti-nausea drugs (Kim 2012). Whether delivered intravenously, orally, transdermally or epidurally, a lock-out interval avoids overdosing, and patients are advised to use the device freely.

The **epidural** route alters spinal processing by delivering drugs to the epidural space using a catheter inserted in the operating theatre and left in situ. Patients should be advised that postoperative epidurals are not the same as those given during childbirth and they will not be numb below the catheter. In increasing order of efficacy, administration is by intermittent blockade, continuous infusion or PCA (Kim et al 2013).

Advantages of epidurals are improved pain control (Kim 2013), earlier mobilization, restored lung volumes (Slinger 2013) lower mortality (Pöpping et al 2013) and reduced risk of DVT (Shouhed et al 2013).

Disadvantages are the risk of nausea, vomiting, hypotension, urinary retention and sometimes partial sensory or motor loss (Kim 2013). Patients receiving intermittent dosage may need to lie down for 30 minutes after a top-up to avoid hypotension, although lying flat for too long may allow the drug to move up the epidural space to the brain, causing respiratory depression. Respiratory function may also be impaired by a block higher than T4, and mild motor impairment is expected with a lumber epidural. High blocks are most associated with hypotension, while low blocks may cause urine retention. Capnography can be used to monitor respiratory depression (Whitaker 2011).

The **intrathecal** or **spinal** route delivers 'one-shot' drugs to the subarachnoid space below L2, producing profound analgesia without motor, sensory or sympathetic blockade (Hein et al 2012). Complications include 'spinal headache' due to leak of cerebrospinal fluid (CSF) through a punctured dura, leading to loss of the intracranial CSF 'cushion' (Arevalo-Rodriguez et al 2013).

The **transdermal** route is useful for local procedures such as taking blood. Anaesthetic cream causes topical anaesthesia when applied to the skin 30–60 minutes beforehand (Wiles et al 2010). No child should be submitted to venipuncture, lumbar puncture or, indeed any injection without prior application of their 'magic cream'. Needle-phobic adults also benefit. As well as skin anaesthesia, systemic analgesia can be delivered transdermally (Thakkar et al 2014).

The **transmucosal** route uses 'fentanyl lollipops' or tablets under the top lip for rapid analgesia (Arthur & Holder 2012), mucous membranes imposing less of a barrier than skin, as cocaine users have discovered.

The **intramuscular** route is rarely used because it is relatively ineffective, especially if given 'p.r.n.' (otherwise known as 'pain relief never').

The physiotherapist may take more direct action by using acupressure (Chung et al 2013), acupuncture (Taghavi 2013) or TENS (Silva 2012).

> *Freedom from pain should be a basic human right.*
> Liebeskind & Melzack (1987)

POSTOPERATIVE PHYSIOTHERAPY

Is physiotherapy necessary postoperatively? Research has shown positive outcomes when delivered accurately (Agostini & Singh 2009, Souza et al 2013) but not when applied routinely (Pasquina et al 2006). Respiratory complications are the leading cause of morbidity and mortality (Westwood et al 2007) and most patients gain from physiotherapy input to the team management of positioning and mobility, but those with the risk factors in Box 16.2 are most likely to need direct intervention. Risk scoring models also help to identify suitable patients (Anderson et al 2010, Bruton et al 2000).

Postoperative physiotherapy is based on techniques to increase lung volume and clear secretions (Chapters 6–8). Modifications specific to surgery are discussed below.

BOX 16.2

Risk factors for postoperative complications

- Surgery to the upper abdomen or chest, or comorbid cardiorespiratory disease (Smith et al 2010)
- Smoking history (Musallam et al 2013)
- Obesity (Stein & Matta 2013)
- Malnutrition (Kuppinger et al 2013)
- Old age (Deyo et al 2013)
- Emergency surgery (Alcock & Chilvers 2012)
- Postponed surgery (Kim & Park 2013)
- Drugs such as insulin and steroids (Deyo et al 2013)

Mobility

> **PRACTICE TIP**
>
> Patients are encouraged to sit with their legs dangling over the edge of the bed as soon as they are willing.

Early mobilization improves outcomes (Sunil 2013), including increased lung volume, improved S_pO_2, easier chest clearance (Stiller *et al* 2004) and shortened hospital stay (Haines *et al* 2013). If surgically and medically acceptable, this should be on the first postoperative day (ASGBI 2009). Patients can have targets such as walking along increasing lengths of a coloured line painted along the corridor.

Intravenous equipment that is plugged into the mains can usually be temporarily unplugged, so long as the battery is functioning. For patients with a urinary catheter, leg bags are more dignified than loose catheter bags. Posture correction is incorporated as soon as discomfort has eased. Safety aspects are on p. 476, with specific precautions for epidurals below:

- Check local protocol to identify if two staff members are required for mobilization.
- Check lower limb strength to ensure that there is no motor block.
- Check blood pressure (BP) to ensure that there is no sympathetic block.

Positioning

If pain, surgical procedure or instability delay mobilization, emphasis should be on accurate and comfortable positioning, as upright as possible (Mynster *et al* 1996) or side-lying. Sitting shows better gas exchange than supine (Duggan 2005) and, in half the research surveyed by Nielsen (2003), side-lying was preferred to supine. Regular position change, including alternate side-lying, helps prevent atelectasis. If side-lying pulls on the incision, the position may be modified, or a pillow can be supported against the wound.

Clinical and radiological assessment assists in decisions about positioning. Fig 16.8 would suggest lying the patient primarily on the left so that the collapsed lobe (R) is uppermost, but also to spend time on the right side to avoid the consolidation (L) developing into collapse.

Breathing exercises

Breathing exercises have not been indicated for uncomplicated surgery since Stiller *et al's* seminal work in 1994, but if mobilization is delayed, positioning limited, or atelectasis develops, deep breathing may be beneficial (Duggan 2005). Following high risk procedures such as oesophagectomy or upper abdominal surgery, regular prophylactic deep breathing is advisable, though this suggestion comes from physiological reasoning and auscultatory outcomes rather than research. For these patients, the ten deep breaths an hour advised by Bartlett *et al* in 1973 still make physiological sense today.

FIGURE 16.8 Upward shift of R hemidiaphragm suggests lower lobe collapse, and loss of the R heart border indicates some middle lobe involvement. Opacity of the L lower zone could be the breast shadow, especially as it is not possible to compare it to the R, but clinical assessment revealed bronchial breathing, indicating consolidation. *R*: right, *L*: left.

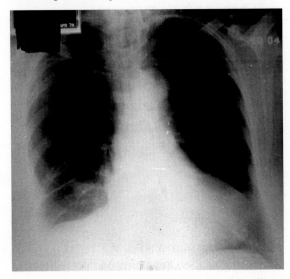

Pain must first be minimized (Lunardi et al 2013), then deep breathing done in a position that achieves a balance between comfort and optimal ventilation, usually well-forward-side-lying. For patients who cannot achieve this, upright sitting is the next option, but this tends to compress the lower chest and is unlikely to inflate dependent lung regions. Patients who are able to stand and lean against a wall can take relaxed deep breaths from there (p. 180).

Incentive spirometry augments deep breathing and has been shown to reduce pulmonary complications and length of stay after major abdominal surgery (Westwood et al 2007). Zarmsky (2001) calls incentive spirometry 'the number one best tool for preventing postoperative complications'. Even so, it is only required for patients, who need the incentive to achieve the quality or quantity of breaths required.

Accumulated secretions are usually cleared without assistance postoperatively as mucociliary transport regains its momentum, but if sputum retention occurs, ACBT/AD can be effective if pain does not dampen the huff. Coughing, percussion, vibrations and unnecessary forced expiration are not used routinely because they may cause pain and muscle splinting. If coughing is required, patients may prefer to remain in side-lying, but if they are willing, sitting over the edge of the bed is mechanically efficient and allows maximum support (Fig 16.9). Pressing on the incision with a pillow is less effective than sensitive and accurately-timed manual support, but when patients are on their own, they may find a pillow, towel or cough belt (Fig 16.10) helpful.

If patients are too weak, fatigued or drowsy to co-operate, mechanical aids may be useful, such as continuous positive airway pressure (CPAP) for hypoxaemia (Squadrone 2005), intermittent positive pressure breathing for reduced lung volume or sputum clearance, and non-invasive ventilation (NIV) for excess work of breathing or low oxygenation (Mathai 2011).

PRACTICE TIP

Practice Fig 16.9 in pairs, the 'patient' giving feedback on the timing and pressure of the manual support.

FIGURE 16.9 Manual support for postoperative coughing after laparotomy. For thoracotomy, the physiotherapist sits beside the patient on the opposite side to the wound in order to support the wound while providing counterpressure to the patient's body. Gentle firm pressure is directed at holding the wound edges together (This is a historic picture: the physiotherapist would now kneel on a plastic apron and use gloves)

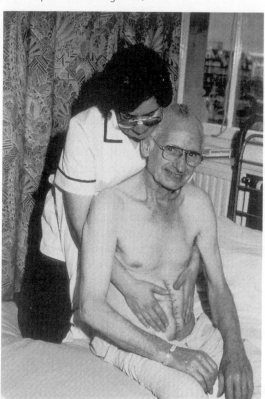

Prevention of deep vein thrombosis

There is no evidence that postoperative leg exercises have any place in the prevention of deep vein thrombosis (DVT) and clinical reasoning suggests that near-continuous ankle exercises would be required during and after surgery. There is also no evidence that getting a patient out of bed prevents DVT, especially as most cases become apparent after discharge (Dahl 2012). This does not apply to other situations such as long haul flights. A systematic review suggests that

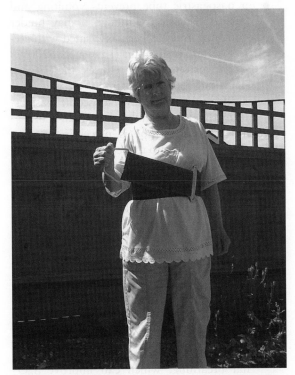

FIGURE 16.10 The 'Cough lok', designed for chest surgery but also useful for abdominal surgery, can be homemade or bought from www.hawksley.co.uk

patients with a DVT should get up, mobilize and, if ready for discharge, go home (Anderson *et al* 2009) so long as they are on anticoagulant drugs.

Discharge

We may experience them as recovered at discharge but many patients say that they do not understand where their strength has gone.
Allvin *et al* (2008)

Assessment for discharge from physiotherapy can be facilitated by a scoring tool using mobility, breath sounds, secretion clearance, S_pO_2 and respiratory rate (Brooks *et al* 2002).

Discharge advice is to encourage progressive paced activity suited to the individual's lifestyle, along with regular rest because fatigue becomes troublesome mainly

after participants have returned to regular activities (Allvin *et al* 2008). For patients who have been doing breathing exercises, a reminder to stop prevents conscientious patients continuing indefinitely. Wireless monitoring of mobility assists outcome evaluation (Cook 2013).

CLINICAL REASONING TIP

Lung function can be increased significantly when incentive spirometry and specific inspiratory muscle training are used before and after operation.
J Thorac Cardio Surg (1997), 113, 552–7

Reasoning:
● The techniques described are for different problems: incentive spirometry is to increase lung volume, and inspiratory muscle training is to reduce the work of breathing.
● There is a double whammy of variables: which of these modalities is the effective one, and is it before or after surgery that they are effective?
● And that old chestnut again – if lung function is measured with tests of forced exhalation, this does not control for postoperative pain.

ABDOMINAL SURGERY

The effect of an upper abdominal incision seems to strike at the root of normal respiration.
Bevan 1964

Abdominal surgery impinges less on respiration now that most abdominal organs are amenable to the laparoscope, but procedures such as laparoscopic cholecystectomy take longer than open laparotomy and entail tilting the patient head down and pumping CO_2 into the peritoneum. This impairs diaphragmatic function (Lunardi *et al* 2013) and can refer pain to the right shoulder, but this is minimized by two recruitment manoeuvres before extubation (Khanna *et al* 2013). Laparoscopic surgery usually leads to less morbidity and mortality than open laparotomy (Bulus *et al* 2013).

Complications

Pulmonary complications remain the most significant cause of morbidity following open upper abdominal surgery (Branson 2013). In addition to those previously described, the following may occur:

1   Pain tends to be taken less seriously than after chest surgery, even though pain after laparotomy is often worse on movement because most activity requires some abdominal muscle contraction.

2   Abdominal distension and guarding spasm require attention to positioning in order to reduce pressure on the diaphragm. The position chosen best follows patient comfort and auscultation, but head-up at 30° has shown benefit after major surgery such as liver transplant (Cresswell *et al* 2012).

3   Paralytic ileus is a normal postoperative delay in gut motility. It becomes problematic if prolonged beyond the usual one to two days, causing nausea and exacerbating diaphragm dysfunction. Management is by non-opioid pain relief, avoidance of nasogastric tubes, early ambulation, early feeding and chewing gum (Marwah *et al* 2012).

4   Fatigue is a particular problem with abdominal surgery, along with release of inflammatory markers and reduced pulmonary function (Havey *et al* 2013).

5   Malnourishment may occur with abdominal surgery because of:
    - pre-existing gut pathology
    - preoperative fasting
    - the catabolic effects of surgery
    - intestinal handling which affects the delicate mucosal lining
    - postoperative nausea and precarious appetite
    - unfamiliar food.

Nutrition

Preoperative oral carbohydrates are thought to speed recovery (Awad *et al* 2013). Early postoperative enteral nutrition reduces postoperative complications, and most patients can eat normally in the immediate postoperative period, regardless of traditional markers of gastrointestinal function (Kirchhoff *et al* 2010). Enhanced recovery programmes (Kennedy *et al* 2012) encourage the following:

- a **nasogastric** tube prevents vomiting and gastric distension, although it may hinder coughing and has been associated with atelectasis and pneumonia (Lassen *et al* 2009)
- a **gastrostomy** tube reduces these risks, delivering food directly into the stomach via a PEG (percutaneous endoscopic gastrostomy tube) through the abdominal wall
- a **jejunostomy** tube is placed percutaneously directly into the jejunum.

Local anaesthesia during surgery speeds the recovery of bowel function and brings the added benefit of inhibiting cancer dissemination (Votta-Velis 2013).

Physiotherapy

Patients having lower abdominal surgery require no more than a reminder about mobility and posture, unless they fall into a high-risk category. Others benefit from intervention (Mackay *et al* 2005) such as:

- postoperative deep breathing and abdominal breathing, which can improve S_pO_2 (Manzano *et al* 2008), supplemented by incentive spirometry if this is found effective (Alaparthi *et al* 2014)
- positioning and deep breathing (Olsén 2000) with CPAP if gas exchange is inadequate (Ferreyra *et al* 2008).
- mobilization (Silva *et al* 2013, Choi *et al* 2013).

Mobilization may not be accompanied by increased abdominal excursion in the early stages because of diaphragmatic inhibition (Zafiropoulos *et al* 2004).

Suggestions for specific operations are below.

An **abdominal aortic aneurysm** (Ch. 4) is normally asymptomatic, but if found by screening, open or endovascular repair may be required (Piazza 2013). Postoperatively there is a risk of cardiovascular instability, and patients are not usually mobilized for two days.

People requiring **hepatectomy** for liver cancer may improve insulin resistance associated with hepatic impairment by exercising from one month preoperatively to six months postoperatively (Kaibori *et al* 2013).

Bariatric surgery by gastric bypass, sleeve gastrectomy or gastric band can reduce mortality by 30% (Neff 2013) and reverse comorbidities. A preoperative exercise regime of 20 mins/day is advised, increased each day as tolerated (DeTurk & Cahalin 2011, p. 489). Postoperatively, atelectasis is common due to pressure on the diaphragm. Patients with a 'buffalo back' may develop brachial plexus injuries during surgery if elevated arm boards are not used. Follow up includes lifelong calcium and vitamin D supplementation following bypass to prevent osteoporosis (Werling *et al* 2013), and addressing the cause of any accompanying eating disorder to lessen the risk of subsequent substance misuse (Conason 2013).

LUNG SURGERY

The exercise component of enhanced recovery protocols is particularly important in this group of patients to reduce morbidity and length of hospital stay (Jones *et al* 2013b).

Procedures

An open posterolateral **thoracotomy** (Fig 16.1) involves an incision below the scapula, dividing latissimus dorsi and retracting or resecting one or more ribs, leading to restricted shoulder and chest wall movement. Keyhole thoracoscopy can be used for pulmonary (Fig 16.11), pleural, cardiac and oesophageal surgery, reducing morbidity and hospital stay (Sartipy 2013).

To remove a cancerous tumour, a **lobectomy** may be curative if mediastinal lymph nodes are not involved. The vacated space is accommodated by expansion of the rest of the lung and slight reorganization of moveable structures. Limited resection such as **sublobar resection** (Fox 2013), **segmentectomy** or a smaller **wedge resection** may be adequate for early-stage peripheral lesions (Hennon *et al* 2012).

A complete lung is removed by **pneumonectomy**, sometimes accompanied by chest wall resection if a tumour has spread (Lee & Byun 2012). Stretch of the remaining lung stimulates some growth (Filipovic *et al* 2013), but most of the space fills with air, blood and fibrin (Fig 16.12), the quantity of which is regulated by one of the following:

- a chest drain, which is kept clamped except when drainage is required

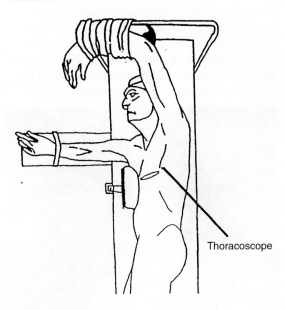

FIGURE 16.11 Patient in position for minimal-access lung surgery. The shoulder joint ligaments are vulnerable to overstretch

Thoracoscope

- a small thoracic catheter
- needle aspiration.

A chest drain allows recognition of haemorrhage and, if sutures break down, prevents a pneumothorax. It must never be attached to suction, nor clamped or unclamped except by instruction of the surgeon. Too much drainage of the vacated space pulls the remaining lung into the space, risking a pneumothorax on the good side, and too little drainage leads to the bronchial stump becoming soggy.

If all goes well, the air is absorbed over four to six weeks. In the ensuing months, the space shrinks by upward shift of the hemidiaphragm, lateral shift of the mediastinum and crowding of the ribs (Fig 16.13). The remaining lung expands, undergoes some remodelling, and its perfusion doubles (Dane *et al* 2013).

A **bi-lobectomy** removes two lobes (Icard 2013) and a **sleeve resection** removes the T-junction of a bronchus with its lobe (Eichhorn *et al* 2013). Sleeve resection is commonly followed by atelectasis and sputum retention due to oedema around the anastomosis and ciliary damage from nerve involvement. Positive pressure techniques such as manual hyperinflation are contraindicated in the immediate postoperative period because of

FIGURE 16.12 One day after
R pneumonectomy showing a horizontal fluid line
below an empty air space without lung markings.
The trachea is shifted towards the vacated space.
Compared to a pleural effusion, the fluid line shows
no meniscus because it is not tracking up the pleura
as the parietal pleura is now in the bin. The speckled
appearance just visible in the soft tissue outside the
R ribcage is subcutaneous emphysema

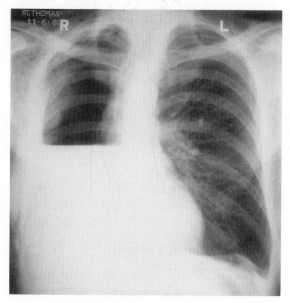

potential damage to the anastomosis and risk of a pneumothorax.

An area of non-functioning lung can be removed
by **lung volume reduction** (Song *et al* 2013) and a
giant bulla by **bullectomy** (Park 2013) in patients with
hyperinflation due to emphysema. This allows the diaphragm to return to a functional dome shape, which,
in one patient, increased exercise tolerance from
dyspnoea at rest to walking a kilometre (Saxena *et al*
2013).

Thoracoplasty is a historic procedure involving rib
resection so that part of the chest wall collapses and
obliterates underlying TB-infected lung so that the tubercle bacillus cannot breathe and dies. The procedure
may make a comeback if drug-resistant strains overwhelm the pharmacological industry, and is still an
option for chronic empyema (Botianu 2012). The space
is sometimes filled with ping-pong balls (App D) to prevent chest wall deformity, which may also be done after
complicated pneumonectomy (Morrow 1998).

FIGURE 16.13 Some months after L
pneumonectomy in a female patient, showing the
vacated space now opaque. The deviated trachea is
clearly visible against the opacity, healed rib and stitches

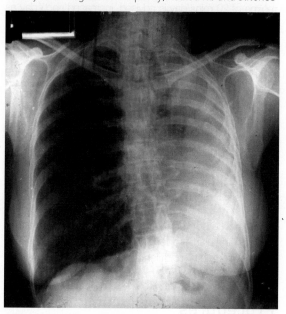

Patients who have an FEV_1 >2 L are considered
suitable for pneumonectomy and those with FEV_1 >1.5
L are expected to tolerate lobectomy (Kallianos *et al*
2012).

Complications

Diaphragm dysfunction occurs if the phrenic nerve is
damaged. During pneumonectomy, some surgeons deliberately cut the phrenic nerve to shrink the residual space.

An **air leak** is escape of air from the lung into the
pleura, then out through a chest drain, as shown by bubbling through the underwater seal drainage bottle. The
chest drain must not be removed until bubbling stops.

Escape of air into subcutaneous tissue may also occur,
causing **subcutaneous emphysema**. This is rarely of
more than cosmetic significance, but patients need reassurance that it is temporary, and when secretions are a
problem, ACBT/AD is preferable to coughing. If it causes
the face to swell and eyes to close, relatives can be shown
how to massage the eyelids to allow temporary vision.

Recurrent laryngeal nerve damage may occur
after left pneumonectomy or upper lobectomy, impairing speech and cough (Gelpke *et al* 2010).

Bronchopleural fistula is a breach between lung and pleura, which has the same effect as a pneumothorax and is often accompanied by **empyema**, the combination bringing a mortality of 16–50% (Chen *et al* 2011). It is most likely if MV is required, and is suspected if there is a spiking temperature, x-ray evidence of a decreasing fluid level after pneumonectomy, or expectoration of bloody-brown secretions, especially when lying down with the fistula upwards. Spread of infected material is minimized by the patient sitting up or lying on the fistula side. Large fistulae need a chest drain, sealing via bronchoscopy, or surgery (Sakar 2010). Positive pressure physiotherapy techniques are contraindicated.

Shoulder pain on the side of the thoracotomy may be caused by positioning during surgery or pleural irritation.

Long term pain lasting more than two months occurs in 30–40% of patients and is best prevented by adequate pre-emptive and postoperative analgesia (Wildgaard *et al* 2013).

Physiotherapy

Preoperative pulmonary rehabilitation improves postoperative exercise capacity (Nagarajan *et al* 2011). Physiotherapists may also be involved in assessing suitability for surgery by exercise tests (Kallianos *et al* 2012).

Postoperatively, patients at risk of sputum retention can be predicted by a history of COPD or absence of regional analgesia (Bonde *et al* 2002). If sputum clearance is not effective by conventional means, high frequency oscillation can be helpful (Park 2012).

Non-invasive ventilation may be needed (Anand 2010), sometimes prophylactically 2012). Concerns have been raised about using positive pressure if there is an air leak through the chest drain, but CPAP has been investigated and does not prolong an air leak (Nery *et al* 2012). Mobilization begins as soon as the patient is agreeable, followed by exercise training (Cavalheri 2013). Shoulder and postural exercises begin once pain allows, and if the shoulder has not achieved full range before discharge, follow-up physiotherapy is required. Park *et al* (2013) claim that the addition of abdominal breathing and inspiratory muscle training reduces pain, but the lack of a control in this study limits its credibility.

Points to note in relation to pneumonectomy are the following:

1 Patients should not lie on the *non-operated* side, to prevent fluid spilling onto the stump. Some surgeons require this to be life-long.

2 After radical pneumonectomy, which entails entering the pericardium, patients should not lie on *either* side in case of cardiac herniation (Gadhinglajkar *et al* 2010).

3 If sputum clearance is necessary, ACBT/AD is preferred to coughing, to avoid pressure on the stump.

4 There should be no head-down tip and, for some patients, no lying flat.

5 Suction, if necessary, should be shallow, as with any surgery involving the airway.

Fast track surgery means that patients may be sent home before complications develop, and a system of symptom monitoring with automatic email alerts to clinicians has proved beneficial (Cleeland *et al* 2011). Post-operative pulmonary rehabilitation is recommended (Sterzi 2013), followed by home-based exercise (Hoffman *et al* 2014).

PLEURAL SURGERY

The commonest indication for pleural surgery is recurrent, bilateral or persistent pneumothorax, caused by a breach in either layer of the pleura. Other indications are problematic pleural effusions or bronchopleural fistula. Pleural surgery leaves a long-term mild restrictive defect.

Pleurodesis introduces irritant chemicals, tetracycline, fibrin glue or laser pulses into the pleura via thoracoscopy, setting up a sterile and intensely painful inflammation, leading to fibrosis and adherence of the two layers of the pleura. Kindly surgeons instil local anaesthetic into the pleura before closure. The procedure relies on an inflammatory response and should not be followed by anti-inflammatory analgesia (Suárez *et al* 2013). Chest drains are used to ensure lung and chest wall apposition.

Pleurectomy strips off the parietal pleura so that a raw surface is left at the chest wall, to which the visceral pleura adheres (Kara *et al* 2013).

Empyema is normally managed by chest tube drainage, but if it is large or loculated, thoracoscopic surgery may be required, entailing debridement or, if infection is not contained, **decortication**, which involves peeling off the restrictive fibrosed visceral pleura and releasing the trapped lung (Christie 2010). The parietal pleura is spared unless longstanding empyema and deformity mean that it will impair lung expansion. Surgical patients are debilitated from extended infection and need attention to graded exercise.

CHEST DRAINS

Simple wound drains are adequate to remove blood from the affected site after most forms of surgery, but if the pleura has been cut, large bore underwater-seal drains are usually required to restore negative pleural pressure. The proximal end is inside the pleura, with one end-hole to drain fluid and air, and several small side-eyes to prevent catheter occlusion. The last side-eye can be identified radiologically by an interruption in its radiopaque line. The distal end, outside the patient, drains into a collection chamber. The airtight system becomes an extension of the patient's pleura and allows air and blood to escape from the pleural space while preventing re-entry, thus allowing the lung to re-expand.

These pleural chest drains may be used after lobectomy, pneumothorax, pleural effusion, haemothorax or empyema. One is traditionally placed in the apex to remove air and the other in the base to remove blood, but both air and blood will usually find the drains, especially when suction is applied. Pleural drains may also be required if the pleura has been cut during oesophageal, kidney or upper abdominal surgery, either by mistake or of necessity. They should be accompanied by eight-hourly intrapleural local anaesthesia (BTS 2003).

An alternative to the underwater seal system is a flutter valve such as the Heimlich, which releases air on expiration but collapses shut by the negative pressure on inspiration (Brims & Maskell 2013). It does not require a bottle system and is cheap, safe, effective unless suction is required, and can stay in situ on discharge.

Non-pleural chest drains may be used after:

- pneumonectomy, when they are placed in the space vacated by the lung to drain blood and debris and prevent excessive displacement of the mediastinum
- heart surgery (although some cardiac surgeons find that simple wound drains are sufficient), when one drain is usually placed inside the pericardium to prevent cardiac tamponade, and one outside the pericardium to drain blood from the mediastinum.

Procedure

All tissues down to the pleura are infiltrated with local anaesthetic, and after this has taken effect, the drains are inserted above a rib, where there are fewest nerves and blood vessels, and within the 'safe triangle' bounded by latissimus dorsi, pectoralis major and a line from the nipple to below the axilla (BTS 2010b).

Mechanism

Chest drain units incorporate one to three bottles or chambers, one for drainage, one to act as a water seal, and a suction-control chamber, sometimes as separate bottles but usually as one system (Fig 16.14):

1. The drainage chamber collects expelled fluid.
2. The water-seal chamber acts as a one-way valve so that air and fluid can escape from the negative pressure inside the chest but cannot return.
3. The suction-control chamber regulates the amount of negative pressure that sucks fluid and/or air from the chest (Leo 2013).

Fluid from the pleura enters the drainage chamber and cannot return so long as the system is below the level of the patient's chest. Air from the pleura enters the drainage chamber and then the water-seal chamber, where it bubbles through the water, which acts as a seal to prevent its return.

Drainage depends on gravity or suction. Gravity drainage occurs when the exit tube is open to the atmosphere. This allows the water level in the tubing of the water-seal chamber to swing, reflecting the change in pleural pressure with breathing. It rises by 5–10 cm on inhalation and falls on exhalation, but goes the opposite way if the patient is on positive pressure ventilation. If a suction system is not in place, the exit tube must be open to allow free drainage.

An air leak is present if air is bubbling through the water, having passed from the lung and through the visceral pleura at each breath. The hole in the visceral pleura should seal in time. If there is any change in air leak after treatment, this should be reported.

If the negative pressure of the patient's breathing is inadequate to reinflate the lung, e.g. if there is excess fluid drainage or large air leak, suction is applied at a pressure of minus 10–20 cmH$_2$O, either from a dedicated pump or from wall suction via an adaptor to avoid too high a pressure. A large air leak may cause a pneumothorax if suction is not used (Cerfolio 2005). Persistent air leaks can be sealed by bronchoscopic insertion of endobronchial valves (NICE 2013b).

FIGURE 16.14 Chest drains, shown as bottle drainage systems (top and middle) and an integrated system (bottom). The chamber on the left receives drainage from the patient. The second chamber provides the water seal. The height of water in the right hand chamber determines the pressure required to expel the unwanted contents from the chest, or this is provided by suction.

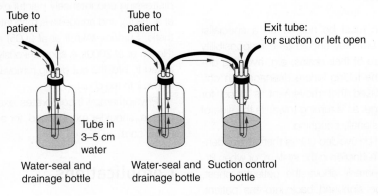

Tube to patient

Tube to patient

Exit tube: for suction or left open

Tube in 3–5 cm water

Water-seal and drainage bottle

Water-seal and drainage bottle

Suction control bottle

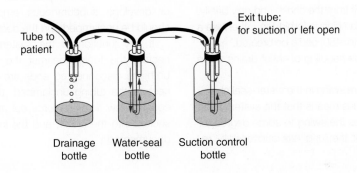

Tube to patient

Exit tube: for suction or left open

Drainage bottle

Water-seal bottle

Suction control bottle

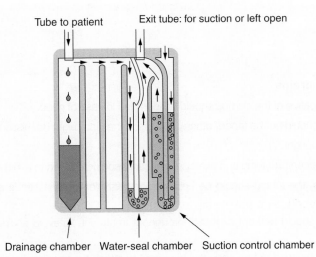

Tube to patient

Exit tube: for suction or left open

Drainage chamber

Water-seal chamber

Suction control chamber

Patients with an uncomplicated pleural effusion, hae-mothorax or pneumothorax usually only require one bottle which acts as both drainage and water-seal chamber.

Management

Patients on suction must be nursed on a specialist ward (BTS 2003), but they should take responsibility for some of the care of their drains, e.g. avoiding dependent loops in the tubing where drainage can collect. They are advised that movement is good for encouraging drainage, as is turning towards the side of the drain, and occasionally coughing.

Clamping should be avoided unless there is accidental disconnection of a junction in the system, or when lifting the bottle temporarily above the patient's chest, when fluid could be siphoned back into the patient. When clamping is required, the tubing should be clamped close to its exit from the chest, and only briefly. If there is an air leak, clamping is forbidden, otherwise a tension pneumothorax (p. 480) could be created.

The principles of safe handling of chest drains are in Box 16.3.

If there is no pressure swing in the water-seal chamber of a pleural drain, this means that the system is on suction, which overrides the swing to some degree, or the tube is blocked. If the lung has successfully re-expanded, the pleural end of the tube will be occluded and the swing is reduced.

Chest drains are removed by nursing staff if drainage is complete, there is no air leak and the lung has fully expanded. This can be experienced as 'the most distressing and intensely painful experience of all' (Fox *et al* 1999), and analgesia is mandatory, e.g. local anaesthetic, Entonox (Akrofi *et al* 2005) and/or EMLA cream (Rosen *et al* 2000). A spontaneously-breathing patient is asked to breathe out during removal to prevent air being drawn into the chest.

Physiotherapy incorporates exercise, posture correction, shoulder mobility and, for some patients, respiratory care.

Complications

If a patient with a clamped drain becomes breathless or develops subcutaneous emphysema, the drain should be unclamped and the doctor informed.

If any junction in the system becomes disconnected, the tubing nearest the patient is clamped, both the disconnected ends are cleaned and reconnected, the tubing unclamped, the patient asked to cough a few times to force out any air that has been sucked into the chest, and the incident reported and documented.

BOX 16.3

Tips on managing chest drains

- Before treatment, the location of the clamps should be identified in case of need.
- Junctions in the tubing should not be taped, otherwise a disconnection might be missed.
- Bottles should be kept upright.
- Drainage is assisted by deep breathing and exercise, but care should be taken to avoid disconnection.
- When handling patients, the tubing should be held in alignment along the patient's chest to minimize discomfort.
- The bottles and tubing should be kept exposed throughout treatment, to avoid accidental knocking or kinking.
- The system should be observed before and after treatment to check for any change in drainage, air leak or swing in water level. Extra drainage is expected after treatment, but excessive loss suggests haemorrhage and should be reported.

If the tubing becomes disconnected from the patient, the following steps should be taken:

1   Ask the patient to exhale and, at the same time, press a hand against the wound at end-exhalation, preferably using a dressing or glove but speed taking precedence over sterility.
2   Ask the patient to breathe normally.
3   Summon assistance.
4   If air is heard leaking from the site, or the drain was previously bubbling, the hand should be removed periodically (with the patient breathing out) to allow air to escape and prevent a tension pneumothorax.
5   Explain to the patient that the drain will probably need to be reinserted and the pressures will then regain their equilibrium.
6   Observe breathing rate and chest symmetry.
7   Give oxygen if S_pO_2 drops.

HEART SURGERY

> *[Waiting for surgery] is like driving a car with no brakes. When I get the pain, all I can think about are those five blocked arteries.*
>   Patient quoted by Fitzsimons (2003)

The anxiety of waiting for heart surgery is reflected in higher death rates for people with longer preoperative waiting times (Sobolev *et al* 2013). Coronary artery bypass graft (CABG) is the commonest heart operation and usually reduces angina and mortality (Tully 2012). Some of the 20% of patients who do not achieve improved quality of life are thought to suffer long term cognitive defects or traumatic memories from their intensive care experience (Schelling *et al* 2003).

Incisions and procedures

Sternotomy (Fig 16.1), if used, divides the aponeurosis of pectoralis major, cuts through and retracts the sternum, then instigates cardiopulmonary bypass to allow surgery on a quiescent heart in a bloodless field. Bypass involves the heart being stopped, the aorta cross-

clamped to separate outflow of the heart from the systemic circulation, the circulating blood removed from the right atrium, filtered and oxygenated outside the body, then pumped back into the ascending aorta. Neither heart nor lungs are functioning during this period, and the lungs are partially collapsed. Some surgeons fill the pericardial sac with chilled saline to reduce tissue oxygen demand and reduce the flow required for bypass.

To replace the diseased coronary arteries, the saphenous vein, radial artery and/or internal mammary artery (IMA) are used (Fig 16.15). IMA grafts last longer (Ennker 2012) but the artery is harvested from the chest wall, usually punctures the pleura (Ghavidel *et al* 2013), and can cause shoulder pain and greater impairment of lung function than saphenous vein grafts (Bonacchi *et al* 2001).

Minimal access surgery avoids cardiopulmonary bypass and reduces the consequent inflammatory response, but the same multimodal analgesia is still required (Sondekoppam *et al* 2014). These off-pump techniques use an 'octopus' to stabilize the beating heart (Wu 2012).

Complications specific to heart surgery

Patients spend varying amounts of time on mechanical ventilation postoperatively, leading to **ventilator-associated pneumonia** being the major independent risk factor for hospital mortality (Tamayo *et al* 2012).

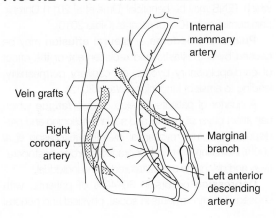

FIGURE 16.15 Grafts to the heart

Haemorrhage is a particularly dangerous complication after surgery if blood is trapped in the pericardium, causing **tamponade** (p. 476).

Postoperative **cardiovascular instability**, although minimized by control of pain, fluids and oxygenation, may contraindicate turning or other forms of physiotherapy. Atrial fibrillation or atrial flutter occurs for 10–60% of the time after heart surgery (Maesen 2012) and is associated with cerebral dysfunction (Stanley et al 2002). Hypotension may impair perfusion to vital organs, contribute further to cognitive dysfunction (Seines et al 2012) and delay mobilization.

Loss of lung volume is ubiquitous (Westerdahl & Tenling 2013) but generally resolves within a few days (Khan et al 2009a). Causes are compression from the heart (Neves et al 2013), the lung deflation that accompanies bypass or trauma/cold injury to the phrenic nerve. This can be treated with a pre-extubation recruitment manoeuvre (Claxton et al 2003). Manual hyperinflation might have the same effect, though not to be done routinely (Paulus et al 2011).

Atelectasis can cause **hypoxaemia**, which may contribute to cognitive problems or acute kidney injury (Alsabbagh 2013). Following bypass, the shunt is typically 25% (Kotani et al 2000), reducing to an average 15% after 48 hours (Rasmussen et al 2006).

Brain complications, ranging from memory impairment to stroke, are due to impaired cerebral perfusion, sleep deprivation, acid base imbalance, anxiety (Bruce et al 2013) and cerebral inflammation (Reinsfelt et al 2013). Cognitive dysfunction is greater if bypass is used and may persist in up to 35% of patients for 12 months (Ricksten 2000). Monitoring brain perfusion reduces the risk (Mohandas et al 2013).

Pain contributes to atelectasis, which can lead to respiratory infection (Tenenbein 2008). Wound pain may be compounded by musculoskeletal pain if the sternum and ribs have been retracted (Mazzeffi & Khelemsky 2011), for which TENS may be beneficial (Lima et al 2011) Chronic pain continues in 10% of patients (Gjeilo 2010).

Pulmonary oedema or **pleural effusion** may be caused by enthusiastic fluid replacement or the effect of cardiopulmonary bypass on capillary permeability, leading to a risk of lung injury (Wang 2012).

A quarter of patients develop chronic **fatigue** which can affect physical, mental and social functioning and predisposes to future myocardial infarction (Barnason et al 2008), indicating the need for graded exercise postoperatively and discharge advice tailored to the individual.

Depression occurs in 30–40% of patients, with subsequent impairments in social, physical and general health, reduced attendance at cardiac rehabilitation and increased risk of the return of angina (Tully 2012).

Patients may also suffer **dyspnoea**, on going **insomnia** or **anxiety**, which can continue for weeks or months. Inability of patients to distinguish postoperative symptoms from the side effects of their new medication may result in reluctance to take their drugs (Schulz et al 2012).

Sternal instability occurs in 1–16% of patients. Risk factors are IMA grafting, diabetes, prolonged mechanical ventilation, obesity, smoking, osteoporosis and use of β-blockers (Al-Ansary et al 2007). If the sternum is heard or felt to click on movement, a cough belt (Fig 16.10) or towel is needed to stabilize the chest wall during deep breathing and coughing. Sternal instability in the first two weeks is usually associated with infection. After six weeks it becomes non-union, which is suspected if the x-ray shows broken sutures or a gradually widening lucent line at the sternotomy site. Unilateral arm movement, or any upper limb movement which increases sternal pain, should be avoided.

Physiotherapy

The following benefits of physiotherapy have been shown:

1 Cardiopulmonary fitness reduces complications (Smith 2013b), and preoperative exercise minimizes atelectasis and pneumonia (Hulzebos et al 2012).

2 Preoperative incentive spirometry, deep breathing and mobilization reduce the incidence of atelectasis in some patients (Yanez-Brage et al 2009).

3 Pre- and postoperative cardiac rehabilitation leads to fewer complications and shorter hospital stay (Herdy et al 2008).

4 Pre- and postoperative inspiratory muscle training may improve functional capacity and quality of life (Savci et al 2011).

The importance of education is underlined by the relation between anxiety and poorer postoperative outcome (Williams et al 2013).

Postoperatively, BP should be observed before, during and after treatment. Diastolic pressure is more significant than systolic pressure because coronary artery perfusion is highest during diastole. The operation notes indicate the limits within which BP should be maintained.

A proportion of patients appear euphoric on the first day, possibly as a reaction to their survival, but then sink into depression. When identified, these patients should be encouraged to take things gently on the first day to help avoid mood swings which interfere with rehabilitation.

Some surgeons request that the patient not be turned immediately after CABG, to avoid a shearing stress on the sternum, and with IMA graft to protect the graft. If side-lying is acceptable to the patient and surgeon, the upper arm should rest on a pillow to maintain symmetry and prevent strain on the sternum.

In patients unable to be active, non-invasive ventilation speeds recovery (Al Jaaly et al 2013).

For spontaneously-breathing patients, deep breathing exercises are not normally required (Brasher et al 2003) so long as the patient is able to mobilize. Urell et al (2011) claim that 30 deep breaths an hour improve oxygenation, but these were against positive pressure so it is not known which variable was beneficial. Positive expiratory pressure was also used by Haeffener et al (2011) as well as incentive spirometry, with the outcome of improved exercise tolerance. Deep breathing or incentive spirometry, if required, may be more effective with manual support of the wound on inspiration to improve comfort and allow greater excursion.

Patients should be assessed for musculoskeletal problems and neurological damage (El-Ansary et al 2000). Frequent musculoskeletal problems require liaison with theatre staff.

Shoulder elevation should be limited to 90° for 24 hours after sternotomy, especially after IMA grafting, and should be performed bilaterally to protect the sternum. If patients have to use their arms to stand up, they should be used bilaterally, and if a walking aid is required, weight bearing must be equal.

Epidural analgesia speeds up mobilization (El-Morsy 2012), and within the limits of fatigue, patients without complications should aim at gentle walking the day after surgery. Precautions to mobilization are:

- unstable BP
- complete heart block reliant on external cardiac pacing
- atrial fibrillation with compromized cardiovascular stability
- tachycardia >120 bpm
- heart failure requiring inotropic drugs
- intravenous vasodilator drugs
- pulmonary artery catheter *in situ*
- new myocardial infarct or symptomatic angina
- neurological event.

Before discharge, it is useful to check the breathing pattern and posture to make sure that there are no lingering signs of tension which could become a habit. Patients need to understand the distinction between incisional pain and angina, and receive written information (App. B) and advice on rest/exercise balance. Follow-up cardiac rehabilitation is recommended (Ghashghaei et al 2012).

CABG and angioplasty are effective in reducing angina, but atherosclerosis continues, and these are still generally considered palliative treatments of a progressive disease (Van Domburg et al 2009). Patients are well advised to cultivate a lifestyle that retards the disease process in the grafted vessels, including regular exercise, which continues to improve the quality of life five to six years after surgery (Diane 2007).

TRANSPLANTATION

Each new day is welcomed with open arms come sun, rain or snow. Gone are the excuses for putting off activities until the weather is better or the time more opportune.

Marsh (post-transplant patient) 1986

Receiving a transplanted heart, lung or both sometimes causes profound change in a patient's attitude to life. Postoperative feelings of resurrection are not unusual but the patient's mood may swing between euphoria and depression (Xu et al 2012b), sometimes complicated by conflicting emotions including 'recipient guilt' and being in possession of part of someone else. However, for many who survive the waiting list, operation and complications, each day is precious and life is usually sweet.

The indication for transplantation is end-stage organ disease. Examples are:

- heart transplant for cardiomyopathy
- double lung or heart-lung transplant for cystic fibrosis (CF)
- single lung transplant for non-infective lung disorders such as pulmonary fibrosis or COPD.

Pre-operatively, smokers must have given up for six months, and family members are also exhorted to stop. Nutrition should be optimized and steroids minimized (Mahida et al 2012).

The operations are no longer technically awesome, and now that immunosuppressive therapy is better able to prevent organ rejection, the main limiting factor is lack of donor organs. Lobar transplants are easing this problem for lung surgery (Inci 2013). Delays can sometimes be bridged by a left ventricular assist device for heart transplant (Jung *et al* 2012) and extracorporeal membrane oxygenation for lung transplant (Nosotti *et al* 2013).

Procedures

Cardiopulmonary bypass is used for heart and occasionally double lung transplant. For single lung transplant, a thoracotomy incision is required. For double lung transplant, a massive transternal bilateral thoracotomy (clamshell incision) allows sequential single-lung procedures.

To retain the collateral circulation with lung transplant, both heart and lung may be transplanted, with the recipient's healthy heart donated to a second recipient. To maximize the donor pool, living-related donation allows a lower lobe to be given, for example, by both parents and used as two full lungs by the recipient. This brings the added benefit of elective surgery, well-tested donors and well-perfused donor organs.

Complications

All transplants are complicated by the side effects of lifelong drugs to inhibit organ rejection, which bring risks of infection (O'Shea 2013), malignancy and muscle weakness (Dudley 2012). Uchiyama *et al* (2012) claim that listening to Mozart helps prolong graft survival.

Heart

Complications include emotional repercussions specific to heart transplant (Conway *et al* 2013). Acute rejection is suspected if there are temperature or ECG changes and confirmed by biopsy. Chronic rejection accelerates atherosclerosis of the transplanted arteries and is identified by annual angiography or biopsy (Strecker *et al* 2013). The only treatment for chronic heart rejection is re-transplantation.

Lung

The lung is the only organ in contact with the atmosphere and has evolved a strong protective immunity to anything foreign. This mechanism is compromized by transplantation, and the risk of infection is increased by immunosuppression, lymphatic interruption, hilar stripping during surgery, smoking history of the donor and the insult of retrieval surgery (Glanville 2013). However, successful transplantation leads to positive and durable benefits in physical function (Genao *et al* 2013).

Denervation of the lung contributes to mucociliary transport being reduced to <15% of normal (Caster *et al* 2011) and may lower the patient's awareness of the presence of secretions, which people with CF have developed to a fine art. Excess secretions continue to be produced from the native airway of CF patients above the anastomosis. A short term hindrance to secretion clearance is oedema around the anastomosis, and more long term is a 50% incidence of gastro-esophageal reflux (Davis *et al* 2010). Denervation is often permanent but the bronchial arteries and lymphatic system are thought to regenerate in some weeks (Oh 2009 p. 1079).

Pulmonary oedema can be caused by loss of lymphatic drainage or the ischaemic insult of surgery followed by reactive reperfusion. 'Reperfusion pulmonary oedema' peaks 8–12 hours postoperatively, causing hypoxia and reduced lung compliance. Treatment with fluid restriction and diuretics may bring the side effect of thick airway secretions and dry mouth.

Hypercapnia may endure in people with preoperative CO_2 retention because the new normal oxygenation suppresses their hypoxic respiratory drive. This normalizes within a week.

Prolonged air leak may occur, especially if the new lobe or lung does not fit snugly into the chest, and empyema can develop. Cardiac, renal and neurological problems may arise (Wigfield 2014).

Acute or chronic rejection can occur from a few days to several years postoperatively. FVC and FEV_1 should rise to a plateau some months after surgery and then remain stable, but a subsequent reduction of 10–15% is a warning of possible rejection. Suspicions are confirmed if there is fever, breathlessness, hypoxaemia and fine crackles on auscultation, Radiological signs are similar for both rejection and opportunistic infection, and gentle bronchoscopy is needed to distinguish the two. Treatment of rejection is by steroids. Rejection indicates that exercise training should be temporarily ceased or modified.

Obliterative bronchiolitis may follow repeated episodes of rejection (Gillen *et al* 2013). The small airways become obstructed by inflammation and then obliterated by granulation tissue, which then fibroses. It can extend into alveoli and develop into pneumonia or 'BOOP' (Ch. 3). Re-transplantation may be required, but carries high mortality.

Five year survival is 52%, but exercise capacity relates to survival (Armstrong et al 2012), and exercise training brings sustained gains in quality of life (Wickerson 2013).

Physiotherapy

> *Think transplant ... think pre-hab!*
> Bindoff (2011)

Preoperative physiotherapy takes place at the pre-assessment clinic because there is little time once a donor has been found. An individualized exercise programme is needed because of the inactive lifestyle of most patients (Langer et al 2012), but it may need significant modification for those who are debilitated, as well as liaison with the dietician. Non-invasive ventilation may be needed while awaiting a donor organ (Riha et al 2012).

The wait for an organ is a feat of endurance, during which patients feel in limbo. Active preoperative care needs to be integrated with palliative care (Colman et al 2013) because many patients will not reach the front of the queue.

Postoperative treatment is similar to other forms of chest surgery, with extra attention to prevention of infection, plus the specific considerations below.

Following lung transplant, secretions below the anastomosis do not elicit a cough reflex and continuous humidification and sometimes other techniques may be needed at first, but long term chest clearance is not usually required. If manual hyperinflation or other positive pressure technique is needed, the operation notes should be checked for the pressure to which the anastomosis has been tested, and pressures during physiotherapy kept well below this. Suction, if needed, should not allow the catheter to reach the anastomosis, which in ventilated patients is just below the end of the endotracheal tube.

Progressive exercise continues after discharge, with the following precautions:

1 Following heart transplant, 12 weeks of aerobic and strength training reduce the persistent exercise intolerance commonly encountered in this population (Tomczak et al 2013), but transplanted hearts denervated so that the transmission of angina is impaired, the pulse is not a reliable monitoring tool and there is a delayed heart rate response to exercise, requiring ample warm-up and cool-down periods. After 6–12 months of exercise, responses may become near-normal, although the intensity and duration of exercise will be limited.

2 Patients are at risk of secondary osteoporosis because of anti-rejection drugs (Miazgowski et al 2012).

Attention is focused on the recipient, but the donor's relatives are vulnerable at this time. The wife of one donor, herself a health professional, described her concern about staff 'not being nice to him' (Fulbrook et al 1999). Respiratory physiotherapy may be requested to maintain oxygenation to the organ, and even if the donor is brain-dead, they must be cared for as any moribund patient, especially as physical responses to painful stimuli have been identified (Wu 2013). Conversation with relatives must avoid terminology such as 'harvesting' the organs, or comments on the importance of maintaining vital signs.

REPAIR OF AORTIC COARCTATION

Coarctation of the aorta is a congenital and localized narrowing of the vessel, but it may not be picked up until routine imaging shows an abnormal aorta or inferior notches on ribs three to eight. Surgery is advisable before hypertension wreaks damage in later life. Repair is by resection of the narrowed segment, insertion of a graft or stent placement (Bentham et al 2013).

The following precautions are needed postoperatively to avoid a sudden rise in BP that might strain the anastomosis:

1 The head-down tip should be avoided. Some surgeons prefer the patient not to lie flat.

2 Mobilization should be slow and fatigue avoided. Extra care is needed when patients are beginning to feel well enough to exert themselves.

3 Vigorous exercise should be discouraged for several months.

After this, benefit is gained from regular exercise but patients remain at risk of hypertension because abnormalities in vascular structure and function persist throughout life. Exercise testing is advised (Krieger 2013) to identify patients who can participate in sports without restriction (Buys et al 2013).

OESOPHAGECTOMY

Patients who do not recover physical function, pain and fatigue scores within 6 months … are at significant increased risk of shorter survival.

Lococo et al (2012)

The above is a reminder of the importance of rehabilitation for this debilitated group of patients. Risk factors for oesophageal cancer are, for the squamous cell variety, tobacco and alcohol and, for adenocarcinoma, Barrett's oesophagus (p. 122) or drugs which relax the lower oesophageal sphincter such as anticholinergics (Lagergren 2000).

Oesophagectomy is a harrowing operation, with open access by thoracolaparotomy, thoracotomy and laparotomy, or thoracotomy with neck incision. Keyhole surgery reduces pulmonary complications (Maas et al 2014) and basal atelectasis is reduced if the prone position is used (Kim et al 2012b).

Five-year survival is 15–25% (Pennathur 2013), but short-term outcomes can be improved by a multidisciplinary pathway, including titration of the epidural to facilitate mobilization while maintaining mean arterial pressure >70 mmHg. For inoperable cancer, a stent helps to maintain patency and relieve some symptoms (Hindy et al 2012).

Patients are weak after protracted preoperative malnourishment, and pulmonary complications occur in 25–57% of patients (Dettling et al 2013), including:

- significant atelectasis because the stomach is pulled up into the chest and anastomosed to the oesophageal stump

- leakage or dehiscence at the anastomosis
- pleural effusion
- aspiration pneumonia, reduced by a swallowing evaluation prior to initiating oral feeds (Berry et al 2010)
- recurrent laryngeal nerve damage (Gelpke et al 2010)
- chronic pain in approximately half of patients, reinforcing the importance of acute pain management (Olsén et al 2009)
- empyema (Fig 16.16) or abscess.

Postoperative precautions are:
- avoid the head-down tilt in case reflux of gastric contents damages the anastomosis (some surgeons prefer patients to maintain head elevation)
- avoid neck movements that might stretch the anastomosis
- with a high resection and after extubation, avoid deep suction because the catheter might accidentally enter the oesophagus
- high flow nasal oxygen provides low level continuous positive airway pressure (CPAP) but positive pressure techniques such as full CPAP or non-invasive ventilation should first be discussed with the surgeon due to possible stomach insufflation or damage to the anastomosis (Pedoto 2012).

Preston et al (2013) suggest the following regime:
- evening of surgery: sit up in bed, optimize fluid status
- day 1: walk two to three times a day as far as the patient is able, instigate jejunal tube feeding
- day 2: walk three to four times a day
- day 3: walk four times a day
- follow-on: progressive rehabilitation and intensive dietetic input.

Sputum retention is common and a request for early minitracheostomy is advisable in selected patients. Soon after discharge, a multidisciplinary pulmonary rehabilitation programme leads to improved quality of life and long-term outcome (Lococo et al 2012). Ongoing nutritional support is required, otherwise survivors continue to lose weight for an average three years (Martin et al 2009).

FIGURE 16.16 Opacity in the L upper zone represents empyema which developed after oesophagectomy in this 17 year old. A rib was cut for the thoracotomy, and the colon, containing fluid, was transplanted in place of the oesophagus.

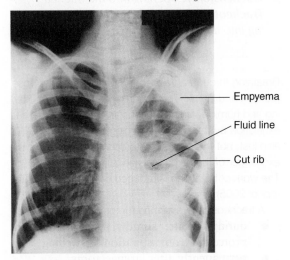

Empyema

Fluid line

Cut rib

BREAST SURGERY

Breast cancer is the most common cancer in women worldwide, with the highest incidence in the West (Adriaenssens *et al* 2012). Any surgery to the breast is distressing, and this distress affects postoperative outcomes (Montgomery *et al* 2010), so preoperative care should provide individualized information.

Breast conservation is usually feasible, but some women require mastectomy, preferably with immediate breast reconstruction (Serra *et al* 2013). Postoperative complications of mastectomy include lymphoedema, joint stiffness, muscle weakness and shoulder pain, especially after axillary node dissection. The risk of developing a neuropathic 'post-mastectomy pain syndrome', characterized by burning and stabbing sensations, may be reduced by using a paravertebral block, which also reduces nausea (Bansal *et al* 2012).

Patients require upper limb exercises and posture correction but after axillary node dissection, the shoulder is best not elevated beyond 90° for the first seven days (Todd *et al* 2008). On going exercise then helps increase shoulder movement and reduce

breast and chest-wall pain (Wong 2012a), with extra benefit when balance and posture are emphasized (Winters-Stone 2011). Interactive games help maintain motivation (Chang & Chang 2012), and yoga can improve sleep, anxiety, depression and distress (Stan *et al* 2012). A stiff shoulder may not become evident for some weeks, so prevention and follow up are required (Campbell 2012, Singh *et al* 2013b), including attention to the opposite shoulder which shows above-average morbidity (Adriaenssens *et al* 2012).

HEAD AND NECK SURGERY

> *Patients are often faced with physical disfigurement and altered abilities to breathe, speak, smell, taste, chew, or swallow, while simultaneously enduring pain and fatigue.*
> Eades *et al* (2013)

Head and neck cancer is the fifth commonest cancer worldwide, the main causes being tobacco and alcohol use (Guru *et al* 2012). **Selective** neck dissection aims to excise the cancer, and **radical** neck dissection also removes malignant lymph nodes. Transoral laser techniques bring improved cosmetic outcomes (Abdurehim *et al* 2012).

Complications include shoulder pain and limited neck movement, which can become long term (Guru *et al* 2012), and difficult or painful swallowing, which can lead to dehydration, malnutrition and a 50% incidence of aspiration (Jung *et al* 2011). Positions which minimize aspiration can be identified by fluoroscopy, and exercises for dysphagia are detailed by Pauloski (2008).

Distressing features include mucous discharge, difficulties with breathing and nose-blowing, and limited ability to express feelings. Gilbert (2012) reports depressive symptoms in 40–50% of patients. Frustration, social withdrawal and problems with close relationships are common, women being the most vulnerable (Katz *et al* 2003).

For disfiguring surgery, a mirror should be given to patients only with prior explanation, and they should not be alone for their first view. Relatives also need preparation before their first visit. Women may have difficulty adapting if their voice has become low-pitched.

Laryngeal cancer

Smoking and inactivity are risk factors for head and neck cancers (Hashibe *et al* 2013), which include those of the larynx, pharynx, tonsils, salivary glands, oral cavity, lip, nose, sinuses and middle ear. Cancer of the larynx is the commonest (Ying *et al* 2012), but it can be identified early by voice changes, and 70% of patients are cured (Chen *et al* 2010). Surgery preserves the larynx when feasible (Ambrosch & Fazel 2012), but if it is lost, voice restoration may be possible surgically (Robertson *et al* 2012).

Physiotherapy

Head and neck cancer rehabilitation is preventive, restorative, supportive and palliative (Guru *et al* 2012). Postoperatively, patients need posture correction and advice to avoid traction to the brachial plexus. If grafts allow, an exercise regime begins with gentle range of motion exercises, along with advice on supporting the shoulder and arm. A comprehensive exercise programme begins at 10–14 days, after liaising with the surgical team to ensure there is no risk of delayed wound healing, fistula formation or carotid 'blowout' (Guru *et al* 2012).

Surgery or radiotherapy may lead to spinal accessory nerve dysfunction, requiring attention to trapezius strengthening and functional scapula movements (McGarvey *et al* 2013a), with the potential compensatory role of rhomboid and serratus anterior accessory muscles being considered (McGarvey *et al* 2013b). If the sternocleidomastoid muscle has been excised, the patient's head will need support during activity. Connecting tubes must be supported activity so that they do not drag on the wound. Patients need to keep their head up to minimize oedema for the first few days.

If there is a tracheostomy, ACBT/AD can still be performed, an incentive spirometer can be attached with a connector, and inhaled medication can be delivered by MDI, paediatric face mask and small volume spacer (Nandapalan 2000).

After discharge, multidisciplinary rehabilitation helps prevent social isolation and empowers patients to improve their quality of life (Eades *et al* 2013).

TRACHEOSTOMY

> **Stoma:** *surgical opening from the inside to the outside of the body*
> **Tracheostomy:** *opening into the trachea*
> **Tracheotomy:** *surgical creation of an opening into the trachea.*

Breathing through a tracheostomy bypasses the nose, pharynx and larynx. The cough is weakened, and filtering and humidification functions are lost. Resistance to exhalation by the nose ('physiological PEEP', Ch. 1) is also lost, but this can be restored with a heat-moisture exchanger of the same resistance (McRae *et al* 1996). The work of breathing is reduced on inspiration (Christopher 2005).

A tracheostomy is formed for the following reasons:

- during and after surgery, if the airway needs protection from aspiration or swelling
- permanently after laryngectomy
- to provide airway access for patients on ventilators or after facial trauma.

Full surgical tracheostomy is done in theatre, but percutaneous dilatational tracheotomy causes less trauma and can be done under local anaesthesia at the bedside.

Fig 16.17a shows the location of a tracheostomy with its tube, and 16.17b shows a permanent stoma following laryngectomy.

Tracheostomy tubes

For the first few days after surgery, there is an inflated cuff which encircles the tube within the trachea to minimize aspiration (Fig 16.18a).

For non-laryngectomy patients, the cuff is deflated as soon as there is a cough reflex and swallowing is adequate. If the tube is to be removed, it will then be plugged, with the cuff deflated so that the patient can breathe, for lengthening periods until the plug can be left in situ for four hours without distress. When plugged, oxygen, if required, needs to be delivered by face mask and not the tracheostomy mask.

FIGURE 16.17 (a) Tracheostomy tube in situ, (b) Tracheostomy and laryngectomy

(a)   (b)

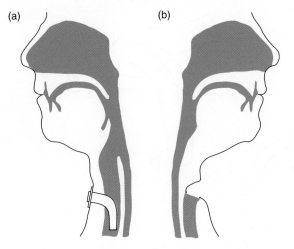

For laryngectomy patients, the cuffed tube is removed after about 48 hours, when haemorrhage is no longer a risk, and replaced with an uncuffed tube (Fig 16.18b).

A silver tube (Fig 16.18c) is uncuffed and hypoallergenic, and is used for people needing a permanent tracheostomy.

Most tubes have an inner cannula (Fig 16.18d), which more than doubles the resistive work of breathing (Carter 2013) but helps prevent blockage and trauma from repeated tube changes. It is left in place for suction, but needs to be removed and cleaned regularly.

For people without a laryngectomy but requiring long term tracheostomy, speech is possible with a fenestrated tube (Fig 16.18d). This has inner and outer cannulae with matching windows (fenestrations) on their posterior curves. With the cuff deflated and stoma occluded by a plug or gloved finger on expiration, the patient can speak on breathing out because the breath is directed out through the holes and up through the larynx. An unfenestrated inner cannula is used for suction and when eating or drinking. Fenestrated tubes should not be used with mechanical ventilation.

A tracheostomy button (Fig 16.18f) acts as a stent to maintain the patency of a mature stoma. It is usually kept closed and does not extend into the tracheal lumen, so if frequent suction is required it should be replaced with a tracheostomy tube to protect the back of the trachea. It is used for neurological patients who may need repeated tracheostomies, or as a step to decannulation, or during rehabilitation.

Mini-tracheostomies are used for suction rather than to facilitate breathing (Ch. 8).

Complications

> *We can never make the sounds of crying, shouting or laughter.*
>   Patient quoted by Ulbricht (1986)

Unavoidable complications of a tracheostomy tube are the following:

- communication difficulties
- impaired cough because there is no closed glottis behind which pressure can build up
- impaired swallow because of reduced muscle co-ordination, upset pressure gradients, compression of the oesophagus and anchoring of the larynx so that swallowing feels like there is a lump in the throat, especially with an inflated cuff
- loss of taste and smell.

Other complications are below (Mitchell *et al* 2013):

1. Occlusion, most likely from a mucous plug.
2. Haemorrhage from tracheal erosion into an artery. This may be obvious, or indicated by pulsation of the tracheostomy tube synchronous with the pulse. If suspected, the airway should be suctioned and cuff inflated. This will temporarily limit aspiration of blood into the lungs until medical attention arrives and bronchoscopy instigated.
3. Displacement, especially if there is uncontrolled coughing, loose tracheal ties or excessive movement of the tube in the immediate postoperative period.
4. Subcutaneous emphysema (Powell *et al* 2011).
5. Aspiration, often without symptoms but sometimes accompanied by an unstable breathing pattern (Martin-Harris 2012). Secretions can trickle past an inflated cuff, but aspiration is more common with the cuff deflated. A deflated cuff may be necessary during eating, but patients with neurological disorders should be assessed by a speech language therapist before cuff

FIGURE 16.18 (a) Cuffed tracheostomy tube (b) Uncuffed tracheostomy tube (c) silver Negus tube (d) inner cannula, (e) fenestrated tube, (f) tracheostomy button

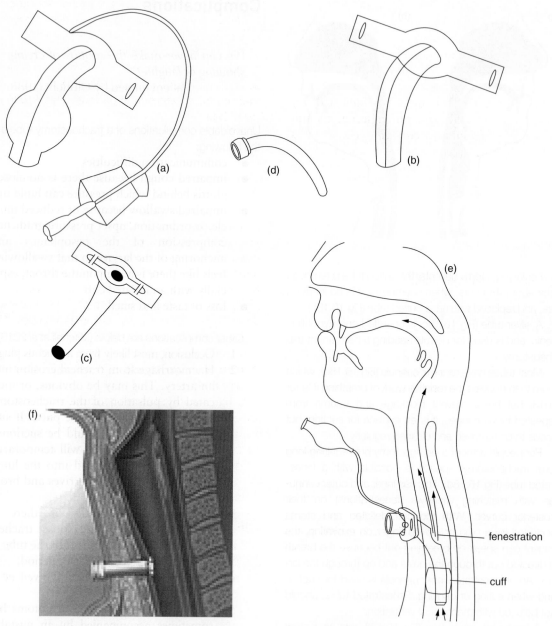

deflation, which is best preceded by suction above the cuff, i.e. via the mouth.

6   Dysphagia, nausea and vomiting if pressure is exerted on the posterior wall of the trachea and oesophagus by the wrong sized tube.

7   Weight loss due to dysphagia, reduced appetite and impaired taste and smell.

8   Infection, partly because the oropharynx is teeming with bacteria and partly because poor suction technique is widespread.

9   Tracheoesophageal fistula, which is suspected if suctioned secretions contain food or drink.

10 Damage to the trachea, increased by pull on the tube if connected to a ventilator, or by mishandling.

11 Late onset stricture following damage to the trachea, due to granulation tissue as eroded areas heal.

12 Stenosis. This may be indicated by cough, difficulty clearing secretions and breathlessness, occurring weeks, months or years after decannulation (Crooks *et al* 2012). Laser treatment or surgery may be required.

Management

KEY POINT

The greatest fear of tracheostomy patients during their early postoperative days is an inability to summon help, and a bell must always be within reach.

Most protocols stipulate that patients should be in sight of the nurses' station and not in a side room. Questions are best framed for a yes or no answer, and time is needed for lip-reading and deciphering written requests.

Sterile gloves should be worn for all contact with the tracheostomy site. The neck plate must be supported when coughing or sneezing.

It takes about a week after tracheostomy for fascia and muscle to fuse and form a tract from the skin to the trachea, during which time tracheal dilators are on hand in case the tube becomes dislodged. The tape securing the tube around the neck is best secured with Velcro and should be loose enough to fit one or two fingers between the tape and neck, depending on local protocol.

Two spare tracheostomy tubes must be available, one the same size and one a size smaller in case a tube change is needed urgently. At the bedside there is also an obturator, a solid insert which assists insertion of a new tracheostomy tube but which must be removed immediately after tube change so that the patient can breathe. Tracheostomy tubes should only be changed by a specifically-trained nurse, physiotherapist or doctor.

With long term tracheostomy, patients are taught to huff out their secretions, but a suction unit at home is required, with instructions to the patient and their carers on its use, and how to deal with a blocked tube (see p. 399).

Humidification

A heat-moisture exchanger is inadequate in the acute stage, especially if oxygen is added (Chikata 2013), and continuous hot water humidification is needed for the first 48 hours, connected to a T-piece or tracheostomy mask. If the tracheostomy is permanent, the airway acclimatizes to its new exposure by metaplasia of the airway lining from respiratory to squamous epithelium. Patients will then need to maintain adequate fluid intake, and are supplied with a Swedish nose or bib over the stoma to filter out large particles (Fig 16.19). Humidification is restarted if infection occurs, and people with chronic lung disease may need a nebulizer at home to use with saline if secretions become thick.

Liberal mouthwashes are required after head and neck surgery, even for patients with excess salivation, and sometimes suction of the mouth is needed, using low pressures. Tracheal suction, if needed, should be with the inner tube in situ. Difficulty passing the catheter should be reported.

Communication

The majority of patients having a laryngectomy can regain communication with speech therapy, preferably begun preoperatively (Gordon 2011). Examples are:

* an electrolarynx held at the neck which produces a tone shaped into Dalek-like speech as the user mouths the words

* oesophageal speech, in which the patient learns to compress air into the oesophagus and release it, creating a more normal sound than the electrolarynx

* a valve inserted into a surgical tracheo-oesophageal puncture through which

FIGURE 16.19 (a) 'Swedish nose' heat moisture exchanger to fit over the tracheostomy tube, and (b) bib to tie round the neck and hang over the stoma

(a)   (b)

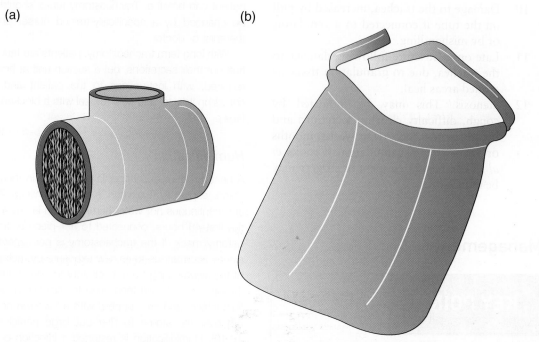

patients can learn to generate oesophageal speech
- laryngeal transplants
- text messaging, iPod touch and laptops, with which patients become expert.

Speaking valves such as the Passy-Muir or Blom (Leder *et al* 2013) can be used with patients who have not had a laryngectomy, including those on a ventilator.

Practical points when using the Passy-Muir valve are to:
- Monitor humidification and FiO_2
- Before connecting the valve, suction the airway, then suction above the cuff, then let the cuff down slowly, with another suction catheter prepared in case of need.
- If the patient finds it hard to breathe, or they are unable to speak or they begin to sound wheezy, remove the valve and identify the cause of the problem.

- Ensure that the valve is removed for sleep to avoid impaired gas exchange due to extra dead space, and ask the patient to take precautions against falling asleep with the valve in situ.
- Increase tolerance gradually to allow accommodation to the dead space.

Nutrition

The speech language therapist assesses for swallowing with cuff inflation and deflation. When eating, the patient sits up if possible, flexes their neck slightly and the cuff is deflated if safe to do so. Sips of sterile water are initially given, and if tolerated without coughing, desaturation, fatigue or signs of aspiration, then thickened fluids may be introduced, followed by a soft diet (ICS 2008). The patient should stay sitting upright for 20 minutes after eating. Patients most at risk are those with mouth and throat tumours, who achieve <50% of their required oral intake (Kalavrezos *et al* 2014) and chronically ill patients with tracheostomies, 80% of whom experience thirst (Arai 2013).

Inner tube change

Local policy varies about frequency of change. A suggested procedure is to:

- explain the procedure, preoxygenate and suction if required
- ask the patient to slightly extend their head
- support the neck plate with one gloved hand
- unlock or unclip the inner cannula with the other gloved hand, then remove the inner tube outwards and downwards, while stabilizing the tracheostomy tube
- insert a new inner cannula and ensure that it is locked or clipped in place

- discard the old inner cannula, or clean with sterile water or normal saline and foam sponges, then leave to air dry.

Blocked tracheostomy tube

If a tracheostomy tube becomes blocked with thick secretions, blood or a foreign body, as shown by difficulty breathing or respiratory arrest, the steps in Box 16.4 should be taken (ICS 2008):

The crash team should have arrived before this is completed, but the steps may be needed in quick succession.

Once the patient is stabilized, a new tracheostomy tube can be reinserted by a suitably experienced member of the team, or a nasopharyngeal tube can be used temporarily.

Information for clinicians, including algorithms for managing tube emergencies to hang above patients' beds, is in App. A.

BOX 16.4

Management of a blocked tracheostomy tube

1 Press the crash button and call for help.
2 Explain to the patient what is happening, while encouraging them to cough.
3 If this is not sufficient, remove the inner cannula.
4 If this is not sufficient, suction the airway.
5 If this is not sufficient, deflate the cuff.
6 If this is not sufficient, move the patient's head in case this relieves the obstruction.
7 If the patient is breathing apply oxygen to the tracheostomy, or to the nose and mouth if the natural airway is patent (and there is no inflated cuff), or to both, which may require oxygen from the crash trolley as well as the wall.
8 If the patient is not breathing, ventilate by attaching the resuscitation bag to the tracheostomy tube, or by blowing down the stoma, using a paediatric facemask or laryngeal mask airway if available, while occluding the nose and mouth (or use a resuscitation bag and mask to the nose and mouth if patent, while occluding the stoma).
9 If oxygenation is inadequate, remove the tracheostomy tube:
  - cut the securing tape or undo the Velcro
  - insert a suction catheter to allow oxygen administration
  - slide out the tube over the catheter, using tracheal dilators to maintain patency of the stoma
  - continue ventilation, keeping tracheal dilators *in situ,* and either encouraging the patient to breathe spontaneously, or blowing down the stoma
  - if the airway is still blocked, suction with a Yankeur or other large bore suction catheter.

Discharge

Patients with permanent tracheostomies should receive a full checklist of emergency supplies and the following information:

- how to remove a blocked tube and replace it in an emergency
- sterile suction procedure
- protecting the stoma from water and dust

- the importance of winter flu vaccination, and avoiding people with chest infections
- instructions for carers on mouth-to-stoma resuscitation
- a contact number in case of problems
- information on support groups (Appendix B).

Decannulation of a tracheostomy tube is described on p. 431.

CASE STUDY : Mr LS

Identify the problems of this 74 y.o. man from Muscat two days after left upper lobectomy for small cell carcinoma.

Subjective

- Pain on coughing.
- Bringing up thick green phlegm.
- Unable to sleep.

Objective

- Notes: *pseudomonas* chest infection.
- Charts: intermittent intramuscular analgesia, pyrexia, S_pO_2 94%, no target saturation documented.
- Patient slumped in bed, on 40% dry oxygen.
- Rapid shallow breathing pattern.
- Auscultation: ↓ BS LLL, coarse crackles.
- Antero-posterior film shows two fluid-filled cavities in left upper zone (Fig 16.20a) which the lateral film shows to be in the left upper lobe (Fig 16.20b). Scan at tracheal level identifies largest cavity (Fig 16.20c). Radiology report states that these may relate to an abscess, empyema or a bronchopleural fistula.

Questions

1 Analysis?
2 Patient's problems?
3 Precaution?
4 Plan?

BS: breath sounds, *LLL:* left lower lobe

FIGURE 16.20 Mr LS

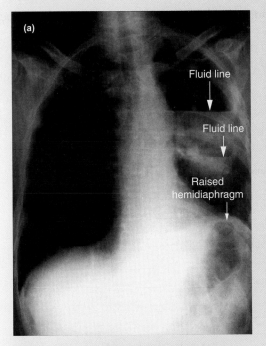

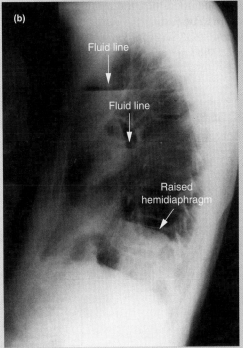

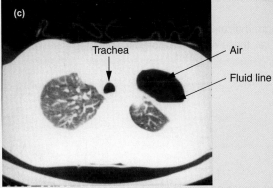

CLINICAL REASONING

A trial concluded that 'the routine use of respiratory physiotherapy after abdominal surgery does not seem to be justified'.

Methods: *'trials were included if they investigated prophylactic respiratory physiotherapy'*.

Search: *The key words excluded 'positioning' and 'exercise'.*

Chest (2006), 130, 1887–99

Response to Case Study

1 Analysis

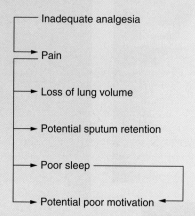

- ↓ BS over LLL and raised L hemidiaphragm indicate atelectasis (the lower lobe would expand to fill most of the space from the lobectomy, i.e. these signs are not just attributable to removal of the upper lobe).

2 Problems

- Pain
- Poor sleep
- ↓ lung volume LLL → poor gas exchange
- Sputum retention → poor gas exchange

3 Precaution

- Avoid right side lying to prevent infected fluid spreading from abscess or bronchopleural fistula.

4 Plan

- Liaise with team to optimize analgesia, instigate pain chart and documentation of both target S_pO_2 and its monitoring.
- Identify cause of poor sleep, e.g. pain/anxiety/noise, then remedy with the team.
- Humidify oxygen.

- Identify goals with patient, then initiate, according to patient preference:
  - controlled mobilization
  - sitting out in chair
  - deep breathing, end-inspiratory hold, incentive spirometry
  - ACBT or positive pressure device or both, to clear secretions
  - when drip is down, monitor fluid balance
  - progressive exercise programme to include shoulder range of motion, posture and exercise tolerance, using tick chart and involving family.

Response to Clinical Reasoning

The authors appear to be confusing 'prophylactic' with 'routine'.
Positioning and exercise are techniques that might be used prophylactically after surgery (and selectively, not routinely).

RECOMMENDED READING

Bagan P (2013) Nutritional status and postoperative outcome after pneumonectomy for lung cancer. *Ann Thorac Surg;* **95**(2): 392–6

Besiege EB, Dongo A, Ezemba N *et al* (2012) Tube thoracostomy: complications and its management. *Pulm Med*; 256878.

Bouyer-Ferullo S (2013) Preventing perioperative peripheral nerve injuries. *AORN J;* **97**(1): 110–124

Bridevaux PO, Aubert JD, Soccal PM *et al* (2014) Incidence and outcomes of respiratory viral infections in lung transplant recipients. *Thorax*; **69**(1): 32–38

Cereda M, Neligan PJ, Reed AJ (2013) Noninvasive respiratory support in the perioperative period. *Curr Opin Anaesthesiol*; **26**(2): 134–40

Cregg R, Anwar S, F-S Paul (2013) Persistent postsurgical pain. *Curr Opinion Supportive Palliat Care;* **7**(2): 144–52.

Davis-Evans C (2013) Alleviating anxiety and preventing panic attacks in the surgical patient. *AORN J;* **97**(3): 355–63

Drummond GB (2013) Characterization of breathing patterns during patient-controlled opioid analgesia. *Br J Anaesth;* **111**(6): 971–8

Faintuch J (2013) Rehabilitation needs after bariatric surgery. *Europ J Phys Rehab Med*; **49**(3): 431–7

Galantino MS (2013) Exercise interventions for upper limb dysfunction due to breast cancer treatment. *Phys Ther*; **93**(10): 1291–7

Gan TJ, Diemunsch P, Habib AS *et al* (2014) Consensus guidelines for the management of postoperative nausea and vomiting. *Anesth Analg*; **118**(1): 85–113

Harrington S (2013) Upper extremity strength and range of motion and their relationship to function in breast cancer survivors. *Physiother Theory Pract*; **29**(7): 513–20.

Kao J-H, Kao H-K, Chen Y-W *et al* (2013) Impact and predictors of prolonged chest tube duration in mechanically ventilated patients with acquired pneumothorax. *Respir Care;* **58**(12): 2093–2100

Maxwell C, Nicoara A (2014) New developments in the treatment of acute pain after thoracic surgery. *Curr Opin Anaesthesiol*; **27**(1): 6–11

McGrath BA, Bates L, Atkinson D *et al* (2012) Multidisciplinary guidelines for the management of tracheostomy and laryngectomy airway emergencies. *Anaesth*; **67**(9): 1025–41

Qiu T (2013) External suction versus water seal after selective pulmonary resection for lung neoplasm: a systematic review. *PLoS One*; **9;8**(7): e68087

Raber-Durlacher JE, Brennan MT, Verdonck IM *et al* (2012) Swallowing dysfunction in cancer patients. *Support Care Cancer,* **20**(3): 433–43

Rehder KJ (2013) Active rehabilitation during extracorporeal membrane oxygenation as a bridge to lung transplantation. *Respir Care,* **58**(8): 1291–8

Rialon KL, Abernethy AP, Mosca PJ (2012) Integration of palliative surgery into the palliative care delivery team. *J Palliative Care Med*, **2**: e115

Rocco G (2013) Remote-controlled, wireless chest drainage system. *Ann Thorac Surg;* **95**(1): 319–22

Russell IF (2013) The ability of bispectral index to detect intra-operative wakefulness during total intravenous anaesthesia compared with the isolated forearm technique. *Anaesthesia*, **68**: 502–511

Sander AP (2012) Factors that affect decisions about physical activity and exercise in survivors of breast cancer. *Phys Ther*, **92**(4): 525–36

Shah N, Hamilton M (2013) Clinical review: Can we predict which patients are at risk of complications following surgery? *Crit Care*, **17**: 226

Takahama M, Mimura Y, Matsuda E (2013) Complications influence ambulation in patients undergoing extrapleural pneumonectomy. *Hong Kong Physiother J*, **31**(1): 52–53

Wanten GJ, Kaanders JH, Merkx MA *et al* (2014) Nutritional status, food intake, and dysphagia in long-term survivors with head and neck cancer treated with chemoradiotherapy. *Head Neck*; **36**(1): 60–5

Watanabe Y (2013) An extremely elderly patient with lung cancer who underwent surgery. *Ann Thorac Cardiovasc Surg;* **19**(5): 382–5

PART IV PHYSIOTHERAPY IN CRITICAL CARE

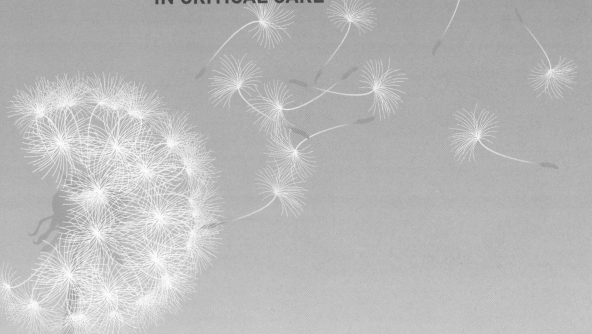

PART IV

PHYSIOTHERAPY IN CRITICAL CARE

CHAPTER 17
Critical care, support and monitoring

LEARNING OBJECTIVES

On completion of this chapter the reader should be able to:

- understand how the ICU environment can affect the patient

- describe the principles and complications of mechanical ventilation

- understand the relevance of fluids, nutrition and medication to patient stability and their relation to physiotherapy

- understand how advanced life support systems modify physiotherapy

- interpret monitor readings.

INTRODUCTION

He may cry out for rest, peace, dignity, but ... he will get a dozen people around the clock, all busily preoccupied with his heart rate, pulse, secretions or excretions, but not with him as a human being.

Kübler-Ross (1973)

Critical care is for patients who require intensive therapy, intensive monitoring and/or intensive support. They are not necessarily critically ill (and the term 'Critical Care' can be worrying for relatives) but they are at risk of failure of one or more major organs. Their needs range from observation of vital signs after major surgery, to total support of physiological systems. Of those who survive the experience, 5–10% become chronically unwell (Bahadur *et al* 2008). There is a growing awareness that survival alone is not enough to demonstrate success, and physiotherapy is playing an increasing role in enabling patients to return to a meaningful life.

Level of care in the UK is allocated according to clinical need:

1   Level 3 is provided in the Intensive Care Unit (ICU), where patients require one-to-one nursing and either mechanical ventilation or support of two or more organ systems.

2   Level 2 involves monitoring or support of a single system and acts as step-down or step-up between levels of care. Patients are nursed in an ICU or a dedicated high dependency unit.

3   Level 1 is 'Critical care without walls' for those at risk of their condition deteriorating or who have recently relocated from a higher level. Their needs are met on an acute ward with support from a proactive 24-hour multidisciplinary outreach team (Table 17.1).

4   Level 0 is for patients whose needs can be met through normal ward care in an acute hospital.

Non-invasive ventilation is provided at Level 1 or 2 (McNeill & Glossop 2012).

ENVIRONMENT

Effects on the patient

> *The environment was interpreted as 'being in the middle of an uncontrollable barrage of noise, unable to take cover'.*
> Johansson & Bergbom 2013

Critically ill people find themselves in an environment that can exacerbate stress and sap their energy. It is not an optional extra to give attention to the human aspect of patient management, but an integral part of physiotherapy. The physiological effects of stress are in Ch. 1.

Pain, lack of sleep and intubation are the three major causes of distress (Kamdar et al 2012), the severity of the stress response varying with the patient's ability to control their situation. Autonomy is hindered by dependence on others for the most basic care decisions, leading to fear and sometimes nightmares which may last for years (Schelling et al 2003). Sensory and sleep deprivation, psychotropic drugs, prolonged immobility, isolation and reduced communication are classified as psychological torture by Amnesty International. These conditions are found in the ICU, albeit without intent. Examples are over the page.

TABLE 17.1 Typical call criteria for a critical care outreach team

Vital sign	Criteria
Airway	Threatened airway, e.g. excessive secretions or stridor.
Breathing	RR <8 or >25 breaths/min.
Circulation	• HR <50 or >150 beats/min. • Systolic BP < 90 mmHg, >200 mmHg, or drop of >40 mmHg. • Systolic BP less than patient's normal value.
Consciousness	• Sustained alteration in GCS of >2 in past hour.
Oxygen	• S_pO_2 <90% on >.50 F_iO_2.
Urine output	• <30 ml/h for more than two hours (unless normal for patient).
General	• Clinically causing concern. • Not responding to treatment.

BP: blood pressure, *F_iO_2*: fraction of inspired oxygen, *GCS*: Glasgow Coma Scale, *HR*: heart rate, *RR*: respiratory rate

1   **Communication problems.** Inability to communicate leads to a high level of frustration (Patak 2004) due to intubation and, for some patients, sedation and analgesia which also affect concentration and short term memory.

2   **Sleep fragmentation.** Most patients lack sleep (Day 2013). This impairs immune function, slows protein synthesis, hinders rehabilitation, impacts physical recovery (Kamdar 2012) and has a greater influence on post-traumatic stress symptoms than severity of illness (Weiner & Sprenkle 2008). It also predisposes to delirium (Roussos 2010) and multisystem failure (Allen *et al* 2012). A full sleep cycle (Ch. 1) is rare in the ICU but is needed to achieve the restorative benefits of sleep (Kamdar 2012). The more ill the patient, the more sleep they need and the less they are likely to get. Sleep disruption is due to lights, anxiety, pain, reversal of the day-night cycle, difficulty in finding a comfortable position, fear of falling asleep and not waking again, and noise, much of which is avoidable (Tegnestedt 2013) but which averages nearly twice the recommended maximum (Kamdar 2012). Drugs which disturb sleep include β-blockers and theophylline (Richards *et al* 2003). Suggested strategies are:

- noise reduction, diurnal lighting, clustering of nocturnal activities and relaxation (Porter & McClure 2013)
- noise-cancelling headphones or the patient's favourite music (Chlan *et al* 2013)
- massage (Richards *et al* 2003), shown to relatives
- a background of white noise such as ocean sounds, which reduce arousals (Fig 17.1).

3   **Fear.** Patients face fears which are compounded by helplessness and the confusing effect of some drugs. They try to assess their progress by watching staff and family reactions and comparing

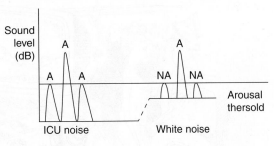

FIGURE 17.1 Arousals from sleep without and with white noise. *A:* arousals, *NA:* no arousals

themselves to others on the unit. Anxiety is highest in patients with respiratory disease (Chlan 2008).

4   **Sensory deprivation.** A form of emotional solitary confinement can be caused by social isolation, loss of non-clinical touch and the patient's familiar social media, immobilization, certain drugs, a limited visual field and removal of hearing aid or glasses. This can leave patients feeling intense loneliness despite constant attention. Sensory deprivation is amplified three-fold in the absence of windows (Criner & Isaac 1995). Virtual reality systems can provide implied environments to help ameliorate this effect (Turon 2013).

5   **Sensory overload** (Fig 17.2). Patients find themselves lost in a sea of electronic wizardry, bombarded by unfamiliar beeps, alarms, lights, confining equipment, painful procedures (sometimes without warning), tubes in various orifices and incomprehensible conversation over their heads. Noise can be damaging (Alway 2013) and predisposes to delirium (Olson *et al* 2013).

6   **Disorientation, depersonalization** and **delirium.** Combined sensory deprivation and overload can cause perceptual distortion, in which hallucinations arise from false perceptions of sensory input, often after the first two or three lucid days. Hallucinations lead to some patients perceiving their body boundaries as permeable and the equipment as part of

FIGURE 17.2 Sensory overload

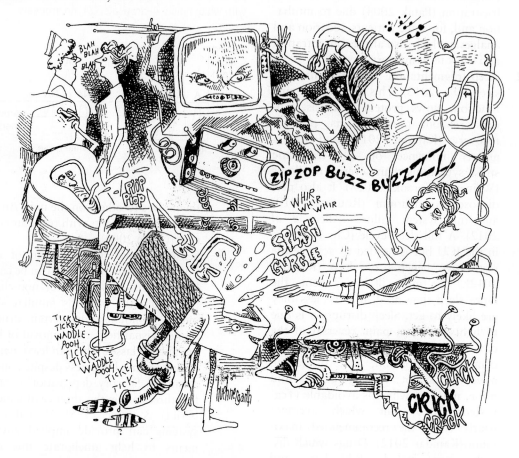

their body (Johansson 2005). Over half of patients develop delirium, which increases morbidity, mortality and length of stay (Porter & McClure 2013), but most cases are missed, partly because 95% of patients manifest the hypoactive rather than hyperactive type (Hipp & Ely 2012). Patients report nightmares of being trapped (Karlsson & Forsberg 2008) and delusional memories of people trying to kill them (Garrouste-Orgeas 2012). These persist longer than factual memories (Carr 2007) and worsen the experience of pain (Azzam & Alam (2013). Delirium may trigger the re-emergence of fearful memories of past

events such as wartime bombing or being sent to boarding school (Hazzard 2002). Depersonalisation is worsened by inappropriate joking between staff, which can be misunderstood by patients or relatives (Reader 2008). Appropriate joking is fine, indeed often welcomed, so long as the patient is included.

7 **Sensory monotony** and **loss of time sense.** Patients struggle to keep track of time through a tranquillized haze, which is worse when there is no day-night sequence in lighting or routine. This compounds disorientation, or, for more alert patients, causes boredom. Boredom is usually a negative experience, but

occasionally the empty time gives patients an opportunity for reflection, and some emerge with a sharpened perception of what is important in their life.

8   **Discomfort.** Patients may experience immobility, gagging on the endotracheal tube, dribbling, a dry mouth, distended abdomen, unscratchable itches and asynchrony with the ventilator. Discomfort is increased with paralysis or other forms of restraint. Physical restraints stimulate inflammation (Tymen *et al* 2013), impede communication, increase both anxiety and depression (Happ 2004), and are banned under many protocols.

9   **Pain.** Pain worsens outcomes and is under-assessed and under-treated, with a 50% incidence of moderate to severe pain identified (Jong *et al* 2013).

10   **Helplessness, dependency** and **depression.** The less patients are able to do for themselves, the more frustrated they feel. This may become internalized as depression, especially as they feel inhibited in expressing feelings when dependent on those who care for them. Depression can hinder rehabilitation, particularly in the recovery period, and continues in 28% of patients over the following year (Kamdar 2012).

11   **Loss of privacy, dignity** and **identity.** It is easy for us to forget how people feel when they lose their clothes, teeth, personal space and surname. Patients who are elderly or from a different culture are particularly vulnerable to this form of depersonalization, and their experiences can haunt them long after discharge (Scragg *et al* 2001). Sometimes patients want privacy from their own relatives, and their permission should be obtained before visitors are ushered in willy-nilly.

Patients' preferences for visiting varies. Gonzalez (2004) found that a third of patients preferred unlimited visiting, a third once a day, and many did not want visitors during procedures, when needing to rest, or either early or late in the day.

> ## KEY POINT
>
> Unless we nurture empathy in understanding a patient's experience, we will not be fully effective with our treatment.

Long term effects vary. Granja (2005) found nearly half of ICU survivors experiencing sleep disturbance six months later, a third reported poor concentration and memory, and over half suffered fatigue. Rates of post-traumatic stress disorder (PTSD) averaged 14% (Modrykamien 2012), which can lead to years of memory dysfunction, panic attacks and depression, as well as the re-experiencing of traumatic ICU events (Carr 2007). Cognitive impairment has been found in up to 70% of patients (Hopkins *et al* (2012) and in 47% of survivors two years later (Modrykamien 2012), which is thought to be missed in half the patients (Hopkins 2009).

Use of a diary, with contributions from staff and relatives, helps link memories with reality, improve quality of life, reduce PTSD symptoms and assist the family (Perier 2013). Anxiety, depression and PTSD symptoms can also be reduced by the inclusion of a clinical psychologist on the team (Peris *et al* 2011).

> *Knowing what to expect gives some control back to a vulnerable person who feels like everything is happening in a haphazard fashion.*
>
> Hipp & Ely 2012

Effect on relatives

Relatives can do much to ease a patient's stress, so long as they in turn are given support. They may feel bewildered, daunted by the environment, reluctant to voice their concerns, and some develop PTSD if they are not kept informed (Azoulay 2005). They benefit from:

●   information about the patient's condition, equipment and the reason for physiotherapy

- visible evidence that staff care about the patient
- a share in decision-making (Happ 2008)
- the opportunity to say what they are thinking or feeling
- reassurance that touch and conversation are welcomed by most patients
- advice that children usually benefit from visiting (Jones & Griffiths 2002 p. 134)
- encouragement to become involved in patient care, e.g. foot massage, certain passive movements, hair brushing and mouth care
- a leaflet describing the ICU layout, machines, terminology and the different staff responsibilities.

If acceptable to staff, relatives may be allowed to join ward rounds (Santiago 2014) or witness resuscitation attempts (Jabre et al 2013), with appropriate support, which helps them realize that everything possible is being done.

Occasionally the needs of patients and relatives diverge, as illustrated by two opposing examples for the same patient:

- 'My mother … cries and gets all dramatic. She grabbed my hand and I got angry and the machine started to go beep beep beep and they took her away …'
- '… Laurie was holding my hand. She was talking to me … she is strong and calm' (Chlan 1995).

Effects on staff

Emotional responses can become dulled by the frequency with which they are elicited. People working in an ICU need defences against the suffering around them, but these are not incompatible with sensitive patient care.

Staff who become stressed are not only less able to identify with the experience of the patient, they are more likely to make mistakes. Reactions to working in the ICU include over-detachment, anxiety due to the responsibility, frustration at communication difficulties and inability to relieve suffering, and burnout (Papadimos et al 2011).

Strategies to reduce stress include:
- involvement of all staff in decision-making

- multidisciplinary training to increase confidence
- feedback, sharing of ideas, debriefing after traumatic incidents and recognition that doubts are acceptable.

Relatives can be asked to bring photographs of patients from when they were well, which when put on the locker act as a reminder to staff of the human side of the patient.

Patients' rights

Consent

The following are currently valid in Britain and are taken from Richardson (2013), CSP (2012), Dimond (2009), and Delany & Frawley (2012). They relate to treatment, teaching and research.

A patient is assumed to have the capacity to refuse treatment even if the treatment is life-saving or if the reasons for withholding consent are irrational, unknown or non-existent. It is illegal to force physiotherapy on patients who resist or who are unable to resist but have made their wishes clear by words or gesture, or have made their wishes clear prior to losing capacity. Patients may withdraw consent during treatment.

The elements of informed consent are:
- Explanations, to include risks and alternative options.
- Voluntariness, i.e. patients take their decision without undue influence.
- Capacity, i.e. the patient's ability matches the required decision-making.
- Consent itself, i.e. voluntary agreement based on relevant understanding.

If patients do not know that they have these rights, they should be informed. In the face of refusal, physiotherapists should seek a change of mind but must not use duress or deceit. The following allow treatment without consent:
- emergencies
- statutory authorization, e.g. the Mental Health Act 2007
- lack of capacity.

Generally a patient is considered to lack capacity to give or withhold consent if they are incapable of one of the following:

- comprehending and retaining treatment information, e.g. deep sedation or cognitive impairment
- believing such information
- weighing such information and arriving at a choice.

Panic, indecisiveness, irrationality, mental illness or intellectual disability do not amount to incapacity. However, if mental incapacity from medication or illness renders patients incapable of understanding or retaining information so that they are unable to make a decision and assess risks, this constitutes incapacity to consent. Relatives cannot give or withhold consent for adults even if the patient is unconscious, but their opinion should be considered.

The medical notes provide information on the patient's wishes, 'presumed consent', difficult decisions discussed with the team, refusal of treatment and subsequent action. Physiotherapists must be able to justify their decisions, which have to be acceptable to the majority of their peers.

Moral rights

> I could think and I could hear. But I could not move and I could not talk or open my eyes.
>
> Patient quoted by Lawrence 1995

Patients have the right to know the truth, to participate in decision-making, to refuse to be used for teaching, and to be given full care even when their choice differs from ours. These rights should not be violated if they are young or have learning disabilities.

End-of-life decisions

> Ethics is the exercise of moral reasoning in circumstances where strong feeling is not always the surest guide to action nor procedural powers the surest way to justice.
>
> Dunstan quoted by Branthwaite (1996)

The notes need to be checked for a 'Do not attempt resuscitation' (DNAR) order, which is based on medical judgment that resuscitation would lead to a high probability of death or severe brain damage, plus if possible the patient's judgement on their quality of life. The British Medical Association directs that DNAR orders be made in consultation with the patient unless this is impossible, because physicians rarely predict accurately a patient's perception of their quality of life (Papa-Kanaan et al 2001). Patients may or may not want their families involved in the decision. Physiotherapists need to be involved in the team discussion of end-of-life decisions in order to avoid possible legal complications (Raper & Fisher 2009 p. 62).

Advance directives, or living wills, allow individuals, when competent, to express a wish to be spared life-sustaining treatment in case of intractable or terminal illness. These are not legally binding in many countries, and may not be available, retrieved or honoured during acute hospital care.

A decision to withdraw mechanical ventilation from a dying patient usually begins a process of 'terminal weaning', in the knowledge that it will be followed by death. This should be accompanied by titrated narcotics and non-invasive monitoring (Billings 2012).

Infection control

Critically ill patients, often in a state of immune exhaustion (Cabrera-Cancio 2012) have their upper airways bypassed, multiple catheters inserted and broad spectrum antibiotics administered. Measures to prevent infection include:

- Hand cleaning, because gloves frequently have undetectable holes, one study finding that anaesthetists' gloved finger tips were contaminated in 83% of cases (Kocent et al 2002).
- Plastic aprons, colour-coded to ensure a change between patients.
- Fastidious attention to sterile suction technique, e.g. resting the disconnected catheter mount on the glove paper to avoid it touching the sheets.
- Respect for tracheostomies as the surgical wounds that they are.
- Doors to the ICU opening only on activation of the hand wash dispenser.

An infection risk is created by each change of invasive equipment and each break in the ventilator circuit.

Teamwork

Communication problems, along with hierarchical and cultural barriers, are major causes of errors (McCulloch et al 2011), augmented by what has been termed 'the tyranny of busyness' (Manias 2000). Teamwork is enhanced by mutual respect and assertiveness, mutual teaching and learning, flexibility and multidisciplinary rounds (Vazirani 2005), to include occupational therapists and speech-language therapists (Brown 2013).

Problems may arise over boundaries and autonomy. If physiotherapists would like to ask for review of a medical therapy that is not their direct responsibility, they can raise the subject diplomatically by asking for advice about it, or by clarifying the link between medical management and rehabilitation. If physiotherapy is medically prescribed, physiotherapists can thank the doctor for their advice and explain that the patient will be assessed and treated as appropriate. Results are likely to be positive when communicating in a way that makes it easy for others to agree.

Communication between physiotherapists and nurses is facilitated by the physiotherapist offering to help change sheets when it fits in with turning the patient during treatment, and the nurse incorporating regimes such as hourly incentive spirometry into the nursing plan. Turning for physiotherapy should be co-ordinated with turning for pressure area care.

MECHANICAL VENTILATION

> *[Some] patients ... resented health professionals touching their ventilators ... [others] perceived the surrounding machinery as reassuring. Patients reported a need for repeated explanations.*
> Patient quoted by Jablonski (1994)

The need for invasive mechanical ventilation is the commonest cause of admission to the ICU, with respiratory disease accounting for 79% of patients (Crooks et al 2012). The ventilator augments or replaces the function of the inspiratory muscles by delivering gas to the lungs under positive pressure. This substitutes for the respiratory pump but is not beneficial for lung tissue, and there is a narrow range of pressures and volumes within which the lungs are safe from either overdistension or atelectasis.

Mechanical ventilation (MV) is supportive, not curative. It helps control gas exchange and acid-base balance by manipulating inspired oxygen, minute ventilation ($\dot{V}_E$), pressure, volume, inspiratory:expiratory (I:E) ratio and positive end-expiratory pressure (PEEP). It is less about the application of a machine to a passive patient and more about the complex interaction between patient and machine.

Indications

Patients may not have respiratory disease but are in impending or established respiratory failure, i.e.:

- They are unable to ventilate adequately, oxygenate adequately, or both; examples are inspiratory muscle weakness due to neurological impairment, severe hypoxaemia due to lung parenchymal disease, or inspiratory muscle fatigue due to exacerbation of COPD.
- They are able to breathe adequately but this is deemed inadvisable, e.g. with acute brain injury, in which case they are sedated to the point of requiring ventilatory assistance.
- They require intubation for airway protection or to overcome upper airway obstruction and need added ventilatory support to compensate for the work of breathing (WOB) through the tubing.

Airway

> *... like a toilet paper roll ... a hard rubber tube ... a soggy cigar ... like you were gagging on something.*
> Patient quoted by Jablonski (1994)

Patient and ventilator are connected through a sealed tracheal tube (endotracheal or tracheostomy tube, Fig 17.3), which reaches just beyond the vocal cords.

An **endotracheal tube** (ETT) through the mouth or nose can be used for up to two weeks, but causes discomfort and distress. A nasal tube causes less movement-related injury to the larynx but creates more airflow resistance and increases the risk of sinusitis.

A **tracheostomy tube** is more comfortable than an ETT, causes less resistance, is easier for suctioning, may improve oxygenation and ventilation (Bellani *et al* 2013), facilitates weaning (Jubran *et al* 2013) and allows speaking and oral intake (Fisher *et al* 2013). Tracheostomy should be considered as soon as the patient is stabilized on the ventilator if it becomes apparent that prolonged MV will be required (AARC 2002c). When performed 3–7 days after intubation this has reduced mortality and hospital stay (Shan *et al* 2013).

Airway irritation is caused with any neck movement (Olympio *et al* 2000). A newly-created tracheostomy indicates the need for extra care during patient handling and suctioning, although once established, it is more secure than an ETT and allows freer mobilization. Tracheostomies (Ch. 16) in the ICU are usually percutaneous, which entails minimal incision and dissection (Maxwell *et al* 2013). They should not be fenestrated because of the risk of subcutaneous emphysema with positive pressure ventilation (Powell *et al* 2011).

The main disadvantage of tracheal tubes is in providing a gateway for ventilator-associated pneumonia (VAP), defined as hospital acquired pneumonia that develops 48 hours after intubation (Chang 2014 p.497) and precipitated by the following:

- a biofilm which develops inside the tube within hours of intubation and acts as a bacterial reservoir (Zolfaghari 2012)
- positive pressure in the chest, which is transmitted to the abdomen and precipitates gastroesophageal reflux
- inability of the vocal cords to close, allowing microaspiration of refluxed and biofilm secretions to trickle past the cuff and into the lungs.

The risk is not lessened by using a head-moisture exchanger (Auxiliadora 2012) but may be reduced by a 'VAP bundle' of strategies such as regular turning, either manually (Schallom *et al* 2005) or by a kinetic bed (Simonis *et al* 2013), antimicrobial photodynamic therapy (Biel 2012), coated ETTs to prevent biofilm formation, oral care, enteral nutrition and continuous

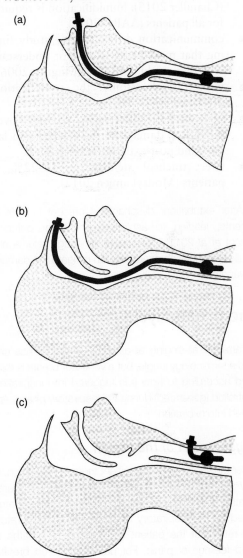

FIGURE 17.3 Tracheal tubes. (a) Oral endotracheal tube. (b) Nasal endotracheal tube. (c) Tracheostomy tube

(a)

(b)

(c)

aspiration of subglottic secretions (Chang 2014 p.499).

The optimum cuff pressure to maximize mucosal perfusion and minimize aspiration is 20–30 cmH_2O (Lizy *et al* 2014), which should be kept stable because fluctuations can trigger an ischaemia-reperfusion cycle (Huckle & Hughes 2010). Squeezing to 'test' the pressure is banned.

Other complications of tracheal tubes are:

- loss of the warming and humidifying functions of the upper airway, which could cause thick secretions and ciliary damage (Chandler 2013); humidification is required for all patients (AARC 2012)
- communication difficulty, one study finding that most patients did not understand why they could not speak (Magnus 2006)
- with a tracheostomy: the complications described in Ch. 16
- with an ETT: discomfort, retching, over-salivation, damage to the trachea and larynx, and post-extubation hoarseness
- later: tracheal stenosis in 10–22% of patients (Modrykamien 2012).

After extubation, dysphagia is present in 84% of patients, leading to aspiration and poor outcome (Macht *et al* 2011), but speech-language referral and swallow-stimulation exercises can mitigate the damage (Hwang *et al* 2007).

The breath cycle

An array of all-singing all-dancing ventilators has created a terminology jungle, but a ventilator breath is classified according to how it is triggered into inspiration, controlled (generated) during the inspiratory phase, and cycled into expiration.

Trigger: start of the breath

Either the ventilator or the patient triggers inspiration, or they attempt to work together. For ventilator-triggered breaths, the trigger is set according to **time**, determined by the respiratory rate or inspiratory:expiratory (I:E) ratio, but the patient can take extra breaths to avoid feelings of panic. For patient-triggered breaths (Fig 17.4a), the ventilator delivers the breath as soon as it senses the beginning of the patient's inspiration, either by **flow**, with a sensitivity of about 3 l/min, or less often by **pressure**, which is harder work for the patient, who has to generate about $-3\,cmH_2O$.

Control: delivery of the breath

This describes how the ventilator delivers gas to the patient. The driving mechanism remains constant while the other parameters vary according to ventilatory load.

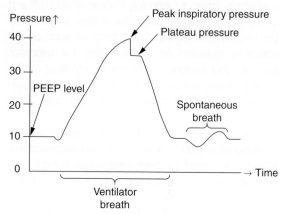

FIGURE 17.4a Pressure-time waveform showing a ventilator breath and a spontaneous breath, both being patient-triggered as identified by the negative pressure deflection. The ventilator breath is larger to make up for the $\dot{V}_A/\dot{Q}$ mismatch inherent in a positive pressure breath. A high PEEP level of $10\,cmH_2O$ is shown

Thus the ventilator can be set as a pressure or volume controller, or a mix. A cycling pressure limit is set for safety, at about $10\,cmH_2O$ above the peak inspiratory pressure (PIP) (Cairo 2012 p. 37).

Volume control (volume-constant) (VC) ventilation delivers a pre-set tidal volume (V_T) at a constant flow rate. The operator sets the V_T, flow, respiratory rate (RR) and I:E ratio. Airway pressure rises slowly during inspiration to a peak pressure that varies with airway resistance and lung compliance, so that if the airways narrow or the lung stiffens, the pressure rises (Fig 17.4b). VC may be used for adults because:

- it can be relied on to deliver a consistent $\dot{V}_E$ regardless of lung characteristics
- it maintains steady P_aCO_2 levels when this is imperative, e.g. with acute brain injured patients.

Flow control is similar to VC but derives volume from flow measurements (Chang 2014 p.59) and maintains a more consistent flow waveform.

Pressure control (pressure-constant) (PC) ventilation delivers a pre-set target pressure during inspiration (Fig 17.4c). The operator sets the peak inspiratory pressure, inspiratory time and RR to achieve a target P_aCO_2. Tidal volume varies with airway resistance, lung

FIGURE 17.4b AND 17.4c Pressure-time waveform: (b) volume control ventilation, the second breath showing increased pressure (arrow), indicating the development of airflow obstruction or stiff lungs; (c) pressure control ventilation. Lack of negative pressure deflection in both waveforms indicates ventilator triggering rather than patient triggering

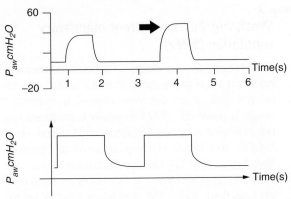

Other names are Autoflow, Pressure Regulated Volume Control and Volume Control Plus.

The above control parameters are sometimes called modes of ventilation in the literature, which can cause confusion because they are different variables within a mode. The mode is maintained independently of the control mechanism.

Cycle: end of the breath

Cycling into expiration occurs according to time, flow, volume or a mix. **Time-cycling** is used for pressure control ventilation, gas delivery being maintained until a pre-set pressure is reached and then maintained for a pre-set time. **Flow-cycling** is used in pressure support mode, when a reduction in peak inspiratory flow cycles the ventilator into expiration. **Volume-cycling** causes the ventilator to cycle at a pre-set tidal volume, but if an inspiratory pause is added, the breath will be classified as both volume and time cycled.

Modes of ventilation

> **Mandatory breath**: triggered and cycled by the ventilator
> **Assisted breath**: triggered by the patient, cycled by the ventilator
> **Spontaneous breath**: triggered and cycled by the patient

compliance and patient effort, and atelectasis is more of a risk. In a supine patient, there is often little ventilation to the lung bases (Zoremba et al 2010), but PC is useful in patients with acute respiratory distress syndrome (ARDS) to control the amount of pressure delivered to damaged alveoli, or for children to compensate for the leak through their uncuffed ETT.

Dual control provides the advantage of PC (limiting peak inspiratory pressure to protect the alveoli) while maintaining the advantage of VC (delivering a constant volume even if lung mechanics vary). It switches between the two as required, varying between breaths or within a breath, but can only control one variable at a time. Various confusing names are used, e.g.:

- Volume Support, which pressure-controls inspiration but adjusts the pressure limit to achieve a target V_T at each breath.
- Volume Assured Pressure Support which switches between pressure and flow control depending on whether the pre-set V_T has been met.
- Adaptive Support Ventilation which adjusts V_T and RR to achieve a pre-set $\dot{V}_E$.
- Volume Assured Pressure Support which automatically adjusts pressure in order to provide a consistent V_T.

In a spontaneously breathing patient, the WOB normally represents less than 5% of total oxygen consumption ($\dot{V}O_2$), but it can rise to 30% in the catabolic critically ill patient (Leach & Treacher 2002). A ventilator can take over all the WOB with controlled mandatory ventilation (CMV) or the work can be shared between ventilator and patient using a variety of ventilatory modes. These create the pressure, flow and volume that allow ventilatory support to be adjusted to the individual so that less sedation is required and less complications ensue than with full CMV.

Modes have to be matched skilfully to the patient because asynchrony is common, leading to unnecessary WOB, discomfort, extra sedation, a longer stay and sometimes a tug of war between patient and machine (Epstein 2012). At night, a mode should be chosen that provides more support (Andréjak 2013).

Names for each mode vary with country and manufacturer, each new machine seeming to pour more confusion into the terminology soup, leading to a 'calamity of ventilation research' because modes are not accurately defined (Henzler 2011, Adams 2012). However the following terms are generally recognized.

Controlled mandatory ventilation (CMV)

This fully controlled mode is ventilator-triggered and only used for patients who are unable to breathe at all or for whom complete control is necessary (Fig 17.5). It is an unforgiving mode which mandates the depth and frequency of each breath and time-cycle into exhalation. Patients do not like to be controlled, and heavy sedation is required. Risk of intrinsic PEEP and other complications is significant. Minute volume is set high enough to maintain a mild respiratory alkalosis so that spontaneous breathing is inhibited.

Assist-control

Assist-control is patient-triggered CMV. Breaths are triggered or imposed according to patient effort. With some ventilators the only difference with CMV is the trigger sensitivity, and indeed the two terms are sometimes

used interchangeably. Hyperventilation and respiratory alkalosis are risks.

Intermittent mandatory ventilation (IMV)

The IMV mode allows patients to breathe spontaneously between a pre-set number of mandatory breaths, without regard to the patient's breathing pattern.

Synchronized intermittent mandatory ventilation (SIMV)

SIMV breaths are mandatory or spontaneous according to the stage of the cycle, so that if patients do not breathe after a pre-set time interval, a mandatory breath is delivered. SIMV has largely superseded IMV because synchrony with inspiratory effort is more comfortable and breath-stacking is avoided. However, asynchrony may still develop (Robinson 2013), and Hess (2002) claims that the respiratory muscles contract as hard during the mandatory breaths as the spontaneous breaths. Pre-set variables include RR and V_T. Cycling is by pressure or time, whichever comes first. The spontaneous breaths of SIMV are usually pressure-supported (see below) in order to overcome the resistance of the tubing (Fig 17.6a).

Pressure support ventilation (PSV)

Also known as assisted spontaneous breathing (ASB), PSV is a patient-triggered mode which provides a pressure boost to each inspiratory effort, the pressure support level above PEEP reducing WOB in proportion to the pressure delivered. Epstein (2002) claims that 3–14 cmH$_2$O offsets the WOB through the tubing, and Tobin (2012) suggests pressures of 5–10 cmH$_2$O to decrease WOB by 31–60%. Aliverti et al (2006) suggests fine tuning the pressure by titrating it to the most synchronous breathing pattern. Even better, the patient could be asked which suits them best.

This pressure continues on a plateau until inspiratory flow reduces to <25% of its peak, when cycling into expiration occurs. Patients must be able to reliably trigger the ventilator and can determine their own RR, V_T and I:E ratio (Fig 17.6b). The pre-set variables are trigger sensitivity and pressure support level.

PSV is relatively comfortable and facilitates synchrony because the patient is in control. It acts like IPPB (Ch. 6) but is flow-triggered rather than pressure-triggered, thus eliminating excess work to trigger the breath.

FIGURE 17.5 Pressure-time curve representing controlled mandatory ventilation

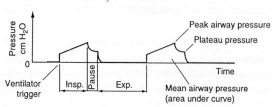

PSV is similar to the BiPAP mode in non-invasive ventilation, where IPAP equates to the pressure support level and EPAP (Ch. 7) relates to PEEP. The terms 'Assist Mode' or 'Continuous Spontaneous Ventilation' are sometimes used for this mode.

Proportional assist ventilation

This is similar to PSV but the supporting pressure provides a positive feedback system by varying in proportion to patient effort, providing a form of 'power steering' so that the harder the patient pulls, the more the ventilator pushes (Carteaux et al 2013) (Fig 17.6c). On some ventilators it is a useful weaning mode because it knows how much work the patient is doing, but there may be some expiratory asynchrony if the machine does not match cycling to the patient.

Assist mode

This is also similar to PSV and the terms are sometimes used interchangeably, but the breathing pattern is more dependent on the characteristics of the machine.

Neurally adjusted ventilatory assist

This mode detects electrical signals from the diaphragm to co-ordinate inspiration with spontaneous breathing, the ventilator acting like a muscle under patient neural command. It has shown better patient-ventilator synchrony and oxygenation than PSV (Richard 2011).

Bilevel positive airways pressure (BiPAP)

BiPAP through the ventilator is equivalent to the support provided by non-invasive ventilation used with spontaneously-breathing patients (Ch. 7).

Biphasic positive airways pressure (BIPAP)

The term BIPAP, with a capital 'I', was invented by someone with an interesting sense of humour. It is not BiPAP with a small 'i', as above, but allows spontaneous breathing at pre-set high and low levels (Fig 17.6d) and may help reduce intrinsic PEEP (Gama et al 2010). It has some similarities to airway pressure release ventilation, below.

Airway pressure release ventilation (APRV)

This is pressure-controlled and time-cycled, with unrestricted spontaneous breathing throughout the cycle.

High and low pressure levels are pre-set, as with BIPAP, but the low level pressure lasts for just a second or so to allow CO_2 to escape and fresh gas to fill the alveoli (Fig 17.6e), leading to an I:E ratio of about 8:1. Pre-set parameters are the high and low pressures, and the time at each pressure level. Expiratory release time is set short enough to prevent alveolar derecruitment and it may prevent the development of ARDS in vulnerable patients (Roy et al 2013). Unlike BIPAP, the I:E ratio is always inverted and there is rarely time for spontaneous breathing to occur at the lower level. Porhomayon (2010) claims that optimum benefit occurs approximately eight hours after implementation.

Problems with APRV are that:

- the long inspiratory time inhibits venous return so the mode is unsuited to haemodynamically-unstable patients
- the short expiratory time facilitates gas trapping.

Continuous positive airway pressure (CPAP)

CPAP (Fig 17.6f) provides a level of positive pressure, devoid of mandatory breaths, within which the patient breathes spontaneously. For intubated patients, CPAP follows the same principle as non-invasive CPAP (Ch. 6) but without the complications of a mask.

CPAP is suited to patients who have poor gas exchange, as with mask CPAP. It is also helpful to reduce intrinsic PEEP because it splints open the airways throughout the cycle to allow trapped gas to escape. Some ventilators confusingly use the term CPAP when inspiratory pressures are greater than expiratory pressures, which is actually BiPAP.

Mandatory minute ventilation (MMV)

This mode provides a guaranteed pre-set minute volume if the patient's spontaneous breathing drops below a pre-set level. Pressure support may be added to ensure an adequate V_T for patients with rapid shallow breathing.

Strategies of ventilation

Inverse-ratio ventilation (IRV)

For patients with refractory hypoxaemia and high peak airway pressures, mean airway pressure can be raised and peak airway pressure reduced by prolonging

FIGURE 17.6 Pressure-time curves showing (a) synchronized intermittent mandatory ventilation, (b) pressure support ventilation, (c) proportional assist ventilation, (d) biphasic positive airways pressure, (e) airway pressure release ventilation, (f) CPAP, in which all breaths are spontaneous

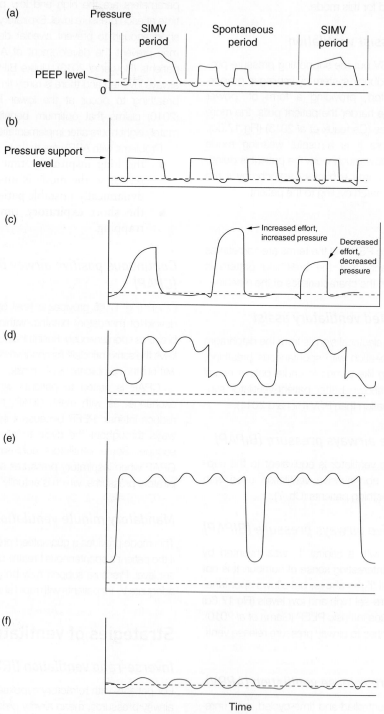

FIGURE 17.7 Pressure-time waveform showing increasing levels of inverse-ratio ventilation

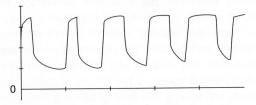

inspiratory time to the point of reversing the I:E ratio (Fig 17.7). This is achieved by slowing inspiratory flow or increasing the inspiratory pause, and encourages recruitment of collapsed alveoli.

An unexpected bonus is that IRV provides an 'expiratory flow bias' because of the faster expiratory time, which encourages mucus to move towards the mouth (Volpe *et al* 2008). Disadvantages of IRV are the risk of intrinsic PEEP, over-stretched alveoli, compromised cardiac output and the discomfort of an unnatural breathing pattern during which the patient is often unable to fully exhale. Heavy sedation is used and no spontaneous breathing allowed.

Lung protective ventilation

Deliberately under ventilating a patient reduces the pressure and volume risks of MV. Blood gas targets are modified and a low minute volume allows P_aCO_2 to rise as far as 8 kPa (60 cmH$_2$O), with pH and oxygenation closely monitored. Acid-base compensation restores pH in the brain and myocardium over several hours, and unacceptable respiratory acidosis can be prevented by decreasing dead space and increasing RR, while cyclic recruitment-derecruitment and hyperinflation are reduced (Retamal *et al* 2013). Some acidosis brings the unexpected benefit of attenuating ventilator-induced lung injury (Contreras *et al* 2012). Hypercapnia is normally tolerated so long as the kidneys are functioning well enough to stabilize the acid-base status. S_pO_2 may be allowed to sink to 88% so long as tissue oxygenation is monitored (Macintyre 2013).

This 'permissive hypercapnia' is used for people with ARDS or acute asthma (Chang 2014 p.379), and may be used to prevent or reduce alveolar inflammation in other patients (Richard 2011).

Patients may feel breathless and suffocated if this strategy is not carefully managed (Vincent *et al* 2002), and there is a risk of atelectasis (Gilbert *et al* 2009) but adequate PEEP may prevent this (Luecke 2004). It is

normally contraindicated in conditions intolerant of hypercapnia such as acute brain injury, severe pulmonary hypertension or congestive heart failure (Gattinoni *et al* 2002).

> **PRACTICE TIP**
>
> Find out which ventilator is used in your ICU, research it online to clarify the terminology, then ask if you can go in pairs to the ICU and sit in front of a spare ventilator with the handbook to correlate what you have learnt.

Settings

> *Sometimes it's going too fast for you, so instead of the machine synchronizing with you, you have to synchronize with the machine.*
> Patient quoted by Jablonski (1994)

Ventilation and oxygenation are matched to the patient according to P_aCO_2 and P_aO_2 respectively. Minute ventilation ($\dot{V}_E$) is adjusted according to P_aCO_2, V_T being adjusted for a small change and RR adjusted for a larger change. Normal values for $\dot{V}_E$ vary widely: a mechanically ventilated COPD patient with chronic hypercapnia requires a great deal less than a hypermetabolic septic patient. The trend is towards low tidal volume lung protective strategies to minimize complications (Kilickaya 2013). Ventilator settings can be adjusted to reduce dyspnoea in the 35% of patients suffering this symptom (Schmidt *et al* 2011), or to influence flow bias by manipulating flow rate, I:E ratio and PEEP (Graf & Marini 2008).

Inspired oxygen concentration (F_iO_2) is adjusted according to P_aO_2, although the relationship between F_iO_2 and P_aO_2 is less direct than that between $\dot{V}_E$ and P_aCO_2 because P_aO_2 is subject to more variables.

Inspiratory flow rate is set from about 40 l/min (e.g. with ARDS in order to prolong inspiration and the time for gas exchange) to about 100 l/min (e.g. with COPD in order to increase expiratory time and limit hyperinflation). **I:E ratio** is normally 1:2 to allow adequate expiratory time for CO$_2$ clearance and to facilitate venous return. Levels as low as 1:4 are used to help prevent intrinsic PEEP and as high as 4:1 (inverse-ratio ventilation) to help recruit alveoli. It is manipulated by the flow rate, RR, $\dot{V}_E$ and/or inspiratory time.

Inspiratory pause (plateau) provides an end-inspiratory-hold which enhances gas distribution by allowing time for recruitment of poorly ventilated alveoli.

Alarms are set for pressure, volume, flow and levels of oxygen and CO_2. It is useful to learn the characteristics of the alarms for each machine, including reset time.

The **100% oxygen** button can be used freely by physiotherapists and has a timed cut off. Experienced physiotherapists may use other buttons, e.g. for ventilator hyperinflation, as part of the team.

Complications

The adverse effects of MV are of particular interest to the physiotherapist because some effects are increased by the extra positive pressure of manual hyperinflation. Added to the complications of intubation are those described below.

Impaired cardiac output

The heart is a pressure chamber within a pressure chamber. Positive pressure in the chest impedes venous return, leading to decreased cardiac output and sometimes reduced blood flow to insatiable organs such as the kidney, liver and brain (De Beer 2013). Compensatory peripheral vasoconstriction normally maintains BP, but this is less viable in patients who are elderly, or who suffer autonomic neuropathy such as with Guillain-Barré syndrome, or are hypovolaemic, either absolutely or functionally due to the vasodilation of septic shock. These patients may become hypotensive at the initiation of MV or on repositioning (Vollman 2013).

Haemodynamic compromise is most likely with high mean airway pressures, prolonged inspiratory time or high PEEP levels. Haemodynamic stability can be facilitated by fluids, inotropic drugs or reduced I:E ratios so that expiratory time is longer and the heart has time to fill. Patients with poorly-compliant lungs suffer less haemodynamic compromise because pressure is transmitted less easily through stiff lungs.

Barotrauma

Barotrauma related to MV is when air gets into the wrong place, e.g. pneumothorax, subcutaneous emphysema, pneumopericardium or pneumomediastinum

(Kim *et al* 2013c). The prefix 'baro-' arose from assumptions that the cause was excess pressure because these complications are associated with high plateau pressures. But it is now understood that excess volume, specifically end-inspiratory volume, is the main culprit because sustained alveolar distension stretches and ruptures the delicate alveolar-capillary membrane. This explains why coughing, when pressure increases massively but volume is stable, rarely causes barotrauma. The term 'volutrauma' rather than 'barotrauma' is sometimes used to describe extra-alveolar air in this context, but the two concepts are linked via the pressure-volume curve (Ch. 1).

Box 17.1 indicates the process, air first squeezing out from distended alveoli (Fig 17.8) especially if the lungs are hyperinflated or unevenly damaged, then tracking centrally along the bronchovascular sheaths and getting into the interstitial spaces, where it is known as **pulmonary interstitial emphysema**. This is difficult to detect radiologically in adults unless contrast is provided by a background of generalized opacification (air bronchogram) such as with ARDS, but it may show in infants as a mottled opacity. This can lead to **pneumomediastinum**, i.e. air around the mediastinum, which can dissect up into the neck. This is rarely dangerous but may be the first warning to avoid manual hyperinflation. Air may then creep under the skin, causing **subcutaneous emphysema** (Fig 17.9), or into the pleura, causing **pneumothorax** (Postmus 2013) (see Figs 2.21, 20.5a).

BOX 17.1

Development of baro/volutrauma

extrusion of gas into bronchovascular sheaths
↓
pulmonary interstitial emphysema
↓
proximal dissection into mediastinum
↓
pneumomediastinum
↓
decompression through other fascial planes
↓
subcutaneous emphysema   pneumothorax

Pneumopericardium is a form of barotrauma but is more likely to be observed after heart surgery, chest trauma (Plurad *et al* 2013), in neonates with stiff lungs or with recreational drug use (Vargas *et al* 2013). It shows as a dark outline contouring the heart and sometimes crossing the midline above the diaphragm, the 'continuous diaphragm' sign (Fig 17.10). The air does not dissect up into the neck.

Ventilator-induced lung injury

Injury to the alveoli can be caused by the abrasive stress of cyclic opening (recruitment) and closing (derecruitment), particularly at low lung volumes (Dickson 2013). Healthy lung can usually withstand this, but repetitive stretch and collapse of alveoli in patients with injured lungs can provoke inflammation, pulmonary oedema and ventilator-induced lung injury, also known as atelectrauma (Jacob *et al* 2013). Insult is added to injury if inflammation disseminates via the systemic circulation and sets off multisystem failure, especially if a chest infection increases the risk of bacterial translocation (Fletcher & Cuthbertson 2010).

The risk is reduced by incorporating spontaneous breaths into the breathing cycle, limiting plateau pressure, ensuring adequate PEEP to minimize derecruitment, modifying the waveform to increase surfactant (Amin & Suki 2012), using lung protective strategies such as high-frequency oscillation (Ronchi 2014) or

FIGURE 17.9 Soft tissue shadowing under the skin of the right trunk, indicating subcutaneous emphysema. The patient also has a R chest drain, suggesting a recent pneumothorax. He is also intubated and has a partially calcified aorta, hinting at advanced age

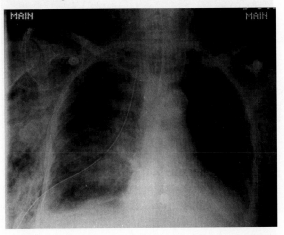

proning the patient to reduce stretch on ventral lung tissue (Gattinoni *et al* 2013).

Gastroesophageal reflux

The more positive the pressure, the more the stomach contents can be pushed up into the oesophagus. Positioning reduces the risk (Ch. 3).

FIGURE 17.8 Development of barotrauma. Left: cross-section of normal alveoli and vessels. Right: overdistended alveoli rupturing through the alveolar-capillary membranes

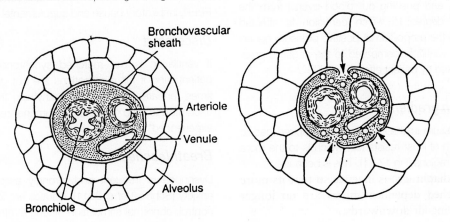

Bronchovascular sheath

Arteriole

Venule

Alveolus

Bronchiole

FIGURE 17.10 Chest trauma following a car accident, showing a continuous diaphragm sign indicating pneumopericardium, fractured ribs anteriorly on the left, and a kinked chest drain

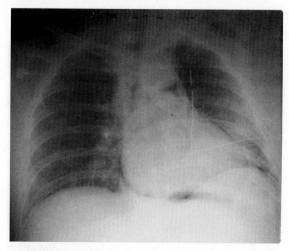

Weakness and muscle damage

Unlike with an actively-contracting diaphragm, perfusion to the muscle is reduced by the passive displacement caused by MV (Davis & Bruells 2012). Full CMV leads to diaphragmatic dysfunction in 6–24 hours (Martin *et al* 2013), which is linked to infection and mortality (Petrof 2013). Patient immobility also promotes generalized muscle weakness (Chen & Lin 2012).

Perfusion gradient

Positive pressure accentuates the perfusion gradient from upper to lower regions (Fig 17.11), leaving nondependent regions cyclically without blood flow (West 2012 p.45), and pushing out blood overall from the chest. The degree to which perfusion is affected depends on the proportion of positive pressure generated by the ventilator compared to the negative pressure generated by patient effort.

Ventilation gradient

Positive pressure in the chest directs inspired gas to take the path of least resistance, which is to the more open upper regions (Fig 17.11). This is because:

- The diaphragm is inactive so that its more stretched dependent fibres are no longer drawing air downwards.

- Dependent lung is less compliant due to compression by the increased perfusion.

Dependent areas therefore receive the least ventilation and are vulnerable to progressive atelectasis. This is ameliorated when a mode of ventilation is used in which spontaneous breathing is encouraged.

Atelectasis

Risk factors for volume loss are reversed ventilation gradient, immobility, a low tidal volume and impaired surfactant secretion (Moloney 2004). This can lead to atelectasis, consolidation and ventilator-induced pneumonia (Ntoumenopoulos & Glickman 2012).

KEY POINT

The main physiotherapy contribution to prevention of atelectasis is regular and accurate position change, and as much activity as is subjectively and objectively feasible.

Increased dead space

Dead space increases because of reduced overall perfusion, and to a lesser extent because of the ventilator tubing.

Ventilation/perfusion ($\dot{V}_A/\dot{Q}$) mismatch

The above complications lead to $\dot{V}_A/\dot{Q}$ mismatch and increased shunt (Vimlati 2012), which would lead to hypoxaemia if not offset by ventilator settings such as PEEP, inspiratory pause and supplemental oxygen.

Discomfort

If ventilation is not matched synchronously to the patient, and if full explanations are not given, sometimes repeatedly, MV can be anything from 'grossly uncomfortable' to 'the most inhumane treatment ever experienced' (Chlan 2011).

Breathlessness

Dyspnoea is frequent and strongly associated with anxiety (Schmidt *et al* 2011). Causes are feeling out of control, abnormal stimulation of lung stretch receptors

FIGURE 17.11 Effect of controlled mandatory ventilation on ventilation and perfusion gradients. The perfusion gradient increases downwards and (compared to healthy young subjects) the ventilation gradient is reversed. See also Fig 1.8

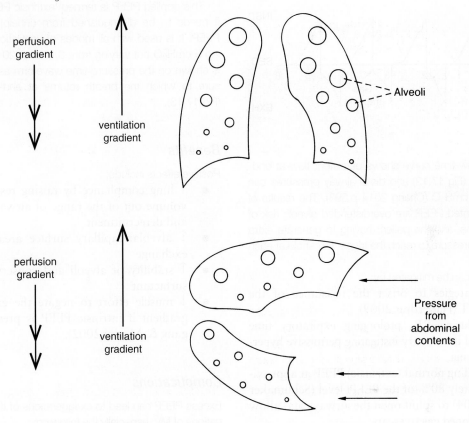

or asynchrony with the ventilator. Asynchrony is indicated by patient report and confirmed by flow or pressure waveforms (Branson et al 2013). After checking for anxiety, secretions and the adequacy of ventilation (by $\dot{V}_E$ or P_aCO_2), the intensivist should be informed so that ventilator settings can be adjusted.

Gut and kidney dysfunction

Splanchnic blood flow does not have autoregulation capabilities and is dependant on BP. It is, therefore, vulnerable to haemodynamic upset, as well as the abdominal distension that is common in ICU patients. Reduced perfusion may increase the permeability of the gut mucosal barrier, facilitating multisystem failure, paralytic ileus, bleeding and ulceration. Haemodynamic compromise triples the risk of acute kidney injury (Akker et al 2013).

Excess secretions

Bronchial secretions are increased due to irritation from the tracheal tube and impaired mucociliary clearance.

Intrinsic PEEP

Gas trapping can be quantified in terms of volume (hyperinflation) or pressure (intrinsic PEEP or PEEPi), though the terms are interchangeable in practice. PEEPi is unwelcome PEEP which occurs unintentionally when exhalation has not finished before the next breath triggers into inspiration (see Fig 3.3). It is commonest with hyperinflation conditions such as COPD or acute asthma, when air is trapped by obstructed airways, or in unevenly damaged ARDS lungs. Lung emptying is also impeded by a narrow endotracheal tube or rapid breathing, which does not allow enough time for expiration.

FIGURE 17.12 Flow-time waveform of IRV with gas trapping as the air starts flowing in before exhalation is finished. $\dot{V}$: flow in litres per minute.

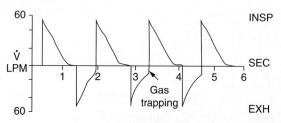

The flow-time curve shows persistent flow at end-expiration (Fig 17.12) and distal airway pressures can reach 15 cmH_2O (Chang 2014 p.393). The results of this unwanted PEEP are overdistended alveoli, risk of barotrauma, and the patient having to generate extra negative pressure to reach the trigger threshold at each breath.

PEEPi can be mitigated by:

- strategies to offset the resistance of the ETT (Haberthur 2009)
- reducing RR, prolonging expiratory time and if necessary instigating permissive hypercapnia
- adding normal (extrinsic) PEEP at approximately 80% of the PEEPi level (Schumaker 2004) to splint open the airways and allow trapped gas to escape
- airway clearance to reduce airway resistance.

Positive End-Expiratory Pressure (PEEP)

There are several ways to boost S_pO_2:

- $\uparrow F_iO_2$
- prolong the plateau (Fig 17.4a)
- $\uparrow$ the I:E ratio
- $\uparrow$ PEEP.

To all intents and purposes, PEEP is CPAP, but the term is used for ventilated patients only and does not require the patient to breathe. PEEP raises functional residual capacity (FRC) and maintains constant positive pressure in the lungs throughout the respiratory cycle so that airway pressure does not fall to atmospheric pressure at end-exhalation. It cannot itself recruit lung

volume without using excessively high pressures (Hess & Bigatello 2002) and if recruitment potential is low, increasing PEEP may simply contribute to over-distention of already open alveoli (Hess 2011b).

This applied PEEP is termed 'extrinsic PEEP' when it needs to be distinguished from unhelpful intrinsic PEEP. It is used with all modes of ventilation, averaging 5 cmH_2O but varying from 3 to over 20 cmH_2O. It is shown on the pressure-time waveform as the pressure to which the breath returns at end-exhalation (Fig 17.13).

Benefits

Positive effects include:

- $\uparrow$ lung compliance by raising resting lung volume out of the range of airway closure and derecruitment
- $\uparrow$ alveolar-capillary surface area for gas exchange
- $\uparrow$ stability of alveoli and conservation of surfactant
- $\downarrow$ muscle effort to negate the expiratory gradient if intrinsic PEEP is present (Pei-gang & Marini 2002).

Complications

Excess PEEP can lead to exaggerations of the complications of MV, especially the following:

1 Continuous positive pressure may impair venous return and cardiac output. This can offset the beneficial effects of PEEP by causing a net decrease in oxygen delivery to the tissues. Haemodynamic compromise usually occurs at >15 cmH_2O PEEP in normovolaemic patients, at higher pressures in patients with stiff lungs and at lower pressures in hypovolaemic patients. Fluid administration can stabilize cardiac output, but may incur pulmonary oedema when PEEP is discontinued. PEEP above 5 cmH_2O should be applied in small increments and titrated against oxygen delivery.

2 High pressure PEEP increases the risk of barotrauma, especially in patients with ARDS (Chang 2014 p.409) or other hyperinflation conditions unless it is being carefully targeted to reduce intrinsic PEEP.

FIGURE 17.13

- Pressure-time waveform for CMV (labelled 'IPPV' on this ventilator).
- Top right shows what is delivered to the patient: F_iO_2 indicates that 21% oxygen (i.e. air) is delivered, P_{peak} shows a peak airway pressure of 30 cmH$_2$O, P_{plat} shows a plateau pressure of 24 cmH$_2$O, MV indicates minute volume of 5.4 l/min.
- The lower half of the screen shows what is pre-set, i.e. oxygen at 21%, V_T at 500 ml, inspiratory time at 1.70 seconds, frequency (RR) at 12 bpm, inspiratory flow at 60 l/min, PEEP at 5 cmH$_2$O.

PEEP showing at 5 cm H$_2$O on the pressure-time curve

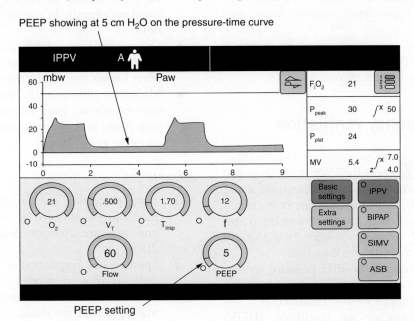

PEEP setting

3 High PEEP may disrupt the alveolar-capillary barrier and redistribute alveolar fluid, leading to pulmonary oedema.

4 Excessive PEEP compresses pulmonary capillaries and decreases compliance by overdistending alveoli.

Raised pressure within the chest increases CVP and PAWP readings (p.440-1) at the same time as the ventricular filling pressure which they represent is declining because of impaired venous return. This is not a complication but allowance is made for this during assessment.

Best PEEP

Optimum PEEP is achieved when it is titrated to ventilation homogeneity through electrical impedence tomography (Chang 2014 p.496), or to maximum tissue oxygenation (Bikker 2013), or to a balance of S_pO_2 and cardiac output. Fig 17.14 shows how best PEEP improves ventilation to the lung bases. When altering

PEEP, time to equilibrium is longer when increasing it than when decreasing it (Chiumello 2013).

FIGURE 17.14 Effect of PEEP on regional pressure and volume relationships, showing how it raises dependent lung onto a steep part of the compliance curve, thereby encouraging basal ventilation.

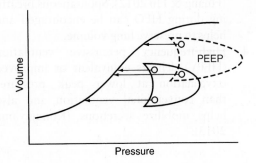

Precautions

High level PEEP is a risk with intracranial hypertension or an undrained pneumothorax, and may be detrimental for patients who have subcutaneous emphysema, bulla, bronchopleural fistula or following lung surgery. Hypovolaemia is a relative contraindication, but if high PEEP is necessary, cardiac output can be supported with fluids and inotropes. At high PEEP levels, manual hyperinflation requires modifications (Ch. 18).

Disconnecting the ventilator circuit for suction is detrimental in PEEP-dependent patients but this risk is eliminated with an in-line suction catheter.

High frequency ventilation

How does the Himalayan mountain shrew maintain oxygenation during copulation? With a RR up to 600 bpm, its tidal volume (V_T) is less than its dead space, but it manages to achieve gas exchange for this important task by a mechanism similar to the intriguing phenomenon of high frequency ventilation (HFV). High RR and low V_T are achieved by the following:

1 High frequency positive pressure ventilation uses time-cycled conventional ventilation at rates of 50–100 breaths/min.
2 High frequency jet ventilation (HFJV) directs short rapid jets of gas through a nozzle into the airways and entrains air by the Venturi principle (Ch. 5). Expiration is by passive recoil and rates of 100–600 breaths/min are achieved (Sutterlin *et al* 2014).
3 High frequency oscillation (HFO) forces mini-bursts of gas in and out of the airway at 3–20 breaths/sec so that both inspiration and expiration are active. It may help patients with refractory hypoxaemia (Huang & Hu 2012). Spontaneous breathing during HFO can be encouraged and helps to preserve lung volume.
4 High-frequency percussive ventilation (HFPV) delivers equivalent or improved oxygenation at lower peak pressures than conventional ventilation and also helps mobilize secretions (Kunugiyama 2013).

Mechanism

With such a meagre V_T, gas exchange cannot rely on bulk flow of gas. The classic concept of 'dead' space is no longer applicable, and this space is in fact thought to play an active part in gas exchange by the following mechanisms:

● High velocity flow creates turbulent mixing in the central airways, which is propagated peripherally by convective inspiratory flow.
● Gas mixing may occur by filling and emptying alveoli independent of each other, an effect known merrily as 'disco lung'.
● Molecular diffusion, the primary mechanism of normal gas exchange in terminal lung units, is augmented, especially by the vibrating gas of HFO.

Advantages

1 Lung protection for patients with acute lung injury is afforded by minimal volume and pressure changes (Siau & Stewart 2008).
2 Spontaneous respiration is inhibited and little sedation is needed. Most patients find the sensation comfortable, as if being massaged from the inside.
3 HFV provides an even distribution of ventilation because diffusion is independent of regional compliance and gas flow does not take the path of least resistance.
4 HFJV via minitracheostomy allows spontaneous breathing through the normal airway.

Disadvantages

1 Shallow breaths hinder lung recruitment.
2 Except with HFO, high inspiratory flows and limited exhalation time risk generating intrinsic PEEP.
3 Noise can be a problem.

Indications

High frequency ventilation tends to be used as a rescue mode when other techniques have failed. The following may benefit:

- patients with vulnerable lungs such as those with ARDS or neonatal respiratory distress syndrome (Sun *et al* 2014), bronchopleural fistula (Wood 2014), large air leak or flail chest
- patients unable to tolerate large pressure swings in the chest, e.g. those with acute brain injury or unstable cardiovascular status.

Physiotherapy

Suction can be performed without interruption of ventilation, and has less adverse effects on oxygenation or heart rhythm than with conventional MV. F_iO_2 must be increased by about 20% for three minutes before and after suction because manual hyperinflation is usually not possible, although a system has been created for its use with HFO (Hickey 2006). Jet ventilation through a minitracheostomy allows patients to take deep breaths and cough.

Weaning and extubation

I was sure I would not be able to breathe on my own. The machine was put to a setting which gave me a couple of breaths and the rest was up to me. I hated that, I never knew when to take my breaths.
Ludwig (patient and physiotherapist) 1984

Multidisciplinary teamwork speeds weaning and can increase survival for long term patients (Black *et al* 2012). The physiotherapist may construct the weaning plan (Danbury *et al* 2013), assisted by protocols (Plani *et al* 2013) and sometimes facilitated by automated closed loop weaning systems (Rose *et al* 2013). It is claimed that some comfortable interactive ventilator modes do not need to be 'weaned' (MacIntyre 2013b).

Weaning should be seamless, and the physiotherapist starts as soon as a patient is intubated, the process being integral to their rehabilitation programme. The first step is a preliminary rest and good night's sleep, then little-and-often exercise is initiated as the patient is able, e.g. squeezing a ball and quadriceps contractions. A graduated exercise programme is then developed, which has shown shortened weaning times (Chen & Lin 2012).

The proportion of patients experiencing difficulty weaning is 25% and rising (Martin *et al* 2013), especially for those with chronic lung disease or neuropathies, and anyone after prolonged ventilatory support. They may benefit from inspiratory muscle training (Smith *et al* 2014); Cader *et al* (2012) report that ventilator manipulations do not provide an effective training stimulus, but the physiotherapist may be able to negotiate a protocol that ensures adequate rest and appropriate inspiratory muscle exercise through the ventilator.

Liberation from the ventilator entails:

- progressive and intermittent reduction in support until the patient is able to sustain spontaneous breathing
- a trial of spontaneous breathing through the tracheal tube using a T-piece, CPAP or pressure support ventilation
- extubation.

KEY POINT

The physiotherapist's contribution to the team management of weaning is to advise on the balance of rest and exercise, to assess the breathing pattern, and sometimes to extubate the patient.

Intermittent reduction in ventilatory support

Reduction in ventilatory support involves periods of decreasing pressure on PSV or decreasing number of breaths in SIMV mode, the latter being considered less effective (Tanaka 2013). This is interspersed with adequate rest, including full ventilator support at night (Chang 2014 p.528), because if the respiratory muscles become fatigued (Fig 17.15) they may need 24 hours to recover (Laghi *et al* 2002). Clear explanations and autonomy are the first priority, and a fan is often helpful.

A daily sedation break enables screening for consciousness, oxygenation, ventilation, airway patency and cardiovascular stability. The following then identify readiness to proceed:

- correction of the underlying reason for MV
- optimum nutrition, fluid, metabolic and cardiovascular status, including adequate haemoglobin

FIGURE 17.15 Failed weaning attempt. Fatigue develops at first, represented by ↑ RR, ↓ P_aCO_2 and alkalosis. Then exhaustion supervenes, represented by ↓ RR, ↑ P_aCO_2 and acidosis

RR: respiratory rate.

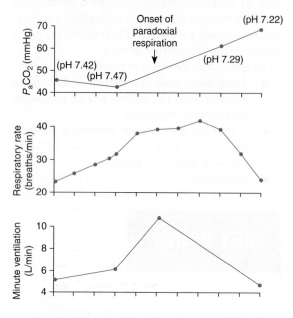

- elimination of unnecessary work of breathing (WOB), e.g. optimum bronchodilation, clear airways, minimum intrinsic PEEP and no abdominal distension
- restoration of normal diurnal rhythm
- minimum pain and reversal of sedation, although certain sedatives may assist weaning once explanations have been given (Shehabi 2010)
- maximum ventilatory reserve and optimum gas exchange: pH and P_aCO_2 related to the individual's premorbid state, vital capacity >10 ml/kg, maximum inspiratory pressure >20 cmH$_2$O, shunt <15%, dead space <60% of tidal volume, P_aO_2 >11 kPa on F_iO_2 of 0.4 and RR <24 (Santos 2013)
- absence of abdominal paradox or rapid shallow breathing (Epstein 2002), which can be monitored objectively by a rapid shallow breathing index (RR/V$_T$) of <100 bpm/litre (Chang 2014 p.526).

Trial of spontaneous breathing

The patient takes up their preferred position (usually sitting upright), suction is applied if required, and spontaneous breathing encouraged, with either (a) support from PSV or CPAP at the same level as would equate to spontaneous breathing without a tracheal tube, or (b), after disconnection from the ventilator, with a T-piece.

For T-piece weaning, high flow humidified oxygen is connected to the inspiratory limb, and for breathless people 30 cm of extension tubing is attached to the expiratory limb in order to avoid entrainment of room air during inspiration. The oxygen flow must be high enough, and extension tubing long enough, to avoid interruption of the mist that should exit throughout inspiration and expiration. Breathing through a T-piece alone is hard work without the support of PSV, CPAP or high flow nasal cannulae (Van Beers *et al* 2012) and also means that the patient is not connected to the bells and whistles of the ventilator for monitoring.

Increasing periods of spontaneous breathing are encouraged, while questioning the patient to ensure that fatigue is avoided, and observing for laboured breathing, desaturation, rising P_aCO_2 or drowsiness. Motivation is helped by liberal praise and the 'exercise' part of the process lasting no longer than promised. A dyspnoea visual analogue scale enables patients to contribute to weaning decisions, and they need a 'day off' if a setback such as infection or diarrhoea occurs.

Continuing problems may be due to weaning strategies which provide neither sufficient muscle work nor sufficient rest (Fig 17.16a), leading to muscle atrophy and/or fatigue. Fatigued muscles cannot be trained, and fatigue may prolong weaning or lead to muscle injury because patients cannot rest their respiratory muscles as they can other skeletal muscles.

Patients undergoing protracted weaning are best given short but increasing periods of significant work during the day (Fig 17.16b), and full ventilator support in between (Epstein 2002).

A hot-water humidifier should normally be used because a heat moisture exchanger causes significant airflow resistance (Uchiyama *et al* 2013). Other difficulties may be undetected diaphragmatic paralysis, obstructive sleep apnoea or fear of suffocation. Fears are managed by providing information and extra ventilatory support when required. Patients unable to wean should be referred to a home ventilation and weaning unit (Danbury *et al* 2013).

FIGURE 17.16 (a) Gradual weaning without periods of rest to replenish the respiratory muscles. (b) Intermittent weaning with periods of complete rest for muscle recovery and periods of maximal work for muscle training.

(a)
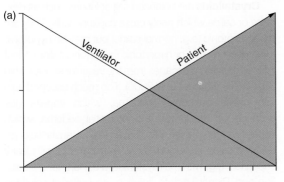

(b)
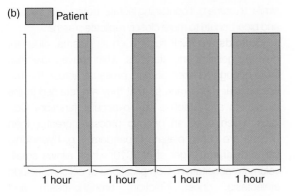

| 1 hour | 1 hour | 1 hour | 1 hour |

PRACTICE TIP

Patients have reported that their primary experience during weaning is exhaustion (Twibell *et al* 2003), which reinforces the importance of taking their views into account throughout.

Extubation

A single, memorable moment of relief.
Patient quoted by
Karlsson & Forsberg 2008

Weaning indices are limited as predictors for extubation (Savi *et al* 2012) but extubation is usually feasible if the reason for intubation has been alleviated, there is a stable breathing pattern, the patient can perform an adequate peak cough flow (Su *et al* 2010), pressure support level is <12 cmH$_2$O, PEEP <7 cmH$_2$O (Grinnan & Truwit 2005) and there is a leak when the cuff is deflated, indicating adequate patency of the upper airway. Inflammation may cause swelling in the upper airway which only becomes apparent by the development of stridor after extubation.

Another problem is the haemodynamic decompensation that can occur when PEEP is removed. Loaded spontaneous inspiration, in particular, can lead to increased venous return and possible pulmonary oedema in people with COPD and a cardiac history (Porhomayon *et al* 2012). It has been suggested that patients are given 30 minutes' unsupported spontaneous breathing through a T-piece before extubation, to ensure that they can cope with the extra cardiac load (Tobin 2012), but longer than this can risk atelectasis (Singer & Webb 2009 p. 16) as well as exhaustion.

The steps for extubation are described by Cooper *et al* (2012) and Chang (2014) p.179. If sputum retention is anticipated, it is sometimes better to request a minitracheostomy than await respiratory distress. Non-invasive ventilation (NIV) is advised in high-risk or hypercapnic patients (Thille *et al* 2013), including those with COPD or neurological disease (Hess 2012).

Emergency reintubation is mostly for respiratory reasons and increases mortality five-fold (Nithya *et al* 2012).

Decannulation of tracheostomy

Weaning for tracheostomied patients incorporates an intermediate step of replacing the cuffed tube with an uncuffed tube (Powell *et al* 2011), which is then plugged for increasingly longer periods to test for adequate breathing and coughing. When plugged, the inner cannula must be removed. The tube is not usually downsized because this increases the resistance to airflow (Valentini 2012). Adjuncts are a Passy-Muir valve to encourage air flow around the tube (Engels *et al* 2009) or alternating with NIV (Duan *et al* 2012).

The tube can be removed when there is a satisfactory cough reflex, cough effectiveness and oxygenation, and minimum secretions (Stelfox *et al* 2008). Neurological patients require peak cough flow testing (McKim 2012).

Once the tube is removed, the patient is taught to hold a sterile dressing over the stoma when coughing. For those leaving the ICU with a tracheostomy, a removable inner tube is essential in case of blockage.

FLUIDS

- **Dehydration:** intracellular and interstitial water deficit, as shown by a dry tongue and low skin turgor.
- **Hypovolaemia** or **volume depletion:** intravascular fluid depletion, due, for example, to severe dehydration or haemorrhage, which affects haemodynamic stability.
- **Preload:**
  - pressure of blood in the ventricles just before systole which stretches the myocardium and assists contraction, determined by venous return and blood volume
  - increased in heart failure or fluid overload, decreased in hypovolaemic shock
  - left preload is monitored by PAWP, right preload by CVP.
- **Afterload:**
  - pressure in large vessels against which ventricles must work during systole, as if opening the door against a wind
  - increased with systemic/pulmonary hypertension or vasoconstriction, decreased with vasodilation e.g. in septic or neurogenic shock
  - left ventricular afterload is monitored by systolic BP and right by pulmonary artery pressure and varies with pulmonary vascular resistance.

Fluid imbalance can arise from hypovolaemia, hypervolaemia, or normovolaemia with maldistribution of fluid. Blood volume determines preload and is the basis of haemodynamic stability, so an adequate circulating volume is the primary consideration before drugs or other forms of support are given. Manual hyperinflation and suction are risky in hypovolaemic patients.

Plasma fluid in the intravascular space (Fig 17.17) is the only fluid compartment accessible therapeutically. Greater than 10% loss of blood volume reduces cardiac output, while more than 20% can reduce BP. Fluid resuscitation must be balanced in order to avoid interstitial fluid overload or, conversely, allowing the kidney to run dry. Fluids may be isotonic, hypotonic or hypertonic in relation to plasma, and electrolytes play an integral role (Overgaard 2013). Administered fluids are either crystalloid or colloid.

Crystalloids are balanced salt solutions such as dextrose or saline which freely cross capillary walls. They are mostly isotonic (e.g. normal saline) but may be hypotonic (dextrose in water) or hypertonic (hypertonic saline). Most infused crystalloid escapes from the vascular space within 30 minutes (Vercueil et al 2006). Too much escaped fluid can cause pulmonary oedema, which impairs gas exchange in the lungs, and interstitial oedema, which impairs oxygen delivery into tissue cells. Enthusiastic crystalloid infusion is particularly risky in patients with leaky capillaries, e.g. with multisystem failure. Hartmann's solution and Ringer-Lactate solution are buffered solutions similar to saline but containing lactate, potassium, calcium and bicarbonate to more closely replicate plasma.

Colloids are thick fluids such as plasma, albumin, dextran, gelatins and starches, which have molecules large enough to exert oncotic pressure across the microvascular membrane so that they are retained in the circulation and stabilize cardiovascular function. Colloids which have an oncotic pressure greater than plasma are called plasma expanders, e.g. hypertonic saline-dextran (Bulger et al 2010) which allows small-volume resuscitation. Complications of colloids include atelectasis, chest infection, bronchospasm and arrhythmias (Canet et al 2013).

FIGURE 17.17 Body fluid compartments in an average adult, showing 3 litres in blood vessels, 11 litres in the interstitial space and the rest in tissue cells. *ICF:* intracellular fluid; *ECF:* extracellular fluid

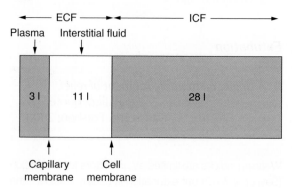

NUTRITION

Nutrition has changed from being an adjunct in critical care to definitive therapy, but malnutrition is common even today (Ramprasad 2012), one study finding 27% of patients to be overfed and 48.3% of patients underfed (De Waele *et al* 2012). Under-nutrition may be due to a hypermetabolic state, not necessarily inadequate calories, but rehabilitation is directly affected, one study showing how extra postoperative nutrition in orthopaedic patients enabled them to be independently mobile five days earlier than controls (Bastow *et al* 1983).

Causes of malnutrition

Many critically ill patients face a cumulative caloric debt during hospitalization because of:

- glucose intolerance or impaired perfusion to the liver or kidney
- gut stasis due to critical illness or surgery, leading to reduced food tolerance, malabsorption, reflux or aspiration (Chapman *et al* 2011)
- lack of recognition of a process as undramatic as malnourishment
- lack of a dietician on ward rounds (Soguel *et al* 2012)
- the patient's lack of hunger, ability to express hunger or capacity to eat normally
- 'critical illness' deranged blood sugar (Marics *et al* 2013)
- systemic inflammation, hypermetabolism or a catabolically stressed state (Plank 2013), in which protein reserves are stripped first from skeletal muscle and then from the viscera, at up to 1% of total body protein per day, particularly with burns or acute brain injury (Hill 2011).

Effects of malnutrition

Underfeeding is associated with muscle weakness, infection, impaired wound healing, increased length of stay and higher mortality (Hill 2011). Of particular interest to the physiotherapist is reduced surfactant predisposing to atelectasis and reduced albumin leading to pulmonary oedema and muscle weakness (Visser *et al* 2005).

Overfeeding with carbohydrate can destabilize blood sugar and increase CO_2 production, which may precipitate respiratory distress during weaning for patients who have little respiratory reserve (Chang 2014 p.406).

Inappropriate feeding facilitates tracheal colonization (Ahmed & Niederman 2001), and lack of antioxidant vitamins such as E and C contributes to oxidative stress and diaphragmatic atrophy (Jaber *et al* 2011). 'Refeeding syndrome' is caused by rapid feeding after starvation, identified first at the liberation of Auschwitz and recently in the anorexia nervosa population. This can occur 2 to 5 days after excess nutrients are administered to patients who have been starved for over 48 hours, leading to cardiopulmonary or neurological complications (Skipper 2012).

Management

Close liaison with the dietician is required because early attention to nutrition reduces the risk of myopathies and aids physical rehabilitation (Confer *et al* 2013). Severe illness requires protein replenishment, and major surgery or other trauma indicates the need for immunonutrition to strengthen the body's defences and dampen down inflammation (Cherry-Bukowiec 2013).

Enteral feeding should be initiated as soon as possible (Deane *et al* 2014). If patients are able, they should sit out and eat at normal times, orally if possible (Martin-Harris 2012), maintaining head and chest elevation at 30° for an hour afterwards. Mastication releases hormones that facilitate gut motility, but if patients cannot swallow, direct feeding beyond the stomach is advised (Deane 2013). A nasogastric tube risks aspiration (Jiyong *et al* 2013) and is placed in the stomach, which is the least tolerant area of the gut (Quirk 2000).

The gut is one of the largest immune systems in the body and needs regular bathing in nutrients to maintain its structural and functional integrity. Parenteral feeding leads to atrophy of the gut lining, which may allow intestinal flora access to the circulation, whence to wreak havoc and risk multisystem failure (Anastasilakis 2013). Enteral nutrition reduces infections (Omata *et al* 2013) and shortens length of stay (Heyland 2012).

To optimize rehabilitation, nutritional support needs to continue after discharge from the ICU (Merriweather *et al* 2014).

CRITICAL CARE DRUGS

Infusion pumps are used to titrate exact drug dosage to the individual because:

- some ICU drugs have a narrow window between effective and toxic doses
- individuals respond differently to complex interactions of multiple drugs
- physiological processing may be affected by the stress response
- ICU delirium has been associated with certain doses of sedatives, opiates, anticholinergics, antibiotics and steroids (Hipp & Ely 2012).
- Drugs may have to be adjusted if they rely on a failing organ for excretion.

Cardiovascular drugs

Cardiac output (CO) depends on heart rate (HR), contractility, preload and afterload. The relationship between heart function, vascular tone and fluid volume can be manipulated to augment CO, reduce myocardial oxygen demand or redistribute blood flow to vital organs.

Diuretics

Blood volume and preload are reduced by diuretics (Ch. 4).

Inotropes

Inotropes boost cardiac output. Fluid status should first be optimized to ensure adequate preload so that the drug is not stimulating an empty heart. Some inotropes have been called a 'necessary evil' because of their association with intrapulmonary shunt, neurological complications (Bryan 2013) and mortality (Shahin et al 2011). They are often given alongside vasodilators to reduce the extra work imposed on the heart (Bracht et al 2013).

Dopamine activates the same brain mechanism as falling in love (Xu 2012), but its less agreeable side effect of peripheral vasoconstriction limits its use, although a small 'renal dose' may selectively vasodilate vessels to the vulnerable kidney (Redfors et al 2012). **Dobutamine** gives a greater boost to oxygen delivery, but can cause myocardial damage, tissue hypoxia, bacterial growth and immunosuppression (Singer & Brealey 2011). **Dopexamine** increases renal and splanchnic blood flow and has some anti-inflammatory properties (Hollenberg 2013).

Adrenaline stimulates the sympathetic system and increases the speed and force of cardiac contraction, dilating coronary and skeletal muscle vessels but constricting peripheral vessels, which risks ischaemia to the kidney, gut and peripheries. **Noradrenaline** causes more generalized vasoconstriction.

Digoxin is a mild inotrope which has been in and out of fashion for two centuries. It helps control atrial fibrillation by strengthening and slowing the HR, but increases the risk of stroke in some patients (Chang et al 2013) and may increase mortality in patients with incident heart failure (Freeman 2013).

Vasodilators

Arterial dilators such as hydralazine reduce afterload and are used for hypertension. Venodilators such as the nitrates predominantly reduce preload.

Vasoconstrictors

Vasoconstrictors boost BP. High doses can reduce CO and sometimes impair brain and kidney perfusion (Müller et al 2008).

Beta-blockers

Beta-adrenoceptor blocking agents, or β-blockers, have a negative inotrope effect by blocking some heart activity (Ch. 4). They are also used for anxiety, migraine and glaucoma.

Pulmonary vasodilators

These drugs are used to treat pulmonary hypertension, e.g. in patients with ARDS (Spieth & Zhang 2014).

Nitric oxide (NO) has an unpromising history as a corrosive gas in bus exhausts, cigarette smoke and welding fumes, but more helpfully it dilates vessels adjacent to ventilated alveoli and reduces $\dot{V}_A/\dot{Q}$ mismatch. When inhaled, its effects are limited to the pulmonary vasculature because it is inactivated by haemoglobin and is powerless by the time it reaches the systemic circulation. Patients should not be removed from their nitric oxide during physiotherapy. If manual hyperinflation is necessary, the gas can be entrained through a rebreathe bag, or ventilator hyperinflation can be used. However, many of these patients are critically ill and PEEP-dependent, and manual hyperinflation may be contraindicated.

Prostacycline is administered intravenously or by nebulizer and is less toxic than nitric oxide, but it has a half-life of five minutes and is not metabolized by the lung so it can affect the systemic vasculature and cause hypotension.

Sedatives

Sedation should not be used as the first line management of anxiety or asynchrony with the ventilator, for which explanations or ventilator management are required. Drugs that cloud consciousness cause delusions if anxiety stems from the patient's realistic perception of their situation. Factual memories, even if disagreeable, assist patients to anchor their ICU experience in reality rather than in a fog of confusion, helping to disperse 'fear memory' and giving some protection from anxiety (Vick 2002) and PTSD (Usuki et al 2012).

Sedation is used with the best of intentions, but it has been claimed that they may not in fact reduce anxiety in ventilated patients (Chlan 2011) possibly because of a loss of time sense and misinterpretation of voices and noises. Side effects include reduced sputum clearance (Savian et al 2006), prolonged weaning, pneumonia, hypotension (Gurudatt 2012), sometimes ventilator asynchrony (Vaschetto et al 2014), delirium, especially with fluctuating levels of the drug (Svenningsen et al 2013) and subsequent cognitive impairment (Brummel 2011).

When sedation is required, the optimal dose is that which offers comfort while allowing for interaction with the environment (Griffiths 2012). Patient-controlled sedation is preferred by patients who can use it (Rodrigo et al 2003).

Commonly prescribed anxiolytics are:

- **diazepam** and **midazolam,** which have a long half-life
- **propofol,** which has a short recovery time and may be useful as a bolus two minutes before physiotherapy
- **dexmedetomidine,** which acts rapidly, does not cause respiratory depression or predispose to delirium, has analgesic and sympatholytic effects (Allen *et al* 2012) and facilitates communication (Jakob *et al* 2012)

- **chlormethiazole,** which can increase bronchial secretions.

Over-sedation can be differentiated from neurological damage by an assay method described by McKenzie et al (2005).

Analgesics

Prior to physiotherapy, a bolus of intravenous analgesia is often indicated, using a short-acting drug such as **fentanyl** or **alfentanil**.

Muscle relaxants

> *You can't scratch your arm if it itches. You can't do nothing. Except lay there in one position. That's very, very uncomfortable.*
> Patient quoted by Jablonski (1994)

Neuromuscular blocking agents are paralyzing drugs which are used if communication or deep sedation are inadequate, e.g. to reduce oxygen consumption in septic patients (Steingrub *et al* 2014), to prevent patients moving after acute brain injury or as a last resort for patients who are resisting ventilation.

These drugs may be frightening for patients if they have not been told that they are receiving a drug that will make them feel weak, and they must not be used as chemical restraints. Patients should be sedated to the point of unrousability beforehand (Oh 2009 p. 919) and appropriate analgesia administered because muscle relaxants may obliterate the only means by which patients can indicate distress.

Neuromuscular blockade may lead to persistent myopathy (Piriyapatsom *et al* 2013), but an unexpected benefit is less painful postoperative suction if patients cannot cough.

Drugs for airflow obstruction

Inhaled bronchodilators are commonly used in ventilated patients without evidence of airflow obstruction (Ari *et al* 2012) and come with some disadvantages:

- tachycardia from β_2-agonists can lead to haemodynamic compromise in unstable patients

- disconnection to attach the delivery device may lead to derecruitment and swings in oxygenation (Grivans *et al* 2009)
- impaction on the artificial airway may reduce deposition of the drug to just 2.9% (Kallet 2013).

Benefit must be demonstrable e.g. by decreased wheeze on auscultation, a drop in peak airway pressure (with VC ventilation), a normalized flow curve (Fig 17.21c) or reduced intrinsic PEEP. If improvement is not evident, it is worth removing the in-line suction catheter, which may impede delivery, and trying again, before abandoning the drug (Manthous 2000). People with severe asthma invariably benefit from inhaled bronchodilators, those with COPD often benefit, but those with parenchymal disorders such as ARDS do not (Matthay *et al* 2011).

Bronchodilators or steroids can be delivered to ventilated patients by small-volume nebulizer or metered dose inhaler (MDI), after removal of any heat-moisture exchanger in the ventilator circuit or removal/bypass of a humidifier. Advantages of nebulizer delivery are near-continuous bronchodilation for status asthmaticus, and no need for co-ordinated administration with the patient's breath. Disadvantages are that they need higher doses of bronchodilator, require more staff time, and are associated with greater risk of infection than an inhaler (Khoo *et al* 2009).

If an inhaler is used, a spacer is required (Schumaker 2004) and the following advised:

- ensure that the ventilator tidal volume is more than 500 ml and that inspiratory time (excluding the pause) is over a third of the total breath time
- shake the inhaler
- insert canister into the actuator of the spacer and into the inspiratory limb of the ventilator circuit (Fig 17.18), about 15 cm from the tracheal tube (Laube *et al* 2011)
- fire inhaler at onset of inspiration
- allow passive exhalation
- repeat after 30 seconds or until the total dose is delivered, usually after four puffs.

The spacer should remain in the ventilator circuit. Dry powder inhalers cannot be used (AARC 1999b).

A nebulizer should be connected to the inspiratory limb of the circuit, and ventilator settings may need adjustment, e.g. increased inspiratory time. It should be removed and cleaned after each use, unless it can be bypassed so that the ventilator circuit does not have to be opened.

ADVANCED LIFE SUPPORT

Advanced cardiac support

When the heart's conducting pathways are damaged, an artificial **pacemaker** can be used to deliver an electrical stimulus to the heart muscle. For temporary use, pacing wires connect the patient's myocardium to an external pacing box. For permanent support, the energy

---

FIGURE 17.18 Metered dose inhaler and spacer

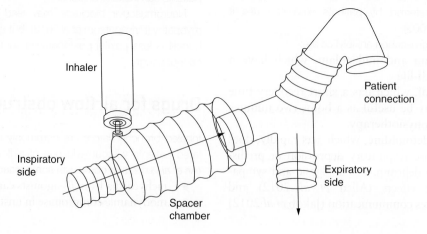

Inhaler

Patient connection

Inspiratory side

Expiratory side

Spacer chamber

source is implanted under the skin (Pastore *et al* 2013). Indications are third degree heart block, arrhythmias refractory to medication and prophylactic support in the days after heart surgery. Insertion of a permanent pacemaker requires the patient to rest afterwards, but they can mobilize fully in 24 hours. A **cardioverter defibrillator** may be implanted in patients who are at risk of ventricular fibrillation (Klein *et al* 2013).

For hospitalized patients in profound heart failure, for whom vasopressor and inotropic support are inadequate, temporary assistance by an **intra-aortic balloon pump** (IABP) provides mechanical support for cardiac output. The pump is connected to a catheter with a deflated balloon at its tip. This is threaded through the femoral or radial artery and up into the aorta (Fig 17.19), and is triggered by the heart's own electrical activity. Diastole causes balloon inflation, which assists aortic valve closure and diverts blood to the myocardium, increasing cardiac output by up to 40% (Macauley 2012). In systole, the balloon deflates, decreasing afterload and assisting cardiac output.

The effect is similar to combined inotropic and vasodilator therapy, increasing myocardial perfusion and reducing workload. Complications include embolism and lower limb ischaemia. Heparinization lessens the risk of thrombosis but increases the risk of bleeding.

Indications for the balloon pump are critically impaired cardiac output, e.g. cardiogenic shock, inability to wean from cardiopulmonary bypass, and occasionally prophylactic use for high-risk surgical patients (Sá *et al* 2012). As patients recover, assistance is reduced gradually from every beat (1:1) to every 8th beat (1:8).

Implications for physiotherapy are the following:

1 The augmented BP should be monitored throughout.
2 With a femoral catheter, hip flexion should be avoided on the cannulated side, and sitting up is limited.
3 Patients are often too unstable to turn, but if turning is indicated, care is required to avoid disconnection of the cannula.
4 If manual hyperinflation is necessary, cardiac output should be closely monitored.
5 Manual percussion or vibrations are unwise because of interference with the ECG, and mechanical percussors and vibrators are contraindicated. If vibrations are needed, one supporting hand underneath the patient minimizes movement.

FIGURE 17.19 Intra-aortic balloon pump

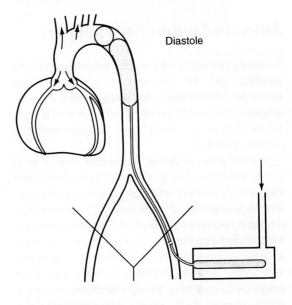

Diastole

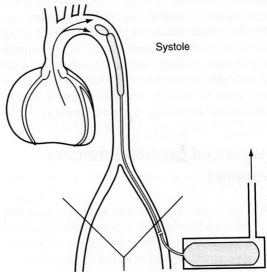

Systole

6 Coughing should be avoided for four to six hours after removal of a femoral catheter, to prevent pressure on the healing femoral artery.

A **ventricular assist device** is a supplementary pump implanted in the abdomen and used for permanent circulatory support or as a bridge to recovery or transplantation (Wells 2013). Precautions for physiotherapy relate to the complications of bleeding or thrombosis (Kurien & Hughes 2012).

Advanced pulmonary support

Potentially damaging volumes and pressures from the ventilator can be reduced by augmenting gas exchange with **intravascular oxygenation**, in which oxygen is delivered to the inferior vena cava via a mop-like two-foot-long bundle of hollow fibres, permeable to gases but not fluids.

Equally exotic is **liquid ventilation** (Murgia *et al* 2012), which emerged as a concept in the First World War, when it was found that gas-poisoned lungs tolerated large quantities of saline lavage. Liquid ventilation is used in neonates to eliminate the gas-liquid interface in dependent lung regions, which are most susceptible to collapse, and sometimes in adults with ARDS to prevent further damage to alveoli. A heavy inert liquid called perfluorocarbon, through which the patient is able to breathe, fills the lungs to FRC, eliminating surface tension, reducing ventilatory pressures and recruiting dependent alveoli by a 'liquid PEEP' effect. Radio-opacity makes densities such as consolidation undetectable on x-ray, although pneumothoraces are crystal clear. Mucus cannot mix with perfluorocarbon and tends to float on top, from where it can be debrided by saline lavage. Suction is forbidden.

Advanced cardiopulmonary support

As a last resort for people with severe but potentially reversible cardiopulmonary failure, extracorporeal gas exchange acts as a modified form of cardiopulmonary bypass and buys time for an injured lung to recover.

Extracorporeal membrane oxygenation (ECMO) supports cardiorespiratory function via a cannula in the vascular system (Turner 2013). Blood is removed, pumped across a membrane oxygenator and returned to the patient, either into the venous system (veno-venous [VV] circuit) or arterial system (veno-arterial [VA] circuit). The VA system requires 80% of the cardiac output to be drained, pumped, oxygenated, rewarmed and returned to the internal carotid artery, with CO_2 transferring back as a secondary effect (Fig 17.20). The VV system relies on some heart function and requires 20% of the circulating volume to be outside the body

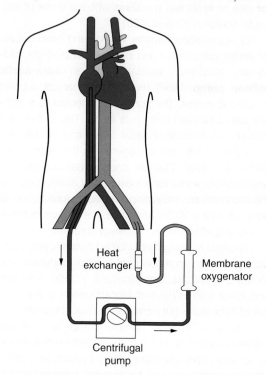

FIGURE 17.20 Extracorporeal membrane oxygenation via veno-arterial circuit. Venous blood passes through a pump to substitute for heart function and a membrane oxygenator to substitute for lung function, then returns to the arterial system

Heat exchanger

Membrane oxygenator

Centrifugal pump

at one time. It is less damaging, removing desaturated blood from the vena cava, oxygenating it outside the body and returning it to the venous system.

For adults, ECMO is normally only used in severe multisystem failure (Ma *et al* 2012) but it is well-established in specialist neonatal units, though there is concern about neurological damage from cannulation of the carotid artery. Analgesic doses should be increased to compensate for loss of the drug through the circuit (Shekar *et al* 2012).

If patients are stable enough for physiotherapy, the ECMO cannulae require careful handling and a technician should stand by in case the machinery needs attention. Reliance cannot be placed on auscultation because of the reduced ventilation. Bleeding during suction is a risk if there is not tight heparin control. Physiotherapy is not likely to cause hypoxaemia because oxygenation is maintained outside the lungs. If ECMO is being used as a bridge to lung transplantation, a dual lumen cannula may allow the patient to mobilize (Rahimi *et al* 2013).

Support systems such as haemodialysis, plasmapheresis and surfactant replacement are discussed with the relevant pathologies.

MONITORING

> *Frankly it feels quite awful to be connected to machines through every available orifice, plus several new medically-made ones, in spite of feeling thankful for all the life-sustaining help and healing ministrations.*
>
> Brooks (patient) 1990

Monitoring differs from measuring: it implies regular observation and a systematic response if there is deviation from a specified range. It is complementary to clinical observation and is necessary to record sudden or subtle changes in a patient's status. False alarms are frequent and can desensitize staff (Hannibal 2011).

Ventilator interactions

The relationship between patient effort and mechanical support is represented by pressure, volume and flow, measured relative to their values at end-expiration (de Wit 2011). Pressure levels are relative to PEEP, volume is measured as lung volume above FRC, and flow is measured relative to its end-expiratory value (usually zero). Details are in Cairo 2012 p. 148, Chang 2014 p.309 or the ventilator manufacturer's handbook. Below is an outline.

The **pressure time curve** shows pressures throughout the respiratory cycle (Fig 17.5). 'Peak airway pressure' (peak inspiratory pressure) is the highest pressure. This settles down to the end-inspiratory 'plateau pressure', termed 'inflation hold' or 'inspiratory pause' on some ventilators, which reflects alveolar pressure (Chang 2014 p.409). 'Mean airway pressure' is represented by the space under the curve and is associated positively with oxygenation and negatively with the haemodynamic side effects of MV.

The **flow time curve** is useful to verify the presence of intrinsic PEEP, as shown by inadequate expiratory time, and the effect of bronchodilators (Fig 17.21).

Gas exchange

Each step of the oxygen cascade can be monitored, as described below for gas exchange in the lungs and on p.447 for oxygen delivery to the tissues.

Arterial blood gas measurements are taken continually from an indwelling arterial catheter rather than by intermittent arterial puncture.

Arterial oxygen saturation (S_aO_2) is also monitored continuously, using pulse oximetry (S_pO_2). If desaturation occurs during physiotherapy, treatment should normally stop and the '100% oxygen' button on the ventilator activated. If S_pO_2 does not return to its baseline within a minute, remedial action should be taken such as re-positioning the patient, increasing F_iO_2, or initiating manual hyperventilation or suction. An ear probe or forehead sensor may be required if there is low cardiac output or poor perfusion, and in the most

---

FIGURE 17.21 Flow-time curves. (a) Normal inspiratory flow above the line and normal expiration below. (b) Intrinsic PEEP, as indicated by expiratory flow not returning to zero before the next inspiration begins. (c) Before and after bronchodilation, shown as prolonged and then normal expiratory flow.

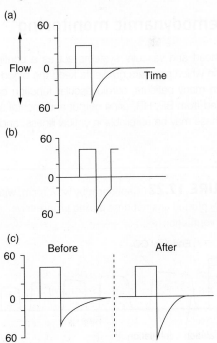

severely ill patients there may be discrepancy between S_aO_2 and S_pO_2.

Capnography indicates CO_2 levels by exhaled end-tidal CO_2 ($ETCO_2$) measurement, providing continuous assessment of the adequacy of ventilation (Fig 17.22). $ETCO_2$ is measured by a sensor between the tracheal tube and ventilator tubing (Pekdemir et al 2013). Normal values are 1 mmHg below P_aCO_2, with an acceptable range up to 5 mmHg difference. Values decrease during manual hyperinflation because this usually incorporates hyperventilation.

Transcutaneous monitoring ($P_{tc}O_2$ and $P_{tc}CO_2$) measures oxygen and CO_2 as they diffuse through the skin, using a heated sensor to increase gas permeability across the skin barrier (Ruben et al 2012). In haemodynamically stable patients, values relate to respiratory status, but measurements vary with cardiac output and capillary blood flow. Neonates show good correlation with arterial measurements, but adults have varying skin thicknesses and results are less reliable. $P_{tc}CO_2$ is useful during weaning (Johnson & Batool 2008).

Haemodynamic monitoring

The heart and vascular systems act as a continuous loop in which pressure gradients keep the blood moving. In many patients, cardiovascular function can be gauged from BP, HR, urine output and mental status, but these may be unreliable in critical illness, and invasive cardiovascular monitoring is then required to identify pressures and assume volumes.

Fluid status

The term 'resuscitation' in the ICU usually relates to fluid resuscitation. Haemodynamic stability depends on intravascular fluids, especially during and after surgery and in the 'golden hour' after trauma. Fluid in the vasculature affects all aspects of the haemodynamic system, i.e. HR, BP, cardiac output, left and right atrial pressures (below), the difference between peripheral and central temperature and, representing the kidney's sensitivity to perfusion, urine output. Fluids in the interstitial and intracellular spaces are more difficult to assess, but dehydration is suggested by thirst and dry mucous membranes, and overhydration may cause increased weight and peripheral/pulmonary oedema. Fluid balance is monitored by the fluid chart, weight change, electrolyte density or fluid challenge. Fluid responsiveness is measured by pulse pressure variation, stroke volume variation, leg raising (Huang et al 2014) or fluid challenge (Hu et al 2013).

Blood pressure

A continuous display of BP is provided by an arterial line in the radial, femoral or brachial artery, so long as it is not kinked or malpositioned. The most relevant reading is mean arterial pressure, which represents perfusion pressure over the cardiac cycle.

Cardiac output (CO)

Reduced urine output may be the first indication of impaired CO. Monitoring is by thermodilution, arterial pressure waveforms, Doppler measurements of blood flow or regional oxygenation (Gilbert 2013). Cardiac output usually reflects BP, but peripheral vasoconstriction may maintain BP in the face of a falling CO. Conversely, a septic patient in a hyperdynamic state may have a high CO but vasodilation reduces BP.

Central venous pressure (CVP)

An extension of the patient's vascular system is created by passing a radio-opaque catheter through a large central vein, usually via the neck or arm, until it is just outside the right atrium, through which all venous blood passes. The pressure within this system (the CVP) reflects right atrial pressure (RAP), which indicates the preload of the right ventricle. CVP is a pressure but relates to circulating blood volume and the

FIGURE 17.22 Capnography waveform, with $ETCO_2$ plotted against time during progressive hyperventilation

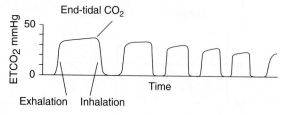

ability of the heart to handle that volume. It is similar to the jugular venous pressure (JVP) and is affected by the interaction between blood volume, right heart function, peripheral venous tone and posture. It also fluctuates with the pressure changes of breathing. High pressure MV or high PEEP levels increase intrathoracic pressure, leading to higher CVP readings, but the trend is relevant.

Single values are less pertinent than the trend, but a high value might indicate heart failure, pulmonary embolism COPD, pneumothorax or over-transfusion of fluid. The CVP also provides early warning of cardiac tamponade, which causes a sudden rise in CVP, or haemorrhage, which causes a sudden drop. CVP is more sensitive to haemorrhage than BP because arterial pressure can be maintained for longer by vasoconstriction.

Multiple functions are serviced by multilumen catheters which infuse fluids, drugs, blood and nutrition while maintaining continuous pressure monitoring. Thick hyperosmolar feeds are needed for patients who need nutrition without too much volume, and these require central rather than peripheral veins for delivery.

Implications for physiotherapy are the following:

1 Cannulation of a large vein near the pleura may cause a pneumothorax, haemothorax or subcutaneous emphysema. After placement of a central line, the x-ray should be examined before considering any positive pressure treatment such as manual hyperinflation.

2 A high CVP may indicate pulmonary oedema, which impairs gas exchange. A low CVP may indicate hypovolaemia, which can lead to adverse haemodynamic responses to positioning, manual hyperinflation or suction.

Pulmonary artery wedge pressure (PAWP)

The CVP usually reflects filling pressures for both sides of the heart. However, left atrial pressure may need to be measured separately because:

- it takes time for the CVP to rise in response to left ventricular failure because the pressure has to back up through the pulmonary circulation and the right ventricle may initially compensate

- the CVP does not reflect left atrial pressure if the compliance of either ventricle is affected by septic shock, ischaemia, vasopressors or vasodilators
- the CVP does not reflect left atrial pressure if pulmonary hypertension pushes up the CVP but the patient is systemically hypovolaemic.

To measure left atrial pressure, a balloon-tipped pulmonary artery catheter is used. Sometimes called a Swan-Ganz, it is passed along the CVP catheter route, then swished through the right ventricle into the pulmonary artery, assisted by the inflated balloon at its tip. Here it measures pulmonary artery pressure (PAP), which reflects the pressure that needs to be generated by the right ventricle to pump blood through the pulmonary vasculature. A raised PAP indicates pulmonary hypertension, pulmonary embolism or fluid overload.

The catheter is then carried into ever smaller pulmonary arterioles until it becomes wedged (Fig 17.23).

Once wedged, the catheter tip is isolated from pressure fluctuations in the right side of the heart and is in communication with the left atrium via the pulmonary capillary bed, so long as there is a continuous column of blood between the two (Fig 17.24). The pressure monitored at this point is the pulmonary artery wedge pressure or left atrial pressure, reflecting pressure in the left atrium via the lung vasculature. The balloon acts as a form of pulmonary embolus so is deflated when not needed, to prevent ischaemia.

The continuous column of blood in the pulmonary vascular bed is tenuous if the catheter is in the upper zone of the lung (Ch. 1) where there may be no perfusion under the positive pressure of MV. Measurements are also compromised if the patient is severely hypovolaemic, changes position, or is subject to high inflation pressures from the ventilator. Values can be affected by valve stenoses, floppy ventricles following serial myocardial infarction or sepsis, or stiff ventricles following sympathetic stimulation caused by hypovolaemic shock. The more ill the patient, the less accurate are single measurements, but the trend is helpful.

PAWP can also be used to calculate cardiac output and systemic vascular resistance, allow fine tuning when establishing optimum PEEP, help to rationalize fluid and drug therapy, and distinguish hypovolaemia

FIGURE 17.23 Passage of the balloon-tipped catheter (a) through the R atrium, (b) into the pulmonary artery and (c) wedged into the pulmonary vasculature.

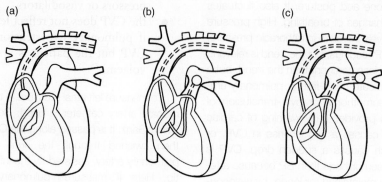

(↓ PAWP) from left ventricular failure (↑ PAWP). Implications for physiotherapy are similar to those with CVP.

PAWP is also known as pulmonary artery occlusion pressure, pulmonary capillary wedge pressure (PCWP) or, on ward rounds, simply wedge pressure. Non-invasive measurements are becoming available (Ali *et al* 2012) which will help reduce the PAWP complications of thrombosis, sepsis, arrhythmias, air embolism, trauma to the delicate pulmonary vessels (resulting in blood stained secretions) and pulmonary ischaemia or infarction.

FIGURE 17.24 Pulmonary artery catheter wedged into a branch of the pulmonary artery, where it is isolated from pressure in the R side of the heart and now picks up pressure transmitted from the L atrium.

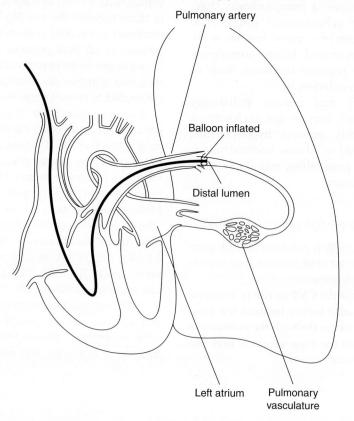

TABLE 17.2

	Vascular pressures		
	CVP	**PAP**	**PAWP**
Normal	0–8 mmHg	Systolic 15–30 mmHg Diastolic 4–12 mmHg	2–15 mmHg
Advanced COPD	↑	↑ ↑↑ during sleep.	N
ARDS	N (but manipulated by treatment)	↑	N (but manipulated by treatment)
Hypervolaemia	↑	↑	↑
Hypovolaemia	↓	↓	↓
Pulmonary oedema/LVF	↑	↑	↑ (>20 mmHg)
Right heart failure	↑	↓	↓

Note: *ARDS:* acute respiratory distress syndrome, *COPD:* chronic obstructive pulmonary disease, *CVP:* central venous pressure, *LVF:* left ventricular failure, *N:* normal, *PAP:* pulmonary artery pressure, *PAWP:* pulmonary artery wedge pressure

Table 17.2 compares vascular pressures for different conditions.

Electrocardiography (ECG)

Disturbances such as hypoxia, physiotherapy, electrolyte imbalance, anxiety or myocardial ischaemia can cause disorders of heart rate (HR) or rhythm. The effects are significant if they affect cardiac output (CO). They are picked up on the ECG, which represents electrical activity in the heart, recorded from the body surface and comprising waves, complexes and intervals.

Sinus rhythm is normal heart rhythm (Fig 17.25) originating from the sinoatrial (SA) node. Supraventricular arrhythmias originate from above or in the atrioventricular (AV) node and are known as atrial or nodal arrhythmias respectively. **Sinus tachycardia** or **supraventricular tachycardia** is HR over 100 bpm, recognized by a rapid rate, regular rhythm and normal QRS complex. Causes include sympathetic activity, electrolyte imbalance or excess β_2-agonist medication. CO is rarely compromised. **Sinus bradycardia** is HR under 60 bpm with normal rhythm.

Ventricular tachycardia is distinguished from supraventricular tachycardia by a lost *P wave* and broad and bizarre QRS complex. It usually impairs CO, BP and tissue perfusion, and can lead to pulmonary oedema or ventricular fibrillation.

Nodal rhythm occurs when the AV node takes over from a non-functioning or slow SA node. This causes lost P waves and a variable or absent PR interval. CO may fall because atrial contraction is out of synchrony with the ventricle, which loses its 'atrial kick'.

FIGURE 17.25 Normal ECG trace of one heart beat. *P wave:* atrial depolarization, *PR interval:* atrioventricular conduction time, *Q:* ventricular depolarization, *R:* first positive deflection during ventricular depolarization, *S:* first negative deflection during ventricular depolarization, *QRS complex:* total ventricular depolarization, *T:* ventricular repolarization (recovery period)

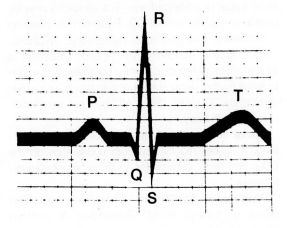

The SA node is the natural pacemaker, but if it does not initiate an impulse at correct intervals, an ectopic (abnormal) focus outside the SA node may take the initiative. These 'ectopics' are seen as premature beats followed by a compensatory pause, sometimes felt as missed heart beats by the patient. They are common and do not contraindicate physiotherapy unless they increase in number or cause haemodynamic disturbance. However, they may signal the onset of more significant arrhythmias.

Atrial ectopics manifest as occasional abnormal *P waves* or an early normal beat, and are of little significance unless frequent. **Ventricular ectopics** are caused by an irritable focus in the ventricle, producing an absent *P wave*, wide and wayward *QRS complex* and inverted *T wave*. They occur in smokers, in those suffering from hypoxia or low potassium levels, or following heart surgery or myocardial infarction (MI). **Bigeminy** means that every other heart beat is ectopic, and **trigeminy** means that every third beat is ectopic.

ST segment elevation suggests pericarditis, coronary artery spasm or MI which will respond to thrombolytic drugs. **ST segment depression** indicates myocardial ischaemia or infarction which is unresponsive to thrombolytic therapy.

Atrial fibrillation (AF) occurs when ectopic foci throughout the atria discharge too fast for the atrial muscle to respond other than by disorganized twitching out of sequence with ventricular activity. It appears as a rapid rate, irregular rhythm and the replacing of *P waves* with a chaotic baseline (Fig 17.26a). It may be triggered by sympathetic stimulation, hypoxia, over- or underhydration, theophylline toxicity, pulmonary embolism, low potassium or magnesium levels, myocardial ischaemia, heart surgery, heart failure or advanced age. The ventricles may be unable to sustain normal CO. Patients may have no symptoms or they may suffer palpitations, dyspnoea, fatigue, angina, hypotension or stroke. Treatment is by correction of the cause when possible, conversion to sinus rhythm using antiarrhythmic drugs, or cardioversion by DC shock. Slow AF does not contraindicate physiotherapy.

Atrial flutter is less common than AF and short-lived. It causes regular sawtooth undulations on the ECG, and either deteriorates to AF or spontaneously recovers.

Ventricular fibrillation (VF) is the commonest cause of cardiac arrest. Breakdown of ordered electrical activity causes an ineffectual quivering of the ventricles, appearing as a chaotic line and providing no CO (Fig 17.26b). **Asystole** is ventricular standstill, i.e. cardiac arrest. It is caused by VF which has burnt itself out, or a bradyarrhythmia that grinds to a halt. It shows as a straight line with occasional minor fluctuations. VF and asystole can be misdiagnosed when similar traces are produced by manual techniques to the chest or disconnected electrodes respectively.

Heart block (HB) is an anatomic or functional interruption in the conduction of an impulse, shown as a disrupted relationship between the *P wave* and *QRS complex*. Causes are hypoxia, MI, digoxin therapy, heart disease or complications from heart surgery. First degree HB shows a prolonged PR interval, but there are no symptoms or need for treatment. Second degree HB shows dropped beats, and if it causes dizziness, fainting or reduced CO, a pacemaker is required. In third degree HB, atrial and ventricular rhythms are independent of one another (Fig 17.26c). This requires a pacemaker to avoid a form of syncope called a Stokes Adams attack. **Bundle branch block** disturbs intraventricular conduction and widens the *QRS complex*.

Changes in rhythm that occur during physiotherapy indicate that treatment should be stopped until it settles or until action is taken by the team to stabilize it.

FIGURE 17.26 ECG traces indicating, (a) atrial fibrillation, (b) ventricular fibrillation, (c) complete (3rd degree) heart block.

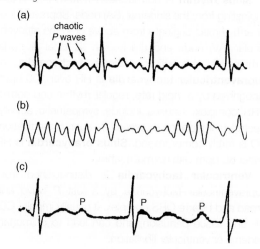

Tissue oxygenation

Oxygen delivery to the tissues (DO_2) is more relevant to cardiorespiratory function than its two main contributors (SpO_2 and CO) separately, in the same way that a bus journey is best monitored by its arrival rather than when it leaves the bus station.

Mixed venous oxygenation ($S_{\bar{v}}O_2$)

Directly related to patient outcome is the oxygen saturation of haemoglobin in the pulmonary artery ($S_{\bar{v}}O_2$), which indicates the amount of oxygen left in the blood at the end of its journey (Svenmarker *et al* 2013). It reflects the extent to which oxygen supply (CO, haemoglobin and SpO_2) has met demand (oxygen extraction at tissue level). Both haemodynamic and gas exchange components of the oxygen cascade are thus included.

The oxygen saturation of venous blood leaving different organs varies, but the mixed venous blood in the pulmonary artery comprises an average of the individual streams from a multitude of capillary beds which, having been mixed further in the right ventricle, now return to the lungs for refuelling (Fig 17.27). Although in the pulmonary artery, it is venous blood because it has given up all the oxygen required for metabolism.

$S_{\bar{v}}O_2$ values are on average 65–75%, and should be more than 10% below SpO_2 to prove that oxygen has been delivered to the tissues.

A low $S_{\bar{v}}O_2$ indicates:

- ↓ DO_2, e.g. from suction, anaemia, low CO, hypoxaemia or haemorrhage
- ↑ oxygen consumption ($\dot{V}O_2$), e.g. from suction, exercise, pain, fever, anxiety, agitation, laboured breathing or hypermetabolic states.

$S_{\bar{v}}O_2$ does not pinpoint which variable is responsible for any change, and acts more as an early warning system. Cardiac output and SpO_2 are simultaneously monitored in order to identify their contributions.

Values below 50% are associated with anaerobic metabolism, and those below 40% are incompatible with life. People with chronic heart failure are more tolerant of low levels. Excessively high values above 85% are, paradoxically, not a good sign. This 'luxury perfusion' means that sepsis has released inflammatory mediators which have damaged the microvasculature so that capillary beds are bypassed and oxygen not supplied to the tissues.

$S_{\bar{v}}O_2$ can be improved by increasing F_IO_2 or CO, reducing stress, or addressing other factors hindering DO_2. During physiotherapy, if $S_{\bar{v}}O_2$ varies by more than 10% from baseline for more than three minutes, treatment should be stopped (Hayden 1993).

Central venous oxygenation

Oxygen in blood from the vena cava represents central venous oxygenation, which reads slightly higher than $S_{\bar{v}}O_2$, with normal values at 73–82% (Kocsi *et al* 2012).

Gastric tonometry

The gut is the crystal ball of tissue hypoxia, having a notoriously poor tolerance for even brief hypoxia due to its tendency to vasoconstrict in response to circulatory failure because of its rich innervation by sympathetic nerves. Using the gut as the 'canary in the mine', a saline-filled balloon in the stomach measures the CO_2 that passes across the membrane (Correa-Martín 2013).

Cerebral oximetry

Cerebral oximetry monitors brain perfusion non-invasively (Udy *et al* 2013).

FIGURE 17.27 Measurement of oxygen saturation of haemoglobin in mixed venous blood via the pulmonary artery catheter

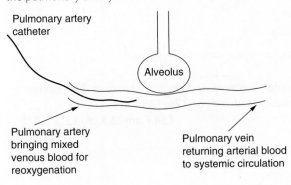

Pulmonary artery catheter

Alveolus

Pulmonary artery bringing mixed venous blood for reoxygenation

Pulmonary vein returning arterial blood to systemic circulation

CASE STUDY : Mr FA

Identify the problems of this patient from London who collapsed in the emergency department, then was intubated and ventilated.

Relevant medical history
- Alcoholism
- Epilepsy

On examination
- On SIMV and PSV with 5 cmH_2O PEEP
- Heavily sedated
- Stable

Questions

1. Auscultation and percussion note (Fig 17.28a)?
2. Analysis?
3. Problems?
4. Goals?
5. Precaution?
6. Plan?
7. Passive movements?
8. Outcome (Fig 17.28b)?

FIGURE 17.28a

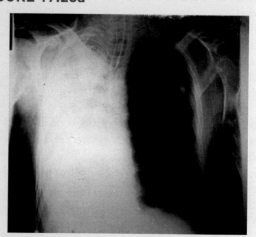

CLINICAL REASONING

Chest physiotherapy may cause cardiac arrhythmias, bronchospasm and transient hypoxemia, and may prolong the duration of mechanical ventilation [references 126-128].

Crit Care (2008), 12, 2, 209

Those references need checking out . . .

Response to Case Study

1 Auscultation and percussion note

- Reduced breath sounds on right, percussion note dull on right.

2 Analysis

- Patient collapse probably due to a seizure.
- Fig 17.28a suggests aspiration to right lung.
- Possible alcohol intake increased the risk of aspiration.

3 Problems

- Loss of lung volume on the right.

4 Goals

- Short term: restore functioning lung volume.
- Medium term: mobilize.
- Long term: team management of follow-up support and rehabilitation.

5 Precaution

- No head-down postural drainage due to recent seizure.

6 Plan

Review radiologist report in case of hidden rib fractures due to fall. If all clear:

- optimize analgesia
- position in left side-lying
- manual hyperinflation
- percussion and vibrations
- suction

Continue until breath sounds are clear, adding saline instillation if required.

7 Passive movements

Unsafe until patient is able to report pain and orthopaedic team has assessed fractured left humerus, head of right humerus and right clavicle (fractures were not identified by ICU medical team, indicating the importance of physiotherapists taking responsibility for the safety of their treatments). Fractures turned out to be old and pain free, and were non-united due to malnutrition related to alcoholism.

FIGURE 17.28b

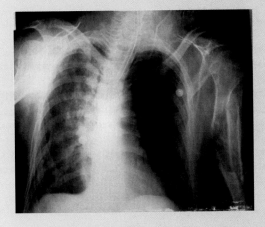

8   Outcome

- Figure 17.28b: short term goal achieved.
- Long term: patient agreed to alcohol and physical rehabilitation.

Response to Clinical Reasoning

Ref. 126 – Cardiac arrhythmias during postural drainage and chest percussion of critically ill patients. Chest (1992) 102, 1836–41
The authors persuaded their physical therapists to treat haemodynamically unstable patients who had pulmonary emboli, pulmonary oedema and ARDS (none of which are hypersecretory disorders) using head-down postural drainage and ten minutes of percussion (described as 'a chest thump given to convert asystole'). The outcome, unsurprisingly, was further haemodynamic instability. This is an oft-quoted study 'proving' the dangers of physiotherapy in the ICU.

Ref. 127 – Chest physiotherapy. BMJ (1989), 298, 541–542
This did not relate to ventilated patients.

Ref. 128 – Chest physiotherapy prolongs duration of ventilation in the critically ill ventilated for more than 48 hours. Int Care Med (2007), 33, 11, 1938–45
This study compared patients who did and did not receive physiotherapy. 'Physiotherapy' was not standardized and included undefined 'respiratory muscle exercise'.
Half the control patients required 'rescue physiotherapy', thus invalidating the results and, incidentally, showing the benefit of physiotherapy.
The value of physiotherapy was confirmed by more patients in the control group being re-ventilated or dying, but this was noted quietly in Table 3 and not mentioned in the text.
'Overwhelming illness' was described as a contraindication for 'physiotherapy', without either being defined.
The authors could not spell 'physiotherapist'.

RECOMMENDED READING

Arai S (2013) Thirst in critically ill patients: from physiology to sensation. *Am J Crit Care*; **22**(3): 328–36

ACCCM (2013) Clinical practice guidelines for the management of pain, agitation, and delirium in adult patients in the intensive care unit. *Crit Care Med*; **41**(1): 263–306

Brummel NE, Girard TD (2012) Preventing delirium in the intensive care unit. *Crit Care Clin*; **29**(1): 51–65

Calzia E, Dembinski R (2013) Preserving spontaneous breathing during mechanical ventilatory support. *Crit Care*; **17**(6): 1013

Cox C (2012) Development and pilot testing of a decision aid for surrogates of patients with prolonged mechanical ventilation. *Crit Care Med*; **40**(8): 2327–34

De Prost N (2013) Effects of ventilation strategy on distribution of lung inflammatory cell activity. *Crit Care*; **17**: R175

Dermitzaki D, Tzortzaki E, Soulitzis N *et al* (2013) Molecular response of the human diaphragm on different modes of mechanical ventilation. *Respiration*; **85**(3): 228–35

Flaatten H (2014) The impact of age in intensive care. *Acta Anaesthesiol Scand*; **58**(1): 3–4. doi. 10.1111/aas.12221

Rafiei H, Abdar ME, Amiri M *et al* (2013) The study of harmful and beneficial drug interactions in intensive care. *J Intens Care Soc;* **14**(2): 155–8

Gingell E, Rushton CY (2012) Ethics in critical care: preventive ethics in the intensive care unit. *AACN Adv Crit Care*; **23**(2): 217–24

Gunther AC (2013) Palmar skin conductance variability and the relation to stimulation, pain and the motor activity assessment scale in intensive care unit patients. *Crit Care*; **17**, R51

Hsieh E (2014) Management of autism in the adult intensive care unit. *J Int Care Med*; **29**(1): 47–52,

Keenan JC (2013) PEEP titration: new horizons. *Respir Care*; **58**(9): 1552–4

Kettles L (2013) Hypovolaemia. *Anaesth Int Care Med*; **14**(1): 5–7

Mahmood NA, Chaudry FA, Azam H (2013) Frequency of hypoxic events in patients on a mechanical ventilator. *Int J Crit Illn Inj Sci;* **3**(2): 124–9

McDermid RC, Bagshaw SM (2011) Octogenarians in the ICU. *Crit Care*; **15**(1): 125–8

Mireles-Cabodevila E, Hatipoğlu U, Chatburn RL (2013) A rational framework for selecting modes of ventilation. *Respir Care*; **58**(2): 348–66

Monroe VD (2013) Blood pressure lability. *Crit Care Nurs Quart;* **36**(4): 425–32

Myburgh JA, Mythen MG (2013) Resuscitation fluids. *N Engl J Med*; **3 69**(13): 1243–51

Ramprasad R, Kapoor MC (2012) Nutrition in intensive care. *J Anaesthesiol Clin Pharmacol*; **28**(1): 1–3

Rezende-Neto JB (2013) Abdominal catastrophes in the intensive care unit setting. *Crit Care Clinics*; **29**(4): 1017–1044

Schindler AW (2013) ICU personnel have inaccurate perceptions of their patients' experiences. *Acta Anaesthesiol Scand*; **57**: 1032–40

Sjöberg F, Svanborg E (2013) How do we know when patients sleep properly or why they do not? *Crit Care*; **17**: 145

Stocchetti N, Roux PL, Vespa P (2013) Clinical review: neuromonitoring. *Crit Care*; **17**: 201

Tonnelier A (2013) Impact of humidification and nebulization during expiratory limb protection: an experimental bench study. *Respir Care*; **58**(8): 1315–22

Volpe MS, Adams AB, Amato MBP (2008) Ventilation patterns influence airway secretion movement. *Respir Care*; **53**(10): 1287–94

CHAPTER 18
Physiotherapy for critically ill patients

LEARNING OBJECTIVES

On completion of this chapter the reader should be able to:

- understand how to assess and handle a critically ill patient

- implement measures to minimize oxygen consumption

- formulate a treatment plan to increase volume and clear secretions, while integrating rehabilitation throughout

- identify and manage emergencies that may arise

- understand the teamwork and application of an on call service.

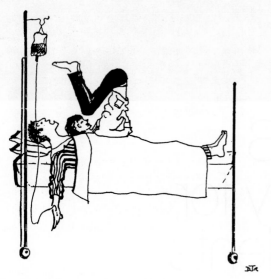

'The physiotherapist will come and do exercises on his chest.'

INTRODUCTION

The major long-term complication for Intensive Care Unit (ICU) patients is deconditioning, which underlines the importance of early rehabilitation, leading to lower mortality and reduced readmission rates (Vollman 2013). Outcomes of physiotherapy combined with occupational therapy include less delirium, shorter time on mechanical ventilation (MV) and increased return to independent function at discharge (Piriyapatsom *et al* 2013). This is reinforced by the findings of Hanekom *et al* 2012) that a specialist physiotherapist allocated to the ICU improves patient outcomes. As well as deconditioning, physiotherapy has been shown to reduce sputum retention, atelectasis, need for intubation, weaning failure (Gosselink *et al* 2008) and brain dysfunction (Girard 2012). The more frequent the treatments, the shorter is the average patient's length of stay (Castro *et al* 2013).

ASSESSMENT

Modifications to the assessment described in Chapter 2 are below.

Notes and charts

Blood sugar, lactate, white cell count and urea/electrolytes can affect treatment. The implications of abnormal values are in Ch. 2 and the Glossary, with some examples relevant to the ICU below.

1 Low or high potassium levels predispose to arrhythmias, as does low magnesium (Parikh 2012), contraindicating most forms of physiotherapy.

2 Low albumin is common in ICU patients because of fluid and membrane permeability problems, leading to metabolic alkalosis and systemic and pulmonary oedema.

3 Neutropaenia can be caused by malnutrition, immune deficiency or anti-cancer drugs, leaving a patient vulnerable to infection.

4 Anaemia is found in up to 95% of patients, compromising oxygen delivery (Kocsi *et al* 2012) and mobilization.

5 Impaired clotting occurs with disseminated intravascular coagulation, or, less drastically, if a patient is on anticoagulants. This increases the risk of bleeding with suction. Conversely, increased clotting raises the likelihood of deep vein thrombosis, as indicated by elevated levels of prothrombin (Aleman *et al* 2013) or platelets (Zakai *et al* 2013).

The notes also identify patients who are dependent on tobacco or alcohol. This is not a time for cold turkey and patients should be given nicotine replacement (Cartin-Ceba 2011) or medication for alcohol withdrawal (Sarff & Gold 2010). Increased morbidity is associated with unmanaged withdrawal from tobacco (Lucidarme 2010) or alcohol (Carlson *et al* 2012).

A typical chart is shown in App. C. Increased core temperature indicates that the patient is consuming extra oxygen. Peripheral temperature is normally 2° lower than core temperature, but if the difference is more than 5°, poor circulatory function is implicated. The chart may incorporate assessment scales for mobility (Kasotakis *et al* 2012), sedation (Becker 2012), (Porter & McClure 2013), thirst (Puntillo 2013), agitation (Chanques 2006) and sleep (Bourne *et al* 2008). There is no reliable means of assessing awareness, so it is assumed that patients can hear and understand. A rough test for comprehension is to ask patients to poke out their tongue, which most paralyzed patients are physically able to do.

Routine pain assessment leads to shorter length of stay in the ICU (Paulus *et al* 2013). Scales have been validated for ventilated (Piriyapatsom *et al* 2013), and non-ventilated patients (Azzam & Alam 2013). Multimodal analgesia is advised (Payen *et al* 2013), especially as uncontrolled pain can impair quality of life even after discharge (Payen & Chanques 2012).

Breathlessness can be measured by two standardized questions (Karampela *et al* 2002):

- Are you feeling short of breath right now?
- Is your shortness of breath mild, moderate or severe?

Breathlessness may be due to patient-ventilator synchrony (Branson *et al* 2013) or it may reflect anxiety.

Blood pressure (BP) should be checked on the chart for its response to turning or previous sessions of manual hyperinflation (MH). If BP is low, unstable or sags on inspiration, or if mean arterial pressure (MAP) is <80 mmHg, the patient may be unable to maintain cardiac output during turning or manual hyperinflation (MH). A drop in systolic BP by more than 40 suggests sepsis (Sevransky 2010).

Electrolyte and haematocrit concentration are decreased with fluid excess and increased with fluid loss. Fluid status is disturbed by diuretics, diabetes, vomiting, diarrhoea, heart or kidney failure, burns, ascites or large open wounds. Hydration is difficult to assess clinically because oedema or overhydration can coexist with intravascular depletion in critically ill people, so reliance is best placed on the fluid balance chart and nurse report.

Signs of hypovolaemia or reduced cardiac output are:

- ↑ heart rate (HR)
- ↑ respiratory rate (RR)
- ↓ systolic BP
- ↓ urine output
- dizziness with position change
- sweating
- confusion or altered consciousness.

Hypovolaemia alone is distinguished by:

- ↓ peripheral temperature (usually the first sign)
- dark coloured urine
- ↓ vascular pressures (Ch. 17)
- ↓ pulse pressure.

Decreased cardiac output is distinguished by:

- pallor
- cold extremities.

PRACTICE TIP

Obtain a blank ICU chart and go through it with colleagues.

The patient

An inability to report symptom distress is not synonymous with an inability to experience suffering.

Campbell 2010

Is the patient conscious, confused, agitated, sedated, paralyzed or in pain? What channels of communication are available? Paralysis, whether pathological or pharmacological, indicates the importance of clarity in communication because patients may be trying to make sense of sounds and sensations but cannot give feedback. Agitation may be due to lack of information, the endotracheal tube, fear, awkward positioning, abdominal distension or any of the causes of stress in Ch. 17.

However unconscious a patient appears, it is worth remembering the 'unconscious' victim of the 7/7 London bombings who later reported that he had heard paramedics pass him by with the comment that he could not be saved.

Thirst is reported by 70% of patients (Arai 2014), but it is not routinely assessed, partly because half the nurses in one study did not perceive that mechanically ventilated patients could be thirsty (Puntillo *et al* 2010).

Table 18.1 shows that unrelieved and distressing symptoms are present for the majority of critically ill patients. Breathlessness was found to be the most distressing symptom.

Other points to note are the following:

1 Accessory muscle activity suggests excess work of breathing (WOB), while laboured breathing may indicate an obstructed airway.

2 A distended abdomen is common, for example Mostafa (2000) found that 83.3% of patients were constipated for a median of six days, which reduced lung volume and contributed to weaning failure.

TABLE 18.1 Prevalence of symptoms reported by ICU patients

Symptom	% of patients
Fatigue	74.7
Thirst	70.8
Anxiety	57.9
Restlessness	49.0
Hunger	44.8
Breathlessness	43.9
Pain	40.4
Sadness	33.9
Fear	32.8
Confusion	26.6

3 Lines and tubes, especially femoral lines, haemofiltration lines, pacing wires, chest drains and lines in the feet, should be kept in view throughout treatment.

4 Muscle atrophy may be masked by limb oedema.

5 A wheeze-like sound at the mouth may indicate air leaking around the cuff of the tracheal tube.

6 If manual hyperinflation is to be undertaken, breath sounds can be heard more clearly when the bag is squeezed, and sometimes crackles can be elicited with a sharp release on expiration.

7 An acoustic secretion detector is available which can identify secretions (Lucchini *et al* 2011).

8 Absent or reduced breath sounds over the left lung may indicate right lung intubation (Fig 18.1).

Monitors

Monitors should be observed before, during and after treatment. The arterial line allows continuous monitoring of BP and blood gases. S_pO_2 must be maintained throughout, low levels being a risk factor for subsequent cognitive dysfunction (Modrykamien 2012).

FIGURE 18.1 The ETT has passed into the R main bronchus and beyond the RUL bronchus, leading to absorption of gas in the non-ventilated RUL and atelectasis. The left lung would also have collapsed if the ETT had not been removed. *ETT:* endotracheal tube, *RUL:* right upper lobe

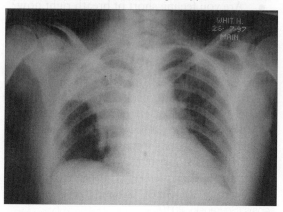

Ventilator

The charts indicate ventilator settings and trends in the patient's response, while the ventilator screen shows events in real time. Interaction between patient and ventilator are represented as waveforms (Ch. 17). Erratic readings may indicate a patient fighting the ventilator or coughing, confirmed by observation of the patient. A high level of positive end-expiratory pressure (PEEP) means that patients are at risk of severe hypoxaemia if they are disconnected from the ventilator. A sawtooth pattern on the expiratory portion of the waveform indicates excess secretions (Fig 18.2).

In volume control ventilation, airway pressure provides the following information:

1 Peak pressure is normally 20 cmH$_2$O above the PEEP level.

2 Peak pressure below normal is usually due to a leak in the circuit.

3 End-expiratory pressure below the baseline suggests excess WOB.

4 Oscillations in airway pressure signify spontaneous breaths between ventilator breaths.

5 Values above 30 cmH$_2$O may be due to airflow obstruction, stiff lungs, pulmonary oedema, pneumothorax, obstruction by upper airway secretions, a kinked tube or clenched teeth (Fig 18.3).

FIGURE 18.2 Expiratory sawtooth pattern on pressure and flow waveforms, suggesting a need for suction

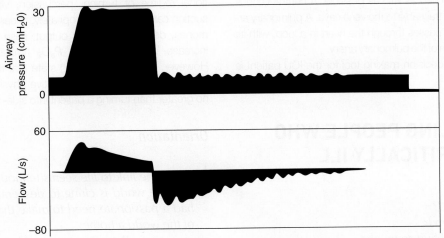

Alveolar pressure is more negative than airway pressure during patient triggering and more positive during a positive pressure breath.

Imaging

Portable x-rays are taken with the patient supine or sitting up as they are able. A supine or slumped position causes a pleural effusion to lose its clear boundary and appear as a generalized opacity on the affected side, with normal vascular markings and no air bronchogram, (App D). Pleural effusions are common because of fluid imbalance or leaky membranes, the lung floating on top of the pleural fluid (Maslove *et al* 2013).

Pneumothoraces are also more difficult to identify on a supine than an upright film because the classic apicolateral location is less common and sometimes the boundary between air and lung is lost.

Close scrutiny of the x-ray is required:

- after unexpected loss of consciousness, in case of aspiration
- after trauma or cardiopulmonary resuscitation, in case of rib or sternal fracture
- after neck line insertion, in case of haemothorax or an apical pneumothorax
- after intubation.

Hardware is deliberately radiopaque. The tracheal (endotracheal or tracheostomy) tube is identified by its opaque line and should extend half-way down the trachea. If it is

FIGURE 18.3 Examples of reasons for increased peak airway pressure in patients on volume-control ventilation. *ARDS*: acute respiratory distress syndrome

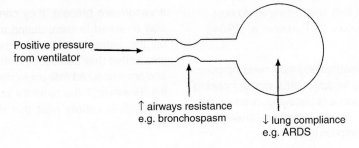

Positive pressure from ventilator

↑ airways resistance
e.g. bronchospasm

↓ lung compliance
e.g. ARDS

too long, unventilated areas collapse (Fig 18.1). If it is too short, it may become dislodged, and the patient's head should be moved as little as possible. A central venous line is usually traceable to the vena cava. A pulmonary artery catheter passes through the heart in a loop, with its tip in a branch of the pulmonary artery.

A clinical decision-making tool for the ICU patient is in App. C.

HANDLING PEOPLE WHO ARE CRITICALLY ILL

> *Who am I?*
> *Where am I?*
> *Why do I hurt so much?*
> *Nursing Times* (1981)

Minimizing oxygen consumption

> **KEY POINT**
>
> Stress increases oxygen consumption and reduces motivation. Treatment is most effective in a motivated patient. Stress is therefore better prevented than treated.

Preliminaries

> *Someone would come near me and would just be working and not saying anything to me. That would be frightening because I didn't know what they were going to do next.*
> Patient quoted by Parker *et al* (1984)

All patients need explanations and most need increased F_iO_2 before and during treatment. All patients, including those who are unconscious or paralyzed, need warning before any physical touch, otherwise anxiety can increase oxygen consumption ($\dot{V}O_2$).

Extra fluids or medication may be required to ensure stable haemodynamics and minimum pain. The traditional regime of turning, percussion, vibrations and suction can, if done inappropriately, release stress hormones, destabilize cardiac output, raise BP and HR, increase $\dot{V}O_2$ and reduce P_aO_2 (Weissman 1993). However, Berney *et al* (2012) state that the metabolic demands of accurate and sensitive physiotherapy are no greater than turning a patient into side- lying.

Orientation

> *When the link to life seems tenuous the immediate world is clung to desperately … I had a passionate need to make that corner of the world a home.*
> Patient quoted by Moore (1991)

Most patients need a visible clock, calendar, family photographs and personal belongings in an area that they can control. They also need information on progress, interpretation of noises and voices, attendance to alarms promptly, explanation of neighbours' alarms, their phone if they are able to talk, and treatment with the same physiotherapist before, during and after admission to the ICU when feasible. We should enter the patient's space gently, introduce ourselves and explain our purpose.

Sleep and rest

Patients should not, if possible, be woken if asleep, especially when flickering eyelids indicate that they are in the REM phase of the sleep cycle when tissue regeneration is at its maximum. Sleep is an essential component of rehabilitation in its function of resting muscles in order to benefit from exercise.

Family

If visitors are present, they can either be invited to stay or asked to leave during treatment, depending on the patient's wish. The presence of relatives means that they can become involved in patient care and are reassured that physiotherapy is not distressing. However, if the patient's wish cannot be ascertained, it is usually best that visitors are asked to leave.

Communication

> *Do not deny the patient their experience. The most helpful conversation I had was with a physician who acknowledged that I was in a 'dark' place ... Immediately, I believed she knew I was suffering ... I trusted this physician.*
>
> Patient quoted by Hipp & Ely 2012

The priority is to establish communication, including:

- clear and explicit explanations, repeated as necessary, including why physiotherapy is necessary, what it will feel like, how long it will last and instructions on how to ask for it to stop
- hearing aid or glasses if used, which reduce the incidence of delirium (Allen *et al* 2012)
- when appropriate, a speaking tracheostomy tube, which also facilitates protective expiration after swallowing to help protect against aspiration (Prigent *et al* 2012)
- referral to speech-language therapy (Radtke *et al* 2011) a lip-reading interpreter (Meltzer *et al* 2012) or a translator, if required
- communication aids such as word or picture charts (Fig 18.4), paper and clipboard, laptop or, for greater privacy, a magic slate
- if unable to write or use picture charts, yes/no questions asked one at a time, e.g.: 'Are you hot? cold? itchy? thirsty? worried? tired? sleepy? nauseous? in pain? Is your mouth dry? Is the tube bothering you? Do you want to turn? raise or lower your head? Do you need more air? less light? less noise? more information? bottle or bedpan?'

Communication should be aimed *at* patients rather than *over* them. Chatting over patients can increase stress more than suction (Lynch 1978). One patient said 'it didn't matter what they talked about, so long as they talked to me' (Villaire 1995).

Anxious patients are not usually helped by being told to relax; the source of anxiety needs to be identified and information provided. If a patient wishes not to communicate, this should also be respected.

Helplessness

> *What do you do when you can't bear it? What are the alternatives?*
>
> Rollin (1976)

Helplessness can lead to depression, so the more helpless the patient, the more important is autonomy. Patients can choose whether they would like treatment now or later, if possible, and their preferred position to be left in. If they request, they should be turned before the allotted time. They can have charge of the TV remote and radio channel, if available, and decide whether they would like to regain their day/night rhythm by being woken in the day or having a sleeping pill at night. Autonomy is particularly important in this situation of unequal power.

Anxiety is reduced by combining factual information with advice that enables patients to be proactive, as much as they are able. Depression is eased by allowing expression of emotion, encouraging independence, using imaginative interventions such as pet visitation schemes (Giuliano *et al* 2000) and ensuring rehabilitation throughout critical illness (Gosselink *et al* 2008).

Touch

ICU patients are extra sensitive to human physical contact as a contrast to the cold clinical procedures to which they are subjected. Therapeutic touch reduces anxiety (Zare *et al* 2010), massage reduces stress (Waldmann 2009 p. 71) and reflexology lessens the need for sedation (Akin *et al* 2014). As always, it should be remembered that individuals and cultures vary and some dislike touch, particularly male/female touch.

Handling unconscious or paralyzed people

> *I heard a lot more than I think they think I heard.*
>
> Patient quoted by Jablonski (1994)

Being moved is a difficult event for ICU patients, and one in three handling procedures is accompanied by cardiac instability, desaturation or ventilatory distress (Jong *et al* 2013). We need to act as the consciousness of the

FIGURE 18.4 Communication chart

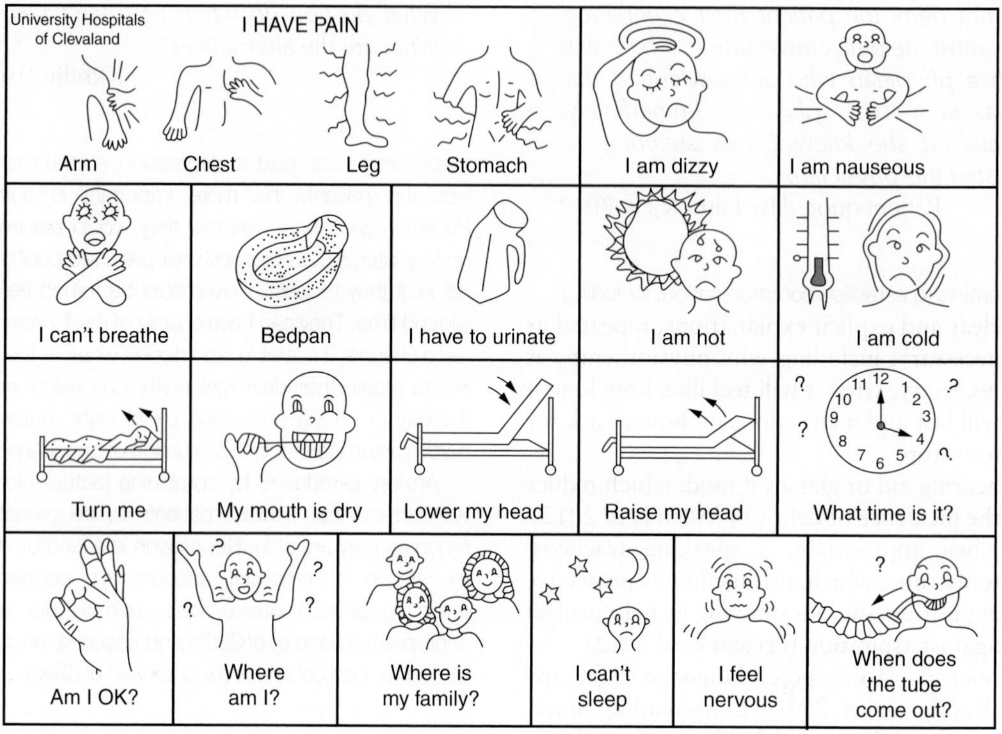

unconscious. It is easy to depersonalize patients who cannot respond to us, especially if we have not had the opportunity to get to know them before they became ill. When handling ICU patients who are paralyzed, unconscious, sedated or weak, forewarning and often a bolus of morphine are required (Ahlers *et al* 2012).

Turning

> To be talked frankly through a complete procedure would help curb the deadly effects of uninformed anticipation.
> Brooks (patient) 1990

The longer a patient has been immobile, the more sensitive their cardiovascular system is to position change. A lateral turn in a critically ill patient can reduce tissue oxygenation by 8–22%, with increased $\dot{V}O_2$ bearing a greater responsibility than reduced oxygen delivery

(DO_2), but monitor readings should return to baseline within five minutes (Vollman 2013). A suggested sequence is the following:

1 Inform the patient, then talk them through each step.
2 Turn off continuous tube feeds.
3 Ensure sufficient slack in lines and tubes.
4 Ensure that glide sheets are in place, the team is following the same manual handling protocol and an individual is responsible for the airway and vulnerable lines.
5 Ensure that the team is co-ordinated in relation to care of the skin and joints (e.g. protect heels from friction, avoid using the leg as a lever).
6 Suction oral secretions, as far as above the cuff, to minimize the risk of aspiration (Gentile & Siobal 2010).
7 Support the tracheal tube. Some trusted patients like to hold an endotracheal tube briefly with their teeth during the turn.

8   Say clearly, so that the team and patient can hear, previously-agreed instructions e.g. 'ready, steady, turn'.
9   Turn smoothly, ensuring that the shoulder joints and head are supported if the patient is paralyzed, and that creases in the sheet are smoothed out.
10 Check lines, patient comfort, monitors, joint positions, re-check cuff pressure (Lizy *et al* 2014).
11 Re-attach continuous tube feeds.

Pressure area care

Pressure sores distress patients and are avoidable. Risk factors are malnutrition, obesity, steroids, vasopressor drugs, diabetes, advanced age and restricted movement due to traction, support systems or patient instability.

Anything can be put on a pressure sore except the patient. Hospitals are full of concoctions for treating them, but better still is prevention by means of:

- adequate nutrition (Dam *et al* 2011), especially vitamin C and protein
- regular turning, without friction, and judicious positioning
- specialized beds
- keeping pressure areas dry
- prevention of hypovolaemia.

A sacral pressure sore that has developed in supine does not preclude sitting out in a chair, so long as a pressure cushion is used and an upright position maintained to prevent pressure on the sacrum. A time limit should be set and there should be meticulous monitoring of the wound before and after.

TECHNIQUES TO INCREASE LUNG VOLUME

No-one explained ... all they said was not to worry about it.
          Patient quoted by Thomson 1973

For spontaneously breathing patients, lung volume can be increased by the techniques in Chapter 6. For ventilated patients, the following modifications can be used.

Positioning

Positioning is the main physiotherapy intervention for critically ill patients, and may be the only treatment for some patients. Spending too long in supine encourages basal atelectasis, especially of the left lower lobe because the heart compresses its bronchus (Khan *et al* 2009b). Turning from supine to side-lying helps clear lower lobe atelectasis, reduce the risk of pneumonia, promote patient comfort, safeguard pressure areas and increase cardiac output (Thomas *et al* 2007). If the patient is lying well forward (Berney *et al* 2012), the abdominal contents are prevented from encroaching on lung volume.

Other effects of positioning have been documented:

1   Kinetic beds turn patients continually along a longitudinal axis and help prevent atelectasis (Ahrens *et al* 2004).
2   As with spontaneously breathing patients, ventilated patients with unilateral lung pathology normally show optimal gas exchange when lying with the affected lung uppermost (Ng & Ong 2010).
3   Miette (2013) found two studies claiming that side-lying reduced bacterial colonization. This position also improves gas exchange, respiratory mechanics and secretion clearance, shortens duration of mechanical ventilation and, so long as the tracheal tube is kept horizontal, appears to reduce aspiration (Mauri *et al* 2010).
4   With the patient horizontal, mucus may be prevented from flowing distally. Bassi *et al* (2008) claim that the head-up position may act as a form of reverse postural drainage, facilitating colonization of the airways and possibly pneumonia.

Evidence for head-of-bed elevation is conflicted (Metheny 2013). Raising the head of the bed is said to prevent ventilator-associated pneumonia by minimizing gastroesophageal reflux (GOR), but the semi-recumbent position encourages pooling of secretions above the cuff, and one study which aimed at a head-up position of 45° found this to be achieved for only 15% of the time (Miette 2013). Unless the whole bed is tipped head-up, skin integrity is put at risk (Grap 2005) and head elevation tends to become the slumped position, with abdominal pressure restricting lung volume and, with enteral feeding, increasing GOR (Leng *et al* 2011). Head of bed elevation to 45° may also reduce BP and oxygen delivery (Gocze *et al* 2013) so monitoring must be continuous.

For patients who are cardiovascularly stable, a tilt table can be used to gradually achieve an upright position. Neurological patients require particular attention to observation and haemodynamic monitoring during this process. When using a tilt table without a manual control, a hoist sling should be placed under the patient in case of malfunction, after checking that the legs of the hoist fit under the tilt table.

Factors which may limit positioning are abnormal muscle tone, pain, neurological instability such as brain or spinal cord injury, fractures, pressure sores, unstable BP and some invasive support systems such as haemofiltration.

Neurological facilitation of respiration

Tidal volume (V_T) and minute volume can be increased by perioral stimulation or intercostal stretch (Ch. 6).

Deep breathing on the ventilator

Most patients are on a mode of ventilation that incorporates spontaneous breathing and they may be able to take deep breaths voluntarily. Deep breathing is particularly successful when patients are motivated by watching the results of their endeavours on the V_T monitor.

Mechanical aids

High frequency percussive ventilation reportedly resolves atelectasis that is unresponsive to bronchoscopy, but clinically meaningful outcomes have not been proved (Kallet 2013).

Manual hyperinflation

> *It was by far the most frightening thing that happened to me.*
> Patient quoted by Rowbotham (1990)

Manual hyperinflation delivers extra volume and oxygen to the lungs via a bag such as a rebreathe bag. Compared to positioning, which is accepted as preventive care for most ICU patients, manual hyperinflation is not used routinely because prophylaxis has not been substantiated, and it comes with a selection of complications.

Terminology

- **Manual ventilation** means squeezing gas into a patient's lungs at tidal volume, e.g. when changing ventilator tubing.
- **Manual hyperventilation** delivers rapid breaths, e.g. if the patient is breathless, hypoxaemic or hypercapnic.
- **Manual hyperinflation** provides deep breaths in order to increase lung volume, e.g. when treating a person with atelectasis or sputum retention.

Physiotherapy is associated with manual hyperinflation (MH). The words 'bag-squeezing' or 'bagging' are also used, but not in front of patients as they can be misinterpreted, e.g. that the patient is to go into a body bag.

Effects

Benefits of MH are:
- reversal of atelectasis (Berney *et al* 2012)
- sputum clearance (van Aswegen *et al* 2013)
- improved oxygen levels (Fig 18.5) and, with suction, temporary improvement in lung compliance (Choi & Jones 2005).

Complications

The complications of MH are an exaggeration of the complications of mechanical ventilation (MV), particularly barotrauma and haemodynamic compromise.

Mean arterial pressure may rise (Grap *et al* 1994) or fall, either of which may reduce cardiac output even in people with normal cardiac function (Anning *et al* 2003). Hypotension is caused by reduced venous return to the heart, and is more pronounced in patients who are hypovolaemic or vasodilated.

For patients on high PEEP, disconnection from the ventilator to attach the bag may not be offset by the benefits of the procedure. In this case, options are to use ventilator hyperinflation or to modify the technique.

FIGURE 18.5 Improved gas exchange immediately after MH and at 10-minute intervals afterwards $P_aO_2:F_iO_2$: oxygen tension in relation to inspired oxygen, *MH*: manual hyperinflation

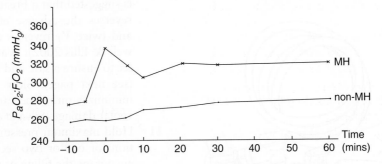

Equipment

A rebreathe Mapleson-C or Water's bag (Fig. 18.6a) is inflated with wall oxygen and comes in 1–3 litre sizes, the 2 litre being used for most adults. It incorporates an expiratory valve which adjusts pressure to the patient, and its compliance allows the clinician to feel the ease of inflation.

Semi-rigid units, e.g. the self-inflating Ambu or Laerdal bag (Fig. 18.6b), use room air with added oxygen and were designed for resuscitation. The flow and pressure are not easily controlled and they are less responsive to techniques such as the end-inspiratory hold. They have a lower peak expiratory flow and do not appear to clear secretions as effectively as the Mapleson's C bag (van Aswegen *et al* 2013). It is also suggested that they are less able to improve respiratory mechanics than ventilator hyperinflation (Savian *et al* 2006). High pressures are avoided by a pressure release valve rather than controlled by the operator. Both bags can be used with a PEEP valve so that pressure is not lost during treatment.

The gas delivered to the patient is usually 100% oxygen. This is safe for patients during the brief period of treatment, but for hypercapnic COPD patients who might be dependent on their hypoxic drive to breathe (p.7), and who are breathing spontaneously with no SIMV back-up, an air source and oxygen entrainment might be preferable, with continuous observation of the S_pO_2 and, if available, end-tidal CO_2.

A heat-moisture exchanger (HME) incorporating a bacterial filter is added to the circuit to ameliorate the inrush of cold air that causes discomfort and sometimes bronchospasm.

Technique

The following method is suggested:

1 Ensure the patient's fluid and cardiovascular status are optimum.

2 Explain to the patient the purpose of the procedure and that it involves several deep breaths; ensure that they know how to communicate if they want the procedure to stop, and obtain consent. Ask if they would like extra analgesia or sedation.

3 Ensure that a manometer and HME are connected to the circuit.

4 Position the patient well forward in side-lying (Fig. 18.7). In supine the bases are unlikely to be responsive to hyperinflation because the positive pressure favours the more compliant non-dependent regions, especially in the larger right lung (van Aswegen *et al* 2013). For patients who cannot turn, close attention to technique (especially nos 10–11, following, may deliver some extra volume to the lung bases in supine. If a different lung region is to be targeted, it is best placed uppermost.

5 Check monitors after the turn. MH should not be started until cardiovascular stability is assured in the new position.

6 Observe chest expansion.

7 Ensure that the patient is free of distractions or nursing interventions.

FIGURE 18.6 Intersurgical Mapleson's-C (a) and Laerdal (b) circuits with pressure manometer and PEEP valve

(a)

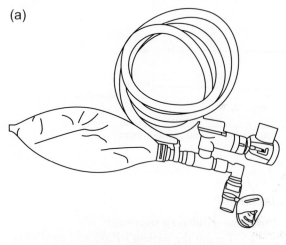

(b)

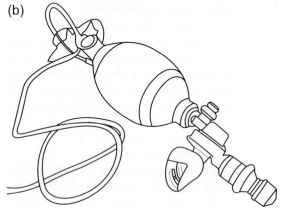

8   Connect the bag to the oxygen with a flow rate of 15 l/min, turn off the low--pressure alarm, turn the ventilator and humidifier to standby, disconnect the patient from the ventilator and connect them to the bagging circuit.

9   Rest tubing on the sheet to avoid pulling on the tracheal tube, tell the patient when to expect ordinary breaths and when deep breaths. Using two hands, squeeze the bag a couple of times at V_T to acclimatize the patient and to assess lung compliance.

10   Then give slow smooth deep breaths, adjusting the valve to increase pressure until expansion is greater than on MV. It is suggested that a breath at 150% of V_T reverses the adverse effects of suction, and twice V_T reverses atelectasis (Maxwell & Ellis 2002). Watch the manometer to ensure a safe and effective pressure (see next page). Slow inspiratory flow minimizes turbulence and the risk of alveolar damage (Silva *et al* 2012).

11   Hold maximum pressure at end-inspiration for one or two seconds in order to encourage the filling of poorly-ventilated alveoli, especially if atelectasis is the problem. This is similar to the plateau pressure in Fig. 17.4a. Haemodynamically unstable patients should not receive this end-inspiratory hold, and are best given one deep breath interspersed with several tidal breaths, or if the patient is able, spontaneous breaths.

12   Release the bag sharply to simulate a huff, especially if sputum retention is the problem.

13   Ensure adequate time before the next inflation to avoid build up of intrinsic PEEP or cardiovascular instability, while watching the S_pO_2 monitor.

14   Throughout, watch the chest for expansion, the face for distress and the abdomen for signs of unwanted active expiration. The more alert the patient, the greater is the need to co-ordinate with their breathing. Stop if the patient's facial expression or the monitors indicate distress, or if crackles indicate that secretions have been mobilized and suction is required. If crackles are heard or the patient coughs, give normal V_T breaths until the patient is suctioned, to avoid pushing the secretions back down. If MH causes no change, stop after about six breaths for re-assessment.

15   Reset the ventilator, advise the patient and reconnect them to the ventilator. Observe chest movement and monitors, auscultate the chest.

FIGURE 18.7 Manual hyperinflation targeting the left lower lobe, which is being palpated to check for optimum expansion

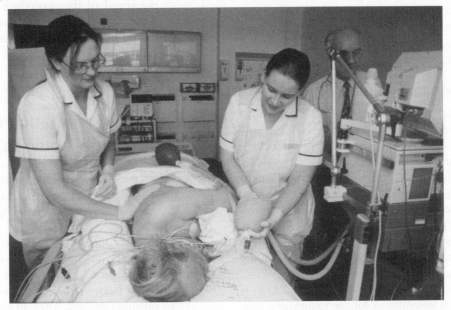

16   Repeat the cycles until auscultation indicates that volume is restored or secretions cleared. If this is not achieved within five to ten minutes of accurate MH, it is unlikely to occur in this session.

17   To maintain the benefits of MH, the side-lying position should be maintained afterwards, ensuring that the tracheal tube is kept horizontal, as long as this position is comfortable for the patient and convenient for nursing procedures.

Pressures

Each bed space should be supplied with its own manometer to ensure effective and safe pressures (Davies & Igo 2004) and to reduce complications (Hila & Ellis 2002). The following are guidelines:

1   For MH to be effective in normal lungs, a sustained inflation to 40 cmH$_2$O is required to reverse atelectasis (Novak *et al* 1987, Rothen *et al* 1999).

2   For MH to be safe in normal lungs, inflation to 50 cmH$_2$O is considered acceptable so long as PEEP is maintained to stabilize the alveoli (García-Fernández *et al* 2013), while just two hyperinflations to a maximum 60 cmH$_2$O have been used safely by Khanna *et al* (2013).

3   For MH to be safe in diseased or damaged lungs, it is impossible to identify a maximum pressure. For people with acute respiratory distress syndrome (ARDS), Gattinoni *et al* (2002) claim that 45 cmH$_2$O is safe and Oczenski *et al* (2005) show no evidence of complications using continuous positive airway pressure (CPAP) at 50 cmH$_2$O for 30 seconds, using the prone position to protect vulnerable lung regions. However few physiotherapists would risk using these pressures in people with such damaged lungs.

All the above studies had limitations, and efficacy should be monitored throughout, to ensure that the minimum effective pressure is used.

Contraindications

MH should be avoided with the following:

- extra-alveolar air, e.g. undrained pneumothorax, subcutaneous emphysema or bulla
- bronchospasm causing peak airway pressures above 40 cmH$_2$0, in particular with acute asthma.

Precautions and modifications

MH should be avoided or modified with the following:

- patients at risk of barotrauma, e.g. those with emphysema, fibrosis, pneumocystis pneumonia or ARDS
- rib fracture because a covert pneumothorax might be present; if MH is essential, the scan should be scrutinized or a radiologist's opinion sought
- pneumothorax with a chest drain
- air leak, as demonstrated by air bubbling through a chest drain bottle
- hyperinflated lungs with intrinsic PEEP; if MH is essential, a longer expiratory time may reduce the risk of further gas trapping
- bronchopleural fistula
- recent pneumonectomy because of the risk of a bronchopleural fistula; the fifth to 10th postoperative days are when the healing stump is most vulnerable
- BP that is low, high or unstable; if MH is essential in hypotensive patients, they should be maximally stabilized first and the technique should be brief, with prolonged expiration and no end-inspiratory hold, in order to facilitate venous return
- hypovolaemia; if MH is necessary, the above modifications are advised
- arrhythmias or frequent ectopics
- during renal dialysis if this destabilizes BP
- acute brain injury, especially if there is no intracranial pressure monitoring
- haemoptysis of unknown cause
- severe hypoxaemia with PEEP above 10 mmHg because disconnection of the patient from the ventilator entails loss of PEEP; if MH is essential, desaturation can be minimized by:
  - incorporating a PEEP valve in the circuit, though this may slow expiratory flow

  - manually preventing the bag fully deflating at end-expiration
  - increasing the flow rate, and increasing the speed of the procedure to prevent deflation and augment oxygenation, but only if the patient is haemodynamically stable
  - ventilator hyperinflation.

Ventilator hyperinflation or recruitment manoeuvres

To reduce some of the complications of manual hyperinflation, alveolar recruitment can be aided by hyperinflation through the ventilator. The following have been described:

1   In volume control, V_T is gradually increased until peak airway pressure reaches 40 cmH$_2$O, then six hyperinflation breaths are delivered before returning the ventilator to its previous settings. After 30 seconds' rest, the process is repeated until the desired outcome is achieved, or complications such as patient distress or haemodynamic instability supervene. This can improve lung compliance and clear secretions, with the assumption that it would increase lung volume similarly to manual hyperinflation. The technique allows the flow pattern to be observed on the screen, to ensure full exhalation before the next breath is delivered, thus reducing the risk of intrinsic PEEP (Berney & Denehy 2002).

2   In pressure control, a stepwise increase in PEEP up to 15 cmH$_2$O and V_T up to 18 ml/kg are administered until a peak inspiratory pressure of 40 cmH$_2$O is reached, then maintained for 10 cycles. This has shown improved oxygenation immediately after heart surgery, with stabilization of newly-recruited alveoli by ongoing PEEP (Claxton et al 2003).

3   The pressure and/or time of the positive pressure breath is increased, e.g. peak pressure of 45 cmH$_2$O and PEEP of 35 cmH$_2$O for one minute followed by PEEP of 10 cmH$_2$O (Halter 2003).

4 Inflation pressure is increased to 30–40 cmH$_2$O for 30–40 seconds, inspiratory pause is extended, three consecutive sighs are delivered at plateau pressure 45 cmH$_2$O, or PEEP raised to 40 cmH$_2$O with pressure control at 20 cmH$_2$O above this level for two minutes followed by on going PEEP at 25 cmH$_2$O (Hess & Bigatello 2002).

5 In SIMV, F_iO_2 is increased to 1.0, inspiratory time adjusted to three to five seconds, RR to 6–8 bpm and V_T to 15 ml/kg body weight, increasing at first by 150 ml per breath until a peak pressure of 40 cmH$_2$O is achieved. Four sets of eight ventilator breaths per treatment are claimed to produce the same outcomes and safety profile as MH (Dennis *et al* 2012b).

6 Inflation pressure is increased to 40 cmH$_2$O for 10 secs (Hedenstierna 2012).

The benefits of these strategies are not sustained unless high PEEP is maintained (Hess & Bigatello 2002).

The following complications of ventilator hyperinflation have been identified:

- haemodynamic instability caused by sustained positive pressure, e.g. 20 second inflations at 40 cmH$_2$O for 8 minutes (Nunes *et al* 2004)
- alveolar overdistension caused by pressure support at 50 cmH$_2$O and PEEP levels above those required for optimal compliance (Villagrá *et al* 2002)
- for patients with acute lung injury, desaturations, arrhythmias and air leaks following 40 cmH$_2$O of CPAP for 40 seconds up to four times a day (Fan *et al* 2012)
- gas trapping, which can be prevented by ensuring that exhaled V_T is no less than inhaled V_T.

Recruitment without overdistension may be achieved by periodic ventilator deep inflations (Allen *et al* 2006). Slow moderate-pressure inflations appear to achieve the same benefit as vital capacity inflations, with less risk of complications (Lowhagen 2011) and thoracic tomography has been suggested for safety (Dueck 2006).

Recruitment manoeuvres were developed to maintain alveolar stability and offset the lost lung volume caused by lung protective ventilation strategies for ARDS (Ch. 19), not primarily to expand collapsed lung units. Most studies do not report on whether complications were documented, and some of the pressures are alarmingly high for patients with damaged lungs. Their safety has been questioned (Hess 2002), particularly after three to five days into the course of ARDS, when the lungs are at their most fragile. Martin (2009) claims that they improve radiographic images of the lungs but not patient outcomes, begging the question as to whether these 'open lungs' are happy lungs or simply pretty lungs.

Manual hyperinflation, which is designed to clear secretions as well as increase volume, has been described as the treatment of choice for physiotherapists (Barker & Adams 2002). However, physiotherapists will probably use both, depending on the outcomes, and further research may tip the balance in favour of using the ventilator rather than a bag to reinflate lungs or clear secretions.

PRACTICE TIP

Set up a test lung with a spare ventilator, using a spontaneous mode with high flow, and display the pressure-volume loop. Practise hyperinflation through the ventilator and relate it to V_T and the pressure attained with MH, including maintenance of manual PEEP. The screen can be frozen to identify details.

TECHNIQUES TO CLEAR SECRETIONS

The most effective interventions to clear thick secretions in intubated patients are hydration, humidification and mobilization (Halm 2008). For intubated people who cannot mobilize, regular turning will help keep secretions moving. Hydration in the ICU is normally aimed at optimum haemodynamic status rather than secretion clearance, but the physiotherapist can have a say on ward rounds. Other interventions are suction as required, and sometimes manual techniques or manual hyperinflation.

Humidification

Humidification is provided by a **hot water humidifier**, with temperature alarms set at maximum 37°C and minimum 30°C. An alternative is a **heat-moisture exchanger** (HME), which may be adequate for short term use in well hydrated patients who do not have excessive or thick secretions. Added to the information in Ch. 8, the following arguments have been made about the two systems:

1   Compared to hot water humidification, HME's are less able to increase mucociliary transport (Nakagawa *et al* 2004). They quadruple the risk of endotracheal tube (ETT) obstruction (Branson 2009) and increase the work of breathing such that Hilbert (2003) suggests the support level for patients on pressure support ventilation be increased by 8–15 cmH$_2$O.

2   HMEs increase dead space and reduce CO$_2$ clearance (AARC 2012) and allowance should be made for a drop in P_aCO_2 when the device is removed (López *et al* 2000).

3   If mechanical ventilation (MV) is expected to last more than a few hours, a heated humidifier has been advised (Ryan *et al* 2002), although one of the authors of this study was employed by a humidifier company.

4   Lucato *et al* (2005) found that resistance increased within hours of applying an HME. They stated that patients with hypersecretory disease will need a hot water humidifier straight away.

5   In contrast, Branson (2007) suggests that a heated humidifier should be used from the outset only if intubation is expected to last more than 96 hours.

Fig 18.8 shows the risk of ETT occlusion with different HME's and a hot water humidifier.

Saline nebulizers are loved by ICU bacteria. If they are indicated, attention should first be given as to why the humidification system is inadequate. A rather balmy scenario is to intersperse an HME with saline nebulizers.

Postural drainage

The side-to-side positioning applied to most patients is usually adequate for postural drainage and has demonstrated increased sputum yield during MH (Berney *et al* 2012). A head-down tilt may be required (Berney 2004) but gravity is thought to have less of an effect on the movement of secretions than flow bias (Graf & Marini 2008), and the position is unwise for most patients on MV, especially if haemodynamics are compromised. Kinetic beds appear to reduce the incidence of pneumonia (Chung & Mueller 2011).

FIGURE 18.8   Level of humidity provided by different systems (see also Fig 8.4). *HME:* heat-moisture exchanger, *ETT:* endotracheal tube

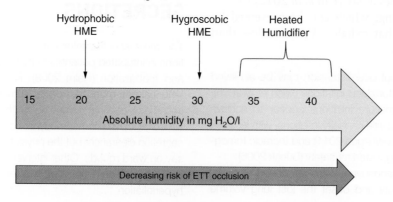

Manual techniques

Percussion or vibrations are not required routinely, and when combined with postural drainage have not been shown to reduce ventilator-associated pneumonia (VAP) or atelectasis (Branson 2007). Vibrations cause less airflow than MH (Fig. 18.9), but manual techniques do not usually cause significant haemodynamic problems (Wong et al 2006) and they may help to clear excessive or thick secretions.

Vibrations with MH may help reduce intrinsic PEEP by ensuring full exhalation before the next hyperinflation, and, when started just before termination of the end-inspiratory hold, they may increase lung volume (Shannon et al 2010).

'Ribcage compression', which may have similar effects to rib-springing, can reduce lung volume, hinder gas exchange and may actually reduce sputum clearance (Unoki et al 2004) though these may not occur if followed by strategies to restore volume.

Flow bias

Expiratory flow greater than 10% above inspiratory flow facilitates mucus movement towards the mouth (Ntoumenopoulos et al 2013). The physiotherapist can discuss ventilator settings with the intensivist if an extra boost to mucus clearance is required.

Manual hyperinflation

If not contraindicated, MH assists sputum clearance, with emphasis on rapid release to reinforce expiratory flow bias (van Aswegen et al 2013).

Mechanical aids

Both bubble PEP (Jones et al 2013c) and the Flutter (Chicayban 2011) can be slotted into the exhalation port. High frequency percussive ventilation may be used with both spontaneous and mechanical ventilation, and an insufflation-exsufflator can be connected to the tracheal tube to facilitate a cough, although disconnection from the ventilator limits its use (Kallet 2013).

Suction

> *The coughing, gagging and choking spasms produced by the sink plunger technique were terrifying.*
> Patient quoted by Day et al (2002)

Suction stops the patient breathing and may cause pain (Paulus et al 2013) but, so long as no 'sink-plunger' technique is employed, it is normally less harrowing than nasopharyngeal suction, especially if the patient is fully informed and talked through the process.

Secretions in peripheral airways are unlikely to contribute to airflow obstruction because of the number of alternative airways, but if stagnant they may contribute to infection. Secretions in the large airways, where there is less collateral ventilation, may interfere with gas exchange or cause plugging. Suction should be carried out when indicated and if secretions are accessible (AARC 2010).

Complications

Suction may cause:
- ↓ lung volume due to the negative pressure and, with open suction, disconnection from the ventilator (Ntoumenopoulos 2013)
- ↑ oxygen demand (White et al 1990)

FIGURE 18.9 Airflow during manual hyperinflation (left) and vibrations (right)

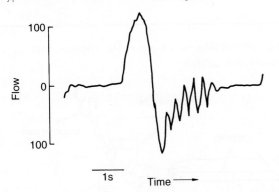

- hypoxaemia, arrhythmias and mucosal injury (Chang 2014 p.174)
- bronchospasm (AARC 2010)
- repeated inoculation of the lungs from the biofilm lining the tracheal tube, releasing up to 60 000 colonies of bacteria with each suction pass (Lewes 2002)
- bleeding (Maggiore *et al* 2013), due to clotting disorder, heparinization or suction that is rough, frequent or with dry airways
- bradycardia in certain patients, which can be attenuated by nebulized atropine (Brooks *et al* 2001).

Most complications can be reduced by preoxygenation, post-suction hyperinflation and optimal technique (overleaf) on page 467.

Catheters

The smallest effective catheter should be used, which must be no more than half the internal diameter of the tracheal tube, a larger size causing more mucosal damage than the suction pressure (AARC 2010). A size >12 FG tends to reduce P_aO_2 and tidal volume, and increase pulmonary artery pressure and P_aCO_2 (Almgren *et al* 2004).

A closed-circuit in-line catheter (Fig. 18.10) is sealed in a protective sleeve and becomes part of the ventilator circuit. It brings the following advantages:

- No disconnection from the ventilator, leading to less desaturation, less volume loss (Maggiore 2003), less airway collapse, maintenance of PEEP and attenuation of pressure changes (Palazzo & Soni 2013).
- Less risk of cross-infection, (Lorente *et al* 2006).

Open suction requires disconnection of the patient from the ventilator but has advantages:

- less likelihood of the preserved PEEP blowing mucus back into the lungs, which could require compensation with higher suction pressures (Branson 2007)
- according to a meta-analysis, shorter time on MV and lower colonization rates (Siempos *et al* 2008)
- ability to use the rocking thumb technique (Ch. 8) rather than obligatory use of intermittent suction to relieve pressure.

Although in-line catheters should reduce cross infection, there appears to be no difference in pneumonia or mortality for the patient (Subirana 2010), and unless there are specific requirements, there is little evidence to favour either type of catheter (Jongerden *et al* 2007).

Preliminaries

Pre-oxygenation is required for all patients (AARC 2010), the '100% oxygen' button being the simplest method. Self-ventilating patients may find it helpful subjectively to hyperventilate beforehand. Indications, contraindications and technique for nasopharyngeal suction are in Ch. 8, with modifications for intubated patients below.

Technique for closed-circuit suction

Each unit will have its own protocol, but some tips are that:

- Extra gloves are not necessary.
- The suction pressure is checked with the vacuum on, i.e. with the vacuum control valve unlocked.

FIGURE 18.10 Closed circuit catheter connected to the tracheal tube via a T-piece. The irrigation port allows the passage of saline for loosening secretions or cleaning the catheter

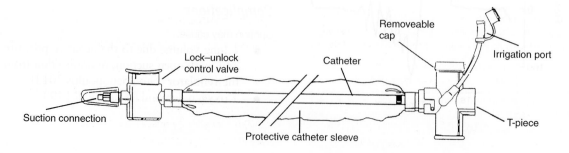

- If the MH bag is connected during suction, its valve must be kept open.
- The T-piece should be supported throughout.

During catheter insertion, it is standard practice to avoid suction in order to minimize mucosal damage, although Lewis (2002) claims that greater risk is caused without suction due to bacteria being pushed further down the airways. Standard practice is advised until further research emerges.

During catheter withdrawal, some patients voluntarily hold their breath longer than necessary, in which case they can be told, once the catheter has been withdrawn back to the tracheal tube, that they can breathe again. Unlike when nasopharyngeal suction is being used, it is not always clear to patients the point at which they can breathe again.

The AARC (2010) claim that shallow suction, i.e. only as far as the end of the tracheal tube, reduces complications, but Ntoumenopoulos (2013) suggests but this is based on neonatal literature and may be counterproductive. If more than one pass is necessary, oxygenation must return to baseline before repeat suction. Suction should be terminated if HR slows by 20 or increases by 40 bpm, if BP drops or arrhythmias develop. The final suction should be outside the endotracheal tube, with the patient's permission, to reach secretions above the cuff, which helps prevent microaspiration and VAP (Hess 2002).

Difficulty passing the catheter may be due to kinking of the tracheal tube, herniation of the cuff over the end of the tube, or the patient biting the tube. Biting requires reassurance and sometimes insertion of a bite block or Guedel airway.

Vibrations are unnecessary during suction because, unless the patient is paralyzed, the enforced coughing accompanying suction overrides outside influences. Occasionally apical vibrations can be used to stimulate a cough.

Modifications for open suction

Open suction entails inserting a sterile catheter directly into the tracheal tube. Aseptic technique should be pristine: the catheter must not touch the rim of the tracheal tube on insertion and sterile gloves are mandatory. Boxed gloves are not sterile and Rossoff (1995) found that half were contaminated. The same catheter should not be used for repeat suction.

For access to the left main bronchus, Branson (2007) recommends turning the head to the right, or using an angled (coudé-tip) catheter with the tip directed towards the left main bronchus. These techniques are used by anaesthetists, but most physiotherapists do not find them necessary because they usually mobilize secretions sufficiently beforehand.

Reducing hypoxaemia

Returning the patient to the ventilator at normal settings between suction passes is not adequate to prevent desaturation, and the following are suggested:

1 Manual hyperventilation or hyperinflation helps reverse hypoxaemia and atelectasis respectively, if not contraindicated.

2 Pressing the '100% oxygen' button whenever the patient is on the ventilator helps maintain oxygenation.

3 During closed suction, the triggering function of the ventilator can be used to deliver pressure-supported breaths at 40 cmH_2O (Maggiore 2003).

4 After suction, ventilator hyperinflation can be used, e.g. 30 seconds of peak inspiratory pressure at 35–40 cmH_2O and PEEP at 15 cmH_2O (Heinze et al 2011).

5 No more than ten seconds should be spent with the patient unable to breathe. If longer is needed, this can be accommodated during open suction by withdrawing the catheter sufficiently to prevent coughing, removing the thumb from the catheter port to release the vacuum, occluding the catheter mount opening (with the catheter still *in situ*), then giving the patient 100% oxygen by the bag or ventilator. Suction can be resumed when the patient has stabilized. This avoids unnecessary removal and reinsertion of the catheter, which increases the infection risk.

Saline instillation

The need for saline suggests that humidification is inadequate. If this has been corrected but secretions are still too thick to clear, normal saline may be instilled into the lungs. This can increase the yield of sputum (Schreuder & Jones 2004) and reduce VAP (Caruso et al 2008), possibly by rinsing out bacteria from the ETT or by stimulating a cough. However, other studies have shown an increased risk of infection, so it should only be done if essential (Roberts 2009).

There are some doubts about the mechanism of saline instillation because mucus does not incorporate water easily (Halm 2008). Its mode of action may be to physically dislodge encrusted secretions or to stimulate a cough.

The procedure should not be prolonged, otherwise gas exchange is compromised (Young-Ra 2002) and breathlessness can persist for up to ten minutes (Halm 2008). The following is suggested:

1   Warm the saline, e.g. by always keeping saline in a pocket so that it is readily available at body temperature.
2   When opening the container, the open ends must not be touched even with gloved hands.
3   Advise the patient, then administer the saline slowly to prevent them feeling as if they are drowning.
4   No more than 5 ml at a time is advised (Bostick & Wendelgass 1987), but more can be used if accompanied by increased ventilator F_iO_2 and if interspersed with manual or ventilator hyperventilation to prevent desaturation.
5   If the aim is to loosen secretions (rather than dislodge debris at the end of the tracheal tube), the patient should be turned after instillation, so that the instilled side is uppermost for treatment. This can be coordinated with the patient's regular turns to avoid unnecessary disruption. Suction performed after the turn, and if required after manual techniques, is then well timed to clear both secretions and saline.

Tips for open suction:

●   Do not allow the saline to splatter over the tracheostomy dressing, or indeed over anything.
●   If saline instillation does not clear the secretions, it can be delivered more distally by injecting it through the catheter.

Tip for closed-circuit suction:

●   hold the T-piece upwards to help the passage of saline, unlock the vacuum control valve, advance the catheter and inject saline through the side port just before inspiration so it is carried distally with the next breath.

Patients who are able can use the yankauer sucker to clear their mouth afterwards. They should not be turned or moved until stable.

PRACTICE TIP

Don't forget the 'Limitations' section in the literature. Fig 18.11 shows a 'positive' outcome from saline instillation, but the authors sensibly point out, in their Limitations paragraph, that the sputum weight included the saline.

EXERCISE AND REHABILITATION

Getting me out of bed has always made me feel like the team and I are working together, not against each other. This simple action helps ground me in the environment and helps my mind, which seems to work overtime to understand the stimuli that bombard it.

Patient quoted by Hipp & Ely (2012)

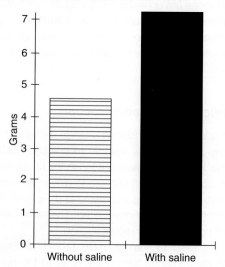

FIGURE 18.11 Mean 'sputum weight' after suction with and without saline instillation

Increasing numbers of ICU patients now survive (Fan 2010), which has raised the profile of rehabilitation. Autonomy is at the heart of rehabilitation, and patients who are involved in their own care have found it easier to move on after discharge (Karlsson & Forsberg 2008). Rehabilitation should be initiated immediately (Mendez-Telle 2012), facilitated by nutritional supplements (Chambers 2009) and the concept of the 'animated ICU' in which sedation is minimized (Hall 2010).

Rehabilitation is recommended for a minimum 45 mins a day (Danbury et al 2013). The importance of exercise is underlined by the detrimental effects of immobility (Ch. 1) and the reported outcomes of ICU rehabilitation:

- brain protection by reducing delirium (Hopkins *et al* 2012)
- lung protection by modulating inflammation in the early phase of acute lung injury (Goncalves *et al* 2012)
- ↑ muscle strength, ↓ length of ICU stay (Renaud *et al* 2013)
- ↑ exercise tolerance and quality of life, ↓ dyspnoea, sedation and re-admission (Adler & Malone 2012)
- ↑ functional outcomes, ↓ days in hospital (Stiller 2012)
- ↑ respiratory muscle strength, sphincter control and ventilator-free time (Porta *et al* 2005)
- ↑ secretion clearance (Morris & Afifi 2010 p. 228)
- ↓ ICU myopathy, systemic inflammation, insulin resistance and microvascular dysfunction (Fan 2010).

Early mobilization, in particular, has shown:

- ↓ lung and vascular complications (Clark *et al* 2013)
- ↓ delirium (Porter & McClure 2013)
- ↓ atelectasis, pneumonia and the cognitive and functional limitation that can otherwise continue for years after discharge (Vollman 2013)
- ↓ ICU stay and ↑ percentage of patients discharged home (Engel *et al* 2013)
- ↓ morbidity and mortality (Hopkins *et al* 2012).

One obese patient had her pre-morbid exercise tolerance of 3 metres increased to 37 metres during her 9-day stay on the ICU (Korupolu et al 2010).

Passive exercise

Clavet *et al* (2008) found that a third of patients who spent more than two weeks in the ICU developed joint contractures sufficient to impair function. This can be prevented by passive movements, which also maintain sensory input and comfort, possibly preserve muscle architecture (Kress 2013) and, if done frequently, reduce the risk of myopathy (Renaud *et al* 2013). Inclusion of the shoulder joint brings a modest increase in minute volume (Loram & de Charmoy 2002).

Special attention is required for the Achilles tendon, hip joint, joints around the shoulder, two-joint muscles and, for long-term patients, the jaw and spine. Continuous passive motion reduces protein loss (Morris 2007), pain and muscle inflammation (Amidei 2013), and a stiff chest wall may respond to stretching exercises including manual rotation of the thorax in time with the ventilatory cycle (Leelarungrayub *et al* 2009), while ensuring that the tracheal tube is stabilized.

A femoral catheter precludes all but minor hip flexion (Perm *et al* 2013). All ICU staff need advice on care of the joints, especially the shoulder, which is the most commonly reported joint affected by subsequent chronic pain (Battle *et al* 2013a).

Patients with fractures, burns or altered muscle tone need input from specialist colleagues, and those with impaired circulation to the peripheries due to septic shock need multidisciplinary intervention. To prevent overstretch of flaccid anterior tibial muscles, a pillow at the end of the bed can be placed against a vertically-placed tray to maintain plantigrade.

There is some limited evidence of benefit from neuromuscular electrical stimulation (Williams & Flynn 2014). For affluent ICUs, whole-bed vibration helps stimulate neuromuscular activity (Ritzmann 2013).

Active exercise

No modern ICU can match the body's sophisticated system for delivery of biochemical compounds during exercise.
Woodard & Berry (2001)

Exercise helps maintain conditioning and reduce inflammation (Winkelman 2007). Benefit has been shown from resistive exercises (Gosselink *et al* 2008), functional exercises such as turning in bed or sitting over the edge of the bed (Chiang *et al* 2006), and Wii (Kho *et al* 2012). Specific effects include the following:

1   Arm strengthening for 20 minutes a day improves strength, mobility and dyspnoea (Porta *et al* 2005).

2   Inspiratory muscle training increases inspiratory muscle strength (Smith *et al* 2014), or, more specifically, when done twice daily up to Borg score 6–8, it can progress exercise tolerance and ADL (Chang *et al* 2005).

3   Stretching, resistance and endurance exercise can improve pulmonary mechanics and functional status (Chen & Lin 2012).

KEY POINT

Active little-and-often exercise is required for all patients who are willing and able.

An exercise programme can be maintained for patients who are on inotropic support (Macauley 2012) but vigorous active exercise should be avoided because of limited cardiovascular reserve. Input from the dietician is advisable (NICE 2009), and patients, nurses and relatives will be motivated by an exercise diary to encourage progression (App. B).

Mobilization

An attempt should be made to stand all patients for whom it is safe (Box 18.1) as soon as they are responsive to verbal stimulation (Kress 2013). With careful management, observation and monitoring, patients can be mobilized with endotracheal tubes (Bahadur *et al* 2008), femoral catheters (Perm *et al* 2013), other central lines, vasoactive drugs, renal replacement therapy, or if they have acute lung injury or delirium (Vollman 2013). Solicitous attention to lines and tubes is required, and wheeled walkers with attachments to carry equipment are helpful.

The following complications of mobilization have been reported in a systematic review that included

mechanically ventilated patients with central lines or on haemodialysis:

- ↓ S_pO_2 (the commonest adverse event)
- unstable BP
- falls
- loss of nasogastric tube
- loss of arterial line
- extubation
- patient-ventilator asynchrony (Adler & Malone 2012).

This list should not prevent mobilization but is a useful reminder of the vigilance required. Although a femoral line can be managed, some physiotherapists encourage their teams to site these elsewhere when possible.

Long term patients may be excited at the prospect of their much-awaited first expedition out of bed, and some are then disillusioned by the extent of their weakness and fatigue, especially if they have lost the comprehension as well as the ability to walk. One patient stated: 'I didn't know how to walk any more' (Strahana & Brown 2005).

Prior to mobilization, the feed is stopped, and increased ventilatory support may be needed at first, with brief sessions to avoid fatigue. The head of the bed is raised before the patient sits up over the edge of the bed, from where they swing their legs. After lowering the bed until their feet reach the floor, the patient stands and their colour and monitors are kept under observation, especially pallor, dizziness, unstable cardiovascular status or reduced S_pO_2. Standing without walking should be brief to prevent venous pooling. Some beds provide a chair position to facilitate mobility.

For patients able to go further than walking on the spot, mobile monitoring and either a rebreathe bag or a portable ventilator on a trolley can be used. Adventurous patients aim to exercise to 50–60% of maximal HR (Stiller 2007). The retinue should be followed closely by a wheelchair.

Getting dressed is a good morale booster, done in a separate session and with the help of the occupational therapist if required. Occupational therapy is feasible from the onset of MV (Pohlman *et al* 2010) and, when combined with early mobilization, leads to earlier functional independence (Hodgson *et al* 2012).

With these precautions, Leditschke *et al* (2012) were able to mobilize their patients on most days, and Nava (1998) showed how a little-and-often but intensive rehabilitation programme led to 'dramatic improvements' even in patients unable to wean (Nava 1998). Clark

(1985) documents a patient describing how visits outside helped to 'maintain my sanity'. The gym is also a useful destination, and even the pool for some patients.

For patients unable to stand, sitting in a chair helps to prevent hypovolaemia, redistribute skin pressure, maintain muscle length, assist orientation and load vertebrae to limit calcium loss and promote cartilage nutrition. Tipping chairs are useful for patients with orthostatic intolerance, and tilt tables can benefit those with low lung volume, muscle weakness, pressure sores and venous pooling (Chang *et al* 2004).

End of treatment session

After treatment, the following are suggested:

1 Check that all alarms are turned back on.
2 Ensure the patient's nurse knows that treatment is finished.
3 Ensure the call bell and other requirements are within reach of the patient.
4 Ensure that lines are in view.
5 Reassure the patient that they are not being left alone and that their lines are safe so that they do not feel inhibited from moving.
6 For a side-lying patient, check that their ear is not folded over.
7 Check any individual concerns, e.g. anxiety about facing a wall.
8 Tell the patient the time and ask if they need further information.
9 If a rest is required, liaise with the nurse about dimming the light and using eye shades.

Transfer from the ICU

You'd gone from this hugely protective critical care to this sort of hit and miss unco-ordinated service.
Patient quoted by Field *et al* (2008)

For longer-term patients who have been under constant supervision, transfer to the ward is a vulnerable time as well as bringing relief at reaching a milestone. Pre-emptive strategies to minimize relocation stress include early identification of risk factors (Hosein *et al*

2013), restoration of sleep patterns, information packs for the patient and family, phased reduction of bedside equipment, a visit from the patient's named ward nurse, an exit interview and follow-up outreach (Field *et al* 2008). Patients may be weaker than either they or the ward staff expect, sometimes leaving them unable to pick up their tablets or press the buzzer. Relocation management is particularly important for older patients, whose ICU mortality is the same as younger patients but post-ICU mortality higher (Christensen 2013).

Premature discharge from the ICU increases mortality (Danbury *et al* 2013), and transition programs reduce the risk of ICU readmission (Niven 2014). Night time discharge should be documented as an adverse incident (NICE 2007).

When I was moved from intensive care to the general ward I felt as if my life support system had been ripped away.
Moore (patient), 1991, p. 12

Follow up

She had offered to peel the potatoes and managed 4 potatoes in 40 minutes, then had to have an hour's rest before peeling the other four.
Jones & Griffiths 2002, p. 54

After discharge, longer-term patients require access to a multidisciplinary follow-up clinic (Danbury *et al* 2013). Physiotherapy input is aimed at musculoskeletal problems and on-going rehabilitation. Without follow-up, the time taken to return to the previous level of activities is typically 9–12 months (NICE 2009), with only half able to return to work (Pawlik 2012). Significant functional improvements can be achieved even for patients who are ventilator-dependent (Sobush *et al* 2012), and structuring rehabilitation on the ICF model helps prevent 'post-intensive care syndrome' (Iwashyna & Netzer 2012).

A dedicated gym class enables patients to find support from others who have been through a similar experience, support which neither professionals nor family can provide. For example, one young man had

BOX 18.1 Precautions when mobilizing ICU patients

System	Factors that may limit mobilization
Cardiovascular	
MAP	<65 mmHg >20% recent variability
HR	<40 or >130 bpm
Cardiac	Cardiac ischaemia, new MI, unstable ECG, unstable angina Arrhythmia requiring new drug Temporary pacemaker
Other haemodynamic	Inotropes, vasoactive drugs especially new vasopressor, β-blockers Bleeding, including oesophageal varices Platelet count <20 000 mm^{-3} PE or DVT not yet medically stable Orthostatic hypotension
Respiratory	
S_pO_2	<88% >4% recent decrease
P_aO_2/F_iO_2	<300
RR	<7 or >35/minute
Ventilator	PEEP >10 cmH$_2$O Asynchrony with ventilator Insecure airway Pressure support >20 cmH$_2$O or SIMV >18 bpm F_iO_2>0.6
Neurological	
Brain injury	Increased ICP or recent surgery
Spinal cord lesion	Unstable injury
Orthopaedic	
	Unstable fracture
Other	
	Limited ability to respond to commands Haemoglobin <7 g/100 ml or acute ↓ in Hb Split skin graft, some vascular operations Blood sugar <3.5 mmol/l Recent eye surgery

Contraindications, or factors indicating that activity should stop

Request by patient to stop, or visible distress

System	Factors that may limit mobilization
Dizziness	
New onset chest pain	
Change in colour	
↓ BP or HR	
RR >35/min sustained for >60 secs	
Change in heart rhythm	
S_pO_2 <85%	

MAP: mean arterial pressure, MI: myocardial infarct, HR: heart rate, PE: pulmonary embolus, DVT: deep vein thrombosis, PEEP: positive end-expiratory pressure, SIMV: synchronized intermittent mandatory ventilation

not been able to come to terms with attempting to hit a nurse while hallucinating, despite reassurance from staff. 'Oh that's nothing to what I tried to do' said a fellow patient on the neighbouring exercise bike, immediately lifting the burden from the young man.

'Strikingly high' rates of psychological morbidity have been found in ICU survivors (Wade et al 2012), including a 25–50% incidence of depression (Vest et al 2011). Anxiety and depression relate to delusional memories (Ringdal et al 2010), and cognitive or emotional difficulties are virtually ubiquitous (Hopkins 2009). Patients who have experienced a life-threatening episode benefit from debriefing (Mishra 2011) and may need help in constructing a narrative of events, facilitated by their ICU diary, which helps the transition from critical illness to normality (Perier 2013).

Patients may also feel that they have been given a second chance in life and experience heightened spirituality (Papathanassoglou et al 2003), each day seeming more precious than before (Walton 2002). Follow them up to give them the chance to process.

On going rehabilitation increases exercise tolerance, reduces anxiety and depression (McWilliams et al 2009), helps patients pace themselves and reduces problems of imbalance, fear of falling, panic attacks and physical, psychological and cognitive difficulties (Aitken 2010). Other complications can be recognized such as visual problems due to hypotensive episodes, sexual dysfunction, chronic fatigue syndrome and polypharmacy (Waldmann 2009 p. 70).

Late rehabilitation can also be successful. One patient described her continued dyspnoea years later, so she hired a trainer 'to brutalize me on the treadmill' and fully recovered after 12 sessions (Misak 2011).

Home visits, telemedicine (Jackson et al 2012) and video teleconferencing can assist rehabilitation (Needham et al 2012) and a self-help rehabilitation manual aids physical recovery and can halve levels of depression (Jones & Skirrow 2003).

Feedback from follow up clinics helps to sensitize ICU staff to the patient experience. For example, a patient who had been described as an ICU success story told how she had experienced lying naked in bed while staff washed her and chatted to each other about their social lives. Every day for the past three years, she said, she 'wished she was dead' (Russell 1999).

Goals and exercise plans should be included in the discharge summary and sent to community physiotherapists and GPs, with copies to the patient.

> Surviving critical illness is only the beginning.
> Batt et al (2013)

Physiotherapy outcomes

Clinical outcomes include:

1 Auscultation
   – ↑ breath sounds, ↓ bronchial breathing, ↓ crackles

2   Radiology
    –   ↑ lung volume
3   Observations
    –   ↑ S_pO_2
    –   with pressure controlled ventilation: ↑ tidal volume
    –   with volume controlled ventilation: ↓ airway pressure.

Functional outcome is aimed at a return to as near as possible the patient's pre-morbid life style, to include cognition, ADL and contentment. For physical function, valid tools are the Chelsea Critical Care Physical Assessment Tool, which includes respiratory function (Corner *et al* 2013) and the Physical Function Test (Denehy *et al* 2013).

> *I suppose it's safe to say that I'm not the same person as before.*
> Patient quoted by Karlsson & Forsberg 2007

RECOGNITION AND MANAGEMENT OF EMERGENCIES

The key to the successful management of emergencies is informed anticipation and recognition. Physiotherapists are not immersed in life-threatening events every day, so it is advisable to review protocols regularly in order to maintain confidence and avoid the indecision that is often evident at the scene of an emergency. It is also useful to know if a patient has an advance directive declining a certain procedure, and if this has been changed subsequently (Loertscher *et al* 2010).

Some emergencies are covered in the text:

- asphyxic asthma, Ch 3
- burns, Ch 19
- chest drains, Ch 16
- fat embolism, Ch 19
- laryngospasm, Ch 8
- shock, Ch 19
- tracheostomies, Ch 16.

Local protocol should take precedence over the information below.

Cardiac arrest

Cardiac arrest is cessation of heart function. It is the normal mechanism of the old-fashioned process of death, but is occasionally reversible. It is followed within seconds by loss of consciousness and then by loss of respiration.

Anticipation

Before starting work on any new ward, the first task is to locate the crash trolley. When seeing a new patient, the medical history will provide evidence of DNAR status and risky conditions such as ischaemic heart disease, severe respiratory disease, drug overdose, metabolic disturbance, arrhythmias or shock. Physiotherapists working in the community or out of reach of a crash trolley need to carry a pocket mask for mouth-to-mask ventilation. Teamwork is assisted by a cardiac arrest risk triage score (Churpek *et al* 2012).

Recognition

Warning signs are a change in breathing, colour, facial expression or mental function. Hypoventilation with altered consciousness is an ominous combination. The ECG then shows pulseless electrical activity, pulseless ventricular tachycardia, ventricular fibrillation or asystole.

After cessation of the heart beat:

- the ECG flatlines
- in 15 seconds, the patient loses consciousness
- in 30 seconds, the pupils dilate fully
- In 90–300 seconds, cerebral damage occurs (Papastylianou 2012), though the brain stem lasts longer.

The patient's colour may be pale, ashen or blue, depending on the cause. No carotid pulse can be felt in the groove between the larynx and sternomastoid muscle. Respiration may become gasping and then stop, unless respiratory arrest has been the primary event.

Action

The time between collapse and initiation of resuscitation is critical, and a false alarm is better than a dead patient. If suspicions are raised by a change in consciousness and colour, call out to the patient, and if they are unresponsive, follow the basic life support stage of cardiopulmonary resuscitation (CPR) as in the Resuscitation Council (UK) algorithm (App. C) and local training.

On arrival of the crash team, advanced life support may include defibrillation, during which staff should stand clear. When no longer needed, the physiotherapist can give attention to other patients who will be distressed at witnessing the event. Survival for in-hospital cardiac arrests is <20% (Chen et al 2013), with survival to discharge dropping to 7.6% (Moulaert et al 2011). Survivors may sustain hypoxic brain injury and benefit from an ICF-based rehabilitation programme (Moulaert et al (2011).

Respiratory arrest

As cardiac arrest leads to respiratory arrest, so does respiratory arrest, if not reversed, lead to cardiac arrest.

Anticipation

Predisposing factors include exacerbation of COPD, airway obstruction (e.g. foreign body, smoke inhalation, swelling or bleeding from trauma) or aspiration. Warning signs are inability to speak, and violent respiratory efforts, laboured breathing or drowsiness.

Recognition

Respiratory arrest is indicated by absence of chest movement, loss of airflow from the mouth and nose, and sometimes cyanosis. This progresses to loss of consciousness.

Action

1 Call for help.
2 Establish a patent airway as for CPR. Sometimes just moving the head will open the airway. If there is no airflow, continue as below.
3 If a foreign body is the likely culprit and the victim is choking, attempt to dislodge it from the throat by suction or by hand. The main causes are the tongue, vomit and blood. If unsuccessful, follow the Resuscitation Council (UK) choking algorithm (App. C) and local training. If the patient is still not breathing, continue as below.
4 Ventilate by a bag-mask system, Laerdal face mask or mouth-to-mouth. Inspiration time is 1½ to 2 seconds. Repeat once

every 6 seconds. Continue for 1 minute, then reassess.

If cardiac arrest ensues, instigate full CPR. If breathing starts, turn the patient into the recovery position because vomiting is common as consciousness lightens. Further details are in the Resuscitation Council algorithms.

Seizure

Anticipation

The medical notes indicate whether a patient has a history of epilepsy. Other causes of fitting are brain injury, alcohol intoxication, or in children, fever. Some patients sense an aura in advance.

Recognition

Seizures vary from transient loss of consciousness to major muscle activity, followed by drowsiness.

Action

1 Patients subject to seizures should have the bed kept low, side rails up and padded, and oxygen and suction available.
2 If there is advance warning, insert a Guedel airway, if the patient consents. Do not attempt this once the seizure is under way.
3 Protect the patient's head and body from injury. Loosen tight clothing around the neck if possible. Do not use restraints or hold the victim down. Keep in side-lying if possible.
4 Afterwards, ensure the patient is in the recovery position. Reassure them as consciousness returns. Request medical assessment.

Haemorrhage

Anticipation

Uncontrolled bleeding can follow surgery, arterial line disconnection or trauma.

Recognition

External bleeding is usually apparent. Internal bleeding is suspected if there are signs of severe hypovolaemia (p.451). BP and HR are the least reliable of these signs because BP can be maintained by vasoconstriction and HR is responsive to other variables. Bleeding into a closed space causes pain.

Action

1   Position the patient supine.
2   Apply pressure to the bleeding point if accessible.
3   Elevate the affected part if feasible.
4   Request assistance.
5   Explain to the patient what is happening.

Riha & Schreiber (2013) describe the medical management of severe bleeding.

Massive haemoptysis

Massive haemoptysis is >200 ml blood loss over 24 hours or enough bleeding to be life-threatening because of hypotension or aspiration of blood.

Anticipation

Predisposing factors are lung cancer, bronchiectasis, abscess or TB.

Action

If the patient can protect their airway, they can sit up and expectorate the blood until bronchoscopy is ready. Other patients should be positioned with the head slightly down, and if the side of the haemorrhage is known, laid on the affected side to prevent aspiration into the healthy lung. Cough suppressants and sedatives should not be given. Patients with depressed consciousness or at risk of aspiration need intubation, suction and sometimes bronchial artery embolization.

Cardiac tamponade

Cardiac tamponade is accumulation of gas or fluid, usually blood, in the pericardium. The pericardium is not distensible in the short term and can only accommodate 100 ml fluid rapidly without affecting cardiac output, after which an additional 40 ml doubles pericardial pressure, compressing the heart and damming back blood into the systemic veins. If this increasing pressure is not relieved, cardiac arrest ensues.

Anticipation

Tamponade can occur in the first 24 hours after heart surgery. Other predisposing factors are trauma, dissecting aneurysm, infection or malignancy.

Recognition

Progressive compression of the heart leads to precipitate loss of cardiac output, and the following may be evident:

- $\downarrow$ BP, $S_{\bar{v}}O_2$ and urine output
- $\uparrow$ HR, CVP and PAWP
- CVP and PAWP approximately equal
- pulsus paradoxus
- distended neck veins
- enlarged heart on x-ray
- restlessness, fear or feelings of impending doom (Ikematsu & Kloos 2012).

Action

Alert the doctor, who will aspirate the fluid (Gumrukcuoglu et al 2011) or take the patient to theatre.

Tension pneumothorax

Gas entering the pleural space on inspiration but unable to escape on expiration causes a tension pneumothorax. Cardiac arrest normally follows within 20 minutes.

Anticipation

In ventilated patients, pneumothoraces may be under tension at the following times:

- immediately after intubation, if inadvertent tube placement into the right main bronchus causes hyperinflation of the right lung
- in the hours following initiation of mechanical ventilation, when air is forced through a previously unknown leak in the pleura.

Predisposing factors are emphysema, and surgery or other trauma to the chest. Subcutaneous emphysema in the neck can be a warning sign.

Recognition

Tension pneumothorax is sufficiently rare to be sometimes mistaken for bronchospasm. Both of these conditions cause respiratory distress, wheeze, increased airway pressure and laboured breathing. The added features of a tension pneumothorax are:

- ↓ amplitude in ECG (often the first sign)
- unequal chest expansion
- hyperresonant percussion note on the affected side
- ↓ breath sounds on the affected side, or both sides if severe
- ↓ S_pO_2
- cyanosis
- distended neck veins and ↑ CVP (unless the patient is hypovolaemic)
- displaced apex beat
- in self-ventilating patients, dyspnoea and tracheal deviation away from the affected side
- in ventilated patients, high airway pressure (in volume control ventilation), and expired minute volume less than pre-set minute volume
- ↓ BP, ↑ HR, progressing to cardiovascular collapse
- radiograph as in Fig 18.12.

Action

Alert the doctor, who will insert a 14G cannula into the pleura at the second intercostal space in the mid-clavicular line to release the pressure. While waiting, an experienced physiotherapist can disconnect the patient from the ventilator, connect to a bag and manually ventilate with 100% oxygen, using high flow and low pressure. Otherwise F_iO_2 through the ventilator should be maximized. Some patients may be able to breathe spontaneously, which will reduce the positive pressure in the chest. These decisions are usually taken by the team.

Air embolism

Anticipation

Air may enter the circulation after cardiac or neurosurgery, or occasionally from a pneumothorax or during insertion or removal of a pulmonary artery catheter or vascath.

Recognition

A large air embolus causes respiratory distress, palpitations, dizziness, weakness and pallor or cyanosis.

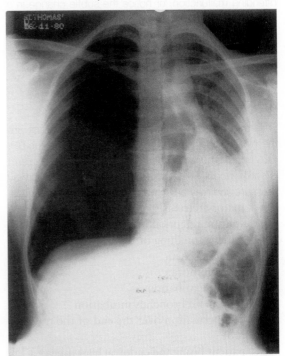

FIGURE 18.12 R tension pneumothorax, as indicated by a black area devoid of lung markings on the patient's right, and mediastinal shift to the left. This is an x-ray that should never be seen because there is not usually time to obtain a film.

Action

Summon help. Place the patient head down in left-side-lying, which diverts air away from the pulmonary artery and pulmonary circulation. Give high-percentage oxygen. An embolus >100 ml may cause cardiac arrest, which requires cardiac compression with heavy and deep pressure to disperse air bubbles to peripheral segments of the pulmonary artery.

Anaphylaxis

Anaphylaxis often manifests as respiratory distress or, with anaphylactic shock, hypotension, occurring minutes to hours after exposure to an allergen. After summoning assistance, the patient should be positioned with legs raised, given high-percentage oxygen (Simons & Sheikh 2013) and asked to cough (Tomori 2013).

Ventilator malfunction or disconnection

Astute eyes and ears pick up the slight hiss of an air leak, identify from an orchestra of alarms which is the offending malfunction, or notice the subtle change in a drowsy patient's demeanour which signifies that something is amiss. Prevention includes reading the manufacturer's handbook in order to understand the workings of the ventilator and distinguish what each alarm signifies.

Alarms

The most relevant alarms for the physiotherapist are the high and low pressure alarms, and those for BP, F_IO_2 and the humidifier heater. The high pressure alarm is set at about 5–10 cmH$_2$O higher than peak airway pressure and may be activated if there is:

- major atelectasis
- sputum retention in a large airway
- patient coughing or fighting the ventilator
- bronchospasm
- pneumothorax
- partial extubation
- right main bronchus intubation
- cuff herniation over the end of the tracheal tube
- patient biting the endotracheal tube (ETT).

If the patient bites the ETT, this requires dissuasion, a bite block or Guedel airway. For a displaced ETT, the doctor will deflate the cuff, reposition the tube, inflate the cuff, listen for equal breath sounds and request a check x-ray.

The low pressure alarm means that pressure has fallen more than 5–10 cmH$_2$O below the desired limit and indicates that there is a leak in the system, confirmed by reduced expired minute volume and airway pressure. A disconnected circuit should be reconnected after a quick alcohol wipe if it has touched anything. The patient's condition should be checked, the cause determined, appropriate adjustments made and the nurse informed.

Alarms are fallible. Patient observation comes first.

Arterial line or central line disconnection

If a major line becomes disconnected at a junction, the patient requires reassurance because of the amount of blood loss, and the nurse may need assistance in reconnecting the line, while ensuring that no air is present in the line.

If a major line comes out of the patient, firm pressure to the site is required and the doctor informed so that it can be reinserted.

Unplanned extubation

Accidental endotracheal extubation can destabilize a patient haemodynamically and compromise the airway. Prevention is assisted by the use of weaning protocols and avoiding restraints (Bouza et al 2007). If extubation occurs, call for help, apply oxygen, re-position the patient, if required, to assist breathing, and advise the patient to breathe steadily. Bag/mask ventilation may be required.

Distress in a ventilated patient

Patient problems causing distress (Figs 18.13/14) include:

- subjective problems (Table 18.1)
- pneumothorax, pulmonary oedema, bronchospasm or mucous plug
- biting the tube.

Ventilator problems include:

- kink (high pressure alarm) or leak (low pressure alarm) in the circuit
- intrinsic PEEP
- inaccurate settings for flow rate, tidal volume, I:E ratio or trigger sensitivity.

Call for assistance, meanwhile check airway pressure/tidal volume and monitors. Ask the patient if they want more air. If the answer is a nod, or the patient is unable to respond, disconnect the patient from the ventilator, after informing them, and connect to the bag with oxygen. Either manually ventilate or allow the patient to self-ventilate through the bag with the valve open for minimal resistance and a high flow rate for comfort.

If distress continues, it is probably a patient-based problem, to be sorted with yes/no questions (p.459) or suctioning the airway. Unilateral air entry raises suspicions of a malpositioned tracheal tube, pneumothorax or mucous plug.

FIGURE 18.13 Physical signs of patient distress

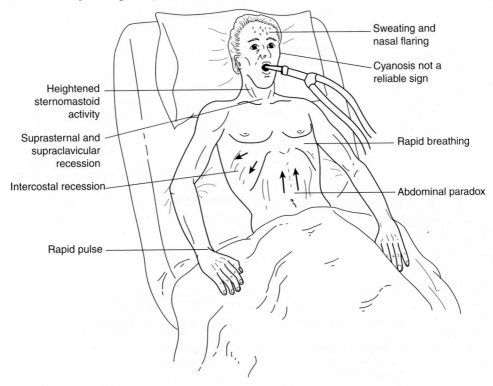

If manual ventilation resolves the distress, it is probably a ventilator problem, to be dealt with as follows:

- leaking tracheal tube cuff: inflate the cuff with air from a syringe, just enough to eliminate the leak, inform the nurse who will measure and record the cuff pressure
- tube disconnection: re-connect after cleaning the disconnected ends
- inability to identify problem: inform the nurse
- tracheal tube malfunction, bronchospasm, ventilator asynchrony unresolved by talking to the patient: inform the doctor.

ON CALLS

A well managed on-call system can sustain many a sick patient through a difficult night. The key to success is education, so that all parties understand the scope and limitations of physiotherapy.

Education of medical staff

All levels of medical staff need information on the indications for out-of-hours physiotherapy, with particular attention to juniors starting a new rotation. Young doctors in a new environment can become anxious with an unfamiliar event and call out the physiotherapist unnecessarily, or not call when it is indicated. Education can be through informal talks, involvement in doctors' continuing education programmes and ensuring that the junior doctors' induction pack contains on-call information. Medical training hardly brushes the subject of physiotherapy and this is an educational opportunity to be grasped gladly.

Education of nursing staff

Nurses and physiotherapists work closely and have an understanding of each others' roles. Day-to-day exchange of information lays the foundation for co-operation, and this can be developed into teaching sessions so that nursing staff know when to advise doctors that the physiotherapist should be called.

FIGURE 18.14 Flow chart to manage distress in a ventilated patient

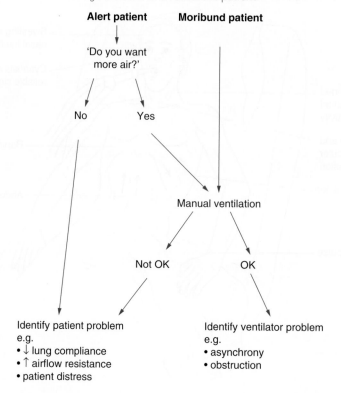

Education of physiotherapists

Junior and non-respiratory senior staff need confidence in making respiratory decisions. Useful time can be spent going through equipment and practising problem-solving with case studies. Competency tools are available (Thomas *et al* 2008) and several steps can be taken to facilitate a sound night's sleep for those on call:

- shadowing a senior colleague on a previous call-out
- time set aside the preceding afternoon for the on-call physiotherapist to see any borderline patient with the respiratory physiotherapist
- a respiratory physiotherapist available at the end of the phone for advice
- after a call-out, discussing with a mentor the clinical reasoning and treatment of the patient
- a hand out to include switchboard arrangements, location of equipment, bleep

information and who is authorized to call out the physiotherapist (example in App. C).

If called to the Emergency Department, it is advisable to check that the patient is not immersed in tests and investigations, and to identify when they will be available for treatment.

The interests of the patient and good relations with other disciplines can be fostered by the physiotherapist taking responsibility for pre-arranging call-outs when appropriate. The physiotherapist can also give advice over the phone.

Many departments organize evening physiotherapy shifts because there is evidence that this can prevent deterioration in patients after major surgery (Ntoumenopoulos & Greenwood 1996) and assist patients with excessive secretions (Wong 2000). Seven-day working has also improved clinical outcomes (Smith & Coup 2011).

An on-call service is particularly helpful for patients with acute COPD (Babu *et al* 2010), and Box 18.2 provides suggestions for the alleviation of dyspnoea in these and other acutely unwell patients.

BOX 18.2   Management of the acutely breathless patient

Tips

- Avoid noise, bright lights and crowding.
- Do not enter the patient's personal space until after introductions.
- Avoid chatter, be specific, talk gently and steadily.
- Offer questions with yes/no answers to minimize the patient's need to speak.
- Identify the patient's view of the cause of their dyspnoea.
- Relatives may have information on the patient's coping strategies.
- Patients may find curtains claustrophobic or need the window open.

Management of symptoms

- Fatigue and SOB: rest, positioning and SOB techniques (Ch. 7).
- Feeling out of control: identify patient's own strategies, suggest others, ensure autonomy.
- Anxiety: identify cause, provide information.
- Lack of sleep: liaise with team re environment, check anxiety, check physical discomfort and positioning.
- Pain: identify cause. If due to coughing, educate on selective cough facilitation and suppression (Ch. 8) as and when appropriate, or wound support. If due to muscle tension, relieve by positioning and relaxation. Suggest or show massage to relatives.
- Exhaustion: monitor P_aCO_2 and pH to identify need for non-invasive ventilation.

Management of objective signs

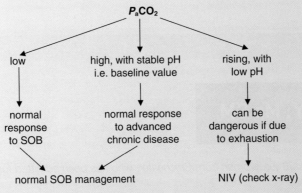

If P_aCO_2 is not available:

- monitor S_pO_2 which is less sensitive to V_E but will decrease if $\downarrow V_E$ is severe,
- monitor symptoms of rising CO_2: headache, flapping tremor, warm hands.

(Continued)

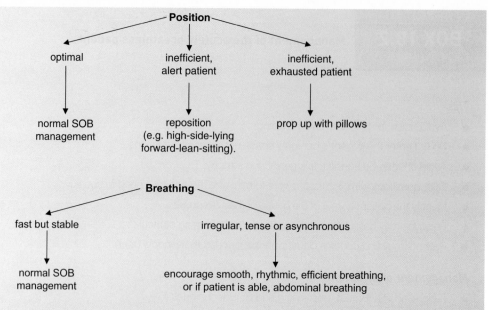

Management of secretions in a breathless patient

- Hydration
- Humidification (warm if bronchospasm)
- Slow rhythmic percussion
- AD or modified ACBT (without slowing RR)
- Cough suppression until secretions are accessible, then cough facilitation

ACBT: active cycle of breathing, *AD:* autogenic drainage, *RR:* respiratory rate, *NIV:* non-invasive ventilation, *SOB:* shortness of breath, V_E: minute volume

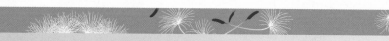

CASE STUDY: Ms CM

Identify the problems of this 58 y.o. woman from Chichester, who has been admitted for mechanical ventilation due to apnoea of unknown cause.

Background

- Several admissions for mechanical ventilation.

Nurse report
- Patient needs regular reminders to breathe at night.

Subjective
- I hate this tube in my throat.
- Tired, not sleeping well.

Objective
- Intubated, on CPAP via the ventilator.
- Patient alert, in side-lying.
- Vital signs, S_pO_2, auscultation and x-ray normal.

Day 2
- Diagnosed with Ondine's curse.

Questions
1 Does the patient have a problem with impaired oxygenation?
2 Does the patient have a problem with impaired ventilation?
3 Does the patient have a problem with her inspiratory muscles?
4 Does the patient have a problem with her respiratory pump?
5 Is the mode of ventilation suitable?
6 Goals?
7 Plan?

Ondine's curse: apnoea caused by loss of automatic control of respiration, usually due to defective chemoreceptor responsiveness secondary to neurological or other disorder.

CLINICAL REASONING

Regarding intubated patients:
Although published guidelines recommend that these catheters be used once only when employing an open technique, this recommendation does not appear to be research-based.

Response to Case Study
1 **Impaired oxygenation?**
   - No, S_pO_2 is normal.
2 **Impaired ventilation?**
   - Yes, Ms M requires regular reminders to breathe at night.

3   Problem with her inspiratory muscles?

- No, she is not complaining of breathlessness and is able to breathe when prompted.

4   Problem with her respiratory pump?

- Yes, the diagnosis implicates the neurological component of her respiratory pump.

5   Mode of ventilation suitable?

- No, CPAP supports oxygenation, not ventilation. Ms M needs a mode that provides mandatory breaths at night for when she does not breathe, e.g. SIMV. No ventilation is required in the day when she can initiate breaths consciously.

6   Goals

- Maintain function while short and long term management is organized, then rehabilitate.

7   Plan

- Liaise with team regarding mode of ventilation; suggest nocturnal NIV.
- Check patient's understanding of diagnosis and agree plan of action.
- Mobilize patient as fully able while ventilated, then when weaned give clothes and advise on self-mobility.
- Liaise with physiotherapist at referral centre to which patient will be sent for initiation of long term home nocturnal NIV.

Footnote – dolphins are also 'conscious breathers' and can only allow half of their brain to sleep at a time.

Response to Clinical Reasoning

If there is no research to justify a technique, then physiological reasoning is required. Re-inserting a used catheter is likely to introduce infection.

RECOMMENDED READING

Asher A (2013) Equipment used for safe mobilization of the ICU patient. *Crit Care Nurs Quarterly;* **36**(1): 101–8

Baldwin CE, Paratz JD, Bersten AD (2013) Muscle strength assessment in critically ill patients with handheld dynamometry. *J Crit Care;* (1): 77–86.

Batt J, Santos CC, Herridge MS (2013) Muscle injury during critical illness. *JAMA;* **310**(15): 1569–70

Brown C (2013) Whither rehabilitation? A call to arms. *J Intens Care Soc;* **14**(2): 110–11

Gagnon MM, Rukstele CD (2013) Making strides in preventing ICU-acquired weakness: involving family in early progressive mobility. *Crit Care Nurs Quarterly;* **36**(1): 141–7

Genc A (2012) Respiratory and hemodynamic responses to mobilization of critically ill obese patients. *Cardiopulm Phys Ther J;* **23**(1): 14–18

Gudzenko V, Bittner EA, Schmidt UH (2010) Emergency airway management. *Respir Care;* **55**(8): 10–35

Hough CL (2013) Improving physical function during and after critical care. *Curr Opin Crit Care;* **19**(5): 488–95

Jackson JC, Ely EW, Morey M *et al* (2012) Cognitive and physical rehabilitation of intensive care unit survivors. *Crit Care Med;* **40**(4): 1088–97

Jain SN (2011) A pictorial essay: Radiology of lines and tubes in the intensive care unit. *Indian J Radiol Imaging;* **21**(3): 182–90

Kelly FE, Hommers C, Jackson R *et al* (2013) Algorithm for management of tracheostomy emergencies on intensive care. *Anaesth;* **68**(2): 217–19

Khan AN, Al-Jahdali H, Al-Ghanem H (2009) Reading chest radiographs in the critically ill. *Ann Thorac Med;* **4**(2): 75–87

Needham DM, Davidson J, Cohen H (2012) Improving long-term outcomes after discharge from intensive care unit. *Crit Care Med;* **40**(2): 502–9

O'Connor MF, Nunnally ME (2013) Expect the unexpected: clinical trials are key to understanding post-intensive care syndrome. *Crit Care;* **17**: 149

Olkowski BF, Devine MA, Slotnick LE *et al* (2013) Safety and feasibility of an early mobilization program for patients with aneurysmal subarachnoid hemorrhage. *Phys Ther;* **93**(2): 208–15

Parker AM (2013) Early rehabilitation in the intensive care unit. *Curr Phys Med Rehab Rep;* **1**(4): 307–314

Richardson V (2013) Patient comprehension of informed consent. *J Periop Pract;* **23**(1/2): 26–30

Robertson LC (2013) Recognizing the critically ill patient. *Anaesth Int Care Med;* **14**(1): 11–14

Russian CJ, Gonzales JF, Henry NR *et al* (2014) Suction catheter size: an assessment and comparison of 3 different calculation methods. *Respir Care;* **59**(1): 32–38

Salisbury LG, Merriweather JL, Walsh TS (2010) Rehabilitation after critical illness: could a ward-based generic rehabilitation assistant promote recovery? *Nurs Crit Care;* **15**(2): 57–65

Smith TL, Coup E (2011) Evaluation of a pilot 7-day cardiorespiratory physiotherapy service. *J Ass Chartered Physiother Respir Care;* **43**: 10–16

Sobush DC, Laatsch L, Lipchik RJ (2012) Restoring functional status: a long-term case report of severe lung and ventilatory muscle pump dysfunction involving recurrent bacterial pneumonias. *Cardiopulm Phys Ther J;* **23**(2): 5–12

Talley CL, Wonnacott RO, Schuett JK *et al* (2013) Extending the benefits of early mobility to critically ill patients undergoing continuous renal replacement therapy: the Michigan experience. *Crit Care Nurs Quarterly;* **36**(1): 89–100

Trotman-Dickenson B (2003) Radiology in the ICU: part 1. *J Int Care Med;* **18**: 198–210

Trotman-Dickenson B (2003) Radiology in the ICU: part 2. *J Int Care Med;* **18**(5): 239–52

Voepel-Lewis T (2010) Reliability and validity of the face, legs, activity, cry, consolability behavioral tool in assessing acute pain in critically ill patients. *Am J Crit Care;* **19**(1): 55–61

Whyte J (2013) Medical complications during inpatient rehabilitation among patients with traumatic disorders of consciousness. *Arch Phys Med Rehabil;* **94**(10): 1877–83

Williams SL (2009) Recovering from the psychological impact of intensive care: how constructing a story helps. *Nurs Crit Care;* **14**(6): 281–8

Wilson JG, Epstein SM, Wang R *et al* (2013) Cardiac tamponade. *West J Emerg Med;* **14**(2): 152

Worrell SG, Demeester SR (2014) Thoracic emergencies. *Surg Clin North Am;* **94**(1): 183–91

CHAPTER 19
Physiotherapy for different disorders in critical care

LEARNING OBJECTIVES

On completion of this chapter the reader should be able to:

- understand the pathology of lung conditions, neurological conditions, trauma and multisystem failure in critical care

- modify treatment according to this pathology

- contribute to the multidisciplinary management of critically ill patients.

INTRODUCTION

This chapter covers mostly non-surgical patients who are mechanically ventilated and require a specific physiotherapy approach in order to maintain oxygenation and promote rehabilitation.

LUNG DISEASE

Chronic obstructive pulmonary disease

Noninvasive ventilation is preferred for patients in ventilatory failure, even with a COPD exacerbation severe enough to alter consciousness, and it has been possible to reduce intubation rates to 15% (Contou *et al* 2014).

But invasive mechanical ventilation (MV) may be required, usually by pressure support (Ch. 17), with extrinsic (applied) positive end-expiratory pressure (PEEP) at about 80% of intrinsic PEEP to counterbalance hyperinflation (Schumaker 2004). High frequency oscillation has also been suggested because it delivers more homogeneously distributed ventilation (Frerichs *et al* 2012). Patients with chronic hypercapnia must have their minute volume titrated to pH rather than P_aCO_2 so that compensatory renal bicarbonate retention will be adequate for buffering during weaning.

A patient who has acclimatized to complex acid-base compensations may find the sudden change to MV destabilizing, leading to serious hypotension in 25% of cases (Schumaker 2004), as well as arrhythmias and the unmasking of hypovolaemia. If physiotherapy is needed within 30 minutes of starting MV, the monitors must be watched closely.

Rest and sleep are required for 24 hours after initiation of MV, interspersed with nutritional support (Sheean 2013), orientation, chest clearance and initiation of modest exercise such squeezing balls and static quadriceps. Bed exercises should be demonstrated to the patient, nurse and family, written down and left with the nursing notes. Once the patient has fully rested, daily standing and walking are added to progressive bed exercises, unless contraindicated or declined. Manual hyperinflation (MH) is not advisable unless essential, because of the vulnerability of hyperinflated alveoli.

Work of breathing can be 10 times normal (Chang 2014 p.41), and weaning can be tiring, protracted and frightening. This is minimized with balanced rest and exercise and, if required, non-invasive ventilation after extubation (Ornico *et al* 2013).

Asthma

Mechanical ventilation is a perilous venture for people with acute severe asthma, but is required if non-invasive support is unsuccessful. High volume positive pressure risks dangerous levels of intrinsic PEEP, barotrauma, impaired venous return, hypotension, arrhythmias and right heart failure due to compressed pulmonary capillaries. Dehydrated patients are particularly vulnerable, and adequate fluid resuscitation and correction of hypokalaemia are required.

Patients will be exhausted from the effort of maintaining hyperinflation in order to keep their obstructed airways open. Their hyperinflated chest means that MV does not necessarily relieve the distressing sensations of breathlessness.

High levels of oxygen and bronchodilators are required, the latter delivered by instillation or continuous infusion (Sellers 2013). Prolonged paralysis should be avoided unless essential because of its association with myopathy when combined with steroids.

The risks of hyperinflation and barotrauma are reduced by:

- permissive hypercapnia (Saulnier *et al* 2012)
- long exhalation times (Rubin & Pohanka 2012) and sufficient extrinsic PEEP to counteract intrinsic PEEP (Caramez *et al* 2005)
- heliox, anaesthetic agents, hypothermia or extracorporeal support (Louie *et al* 2012)
- brief disconnection from the ventilator by the intensivist to allow the trapped gas to escape, which can be facilitated by the physiotherapist performing strong bilateral expiratory manual compressions on the chest (Phipps 2003) during several successive exhalations, using two people in synchrony, or, for one person, applying sustained pressure over ribs 8–10.

Other forms of physiotherapy are inadvisable immediately after initiation of MV because the combination of anaesthesia, hypovolaemia and high airway pressures can cause profound hypotension. β_2-agonists may reduce potassium and further destabilize the cardiovascular system.

However, when airway pressure or volume has settled to normal, treatment to clear mucous plugs may be required. Airway mucus in severe acute asthma is associated with abnormal mucin structure, and fatalities are usually associated with mucous plugging (Rubin & Pohanka 2012). Benefit has been shown by instillation of 2 ml warmed sterile saline every 15 minutes (Branthwaite 1985), nebulized DNase (Chia 2014) or bronchoscopy (Khan 2013). Manual hyperinflation is dangerous while the chest is hyperinflated.

Any sudden deterioration should raise suspicions of a tension pneumothorax. The usual signs (p.480) may be obliterated in a hyperinflated patient on MV.

ACUTE BRAIN INJURY

> *CSF*: cerebrospinal fluid
> *ICP*: intracranial pressure: normal 0–15 mmHg, critical >20 mmHg
> *CPP*: cerebral perfusion pressure: normal >70 mmHg, critical <60
> *GCS*: *Glasgow Coma Scale (Box 19.1)*
> *MAP*: mean arterial pressure (reflects BP): normal 90 mmHg, critical <80 mmHg

Traumatic brain injury (TBI) is the leading cause of death in children and young adults (Haddad & Arabi 2012) and nowhere is accurate assessment and finely-tuned clinical judgement more vital. Methods to control ICP and prevent lung problems may be in conflict, and are often complicated by other injuries.

The effect of most injuries is maximal at onset, but TBI may precipitate a process that converts a moderate injury into a life threatening condition. Primary brain damage at impact is irreversible, but secondary damage affects 35% of patients within minutes, hours or days (Çelik 2004). Oxygen delivery to the injured brain is reduced by any of the following (Haddad & Arabi 2012):

- P_aO_2 <8 kPa (60 mmHg) or S_pO_2 <90%
- P_aCO_2 <4.66 kPa (35 mmHg) or >6 kPa (45 mmHg)
- systolic BP <90 mmHg or >160 mmHg, or MAP >110 mm Hg
- haemoglobin <100 g/l, or haematocrit <0.30
- serum sodium <142 mEq/l
- blood sugar >10 mmol/l or <4.6 mmol/l
- acidosis at pH <7.35 or alkalosis at pH >7.45
- temperature >36.5°C or <35.5°C.

Effect on oxygen delivery

Damage to the respiratory centres may upset the breathing pattern. Hyperventilation and the resulting ↓ P_aCO_2 cause vasoconstriction and tissue hypoxia. Hypoventilation with ↑ P_aCO_2 causes vasodilation and raised ICP, usually as a terminal event. Cheyne-Stokes or ataxic breathing are also signs of severe TBI.

Associated trauma such as facial injury, fractured ribs, haemopneumothorax or lung contusion may compromise the airway or impair gas exchange. Immobility, recumbency or depressed consciousness may cause shallow breathing and impair cough. Pneumonia is the commonest complication (Schirmer et al 2013), especially in the early stages if acute aspiration has occurred at the time of injury or emergency intubation.

The damaged brain releases inflammatory mediators, causing reperfusion injury (p.512), a surge in capillary pressures and leakage, causing a 'blast injury' effect which can lead to acute respiratory distress syndrome (ARDS) in 20–25% of patients (Lee & Rincon 2012) and sometimes neurogenic cardiac injury (Sumidtra et al 2014).

Severe TBI can also release catabolic hormones such as noradrenaline which create a 'sympathetic storm', leading to systemic vasoconstriction and a rush of fluid into the pulmonary circulation, causing neurogenic pulmonary oedema. Other complications include multisystem failure, fat embolism or DIC (Fig 19.1).

Further insult and injury can be added by:

- over-enthusiastic fluid restriction in an attempt to reduce cerebral oedema, leading to hypotension, reduced oxygen delivery and thick secretions; or
- over-enthusiastic fluid administration in an attempt to maintain cerebral perfusion, leading to pulmonary oedema or worsened cerebral oedema.

Transient immunosuppression from the injury may add infection to this formidable list of troubles (Dziedzic 2004).

Effect on the brain

The brain is a hungry organ, requiring 20% of the body's energy to function. Primary injury is caused by bleeding, contusion or shearing forces when the oscillating brain distracts nerve fibres from their bodies (Post & Hoshizaki 2012). Secondary damage includes cerebral oedema, raised ICP, unstable blood pressure (BP) and hypoxia.

The contents of the skull comprise 80% brain tissue, 10% CSF and 10% blood. When damaged, swelling within this rigid container reaches a maximum 24–48 hours after injury but may continue for 72 hours (Roberts 2002). Initially, swelling can be accommodated by displacement of CSF and venous blood into the spinal subarachnoid space and jugular veins. When these

FIGURE 19.1 Effects of acute brain injury on oxygen delivery

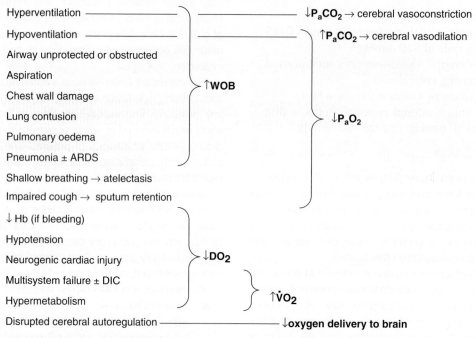

ARDS: acute respiratory distress syndrome, DIC: disseminated intravascular coagulation, DO_2: oxygen delivery to the tissues, Hb: haemoglobin, $\dot{V}O_2$: oxygen consumption, WOB: work of breathing

compensating mechanisms have reached their limit, a small increase in cerebral oedema causes a disproportionate upsurge in ICP (Fig 19.2). Extreme intracranial hypertension may cause coning, in which the brainstem herniates down through the foramen magnum.

FIGURE 19.2 Intracranial compliance curve. ICP is stable at first, but when spatial compensation is exhausted, shown by the inflection point, further swelling causes a steep rise.

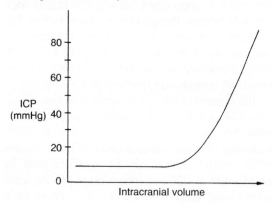

Cerebral perfusion pressure is the driving force of cerebral circulation. Reduced CPP is the principal mechanism by which elevated ICP exerts secondary damage. MAP and ICP are, in effect, competing for space:

- $CPP = MAP - ICP$

CPP is therefore compromised by a high ICP, which prevents perfusion even with high MAP (Cowley 2008). Fig 19.3 shows how a rise in the non-perfusing ICP, without a compensating increase in BP, impairs the perfusing CPP.

The picture is further complicated if loss of autoregulation destabilizes cerebral blood flow, which is normally tightly controlled over a wide range of systemic BP. Cerebral blood flow generally remains constant over a CPP of 50–150 mmHg, due to compensatory vasodilation in response to hypoxia or hypotension. If this mechanism is damaged by brain injury, ICP follows MAP passively rather than remaining independent. BP must therefore be tightly controlled.

Intracranial dynamics are reflected in a vicious circle that exacerbates the secondary effects of TBI (Fig 19.4). Lung complications can cause hypoxia, to which brain

FIGURE 19.3 Monitor showing how a combination of increased intracranial pressure and decreased arterial blood pressure reduces cerebral perfusion pressure.

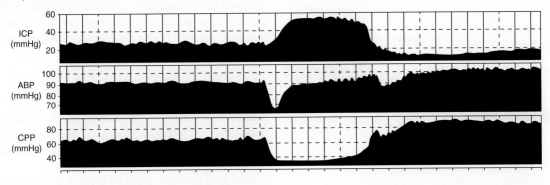

tissue is already sensitive because of its high oxygen requirements and dependence on aerobic glucose metabolism. Hypoxia swells the brain further, and disturbances in P_aCO_2 add to this woeful picture. It is no wonder that TBI has a reputation for being treacherous.

Factors which increase ICP or decrease CPP

Secondary damage can be increased by other factors:

1   Head-down postural drainage increases arterial, venous and intracranial pressures because cerebral veins have no valves. It also impairs compensatory venous outflow and is contraindicated in the acute stage (Lee 1989).

2   Head movement, coughing, suction, manual hyperinflation, and sometimes manual techniques can impede compensatory outflow and raise ICP (Paratz 1993). Outflow is also obstructed by tight tracheal tube tape or cervical collar.

3   Turning the patient increases ICP, much of this due to head movement obstructing drainage from the brain (Fig 19.5).

4   Hypotension reduces CPP, which can double mortality (Cowley 2008). The following carry a particular risk:

   ● on admission, when a patient may be quietly bleeding into the abdomen and losing consciousness because of hypotension rather than TBI

   ● during surgery, when BP may be deliberately kept low to minimize the risk of bleeding.

5   Even deeply comatosed patients show a surprising sensitivity to conversation over their beds. Discussion about their condition increases ICP more than general discussion (Mitchell & Mauss 1978). However, when relatives talk to patients, a reduction in ICP may be seen (Chudley 1994).

6   Continuous sedation must not be interrupted for neurological assessment because this can cause spikes in ICP (Prisco & Citerio 2012).

FIGURE 19.4 Vicious circle set up by acute brain injury, exacerbated by respiratory complications

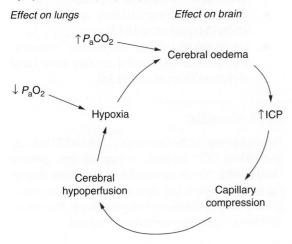

FIGURE 19.5 ICP in a severely head-injured patient, showing prolonged elevation after position change

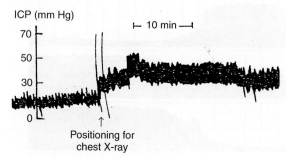

7 Brain injured people show an exaggerated response to the pain of associated injuries (Mirski 1995). ICP also increases with injections, movement of the tracheal tube, yankauer in the mouth, noise, arousal from sleep, restraints, bright lights or emotional upset (Yanko & Mitcho 2001).

8 Transport between or within hospitals causes an adverse event in 40% of patients and increases ICP in 51% of patients (Waldmann 1998).

9 Delayed intracranial hypertension may occur after removal of monitoring devices and is suspected if there is a raised white cell count (Souter *et al* 1999). Systemic infection may exacerbate brain injury (Kochanek 1999).

10 Supposedly minor stressors can cause a spike in ICP such as knocking the bed, using a cold stethoscope, fitting a splint or BP measurement (Ersson *et al* 1990).

Most of these factors warn physiotherapists to keep their distance, but the importance of maintaining gas exchange is a cogent reminder not to stray too far.

General management

Immediate management

All acutely brain injured people are assumed to have an unstable spine until proven otherwise. A CT scan can be transmitted electronically from a general ICU to a neurosurgical unit for advice. Patients with a GCS below eight should be resuscitated, intubated, ventilated, stabilized, scanned and transferred to a neurosurgical unit accompanied by a doctor trained in the handling of such patients, so long as the cause of any unexplained hypotension has been identified (NICE 2007).

Monitoring

Clinical examination is often clouded by coma, sedatives or encephalopathy. Monitoring devices are non-invasive when possible to minimize stimuli that might stir up ICP.

Cerebral perfusion pressure is the main indicator of brain perfusion (Dietrich & Erbguth 2013), and is monitored by Doppler sonography, cerebrovascular reactivity or indirectly by MAP and ICP (Aries *et al* 2012). Mortality increases by about 20% for each 10 mmHg drop in CPP, and the aim is to keep it at 70–80 mmHg by manipulating MAP and fluids (Chang 2014 p.266).

ICP monitoring is needed if GCS falls below eight or the CT scan shows cerebral oedema. Unless contraindicated, the invasive monitor is usually placed in the right side because this hemisphere is non-dominant in 80% of people (Haddad & Arabi 2012). Impending elevations in ICP should be predicted and managed while still within normal limits. Clinical signs of cranial hypertension are not apparent in a patient on paralyzing drugs, but even if evident they indicate that secondary damage has already occurred.

Other monitors are:

● end-tidal CO_2 ($ETCO_2$) as a surrogate for vasomotor stability
● EEG power spectral analysis to identify awareness (Goldfine *et al* 2012)
● direct monitoring of brain tissue oxygenation (Martini *et al* 2013)
● cerebrovascular haemodynamic monitoring, particularly useful to fine tune head elevation (Kim *et al* 2013d).

Head elevation

Raising the head of the bed tends to reduce ICP but may also reduce CPP, especially in hypovolaemic patients. Head position should be established individually according to the monitors, but 10–15° elevation is commonly advised (Cowley 2008), with no neck flexion, the reverse Trendelenberg position being used if required.

BOX 19.1

Glasgow Coma Scale

Best eye-opening response	Spontaneous	4
	To voice	3
	To pain	2
	None	1
Best verbal response	Oriented	5
	Confused	4
	Inappropriate words	3
	Incoherent	2
	None	1
Best motor response	Obeys commands	6
	Localizes pain	5
	Withdraws from pain	4
	Flexes to pain	3
	Extends to pain	2
	None	1
Maximum score		15

Fluid management

Normovolaemia is the usual target so that excess fluid does not rush into the injured brain nor dehydration reduce brain perfusion. Small changes in blood osmolality exert a strong effect on brain water, and initial fluid resuscitation is probably best achieved with hypertonic saline (Eskandari 2013) whose sodium ions do not cross the blood-brain barrier, nor risk brain swelling, nor cause the renal dysfunction seen with repeated mannitol administration. Fluids and drugs aim to keep MAP at >80 mmHg (NICE 2007).

Nutrition

Patients are hypermetabolic, hypercatabolic and hyperglycaemic. Specialist nutritional support is needed because diet modifies brain plasticity (Gomez-Pinilla 2011), vitamin D reduces brain inflammation (Cekic et al 2011) and immunonutrition boosts antioxidants (Khalid & Selim 2012). Resting energy expenditure is 40–200% above normal for about three weeks and mild hypermetabolism can last for a year (Yanko & Mitcho 2001). Paralytic ileus may be a hindrance for the first fortnight, but enteral feeding should be started when possible because IV feeds risk infection and can cause neuronal damage from hyperglycaemia (Yanko & Mitcho 2001). Almost half of patients are injured while drunk (Bombardier 2013) and alcohol dependence may require vitamin B supplements to avoid encephalopathy (Guerrini 2013).

Temperature control

Temperature must be tightly regulated. Damage to the hypothalamus or infection may cause a pyrexia, raising oxygen consumption by 10% for each 1°C rise in temperature (Yanko & Mitcho 2001). Conversely, hypothermia can cause arrhythmias, shift the oxygen dissociation curve to the left, and if it causes shivering, increase oxygen consumption. However, moderate hypothermia may be applied therapeutically if ICP is uncontrollable (Haddad & Arabi 2012).

Drug therapy

The following may be used:

1 Anaesthetic agents can reduce cerebral metabolism or control seizures, which could cause cerebral hypoxia, and a barbiturate coma lowers ICP.

2 Judicious doses of the osmotic diuretic mannitol enhance cerebral blood flow but can cause dehydration.

3 Hypotensive patients who are normovolaemic need systemic vasoconstrictors, which do not also cause damaging vasoconstriction in the brain because cerebral vessels have few adrenergic receptors.

4 Sedatives reduce brain metabolism, but require monitoring to ensure that they do not reduce CPP. Different sedatives, analgesics and anaesthetics have varying effects on the spreading depolarizations that are believed to damage functional neurons. Midazolam, for example, may be counterproductive (Hertle *et al* 2012).

5 Chemical paralysis with neuromuscular blocking agents is not recommended unless necessary for refractory intracranial hypertension because they increase the risk of pneumonia (Haddad & Arabi 2012).

6 Anticoagulation (Joseph *et al* 2014) or glucose stabilization (Matsushima *et al* 2012) are mandatory to avoid thromboembolism or hyperglycaemia.

7 Laxatives may be required because pressure from constipation affects intra-thoracic pressure and inhibits compensatory outflow from a swelling brain.

8 The mechanism of cerebral damage may be counteracted by melanocortins (Bitto *et al* 2012).

9 Hyperbaric oxygen is thought to have neuroprotective properties (Huang & Obenaus 2011).

10 Entonox is contraindicated.

Mechanical ventilation (MV)

Intubation may be needed to maintain a clear airway and MV to regulate an unstable breathing pattern, ensure oxygenation, control ICP or manage chest complications. Alali (2014) recommends early tracheostomy to reduce MV duration, and NICE (2007) suggests that P_aO_2 is kept above 13 kPa (97.5 mmHg) and P_aCO_2 at 4.5–5.0 kPa (33.8–37.5 mmHg) but hyperventilation should not be initiated in the first 24 hours because it may cause cerebral ischaemia (Haddad & Arab 2012). P_aCO_2 levels also need to be balanced with lung protective ventilation which may be required to reduce the risk of ARDS (Go & Singh 2013), while high PEEP impedes outflow from the brain.

Physiotherapy

KEY POINT

The hallmark of physiotherapy is maximum involvement and minimum intervention.

Physiotherapy involvement in the early stages is by:

• frequent assessment to assist delicate risk/benefit decisions
• supervision of handling to minimize ICP disturbance.

Physical intervention is unwise in the presence of cardiovascular instability, hypotension or ICP above 15 mmHg (Paratz 1993). If it is essential for gas exchange, a drug to stabilize ICP should be given beforehand. Quiet explanations are required for all patients, however deeply comatose.

Assessment

Any reduction in S_pO_2 or other signs of impending chest complications requires preventive action. BP, ICP and ETCO$_2$ should be monitored throughout treatment. In the absence of ICP monitoring, clinical signs of intracranial hypertension are:

• ↑ pupil size
• pupil unresponsive to light
• change in GCS

- change in vital signs, breathing pattern or muscle tone
- vomiting.

If the patient is not intubated, a minitracheostomy is advisable if suction is necessary. Nasal suction is contraindicated in the presence of:

- watery CSF leaking from the nose or ear, indicating a connection between the subarachnoid space and nasal passages, thus risking infection
- severe epistaxis.

Close assessment is also important after discharge from the ICU, when patients are less closely monitored and 10% of patients suffer a serious adverse event (Tirkkonen *et al* 2013). Before rehabilitation, bone mineral density should be checked (Banham-Hall *et al* 2013).

Positioning

Turning is safe with ICP <15 (Chudley 1994), one person being responsible for maintaining head alignment.

Accurate positioning in side-lying with neutral head position aids prophylactic chest care, so long as pressure on any postoperative bone flap is avoided. However, for patients with unstable ICP and low risk of lung complications, it is best to leave the patient supine in the early stages if there is a suitable mattress to prevent pressure sores. Neck flexion must be prevented by using a thin pillow or none.

Manual hyperinflation

If MH is essential, this must follow sedation, be brief, and avoid disturbing P_aCO_2. The ETCO$_2$ monitor should be transferred to the MH circuit, and the ETT kept stable throughout.

Manual techniques

Paratz (1993) claim that vibrations and percussion can impede compensatory outflow from the brain and increase ICP, but Neto *et al* (2013) and Figure 19.6 show that careful technique can avoid this complication.

FIGURE 19.6 Effect of physiotherapy on ICP, showing suction to be the most damaging intervention, followed by manual hyperinflation.

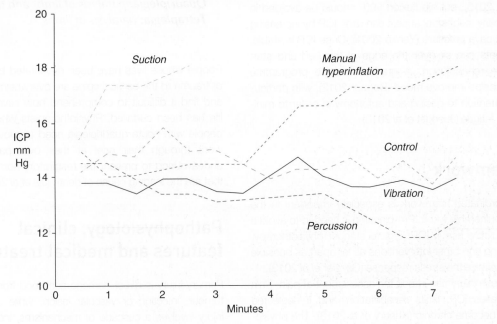

Suction

Elevation of ICP during suction is inevitable (Neto *et al* 2013) and sometimes prolonged. If indicated, the following precautions are advised:

- the patient rested from previous activity
- 100% oxygen delivered before and after
- head kept strictly in alignment
- tracheal tube stabilized throughout
- contact with the carina avoided
- no more than one suction pass at a time, and use of hyperventilation to reduce ICP when necessary.

Exercise

If spasticity develops, appropriate positioning must be maintained and factors which increase tone avoided, e.g. pain, anxiety, pressure under the feet and the weight of heavy bedclothes. If increased tone in the calf or clonus is identified, immediate stretching and splinting to maintain dorsiflexion has been recommended (Mosely 2008) alternating periods with the splint on and off.

If there is no altered muscle tone, it may be best to avoid any movements in the first 72 hours while the brain may be swelling. Thereafter, comfortable passive movements can actually reduce ICP (Thelandersson *et al* 2010) and help promote neural plasticity (Kocan & Lietz 2013), but hip flexion >90° should be avoided in the early stages because it can raise ICP by increasing vena cava pressure (Yanko 2001). Once ICP is stable, patients can sit over the edge of the bed and start active rehabilitation. A graded exercise programme also helps improve mood (Bognor 2012), with particular attention to pacing and autonomy in order to minimize fatigue (Juengst *et al* 2013).

Teamwork

Co-ordinated teamwork is especially important in the first vulnerable week. Pre-planning is needed to avoid a cumulative rise in ICP, e.g. to stagger physiotherapy, nursing and other interventions as far apart as possible to minimize the stress response (Genzler *et al* 2013).

Brain injury can impair the assessment of pain. Pain increases ICP, limits rehabilitation, and if neglected may become chronic (Khoury *et al* 2013). The physiotherapist may be the first team member to detect pain.

Skill in motivation and encouragement of autonomy are also required because of a significant incidence of post-traumatic stress disorder after even mild brain injury (Hoffman *et al* 2012).

Studies have found a progressively increasing incidence of depression in the majority of patients (Fann & Hart 2013) and a 50–80% incidence of fatigue that does not resolve spontaneously (Juengst *et al* 2013). Early rehabilitation and goal-planning, using the contextual factors of the ICF model is particularly useful for this group of patients to co-ordinate their physical, social, emotional and environmental factors (Ptyushkin 2012). Integrating neurorehabilitation treatment into the ICU can benefit even patients in a vegetative state (Eifert *et al* 2013). Absence of consciousness should not preclude referral for specialized rehabilitation (Sommer *et al* 2013).

ACUTE QUADRIPLEGIA

The big things you get used to easier, like not getting up and walking around. The trivial things – like not being able to scratch your nose or feed yourself – they hurt.
  Patient quoted by Stewart & Rossier 1978

Quadriplegia: *paralysis of limbs and trunk*
Tetraplegia: *paralysis of limbs*

People whose lives have been devastated by disease or trauma to the cervical spine are overwhelmed at first and find it difficult to comprehend how savagely their life has been curtailed. Physiotherapists who care for people with acute quadriplegia need to allow them to work through their grief at their own pace, while endeavouring to prevent the respiratory complications that are the leading cause of death (Jia *et al* 2013).

Pathophysiology, clinical features and medical treatment

Primary injury is direct damage sustained from trauma, tumour, infection or vascular lesion, while secondary injury involves a cascade of mechanisms, including inflammation, which release chemicals that can be toxic to spinal cord tissue over hours or days (Boswell *et al* 2013). Respiratory function may be compromised by ascending oedema of the damaged spinal cord shortly after admission, or neurogenic pulmonary oedema caused by vasoconstriction, sometimes exacerbated by overhydration in an attempt to treat shock (Berlly 2007).

The first few hours are when the accuracy, adequacy and speed of management may have an effect on the final outcome (Wing *et al* 2008). Log rolling, for example, should be avoided (Conrad *et al* 2012). As with traumatic brain injury, the first 72 hours are when the maintenance of blood flow and oxygenation are the primary goals (Cook 2003). Patients who cannot be transferred immediately to a spinal unit will need specialist assessment by an outreach team.

Complications include mucous plugging, atelectasis, pneumonia (Galeiras 2013) and, with trauma, a 20–50% incidence of traumatic brain injury (Cook 2003). Later complications include neuropathic pain (Mehta 2013), bladder and gut problems, bedsores, vascular and respiratory disease, sleep disorders and depression (Cristante *et al* 2012), the latter increasing the incidence of physical complications (Krueger *et al* 2013).

Lesions above T6–L1 paralyze the abdominal muscles and impair coughing. Higher lesions paralyze the intercostals so that they are unable to buttress the ribcage on inspiration, causing paradoxical inward motion as negative pressure sucks in the chest. Lesions above C4 denervate the diaphragm, leaving only the sternomastoid and trapezius muscles to shift a trace of air into the lungs.

Paralyzed abdominal muscles impair venous return and risk an exaggerated response to hypovolaemia. Lesions above T6 remove sympathetic control to the splanchnic bed, which is a major reservoir for controlling BP. Hypotension and bradycardia can result, especially during suction of the mouth or airways, and during exertion. Cardiac monitoring is required for the first two weeks, and oximetry should be continued at night. A complete cervical injury is equivalent to a sympathectomy, reducing tone in blood vessels, denervating the cardiac sympathetic nerve supply and leaving parasympathetic tone unopposed. High lesions require MV, often for lengthy periods, and early tracheostomy is recommended (Ganuza 2011). Ventilator adjustments may be required during active exercise to maintain oxygenation. Most patients with a lesion at or below C4 can be weaned, and an initial vital capacity (VC) of more than one litre indicates the likelihood of success, but a compromised hypercapnic drive com-

plicates weaning for some patients (Raurich 2014). For those unable to wean, phrenic nerve pacing can coax the diaphragm to life and gain freedom from the ventilator (Jia *et al* 2013), or the patient may prefer non-invasive ventilation. Ventilator-dependent patients can gain some degree of independence with glossopharyngeal breathing (Ch. 3).

Environmental temperature must be controlled because impaired sympathetic outflow hinders thermoregulation. Bronchodilators may be required to reduce parasympathetic-induced bronchospasm. Deep vein thrombosis risk requires anticoagulation and pneumatic compression boots (Jia *et al* 2013).

Physiotherapy

> *Aggressive management of atelectasis and secretions are the cornerstones of early treatment [and have] been shown to improve outcomes.*
>
> Berlly 2007

The third to fifth days after injury are when associated damage or aspiration may cause cardiorespiratory problems such as hypoxia or hypotension, leading to secondary harm to the spinal cord.

If a halo vest is used to stabilize a fracture, all those involved must know how to open or adjust it in case of cardiac arrest.

PRACTICE TIP

From day one, all the team need to be clear about taking care of the shoulder joints.

Respiratory care

Physiotherapy in the acute stage should take place little and often to avoid fatigue. Regular position change, hourly incentive spirometry, and if necessary intermittent positive pressure breathing can help prevent atelectasis, which is the commonest respiratory complication, while manual techniques and assisted coughing help clear secretions. Excess mucus may be created by loss of sympathetic control and unopposed vagal activity in the days to weeks after injury (Berlly 2007). The head-down position is best avoided, but if essential for postural drainage, care is needed to ensure that tipping is done slowly and not fully, cervical traction is maintained, suction is on hand in case of sudden sputum mobilization, and arterial and venous pressures are monitored because of impaired cardiovascular reflexes.

If MV is not required, early minitracheostomy is advisable if there is a hint of sputum retention, especially as the neck cannot be extended for effective nasopharyngeal suction. If suction is required, whether for an intubated or spontaneously breathing patient, it should be accompanied by increased F_iO_2, close monitoring of S_pO_2, HR and BP, and availability of IV atropine or other drug in case of bradycardia.

Respiratory rehabilitation includes arm exercises and incentive spirometry. Inspiratory muscle training is also advisable because it can improve quality of life (Mueller *et al* 2013), increase lung volumes, cough strength and ability to use voice-activated equipment (Ross 2005), but it may increase spasticity in some patients (Van Houtte *et al* 2008). A mouth trainer, a connector to the tracheal tube or weights on the abdomen (Lin 1999) can be used.

Coughing is assisted by:

- Mechanical assistance with an insufflator-exsufflator (Wong 2012), ending with insufflation to restore lung volume.
- If there is no paralytic ileus, manual assistance using a hand on each side of the lower ribs and one forearm exerting strong pressure upwards and inwards against the abdomen, in synchrony with any expiratory force that the patient can muster (some patients require two physiotherapists for this); care should be taken to avoid disturbing neck traction, jarring the fracture site, exacerbating associated injuries, or pushing towards the spine instead of the diaphragm.
- Expiratory muscle training and electrical stimulation of expiratory muscles (Schilero *et al* 2009).

Quadriplegia at C5 or below allows patients to learn self-assisted coughing when able, leaning forward in their chair and using any strength in their arms to push against their abdomen.

Musculoskeletal care and exercise

Treatment of the limbs involves close attention to positioning and range of movement. A high proportion of

patients develop rotator cuff tears, biceps tendon ruptures and shoulder arthrosis, and regular MRI checks have been recommended (Eriks-Hoogland 2013). Prevention of shoulder problems is by early and frequent full-range movement, scapular stretches and extreme care with positioning, especially if there is cervical traction or a rotating bed. Close attention should be paid to pain prevention, which becomes chronic in an average 78% of patients (Ataoglu 2012).

Patients with complete lesions are best mobilized as soon as possible after surgery. Those with incomplete lesions are usually on bed rest for six weeks to ensure optimum perfusion to the spinal cord. Mobilization takes the form of elevation gradually with a tilt table, monitoring BP with every 10° rise. Standing is less comfortable than supine because the floppy abdominal muscles allow bulging of the abdomen. An abdominal binder for standing, sitting and coughing (Julia *et al* 2011) optimizes lung volumes, expiratory flow, diaphragmatic function and left ventricular function (West *et al* 2012). Diminished venous return and interrupted sympathetic outflow blunt the heart's response to exercise, which can limit exercise capacity. Wheelchair seats positioned parallel to the ground may be a risk factor for shoulder pain (Giner-Pascual *et al* 2011).

Muscle spasticity and flaccidity have a complicated relationship. After the 'spinal shock' period of flaccidity, which varies from a few days to several weeks, the spinal cord below the lesion begins to transmit reflexes. The ensuing spasticity can reduce muscle wasting and risk of osteoporosis, and lung function may improve if spasticity and stiffening thoracic joints provide some compensation for loss of intercostal muscle function. However if spasms cause pain, breathlessness, contractures or impaired mobility, they can be reduced by baclofen or TENS (Chung & Cheng 2010).

Exercise training should be initiated early in the rehabilitation process to improve immunity, autonomic function (Leicht 2013), neuronal plasticity, co-ordination and neurological performance (Cristante *et al* 2012), to minimize the cardiovascular deconditioning and obesity to which patients are prone (Groah *et al* 2012) and to improve bone density (Chain *et al* 2012). This should be on going in order to prevent the continuing decline in lung function that is common in this population (Postma *et al* 2013). Functional electrical stimulation cycling has shown a high level of adherence (Dolbow *et al* 2012). Patients with malignant lesions benefit from rehabilitation (Vishwa 2013) and specialized programmes involving oncology and palliative care teams (Tan *et al* 2012).

ICF categories can provide a structural base for evaluation in early rehabilitation (Nam *et al* 2012):

- Impaired body function and structure, e.g. musculoskeletal pain, lost sensation and motor function.
- Activity limitation, e.g. deficits in activities of daily living or propelling a wheelchair.
- Limited participation, e.g. obstacles to homemaking or social activities.
- Singing therapy can aid all three, including respiratory function, muscle strength, speech intensity, mood and social participation (Tamplin *et al* 2013).

In the ensuring years, annual hospitalization rates of 25%–40% have been reported, with cardiopulmonary causes being strongly related to modifiable risk factors rather than neurological impairment (Waddimba *et al* 2009). This underlines the importance of follow-up physiotherapy, which reduces re-admissions in the first year (DeJong *et al* 2013).

Patients need as much control over their environment and treatment as feasible, and support and encouragement in the early stages enable most patients to find the determination to rebuild their lives, including the ability to enjoy sex and have children (Linsenmeyer 2000). Many patients report that their initial response was that death was better than living with such a disability, but one study found 92% of patients glad to be alive later (DeLateur 1997). Outcomes are best measured by questionnaires (Lindberg *et al* 2013, Fekete *et al* 2013).

> *It is a tribute to the human spirit that 'those who have a WHY to live will put up with almost any HOW'.*
>
> DeLateur (1997)

OTHER NEUROLOGICAL DISORDERS

Neurological conditions may lead to respiratory complications as a result of immobility, respiratory muscle weakness, aspiration pneumonia or neurogenic pulmonary oedema. Weaning may be hindered by reduced respiratory drive (Rialp *et al* 2013). Neurophysiological facilitation of respiration (Ch. 6) may benefit this group of patients.

Intensive care weakness

A quarter of patients who are mechanically ventilated for more than seven days develop muscle weakness beyond disuse atrophy (Li *et al* 2013), leading to prolonged hospitalization, persistent disability and increased mortality (Argov & Latronico 2014). **Critical illness polyneuropathy** is a motor and sensory neuropathy, and **critical illness myopathy** is a primary muscle disease. Both are increasing in prevalence (Novak 2011), both relate to inflammation, muscle proteolysis and deconditioning (Kress 2013), and both persist long after critical illness has resolved (Pawlik & Kress 2013). Other risk factors are hyperglycaemia, intravenous nutrition, renal replacement therapy, sedatives and 'mechanical silence', i.e. lack of the stimulus to muscle that is normally provided by weight bearing or muscle stretch (Renaud *et al* 2013).

Failure to recognize the condition leads to misjudgement of weaning ability and delay in reducing risk factors. It can be identified by electroneuromyography, histology, ultrasound, non-volitional strength measurements (Hough *et al* 2011) or simply hand grip strength (O'Brien *et al* 2008). The physiotherapist may be the first to suspect the condition when a patient is unable to maintain trunk or head control during rehabilitation. If the patient is too weak to move their limbs against gravity, then the diaphragm is probably affected (Santos 2012).

Physiotherapy is through prevention by passive movements or functional electrical stimulation (Parry *et al* 2012), early active exercise and weight-bearing when feasible (Llano-Diez *et al* 2012). Short sessions are required to avoid exhaustion (Novak 2011). Sensory neuropathy requires attention to skin integrity and limb positioning.

Guillain-Barré syndrome

> *I felt as if every tissue in my spine had been superglued together.*
>
> Patient quoted by Savinson 2012

Guillain-Barré syndrome is an autoimmune inflammatory demyelinating polyneuropathy and the most frequent cause of acute flaccid paralysis worldwide. It can occur in children (Ryan 2013) but mainly affects young adults, 20% of whom are left disabled and 5% of whom die (Yuki & Hartung 2012). It often follows an infection and causes a predominantly motor deficit with some autonomic and sensory components. Presenting features vary and include backache, paraesthesia and weakness. Weakness progresses for up to a month, and ventilatory failure develops in 20% of patients, sometimes with alarming speed. This can be predicted by difficulties with speech or swallowing, but reduced VC is the most reliable warning sign. The decision to intubate should be semi-elective to avoid emergency intubation (Mangera *et al* 2012).

Medical treatment is mainly supportive, but patients may benefit from plasma infusion, plasma exchange in which the patient's plasma is replaced by that of a donor (McNair 2013), plasmapheresis in which albumin or other fluids are used for replacement (Cortese *et al* 2011) or intravenous antibodies purified from donated blood (Hughes *et al* 2012).

Physiotherapy

> *The physiotherapist was a most welcome person, as, despite the discomfort endured to have 'dead' limbs stretched and repositioned, this left me comfortable for several more hours.*
>
> Patient quoted by Clark 1985

Physiotherapy at the beginning is aimed at avoiding the contractures that can become major components of disability. Muscle pain is exacerbated at initiation of movement but eased after a few moments of mobility exercises. Exercise should therefore be:

● regular and frequent
● preceded if necessary by anti-inflammatory drugs or accompanied by Entonox
● gentle at the start
● precise, to ensure full range without risking damage that can occur with hypotonia
● brief, to avoid fatigue.

Spinal movements should be included, e.g. double knee-and-hip flexion, knee rolling, and neck movements with due care of the tracheal tube. Relatives can assist with some routine exercises. Extremities may be hypersensitive.

Autonomic involvement leads to unstable BP and heart rate, and sustained hypertension may alternate

with sudden hypotension. The risk of hypotension is reduced by ensuring that turning is gentle, by avoiding any intervention if central venous pressure (CVP) is below 5 cmH$_2$O, which indicates hypovolaemia, and by slow acclimatization to the upright posture with a tilt table. Risk of bradycardia is reduced by oxygenation before and after suction.

Major depression afflicts 27% of patients (Seel *et al* 2003), which hinders rehabilitation. Physiotherapy can incorporate trips outside the ICU and, later, hydrotherapy. Recovery is prolonged (Gupta & Mullins 2013). Self-help groups provide support from the ICU stage onwards (Appendix B).

PRACTICE TIP

Next Sunday morning, on waking, have a cup of tea, go to the toilet, turn on the radio, smooth out the bottom sheet, get back into bed and make yourself comfortable and warm. Then see how long you can remain totally motionless.

Variations are to use an unfamiliar radio station at an unfamiliar volume, leave a crease in the sheet or lie on a damp pad.

Myasthenia gravis

This progressive autoimmune disorder affects the neuromuscular junction and weakens muscles in proportion to their use. Intensive care may be required after thymectomy and sometimes in a myasthenic crisis. Physiotherapy includes clearance of the excess bronchial secretions stimulated by anticholinesterase.

TRAUMA

Trauma may be accompanied by a 'trauma triad' of hypothermia, acidosis and coagulopathy, which needs to be identified early because each compounds the others (McLarty 2012). Following even minor blunt chest trauma, potentially life-threatening complications can develop over the ensuing 72 hours (Battle *et al* 2013). Even sterile injury can set off a systemic inflammatory response, (Hirsiger *et al* 2012), which can sometimes be attenuated by cooling an injured extremity (Ning 2014). A quarter of patients develop pneumonia (Hyllienmark *et al* 2013), sometimes evolving into ARDS (Watkins *et al* 2012). Other complications are thromboembolism (Thorson 2012) or persistent immunosuppression (Vanzant 2014). Intensive physiotherapy has been shown to improve mobility (Calthorpe *et al* 2014).

Rib fracture

> *Medical providers tend to underestimate the presence and severity of pain.*
> Azzam & Alam (2013)

Pain from rib fractures causes a restrictive defect, exacerbated if there is chest wall derangement, pneumothorax, subcutaneous emphysema or haemothorax. Poorly-managed pain may lead to prolonged disability (Fabricant *et al* 2013) and early pain control should be by epidural, which also reduces mortality (Gage 2014) or nerve block (Duggal *et al* 2013). If chest drains are used for pneumothorax or haemothorax, local anaesthetic can be administered through the drain.

The commonest locations are the third to tenth ribs, often laterally where there is no muscle protection. Fractures of the well-protected first three ribs indicate prodigious force and are often accompanied by intra-thoracic injury. Lower rib fractures may be accompanied by intra-abdominal injury. A flail chest results when three or more adjacent ribs are fractured at two different points, causing paradoxical breathing due to an incompetent segment of chest wall (Fig. 19.7). It may not be apparent in the first day or two if muscle spasm stabilizes the chest wall.

Imaging can underestimate the presence and extent of rib fractures, especially if they are anterior, but assessment should not be confirmed by palpation, which elicits exquisite pain.

Each pleural space can hold about two litres of blood, so an adult, can exsanguinate into the thorax if haemorrhage is uncontrolled. Once bleeding has been controlled, haemothorax requires early tube drainage if empyema is to be avoided (DuBose *et al* 2012). Surgical stabilization may be needed (Doben *et al* 2014).

Physiotherapy usually requires liaison with the pain team, especially if intensive treatment is required to avoid pneumonia, a major complication (Byun & Kim 2013). Once pain is controlled, regular incentive spirometry is advisable. If gas exchange is impaired, continuous positive airway pressure (CPAP) provides the added benefit of pneumatic stabilization of the ribcage without impairing cardiovascular function (Schweiger *et al* 2003).

Before mobilizing patients who have a haemothorax, they can first be asked to clear some of the blood from their pleural space by lying with the chest drain dependent, so long as it is not uncomfortable and this does not

FIGURE 19.7 Flail chest caused by fractured ribs. The unstable segment is sucked in on inspiration and pushed out on expiration.

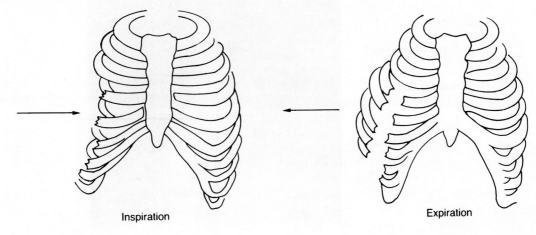

Inspiration

Expiration

block the drain. Extra pain during activity may be eased by Entonox (Ducassé *et al* 2013), if there is no pneumothorax. A cough belt or towel supports coughing. Stab wounds require an exercise programme such as that described by Senekal & Eales (1994).

Lung contusion

Shearing or crushing forces to the chest can lead to pulmonary laceration and a form of 'blood pneumonia' known as contusion. Blood-filled alveoli cause a shunt, ventilation/perfusion mismatch, hypoxaemia and x-ray signs of ground glass mottling, followed by absorption of the infiltrates over three to five days, or progression to ARDS. Patients are breathless and produce bloody secretions. Mechanical ventilation (MV) is needed if hypoxaemia is refractory to oxygen therapy or CPAP. If secretions are present, neither patient nor lungs take kindly to percussion or vibrations, but humidification and, after adequate analgesia, a breathing technique (Ch. 8) may be beneficial. If frank bleeding is present, suction is contraindicated.

Diaphragmatic rupture

Blunt injuries may rupture the diaphragm. Abdominal viscera herniate into the chest, requiring immediate surgical repair. The diagnosis may be missed clinically but can be confirmed by ultrasound, CT scan (Hwang 2011) or X-ray (Fig 19.8).

Burns and smoke inhalation

Immediate management of burns is to:

- remove any clothing that is burning, constricting or covered with chemicals, but not clothing that is stuck to the wound
- cool any burns less than three hours old with cold water, but avoid hypothermia, especially in the young and old
- cover the patient with something clean and dry
- attend to other trauma such as bleeding; monitor perfusion to burn wounds; remove rings
- if available, apply oxygen if there are major burns, and 100% oxygen if carbon monoxide has been inhaled.

The patient will be intubated if there is stridor, hoarseness, facial injury, sooty sputum or burns to the face or neck. Airway swelling develops within hours but obstruction may also occur later (Dries & Endorf 2013). Electrical burns require extra fluid resuscitation and may bring hidden musculoskeletal damage (Sanford & Gamelli 2014).

FIGURE 19.8 Ruptured R hemidiaphragm following trauma, now in its natural resting position.

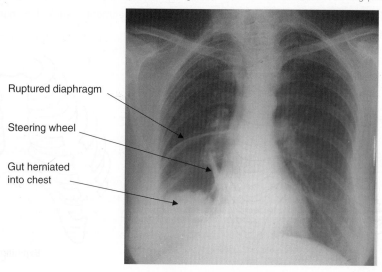

Ruptured diaphragm

Steering wheel

Gut herniated into chest

Pathology and clinical features

Burns cause secondary damage from an exaggerated inflammatory response which can double energy needs (Chang 2014 p.42) and leach skeletal muscle for fuel, just when a sustained supply of amino acids is required for wound healing (Porter 2013). This leads to marked muscle wasting and delayed mobilization (Williams *et al* 2011). Oxygen delivery may be reduced by ARDS due to vascular permeability (Sio *et al* 2010), shock and sometimes inhaled carbon monoxide.

The effects can be prolonged:

1 Increased cardiac work lasts well into the rehabilitation stage.
2 Catecholamine and corticosteroid levels increase 10 to 50-fold for up to 12 months.
3 Glucose metabolism is impaired for up to three years (Williams *et al* 2011).

Other complications include restricted expansion due to a tight armour of scarring around the chest.

The heat from **smoke inhalation** is filtered by the upper airways at the expense of bronchospasm, mucosal swelling, paralysis of cilia and ulceration. Steam, crack cocaine and some other toxins can overwhelm these filtering properties and penetrate to alveoli. Of particular concern to the physiotherapist are atelectasis due to loss of surfactant, and destroyed mucociliary transport (Dries & Endorf 2013).

The stages of lung injury from smoke inhalation are:

- bronchospasm (first 12 hours)
- pulmonary oedema (6–12 hours post-burn)
- bronchopneumonia (>60 hours post-burn).

Wheeze and black sputum may not appear for 24 hours, and x-ray signs of pulmonary oedema are not apparent for some days. Infection is readily transmitted to the denuded airways from the hospital environment, infected burns or endogenous sepsis, and epithelial damage can cause long-term hyperreactivity, tracheal stenosis or bronchiectasis.

Medical management

Medical treatment is by:

- pain management, including opioids, lignocaine (Wasiak *et al* 2012) or for dressing changes, Entonox (Yuxiang *et al* 2012)
- fluid resuscitation with Ringer's lactate or normal saline (Stander & Wallis 2011)
- humidified oxygen, CPAP if the face is not burned, or MV
- modulation of the hypermetabolic response with early excision and grafting of burn wounds, environmental thermoregulation and drugs to stimulate anabolism and oppose catabolism (Williams *et al* 2011)
- early and continuous specialized feeding to promote wound healing, increase resistance to infection and prevent persistent loss of muscle protein, preferably using the gut.

Antithrombin attenuates inflammation and vascular leakage (Rehberg *et al* 2013) and inhaled anticoagulation helps prevent ARDS (Miller *et al* 2013). Prophylactic antibiotics are not recommended, but a sputum specimen should be obtained at the earliest indication of infection. Oximetry may be falsely normal because oxyhaemoglobin cannot be distinguished from carboxyhaemoglobin. Large mucous casts may need bronchoscopy or lavage. Ventilated patients require extubation over a fibre optic bronchoscope in case of oedema.

Physiotherapy

Respiratory care is aimed at maintaining lung volume and clearing the thick and prolific secretions caused by airway damage. Lavish humidification is needed. Precautions are:

- little and often treatment because of the importance of prophylaxis and the inevitable fatigue
- avoidance of percussion and vibrations over chest burns, whether dressed or not; if manual techniques are essential, a vibrator is reasonably comfortable over a sterile towel
- if there is oedema near the head or neck, avoidance of head-down postural drainage
- suction, if it is necessary, to be gentle, scrupulously aseptic, and minimal to prevent further mucosal damage
- attention to communication if facial oedema affects vision or speech

- no nasopharyngeal suction if there is voice change or stridor, which should be reported because intubation will be required.

Two-hourly exercises are needed for burned limbs, especially the hands, using Entonox or other analgesia. Provision of a clean 'burn intensive care gym' provides the opportunity for patients to improve their functional status and take responsibility for self-management.

Fat embolism

Fat emboli occur when fats are released from bone marrow into the circulation. This follows all long-bone fractures and many orthopaedic operations (Kwiatt 2013). Capillary inflammation and the multisystem disorder 'fat embolism syndrome' may develop, which affects organs with high blood flow such as lungs, brain and skin. Respiratory signs are dyspnoea, agitation, tachycardia, pyrexia and cyanosis within 72 hours of trauma, sometimes leading to ARDS. The risk is increased if fractures are not immobilized because movement precipitates intravascular entry of the fat embolus.

Non-fatal drowning

Non-fatal drowning can lead to aspiration, bronchospasm, inactivation of surfactant, blood-stained pulmonary oedema, atelectasis and hypoxaemia, especially with polymicrobial infections as in 'tsunami lung' after the Japanese 2011 earthquake (Kawakami et al 2012). If water is swallowed, there is a high incidence of vomiting, sometimes followed by further aspiration. Frequent chest clearance may be needed for at least 48 hours to prevent atelectasis.

'Dry drowning' accounts for 10% of admissions and is caused by laryngospasm in a panicking victim, leading to apnoea and hypoxaemia. Fluid is not aspirated and the airways rarely need clearance by physiotherapy.

Hypothermia, defined as core temperature below 35°C, commonly occurs with near-drowning or other trauma. It may be difficult to recognize but can cause cardiovascular complications. Resuscitation attempts should be prolonged, with emphasis on the ventilation component (Bierens & Warner 2013) and nobody considered dead until they are 'warm and dead' (Hunger 2013), i.e. until they have been rewarmed to 35°C (Kempainan & Brunette 2004).

Poisoning and parasuicide

Complications of poisoning include arrhythmias, fluid depletion due to vomiting or diarrhoea, and respiratory compromise due to ventilatory depression, upper airway obstruction or pulmonary oedema. Gastric lavage may cause aspiration or laryngeal spasm.

Carbon monoxide is one of the leading causes of poisoning and binds to haemoglobin over 200 times more strongly than oxygen (Pang 2014), shifting the oxygen dissociation curve to the left, hindering loading of oxygen from the lungs and interfering with its unloading to the tissues. P_aO_2 is normal but S_pO_2 is falsely high, and the presentation can mimic common illnesses or exacerbate established disease. Apparent recovery may be followed two weeks later by neurological deterioration which can be permanent. Monitoring is by pulse CO-oximetry (Sebbane 2013) and treatment is with 100% or hyperbaric oxygen (Murad et al 2014).

Some poisoning is accidental but most is self-inflicted. Health staff may show negative attitudes to parasuicide patients, including judgements about attention-seeking (Brockopp et al 2003). However, these patients are often at the extremes of depression or desperation and the professional approach is to withhold personal judgment and care for the patient in such a way that they believe life is worth living after all. Successful suicides are considered a permanent 'solution' to a temporary problem, and bereaved relatives find recovery more difficult than after a normal death. The care they receive in the first hours can have a profound impact on their grief (Odell 1997).

SYSTEMS FAILURE

Disseminated intravascular coagulation (DIC)

The normal response to tissue damage is a contained explosion of thrombin to initiate coagulation and limit blood loss. This may become uncontained after severe damage, e.g. burns, central nervous system injury, fat embolism syndrome, some recreational drugs, transfusion, trauma (Holley 2013) or sepsis (Broomhead & Mallett 2013). This deranged coagulopathy is called DIC, in which liberated thromboplastin activates unrestrained clotting and blocks vessels with clumps of platelets and fibrin, causing ischaemia and organ damage. Once clotting factors have been depleted, bleeding can occur from the slightest trauma, including suction.

Coagulation therapy and treatment of the underlying disorder are required (Schöchl et al 2012). Suction is not contraindicated, but should be minimized. DIC is not usually written in the notes or charts because it is a response to the primary diagnosis.

Acute pancreatitis

Inflammation of the pancreas has a variety of causes including gallstones, alcoholism, drug reaction or eating disorder. Dissemination of the inflammation leads one third of patients to develop ARDS (Litmathe et al 2013).

The acute disease activates enzymes which autodigest pancreatic tissue and may set off a cascade of ischaemia, vasodilation, increased capillary permeability and DIC. Progressive liquefaction of the pancreas may cause abscesses and sepsis. Patients suffer paralytic ileus, which increases the risk of aspiration, a rigidly distended abdomen and continuous epigastric pain, worse in supine. Diaphragmatic splinting often leads to basal atelectasis, consolidation, pleural effusion and respiratory failure.

Medical treatment aims to eliminate the cause, manage complications and prevent progression, e.g. by hydration, epidural analgesia (if not contraindicated by coagulation problems), enteral nutrition within 24 hours (Bakker et al 2011), MV if required and surgery if there is infection.

Physiotherapy is aimed at preserving lung volume, mainly by positioning with the whole bed tilted head-up about 15°.

Collagen vascular disease

These autoimmune disorders may lead to multisystem failure and abnormal clotting. Suction requires extra caution because of the risk of bleeding.

Acute kidney injury

The kidney is central to BP and fluid regulation but is dependent on perfusion pressure while receiving a lower priority than the heart or brain (Hultström 2013). Its sensitivity to impaired perfusion means that acute kidney injury (AKI) is often precipitated by hypovolaemia or sepsis (Prowle 2014). Multisystem failure may be either cause or effect, and AKI and ARDS contribute to each other via 'kidney-lung crosstalk' (Ricci & Ronco 2010).

Kidney function can be supported in several ways:

1   Intermittent haemodialysis circulates the patient's blood outside their body and through a semipermeable membrane, allowing toxins and excess fluid to be removed. Complications include unstable BP, inflammation, wheezing, hypoxaemia due to capillary blockage and bleeding due to anticoagulation. Vascular access is commonly by arteriovenous fistula.

2   Continuous haemofiltration and haemodiafiltration work more slowly and allow control of BP, electrolytes, medication and nutrition. Moderate anticoagulation is required.

3   Sustained low-efficiency daily dialysis is a hybrid therapy combining the advantages of both options (Vanholder 2011).

4   Peritoneal dialysis uses the patient's own semipermeable peritoneal membrane (Wang et al 2014) but risks infection and impairs basal ventilation. Physiotherapy should coincide with the end of the emptying cycle to ensure free diaphragmatic movement.

Patients on specialized nutritional support are ripe for exercise (Magnard et al 2013) but physiotherapists need to develop a healthy respect for the renal vascular catheter or 'vascath' because it is highly sensitive to position change and disconnection leads to major blood loss. Patients with a neck line can sit out in a chair, with extra care taken during the transfer, and those with a femoral line can be mobilized with care (Ch. 18). Other precautions are to be watchful of fluid volume changes, acid-base disturbance or hypertension, and to be aware of the risk of bleeding because of anticoagulation drugs.

Acute liver injury

Liver cells are also vulnerable to hypoxia. Acute liver injury can develop from viral hepatitis, multisystem failure or toxins, such as excess alcohol or paracetamol (Lopez 2014). This may set off coagulopathy, encephalopathy and often respiratory and cardiovascular complications (Wang *et al* 2013d). Handling and suction should be minimal, and brain dysfunction is a warning to take precautions similar to those for acute brain injury. The lungs may suffer a restrictive defect from ascites or pleural effusion.

Support of failing systems either allows the liver to recover or permits survival until a donor organ is available for transplant. Some patients are so poisoned by their own liver that it is removed even if no donor is immediately available. Liver resection can now be done by laparoscope (Mostaedi 2012), but transplantation needs a 'Mercedes-Benz' double subcostal incision and laparotomy, requiring intensive postoperative pain relief and bringing a 50% incidence of lung complications (Jiang *et al* 2012). For survivors, post-transplant recovery is surprisingly rapid once the toxic liver has been removed, but rehabilitation may be slow due to prolonged deconditioning.

Cirrhosis is the final phase of chronic liver disease, which may obstruct the portal vein, transmit back pressure throughout the portal system and cause oesophageal varices. These are a contraindication to most forms of physiotherapy because of the risk of bleeding.

More safeguards for treating patients with liver disease are in Ch. 3.

SEPSIS, SHOCK AND MULTISYSTEM FAILURE

Colonization: *presence of microorganisms*
Infection: *invasion and multiplication of microorganisms*
Bacteraemia: *bacteria in blood*
Septicaemia: *systemic infection in which pathogen is present in blood*
Endotoxin: *toxin released by gram-negative bacteria as they disintegrate*

Sepsis: *systemic response to infection, manifest by two or more of the following:*
- temperature >38° or <36°C
- heart rate (HR) >90/min
- respiratory rate (RR) >20/min or P_aCO_2 <4.3 kPa (32 mmHg)
- WCC (white cell count) >12 000

Systemic inflammatory response syndrome (SIRS): *generalized inflammatory response, manifest by two or more of the above and caused by infection or other insult such as trauma or pancreatitis.*
Multisystem failure (MSF): *systems failure caused by direct insult or SIRS, in which homeostasis cannot be maintained without intervention; also known as multiple organ failure or multiple organ dysfunction syndrome.*
Shock: *tissue hypoxia due to failure of oxygen supply to meet oxygen demand.*

Sepsis

Clinical features of sepsis include fever (or occasionally hypothermia), tachypnoea, and skin which is initially warm from peripheral vasodilatation but may become cold if shock supervenes. Tachycardia and decreased systemic vascular resistance lead to increased cardiac output, which along with fluid therapy leads to a hyperdynamic state, i.e. abnormally increased circulatory volume with decreased BP. Elevated lactate leads to metabolic acidosis, and deranged coagulation is inevitable (Picoli-Quaino *et al* 2014), a third of patients developing DIC (Martin 2009).

Within 48 hours, muscle protein is broken down to provide amino acids for the inflammatory response, and the diaphragm struggles for its share of oxygen, sometimes devouring a quarter of the total body oxygen consumption ($\dot{V}O_2$) (Mager 2009). The process may lead to respiratory failure, circulatory collapse and MSF, each new failing organ adding 15–20% to the risk of death (Martin 2009).

Medical management is based on a 'sepsis care bundle' of timely circulatory and ventilatory support (Jones & Puskarich 2014). Mechanical ventilation should be initiated as soon as rapid shallow breathing is apparent and not await hypercapnia (Magder 2009).

Combination antibiotics (Kumar 2013) may control the infection source but do not reverse inflammatory and clotting cascades, for which immune-enhancing therapy may be beneficial (Sen & Yende 2013).

Impaired cerebrovascular autoregulation means that critical drops in BP are transferred directly to the vascular bed, leading to brain dysfunction (Taccone *et al* 2014) and delirium (Schramm *et al* 2012). On average 33% of patients die (Grover & Handy 2012).

Shock

In contrast to the layperson's shock-horror understanding of the term, shock in medicine occurs when the reserve capacity of tissue respiration is exhausted and hypoxia ensues. If prolonged, this leads to irreversible cellular injury. Once oxygen delivery (DO_2) can no longer satisfy $\dot{V}O_2$, a cascade of events ensues:

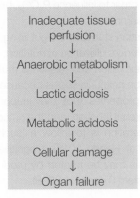

Inadequate tissue
perfusion
↓
Anaerobic metabolism
↓
Lactic acidosis
↓
Metabolic acidosis
↓
Cellular damage
↓
Organ failure

Shock is defined in terms of the cardiovascular component of DO_2, i.e. mean arterial pressure <60 mmHg or systolic BP <90 mmHg, or decrease in systolic BP greater than 40 mmHg (Nebout & Pirracchio 2012).

Hypovolaemic shock is caused by 15% loss in intravascular volume. Reasons may be haemorrhage, burns, severe diarrhoea or diuresis. Early physiological compensation is by redistribution of fluid from extravascular to intravascular space, and selective vasoconstriction to non-vital systems.

Cardiogenic shock is caused by sudden heart failure, as in severe myocardial infarction. It is characterized by high CVP, low cardiac output (CO) and pulmonary oedema.

Septic shock occurs when sepsis-induced hypotension is unresponsive to fluid resuscitation. Peripheral vasodilation depletes perfusion to the viscera and

leaks albumin to the tissues. Damaged organs release endotoxins, which stimulate nitric oxide production and augment uncontrolled vasodilation, leading to a 'functional haemorrhage'. High CO cannot sustain an adequate BP and hypoxic tissues cannot extract sufficient oxygen, as shown by a rise in mixed venous saturation ($S_{\bar{v}}O_2$) above 85% and loss of muscle tissue (Poulsen *et al* 2011). Patients are pyrexial, flushed, tachypnoeic, hypotensive and have a bounding pulse. Skin mottling indicates microcirculatory impairment but is correlated with survival (Ait-Oufella *et al* 2011). Treatment is by vasopressors, 100% O_2 in the first 24 hours (Calzia *et al* 2010) and avoidance of inotropes (Wilkman *et al* 2013), but mortality reaches up to 50% (Huet 2014).

Other types of shock are **anaphylactic** shock, an allergic reaction by more than one system, and **neurogenic** shock, loss of sympathetic tone following nervous system damage. Both are characterized by disordered vascular control and hypotension.

Hypovolaemic and cardiogenic shock lead to reduced CO. Other forms of shock lead to maldistribution of DO_2 between and within organs. Prompt treatment with fluids and vasopressors (Brown *et al* 2013b) during the first hour may prevent progression to MSF.

Multisystem failure

Causes

Multisystem failure may follow sepsis, shock or any process that makes excessive demands on $\dot{V}O_2$, e.g.:

- aspiration
- burns, smoke inhalation or lung contusion
- multiple transfusions, especially of colloid or blood, or cardiopulmonary bypass
- complications of trauma or surgery
- brain injury
- non-fatal drowning ± hypothermia
- pulmonary embolism or fat embolism syndrome
- neurogenic pulmonary oedema
- prolonged hypotension
- poisoning or drug abuse
- peritonitis or acute pancreatitis
- disseminated intravascular coagulation (DIC)
- immunosuppression, e.g. neutropaenic or postoperative states.

Interaction of these predisposing factors can blur cause and effect, e.g. the inflammatory response can activate coagulation, leading to DIC, and shock can initiate immunochaos, whereby homeostasis is lost.

Pathophysiology

If a limb is amputated and then after a delay is reimplanted, the dying tissue releases endotoxins which invade the body and set off an inflammatory domino effect. Re-amputation is then required to prevent the rest of the body becoming poisoned. Similarly with MSF, except the body cannot be amputated. Circulating inflammatory products cause reperfusion injury, with widespread capillary leak, hypovolaemic shock and multisystem damage. This 'rogue inflammation' subverts the normal healing process, a deadly cascade of inflammation escaping the usual control mechanisms and exacerbating rather than repairing injury.

The main culprit is the gut, whose vulnerability to hypoperfusion has earned it a reputation as the 'engine of multisystem failure' by leaking its bacteria into the rest of the body. The main victim is the lung because of its large vascular component, now permeable and poisoned.

Circulating catecholamines increase CO and blood flow, but deranged autoregulation sends the circulating blood to robust tissues such as skin and muscle, at the expense of needy systems such as the brain, gut and kidney. Patients are in effect poisoning themselves, which explains why some patients have no identifiable septic focus.

The resulting hypoxia is due to:

- refractory hypoxaemia
- reduced gas diffusion at tissue level because of interstitial oedema and impaired oxygen extraction due to damaged microvasculature
- excess oxygen consumption due to hypermetabolism (Fig 19.9).

The failing systems most relevant to the physiotherapist are the haematological and respiratory systems, leading to DIC and acute lung injury.

Medical management

Any septic focus needs treatment to prevent further stimulation of the inflammatory response, e.g. excision of dead bowel or stabilization of fractures. The aim is then to restore homeostasis and sustain tissue perfusion rather than focus on a single system.

Glycaemic control and antibiotics are required within one hour of diagnosis, and fluid resuscitation within six hours (Dellinger *et al* 2013), although transfused fluid tends to escape into the leaky lung. Renal impairment complicates the picture, leading to the dilemma of whether to sacrifice the kidneys in order to keep the lungs dry, or increase fluids to restore urine output and risk the complications of more intense respiratory support. On balance, the aim is for a CVP of 10–12 cmH_2O and pulmonary artery wedge pressure (PAWP) of 18 cmH_2O.

DO_2 is supported by oxygen therapy, inotropes and vasodilators, aiming for MAP of at least 65 mmHg, but this brings a similar dilemma of lower values risking acute kidney injury and higher values risking fluid overload (Correa *et al* 2013). $\dot{V}O_2$ is reduced by respiratory support and avoidance of stress or pyrexia. Packed red cell transfusion or haemofiltration may be used to wash out circulating inflammatory mediators. Lactate-induced metabolic acidosis can usually be corrected by manipulation of MV in order to influence P_aCO_2, but a pH below 7.2 requires haemofiltration.

Enteral nutrition stabilizes the gut lining, but the septic response hinders utilization of nutrition, as shown by high nitrogen excretion and relentless muscle wasting. Steroids may be helpful in sepsis because of their anti-inflammatory properties, but they suppress the patient's own adrenal function, and the outcome of much scientific deliberation is to follow a 'suck it and see' policy (Grover & Handy 2012). Cognitive impairment following sepsis may be treated by modulation of the adrenergic system (Tuon *et al* 2008).

Physiotherapy

Treatment should keep $\dot{V}O_2$ to a minimum, but preventive respiratory care is required and judicious exercise to manage the myopathy that will probably arise from inactivity and inflammation (Winkelman 2004).

Meningococcal septicaemia can cause hypoperfusion to the peripheries, leading to severe musculoskeletal and neurological consequences, including necrosis and gangrene. Passive movements require extreme care to safeguard the skin, and if fingers are affected, the hands may need to be splinted, with much padding, in a functional position to optimize circulation and prevent contractures. Teamwork requires a splinting specialist (occupational therapist or physiotherapist) and tissue viability nurse.

Follow up rehabilitation is always required (Poulsen *et al* 2009).

FIGURE 19.9 Effect of imbalance in oxygen delivery and consumption, leading to multisystem failure

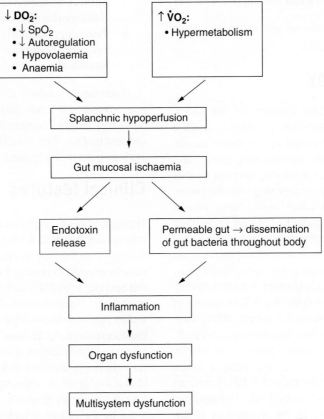

DO_2: oxygen delivery, $\dot{V}O_2$: oxygen consumption, CO: cardiac output

ACUTE RESPIRATORY DISTRESS SYNDROME

Atelectrauma: alveolar damage due to cytokine release as a result of alveoli repeatedly collapsing and reopening during the respiratory cycle
Alveolar recruitment: maintenance of open alveoli in order to (a) prevent atelectrauma and (b) promote gas exchange
Alveolar derecruitment: collapse of open alveoli

Acute respiratory distress syndrome (ARDS) occurs when parenchymal lung damage leads to alveolar-capillary leak and non-cardiogenic pulmonary oedema. It has also been called leaky lung syndrome, or shock lung due to an oft-associated state of shock, or white lung due to its radiological appearance, or Nam lung due to its first description in badly-injured US soldiers salvaged from Vietnam battlefields. The incidence is increasing (Cárdenes 2013) and mortality is around 20% (Kress 2013), being highest for patients with sepsis, pneumonia or aspiration, and lowest after trauma (Ragaller & Richter 2010).

Lungs can be injured directly, for example by aspiration, contusion or smoke inhalation, or indirectly by toxins let loose from multisystem failure. Either way, patients who die usually succumb to multisystem failure rather than respiratory failure (Kreyer et al 2014). Severity is classified according to gas exchange:

- Mild: P_aO_2/F_iO_2 ratio of 200–300 mmHg (27–40 kPa)

- Moderate: P_aO_2/F_iO_2 100–200 mmHg (13.3–27 kPa)
- Severe: P_aO_2/F_iO_2 <100 mmHg (<13.3 k Pa)

Mild and moderate disease are also called acute lung injury (ALI).

Pathophysiology

Both alveolar and vascular functions of the parenchyma are ravaged by inflammatory mediators, and the resulting sieve-like alveolar-capillary membrane causes flooding of the alveoli with fluid containing protein and blood, leading to massive pulmonary oedema so that the patient feels as if they are drowning from the inside. The waterlogged lungs weigh nearly twice normal (Dirkes et al 2012) and begin to collapse under their own weight, leading to compression atelectasis in dependent regions. Surfactant is washed out and hypoxic vasoconstriction (p.16) is lost in the metabolic disarray, leading to a widened P_{A-aO_2} gradient, a shunt that may exceed 25% and work of breathing (WOB) averaging 50% of total oxygen consumption (Martin 2001). Vascular injury leads to pulmonary hypertension (Lai 2013), which exacerbates pulmonary oedema and inhibits right ventricular function. Only a proportion of alveoli are ventilated, just 20% in the case of ALI (Porhomayon 2010), leading to the term 'baby lung'. The resulting restrictive defect worsens as the architecture of the lung, which has been intact during the florid **exudative phase** (days one to five), is remodelled and weakened by the inflammatory process. The lungs may then recover, or over the next week move into the **proliferative phase** when the alveolar exudate organizes. The **fibrotic phase** then dominates for the next few weeks, shown radiologically as cysts and honeycombing.

The functioning alveoli are vulnerable to barotrauma, especially as the non-homogenous loss of compliance causes alveoli to empty at different speeds, contributing to an uneven distribution of ventilation (Cressoni 2014):

1   Dependent alveoli are either consolidated with a proteinaceous fluid and inflammatory cells, or collapsed. Collapsed alveoli are recruitable in the early stages by prone positioning to place them uppermost, but later they become fibrosed and non-recruitable. Consolidated alveoli are non-distensible and therefore protected from atelectrauma, but are not contributing to gas exchange.

2   Alveoli in the middle are closed at end-expiration but recruitable and therefore subject to atelectrauma, so they are more damageable than dependent alveoli.

3   Non-dependent alveoli stay open throughout the respiratory cycle but are overstretched and subject to barotrauma.

When oxygen delivery (DO_2) decreases to a critical level, oxygen extraction cannot increase to compensate, and oxygen consumption ($\dot{V}O_2$) becomes dependent on DO_2, thus reducing linearly with it instead of increasing according to need.

Clinical features

The signs of ARDS begin one to three days from the provoking insult (Bigatello & Hess 2002). Respiratory failure develops over the next 48 hours (Chang 2014 p.493) as patients struggle to breathe through lungs that feel like a wet sponge. Both P_aO_2 and P_aCO_2 drop due to hypoxaemia and hyperventilation. Diagnosis is usually when virulent hypoxaemia develops and, in the spontaneously breathing patient, P_aCO_2 rises as the patient tires. Development of the syndrome is less obvious if MV is already up and running, and the condition is not necessarily identified at the handover, unless specifically queried, because it is not the primary diagnosis. The physiotherapist works it out by the history, intractable hypoxaemia, ventilator manipulations aimed at optimizing gas exchange without further damaging the lungs, and imaging, usually in that order, and then checks it with the team.

X-ray signs lag behind clinical signs by 24–48 hours. Bilateral opacification is at first indistinguishable radiologically from pulmonary oedema, then increasingly dense 'snowstorm' consolidation fills the air spaces, often sparing the costophrenic angles (Fig 19.10). If the patient remains supine, CT scanning shows dense consolidation in dependent regions (Fig 19.11).

Breath sounds are surprisingly normal, with just a harsh edge to them (Rasanen et al 2014). Pulmonary artery catheterization shows high pulmonary artery pressure, reflecting pulmonary hypertension. PAWP is <18 mmHg, in contrast to the high PAWP of cardiogenic pulmonary oedema, because ARDS is not a condition of generalized overhydration. A decision tool is available to distinguish ARDS from pulmonary oedema (Schmickl et al 2012). $S_{\bar{v}}O_2$ is usually reduced because of hypermetabolism, but may be increased if hypoxic cells are unable to extract oxygen.

FIGURE 19.10 Image of lungs affected by ARDS showing diffuse opacification and air bronchograms where airways show up against white background. Endotracheal tube and ECG leads are apparent

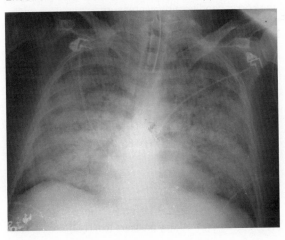

FIGURE 19.11 CT scan of a patient with ARDS, showing dense areas of atelectasis in dependent regions and a pneumothorax in the R anterior region.

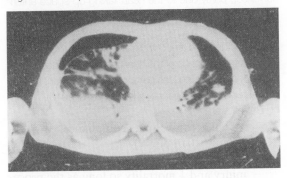

Medical management

Automated screening with electronic alerts from the laboratory and radiology departments helps early detection (Barbas et al 2012). The cornerstone of treatment is then meticulous supportive care. Fluid management is aimed at zero fluid balance if there is no shock or renal failure (Roch et al 2013). A high-fat low-carbohydrate diet minimizes CO_2 production, and immunonutrition may diminish inflammation (Hecker et al 2013). Pharmacotherapy includes hypertonic saline (Wohlauer et al 2012), surfactant, pulmonary vasodilators and muscle relaxants (Spieth & Zhang 2014). Instil-

lation of vitamin D may reduce neutrophil recruitment and aspirin may prevent micro-thrombi.

Mechanical ventilation

The balance between beneficial and damaging ventilatory support is a fine one. MV is both 'friend and killer' (Pelosi & Gattinoni 1996), high tidal volumes maintaining gas exchange but squeezing the bulk of inspiratory gas into the fragile open alveoli, and low tidal volumes protecting lung tissue but risking further hypoxaemia. Target SpO_2 is 88-95% (Blakeman 2013) and following strategies attempt a balancing act:

1. **'Open lung' ventilation** uses recruitment manoeuvres (Ch. 18), e.g. high but judiciously-applied PEEP to stabilize alveoli, reduce intrinsic PEEP, distribute inspired gas more evenly and limit dissemination of inflammatory material (Graf & Marini 2008). High (Sarge 2014) PEEP under CT or ultrasound guidance, and with early extubation to non-invasive ventilation, can reduce non-aerated tissue four-fold, but may cause barotrauma (De Matos et al 2012). Other recruitment manoeuvres are cyclical sighs, inverse-ratio ventilation, sustained inspiratory pauses and increased inflation pressures.

2. **Lung protective ventilation** prevents over-distension of compliant lung by reducing high-pressure high-volume MV, e.g. with pressure control (Ch. 17) to limit peak pressure to <30 cmH_2O (Chang 2014 p.494), low tidal volume, which may also limit the spread of infectious material (Graf & Marini 2008), high-frequency ventilation, extracorporeal gas exchange (Gothner et al 2013) or airway pressure release ventilation, which draws gas into dependent lung during the time-cycled release phase.

Disadvantages of lung protective strategies include retention of secretions (Volpe et al 2008) and loss of volume (Kallet et al 2001), the two core areas of physiotherapy. Disadvantages of recruitment manoeuvres are:

- a tendency to distend already overinflated alveoli (Smetkin 2012)
- promotion of ventilator-induced lung injury (Kallet 2004)

- risks of barotrauma, transient hypotension, ventilator asynchrony and discomfort (Meade *et al* 2008)
- ineffectiveness once fibrosis has set in (Mols 2006).

Benefits of recruitment manoeuvres last no longer than an hour (Benfield *et al* 2007), or seconds if not stabilized with sufficient PEEP (Mols 2006). The potential for recruitment is low if ARDS is caused by a lung condition but higher if it is secondary to multisystem failure (Gattinoni 2002). If these open lung strategies are used, lung damage may be reduced by a slow inspiration (Silva *et al* 2012) or prone positioning (Oczenski *et al* 2005) so that ventral lung tissue is cocooned against the high volume/pressure of the manoeuvre. The limited survival benefit of open-lung strategies may relate to atelectrauma being less damaging than volutrauma (Wakabayashi 2014).

Physiotherapy

KEY POINT

Physiotherapy aims to maximize oxygen delivery while causing the least harm.

Gratuitous increase in stress and energy expenditure must be avoided because of the linear association between DO_2 and $\dot{V}O_2$. The main respiratory problem is reduced functioning lung volume. Excess upper airway secretions caused by intubation should be cleared, but the excess fluids caused by ARDS are not amenable to physiotherapy. Waterlogged alveoli do not respond to physical intervention, and inflammatory biofluids lurking in the deeper airways are best left undisturbed in the early stages (Ntoumenopoulos *et al* 2011).

Positioning

Dependent lung is congested, heavy and collapsed. Prone positioning can open this up (Fig 19.12) and increase gas exchange in 70–80% of patients (Dirkes *et al* 2012). This should be the first option before more complex interventions are attempted (Harcombe 2004).

FIGURE 19.12 Recruitment in ARDS lungs as a function of applied airway pressure, shown by the opening up of lung tissue along the volume–pressure curve. R indicates the % of recruitment occurring at the corresponding airway pressure.

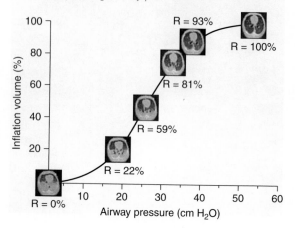

The rationale is that there are more alveoli in the posterior chest, partly due to the heart taking up space anteriorly, and partly due to the configuration of the chest creating greater volume posteriorly. In prone, more lung units are therefore freed from the weight of the dense lungs, with the bonus of the heart being supported by the sternum and causing less parenchymal distortion, leading to greater lung homogeneity (Gattinoni *et al* 2013).

Benefits are:
- ↑ SpO_2 and lung compliance, ↓ $\dot{V}O_2$ (Chang 2014 p.409)
- ↓ barotrauma, ↓ ventilator-induced lung injury and ↓ mortality so long as the procedure is initiated early (Mancebo 2006) and for long enough (Dirkes *et al* 2012)
- ↑ drainage of secretions and ↓ ventilator-associated pneumonia (Dirkes *et al* 2012).

Oxygenation may be greater if pressure against the abdomen is minimized by using an air-fluidized bed, a Respicair bed or support for the chest and pelvis with pillows.

Lack of response may relate to variations in chest configuration or redistribution of blood flow to more diseased lung. Delay reduces success because fibrosis may have set in. For patients who respond, saturation usually improves within 15 minutes, after an initial wobble (Fig 19.13), but if it does not, patients should be left prone to allow them to respond, so long as there is no deterioration, benefits having been shown at 6 and 12 hours (Guervilly 2013). Some take days to respond (Marion 2001). For patients who do not respond, proning may or may not be beneficial if tried again later (Rowe 2004). Adding a recruitment manoeuvre in the prone position is usually beneficial (Pelosi *et al* 2003).

Precautions are spinal surgery/injury, a grossly distended abdomen, unstable fractures, seizure, MAP <60 (Dirkes *et al* 2012), acute brain injury and post-abdominal or eye surgery. Contraindications are intractable intracranial hypertension and haemodynamic instability unresponsive to treatment (Marion 2001). Proning has been used successfully in morbidly obese patients and following subarachnoid haemorrhage (Reinprecht *et al* 2002).

Returning to supine may be required for various procedures, or at night if sufficient skilled night staff are not available to return the patient rapidly to supine in case of cardiac arrest. During periods in supine, the physiotherapist can make a full assessment and maintain range of movement for all joints, including elbows, hips and shoulders, which can develop contractures if prone is prolonged.

Three to five staff are required for the turn, including an intensivist or experienced nurse at the head of the bed to protect the airway and neck lines. A suggested procedure is described below.

FIGURE 19.13 Oxygenation over three hours, showing improvement during prone positioning. The dip during the turn reflects the effort of the manoeuvre. Some improvement is maintained on returning to supine, suggesting that recruitment of alveoli has been sufficiently robust to withstand the burden of the lung that is now weighing down on it.

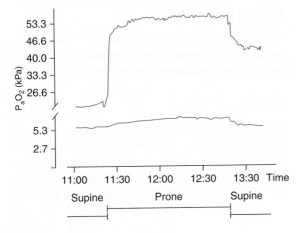

1   Explain to the patient, with reassurance that they will be safe and turned towards the ventilator; obtain consent if they are able to communicate.
2   Ensure that mouth care, eye care and, if required, a chest x-ray have been done before the turn.
3   Stop enteral feed.
4   Close eyes and protect with gel or pad.
5   Ensure reintubation equipment and staff are on hand.
6   Disconnect or plug lines as appropriate, redirect others in axis of body and track them during the turn.
7   Increase oxygen to 100%.
8   Suction.
9   Place the patient's palms against their thighs, thumbs upwards, elbows straight and shoulders neutral, ensuring protection of any arterial lines.
10 Place a clean sheet on top, wrap edges together with the underneath sheet to create a tight sandwich.
11 Slide the patient to the edge using the underneath sheet or glide sheet, according to hospital protocol.
12 Check that team members understand the vulnerability of the shoulders.
13 Roll patient into the lateral position using the underneath sheet, relocate ECG leads to the back.
14 If pillows are to be used for pelvis and chest/shoulder support, place them on the bed, with pillows close enough to avoid lordosis. Anything firmer than a pillow may be counterproductive (Chiumello *et al* 2006).
15 Roll patient into prone, suction the airway.
16 Reconnect lines.
17 If a Respicair bed is used, the abdominal section can be deflated.
18 Ensure that no joint is at end-range. Slight neck flexion can be facilitated by sliding the patient beyond the top of the bed and supporting their head on a cushioned table placed slightly below bed level. A pillow or horseshoe headrest allows the tracheal tube to be unrestricted but secure.
19 Ensure that the brachial plexus is not stretched by elevating shoulder girdles slightly.

20 Shoulder joints and neck should be near neutral. If the 'swimmers position' is used (Fig. 19.14), the elbow to which the head is semi-rotated should be flexed to no more than 90° to avoid ulnar nerve stretch, and the other arm internally rotated by the side (Rowe 2004). If the neck is neutral and the head is on a cushioned table (No 18, above) the arms can be either in the swimmers position or by the patient's side, shoulders internally rotated and palms upwards.

21 Ensure that women's breasts or men's genitals are not compressed.

22 Place two pillows under each shin to prevent peroneal nerve stretch, positioning them to avoid knee and toe pressure from the mattress.

23 Tilt the entire bed head-up to prevent facial oedema and eye damage, to between 30° (Rowe 2004) and 4° (Grant *et al* 2010). This may also improve oxygenation (Robak *et al* 2011).

24 Place gel cushions on pressure areas, reinstitute feed cautiously, return F_iO_2 to original level once S_pO_2 has settled, liaise with intensivist in case ventilator parameters need changing in the new position.

Head and arm positions are alternated two to three hourly. Pressure areas now include ears, cheeks, knees, toes, anterior superior iliac crests and any skin in contact with the tracheal tube (Jackson 2012). Potential cardiac arrest must be planned for and a protocol prepared for rapid return to supine.

Some clinicians find that placing 5 kg sandbags or a 5 l bag of fluid on the chest of a supine patient may have similar effects. It is thought that chest compression reduces the risk of barotrauma to upper lung regions while directing ventilation to dependent lung.

FIGURE 19.14 Suggested position for a proned patient. The head of the patient's L humerus may need support with a small folded towel.

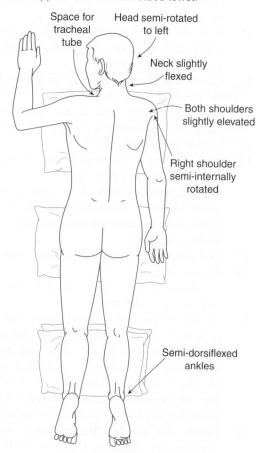

- Space for tracheal tube
- Head semi-rotated to left
- Neck slightly flexed
- Both shoulders slightly elevated
- Right shoulder semi-internally rotated
- Semi-dorsiflexed ankles

CLINICAL REASONING TIP

'Turning can be a frightening experience if the patient is not sedated adequately'.

Dirkes *et al* 2012

Sedation may well be appropriate, but primarily the patient must be given explanations and talked through the procedure, otherwise sedation may leave the patient with a distorted and fearful memory.

Manual hyperinflation

MH is normally avoided, especially in the later stages, because low compliance and heterogeneity of alveolar damage risks barotrauma (Fig 19.15).

Suction

Damaged alveoli are vulnerable to derecruitment during suction, lung volume often falling to below functional residual capacity. Ventilator recruitment manoeuvres may be used after suction, such as pressure support at 40 cmH$_2$O (Maggiore 2003) or CPAP at 45 cmH$_2$O for

FIGURE 19.15 Effect of manual hyperinflation on (left) normal alveoli, and (right) unevenly damaged alveoli

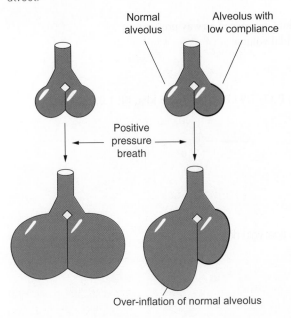

Normal alveolus

Alveolus with low compliance

Positive pressure breath

Over-inflation of normal alveolus

20 seconds (Dyhr 2002). However, these pressures could cause atelectrauma or barotrauma, and many physiotherapists would prefer to simply ensure that closed-circuit catheters are used to avoid loss of PEEP, and F_iO_2 increased until S_pO_2 returns to normal.

Rehabilitation

Muscle strength usually recovers within 12 months but impaired physical function and quality of life continue beyond two years (Fan *et al* 2013). Rehabilitation should therefore begin while the patient is bed-bound and maintained after discharge because of on going exercise intolerance (Herridge *et al* 2011), and, for 50% of patients, respiratory symptoms including breathlessness (Smith & Sinclair 1996).

Cognitive impairment is universal on discharge (Carr 2007), affecting 46% of patients after one year and 25% after six years, probably related to hypoxaemia (Mikkelsen *et al* 2012). Long term depression and memory loss may hinder return to work (Adhikari *et al* 2009), and post traumatic stress has been found in 27% of survivors due to their experiences in the ICU (Schelling 1998).

CASE STUDY : Mr AP

Mr AP was admitted to A & E after inability to sleep due to abdominal pain.

Social History
● Unemployed
● 15 cigarettes/day
● 80 units alcohol/day

On admission
● Distended tender abdomen
● ABGs when self-ventilating on F_iO_2 of 0.6: pH 7.26, P_aO_2 12.3 kPa, P_aCO_2 8.4 kPa, BE 1.5, HCO_3^- 23.2
● ↑WCC

Medical treatment

- Nasogastric tube, analgesia, fluid resuscitation

Progression

- S_pO_2 deteriorated → intubated and ventilated → gradual increase in airway pressure
- Changed to pressure control → gradual reduction in tidal volume

On examination

- ABGs on IRV, F_1O_2 of 0.85 and PEEP of 10: pH 7.20, P_aO_2 7.9 kPa, P_aCO_2 7.5 kPa, BE 1.0, HCO_3^- 25.2
- Breath sounds absent bibasally

Diagnosis

- Acute pancreatitis

Questions

1 What is causing the high airway pressure and then low tidal volume?
2 What is obliterating the breath sounds?
3 What syndrome is probably developing?
4 How is the ventilator set to enhance gas exchange?
5 How is the ventilator set to protect Mr P's lungs?
6 Problems?
7 Goals?
8 Plan?

ABGs: arterial blood gases, *BE:* base excess, *IRV:* inverse-ratio ventilation, *WCC:* white blood cell count.

CLINICAL REASONING

Comment on the rationale and evidence for 'chest physical therapy' in a group of mechanically ventilated patients:

The indications [for chest physical therapy] included . . . lung contusion . . .
Treatment times . . . averaged 67 min . . . [followed by increased] Q_s/Q_t in [50%] of the contusion patients . . .
The long-term clinical effect of these changes is unknown.

Q_s/Q_t = shunt fraction.

Crit Care Med (1985) 13, 483–6

Response to Case Study

1–2 What is causing the high airway pressure, low tidal volume and obliterating the breath sounds?
- Pressure against diaphragm from distended abdomen. Plus answer to question 3

3 What syndrome is probably developing?
- Acute respiratory distress syndrome

4 How is the ventilator set to enhance gas exchange?
- F_iO_2 0.6 then 0.85, IRV, high PEEP

5 How is the ventilator set to protect Mr P's lungs?
- Pressure control ventilation, lung protective ventilation with permissive hypercapnia and PEEP maintaining open lungs

6 Problems?
- Progressive compression atelectasis, with deteriorating gas exchange

7 Goals?
- Reverse and prevent further atelectasis, rehabilitate

8 Plan:
- reverse Trendelenberg positioning (whole bed head up)
- if this does not improve gas exchange, prone after cutting hole in mattress for abdomen (still in reverse Trendelenberg)
- hot water humidification
- suction as required
- musculoskeletal care.

The prone position opened up the lung bases. Mr P survived and the experience motivated him to address his alcohol dependency.

Response to Clinical Reasoning

Over an hour of postural drainage, percussion, vibration and suction is unlikely to be indicated for any condition, let alone lung contusion, i.e. bruising. Indeed, manual techniques are contraindicated with lung contusion because of the risk of bleeding.
Bleeding into alveoli is not cleared by techniques aimed at airways.
Objectively this technique appeared damaging by increasing the shunt in half the patients with contusion.
Subjectively, one can only guess.

RECOMMENDED READING

Atema JJ (2014) Clinical studies on intra-abdominal hypertension and abdominal compartment syndrome. *J Trauma Inj Inf Crit Care;* **76**(1): 234–40

Baldwin CE, Bersten AD (2014) Alterations in respiratory and limb muscle strength and size in patients with sepsis who are mechanically ventilated. *Phys Ther;* **94**(1): 68–82.

Chang WT, Nyquist PA (2013) Strategies for the use of mechanical ventilation in the neurologic intensive care unit. *Neurosurg Clin N Am;* **24**(3): 407–16

Chiumello D (2013) Clinical review: Lung imaging in acute respiratory distress syndrome patients. *Crit Care;* **17**(6): 243

Fan E (2012) Critical illness neuromyopathy and the role of physical therapy and rehabilitation in critically ill patients. *Respir Care;* **57**(6): 933–46

Ganesh S (2013) Medical comorbidities in disorders of consciousness patients and their association with functional outcomes. *Arch Phys Med Rehabil;* **94**(10): 1899–1907.e3

Hellweg S (2012) Effectiveness of physiotherapy and occupational therapy after traumatic brain injury in the intensive care unit. *Crit Care Res Pract*: 768456

Jones MG, Rae W, Lwin AA (2013) Pneumomediastinum leading to respiratory compromise as a complication of acute severe asthma. *Am J Respir Crit Care Med;* **187**(3): e5–6

Koshy K, Zochodne DW (2013) Neuromuscular complications of critical illness. *Handb Clin Neurol;* **115**: 759–80

Mani RK, Schmidt W, Lund LW (2013) Respiratory dialysis for avoidance of intubation in acute exacerbation of COPD. *ASAIO J;* **59**(6): 675–8

Marini JJ (2013) Ventilator-associated problems related to obstructive lung disease. *Respir Care,* **58**(6): 938–47

Qvarlander S, Sundström N, Malm J *et al* (2013) Postural effects on intracranial pressure. *J Appl Phys;* **115**(10): 1474–80

Rabinstein AA (2002) Pulmonary complications in patients with stroke requiring mechanical ventilation. *Crit Care;* **6**(Suppl 1): P49

Stocchetti N, Roux PL, Vespa P (2013) Clinical review: neuromonitoring. *Crit Care;* **17**: 201

Urfy MZ, Suarez JI (2014) Breathing and the nervous system. *Handb Clin Neurol;* **119**: 241–50

Weijs TJ (2013) Strategies to reduce pulmonary complications after esophagectomy. *World J Gastroenterol;* **19**(39): 6509–14

Whyte J (2013) Disorders of consciousness: outcomes, comorbidities, and care needs. *Arch Phys Med Rehabil;* **94**(10): 1851–4

PART V
DOES IT WORK?

CHAPTER 20 EVALUATION OF CARDIORESPIRATORY
         PHYSIOTHERAPY

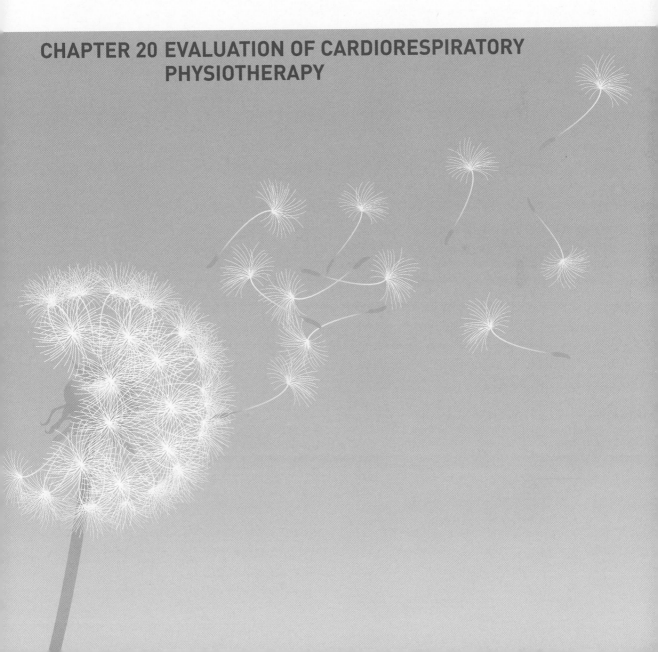

CHAPTER 20
Evaluation of cardiorespiratory physiotherapy

LEARNING OBJECTIVES

On completion of this chapter the reader should be able to:

- summarize the concepts behind outcomes, standards and cardiorespiratory audit

- critically analyze the literature to identify valid research

- supervise students and junior staff to ensure that they work effectively as part of the multidisciplinary team

- apply evidence-based clinical reasoning in the management of cardiorespiratory patients.

INTRODUCTION

There are known knowns: things that we know we know.
There are known unknowns: things that we know we don't know.
There are unknown unknowns: things that we don't know we don't know.

Taleb (2007) quoted by Rumsfeld

If a patient who is having physiotherapy gets better, is this due to the physiotherapy, the physiotherapist, the placebo effect or divine intervention? The credibility of cardiorespiratory physiotherapy is being challenged (Rubin *et al* 2012), which is to be welcomed.

An evidence-based approach is facilitated by clinical reasoning (Manns & Darrah 2006) using the hierarchy of evidence in Ch. 6, but its components can be hampered by several factors:

1   Research is scarce and ambiguous, 'chest physiotherapy' is poorly defined, and

variables such as simultaneous medical input can skew results.

2   There is evidence that:

- one-third of patients adhere to therapy
- one-third reject it outright
- one-third accept it but get it wrong (Lloyd 1998).

3   Lack of recognition of the need to have time for reflection leads to frustration and a lower standard of care, according to Toft (2000), who goes on to quote Huxley: 'fear casts out intelligence, casts out goodness ... in the end fear casts out even a man's humanity'. This could be one explanation for the inhumanity that we sometimes find when time seems ever shorter and fear of not keeping to targets can detach staff from the reason that they chose to work in the health system.

Clinical reasoning incorporates the ability to:

- access an organized knowledge base related to clinical problems
- generate and test hypotheses
- evaluate and use clinical data
- use reflection to self-evaluate
- generate knowledge from the reasoning process (Christensen *et al* 2008).

Communicating this knowledge involves not just the multidisciplinary team but also, to improve outcomes, the patient (Jones *et al* 2008 p. 248).

KEY POINT

The goal of clinical reasoning is wise action.

Jones *et al* (2008)

This chapter will use clinical reasoning to identify how critical evaluation of the research can inform practice, how continuous audit helps ensure that this is acted on, and how education can be used so that evaluation of cardiorespiratory physiotherapy does not become a luxury to be tagged on at the end if there is time.

Clinical expertise is reflected in the more thoughtful identification and compassionate use of individual patients' predicaments, rights and preferences.

Gray *et al* (1996)

DEFINITIONS

Only about 15% of all contemporary clinical interventions are supported by objective scientific evidence that they do more good than harm.

White 1988

Benchmark is an agreed criterion by which a practice can be judged.

Clinical governance is a framework to improve patient care using evidence-based guidelines. It includes audit, accountability and patient satisfaction (DoH 2011b).

Clinical pathways are locally developed, consensus-driven, evidence-based multidisciplinary steps which incorporate national guidelines into the care of patients with a specific clinical problem in order to increase efficiency and timeliness (Rotter *et al* 2010).

Clinical practice guidelines are systematically developed recommendations on the effective management of different conditions or problems. They are consensus-driven but accuracy may be elusive if 'various professional organizations fight over the same meta-analyses and come to different conclusions' (Stern 2013).

Consensus statements are a synthesis of research with implications for re-evaluation of practice.

Criteria identify what should happen for a standard to be achieved.

Evidence-based practice involves clinical decision-making based on the systematic search for, appraisal of, and use of current evidence. Where there is lack of objective evidence, clinical expertise is used, but as a tool to be nurtured mindfully, not used as anecdotal justification.

Guidelines are sets of recommendations that identify management strategies based on the evidence.

They require references, explanation of reasoning and grading of both recommendations and quality of the evidence. For patients with multimorbidity, guidelines may drive polypharmacy (Hughes *et al* 2013).

Outcome measures are subjective or objective changes due to physiotherapy input. They must be appropriate, reliable, valid and responsive.

Peer review is a review of the work of an individual by those who are equal in grade and specialty.

Protocols are precise instructions for a specific clinical problem, developed from a guideline. They are stricter, more explicit and usually shorter than guidelines.

Standards: see next page.

RESEARCH

There are no known facts, only the present theory of the day.

Howell cited by Conway (1992)

The above may or may not be ironic, but Kerry *et al* (2012) claim that the majority of clinical reviews in rehabilitation medicine are not actually true. Another hurdle is identified by Lin & Murphy (2010), who found a 17-year lag between evidence and change in practice, due to lack of time and training. This is compounded by publication bias, which favours trials with positive results (Costa *et al* 2013) while negative results, when they do get published, emerge more slowly.

On the positive side, Hurley *et al* (2012) identified ClinicalTrials.gov as a database of on going clinical trials to help bridge the gap, and Gehanno *et al* (2013) acknowledged PubMed and Google Scholar as adequate general databases. Cochrane is useful but can be somewhat depressing with its almost inevitable conclusion '... there is insufficient evidence' for a physiotherapy technique. This is because many cardiorespiratory physiotherapy techniques have not been subject to the purifying heat of randomized controlled trials.

The paucity of research should not hinder the identification of other components of evidence-based practice. Stolper *et al* (2009) state that results should be tempered by the richness and variety of different patients' needs and that even intuition can be included.

'Bundles' of care have improved the management of patients with complex cardiorespiratory problems, but they have complicated the search for an active ingredient (Wakefield *et al* 2013), and the physiotherapy component may sink from view.

The placebo effect is a constant presence in physiotherapy and cannot be ignored. Indeed it has been described as 'arguably more powerful than any physiotherapy technique has been' (Stack 2006). This can be harnessed, but selectively and honestly, and not as a substitute for research. The placebo effect in animal research suggests that its main driver is the relationship with the health professional (Haselen 2013). The more experienced the physiotherapist, the more the relationship with the patient is understood as the bedrock of effective treatment.

LITERATURE APPRAISAL

Why do kamikaze pilots wear helmets?

A questioning and indeed a suspicious mind is necessary when reading studies because research can prove or disprove almost anything and may be published in the most prestigious journals.

An assessment tool is available to reduce the risk of investigator bias (Farmer *et al* 2012), which tends to occur in favour of sponsors who fund studies (Rubin & Haynes 2012), especially as disclosures are considered 'very rare' (Bindslev *et al* 2013). Government guidelines tend to be funded by drug companies, and in asthma research, 95% of studies report pharmaceutical involvement (Bond *et al* 2012). In the US, pharmaceutical companies have had to pay billions in fines to settle investigations into fraudulent practice related to research (Braillon *et al* 2012).

Beware also of literature that contains:

- limited sample sizes which tend to report greater benefits (Zhang *et al* 2013)
- extrapolation of results from healthy young volunteers, e.g. dynamic hyperinflation simulated by using continuous positive airway pressure on normal subjects
- extrapolation of results from animals; dogs, for example, have a different chest

shape and their pleural space communicates bilaterally

- assessment of more than one technique in one study
- lack of distinction between correlation and causation
- interpretation without consideration of alternative explanations
- uncontrolled variables
- physiotherapists used as handmaidens to collect data rather than as designers of the study
- extrapolation of results from medical research, e.g. the manual ventilation used by anaesthetists is not the same as the manual hyperinflation used by physiotherapists
- lack of precision, e.g. 'chest physiotherapy was of no value', instead of the cumbersome but accurate: 'postural drainage with percussion in this way for this amount of time with these patients showed no evidence of faster mucociliary clearance/greater quantity of sputum/reduced airflow resistance/improved quality of life'
- physiological illiteracy, e.g. one study attempted to evaluate respiratory muscle activity during 'unilateral' chest expansion, but did not distinguish inspiratory and expiratory muscles and used 'subjective observation' to judge this notoriously ambiguous manoeuvre (Ng & Stokes 1992)
- wasted time, e.g. a study described by Decramer (2009) concluded that inspiratory muscle training gave better results in patients with inspiratory muscle weakness than those without inspiratory muscle weakness.

Examples are below.

1 Torrington et al (1984) imposed four-hourly intermittent positive pressure breathing, four-hourly incentive spirometry, two-hourly deep breathing and two-hourly nebulization on their hapless postoperative patients. The authors expressed surprise that additional four-hourly postural drainage and percussion increased cost, discomfort

and fever in one (presumably exhausted) group, without reducing atelectasis. The study has been much quoted to claim that postoperative physiotherapy is ineffective.

2 Weissman et al (1984) did not define chest physical therapy in a paper associating it with major haemodynamic and metabolic stress.

On the positive side, the British Thoracic Society guidelines on acute oxygen therapy are about as good as it gets (BTS 2008).

> All who drink of this remedy recover in a short time, except those whom it does not help, who all die. Therefore it is obvious that it fails only in incurable cases.
>
> Galen, 2nd century

STANDARDS

> The perception is, if chest physiotherapy doesn't help, it won't hurt.
>
> Eid 1991

The above is, hopefully, tongue in cheek, but the concept still hovers over the profession. Evaluation of cardiorespiratory physiotherapy therefore needs standards against which outcomes are measured. Standards define the expected level of performance and must be measurable, understandable, desirable and achievable. They are usually subject to staffing levels. Standards are only useful if audited and if audit leads to positive change in practice. Box 20.1 gives examples for mobility.

Other standards could include identification of which surgical patients are to be assessed, time between referral and assessment for acute and non-acute medical patients, agreement with patients of goals and plans, explanation to patients about limitations and risks of treatment, provision for patient self-management and liaison with the multidisciplinary team.

BOX 20.1

Standards of mobility for all inpatients

1 All patients mobilize daily, independently or with assistance, unless:
   - it is unsafe, e.g. haemodynamic instability
   - it is impossible, e.g. coma
2 For patients who do not mobilize, the reason and action taken are documented, e.g. pain, contraindication, patient unwilling, staff shortage
3 The daily exercise programme is documented:
   - in the patient notes, if given verbally to the patient, or
   - as a hand out for the patient, copied in the notes
4 Documentation demonstrates progress, or reason for lack of progress

OUTCOME EVALUATION

> The most important outcomes in clinical trials are patient-centred outcomes.
> Alifano et al (2010)

Economic austerity renders areas of physiotherapy vulnerable to closure unless outcome is documented (Duncan & Murray 2012). Outcome measures also motivate patients by providing tangible proof of their progress, even if it is slow.

Both subjective and objective measures should show, when possible:

- how effective one outcome measurement is compared to others (validity)
- the extent to which it yields repeatable results on the same person over time (reliability)
- how well it detects a change in an individual (responsiveness).

Unlike research, outcomes can include the complete package of treatment as well as individual components (Dalley 1999).

Subjective measurement

The patient experience is positively associated with clinical effectiveness and patient safety (Doyle 2013)

and is included in quality of life scales and questionnaires.

Objective measurement

Obstacles to measuring cardiorespiratory outcomes include:

- S_pO_2 and other measurements varying with factors other than physiotherapy
- quality not equating with the number and length of treatments
- postoperative atelectasis sometimes being self-limiting
- mouthpieces interfering with measurement
- cardiorespiratory disease often complicated by multipathology.

Some measurements are suitable if taken in the context of the full clinical picture:

- ↑ oxygenation: ↑ P_aO_2 or S_pO_2
- ↑ oxygen delivery: mixed venous saturation
- ↑ ventilation: ↓ P_aCO_2
- in the case of hyperventilation syndrome: ↓ minute ventilation, as reflected by ↑ P_aCO_2
- increase or maintenance of exercise tolerance
- ↑ independence e.g. with activities of daily living
- increase or maintenance of lung volume (Ch. 6)
- ↓ work of breathing (Ch. 7)

FIGURE 20.1 Reduced vibration energy after secretion clearance in the R and L lungs of 15 mechanically ventilated patients.

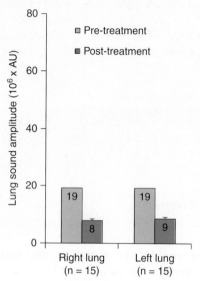

- clearance of secretions (Ch. 8)
- lack of deterioration.

Measurements currently used for research may become bedside outcome measures in the future, e.g. vibration energy computed before and after treatment to monitor secretion clearance (Fig 20.1).

Data collection requires training, administrative support and time. It is best that the choice of outcome measures is not organisationally imposed (Duncan & Murray 2012).

On call criteria (App. C) provide guidance for on-call staff, an indication of the adequacy of training and a means of monitoring the appropriateness of the call. Lack of improvement in the patient does not necessarily mean an inappropriate call-out.

Successes folder

To help compensate for the dearth of research, it is wise to build up a record of objective markers of success, e.g. before-and-after auscultation, S_pO_2 or electronic copies of x-rays (Figs 17.28 and 20.2). This is a crude measure which does not reflect the effects of education and prevention on a patient's quality of life, but is useful for continuing professional development, comes in handy if challenged by budget holders and helps towards outcomes becoming embedded in practice.

COST EFFECTIVENESS

Do no harm – cheaply.

Hughes 1980

Efficiency is allied to effectiveness because time is freed up for other input. Measures to save time include:

- avoiding treatment that is not evidence-based
- journal club to cover more journals than one person can read
- assistants supported and valued

FIGURE 20.2 Clearance of atelectasis after physiotherapy

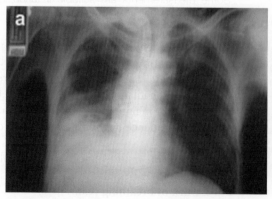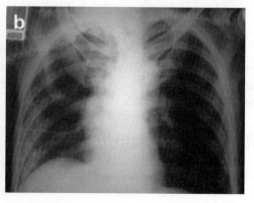

- for inpatients: hand outs to reinforce education, mobility tick charts to involve nursing staff with rehabilitation (App. B), written weekly referral sheet to assist the ward report, filled out by referring staff and checked daily by the physiotherapist (e.g. Box 20.2)
- for outpatients: information sent out before the first appointment, follow-up phone calls for motivation and support when face-to-face contact is not essential
- for ICU patients, early rehabilitation, which in one hospital trust cut almost eight days from the average length of stay and saved over £2 million (*Frontline* 2014)
- information for nursing and medical staff about appropriate referrals, by problem or condition (App. C).

Extended scope physiotherapists improve efficiency by training in skills such as taking arterial or capillary blood gases, supervising weaning, heading up ICU outreach or tracheostomy teams and performing bronchoscopies or minitracheostomies, thus being able to progress treatment without waiting for medical input.

It is cost-effective to spend time individualizing pre-written daily exercise programmes if this motivates the patient. It is cost-effective to reduce a patient's need for medication. It is cost-effective to increase a patient's independence and reduce their need for other services.

An on-call service is cost-effective if it prevents deterioration or avoids the need for more time-consuming interventions. It is not cost-effective if non-respiratory physiotherapists have not developed the competencies to deal with critically ill patients. The credibility of respiratory physiotherapy has been clearly extolled: 'We cannot claim to offer 24-hour care for patients while working only eight of them' (Nicholls 1996).

Short-termism must not intrude on cost-effectiveness. Prevention and rehabilitation are central to efficient respiratory care.

> *If you go for cost, you will lose quality.*
> *If you go for quality, you will save money.*
> Taylor & Odell (2011)

THE AUDIT CYCLE

> *People do not resist change. They resist being changed.*
> Lloyd 1998

Research and patient feedback tell us the right thing to do. Audit tells us if we are doing the right thing right. It entails clinically-led peer review, which systematically analyzes practice and outcome against agreed standards, then modifies practice where indicated.

Protected time, simple topics and minimal documentation are advised. Liaison with the clinical audit

---

BOX 20.2

Referrals for physiotherapy

Week:	Ward:	Physiotherapist:	Bleep:
Date	Name of patient	Referrer (print name and designation)	Physiotherapy problem for which assessment is requested

FIGURE 20.3 Notes audit cycle

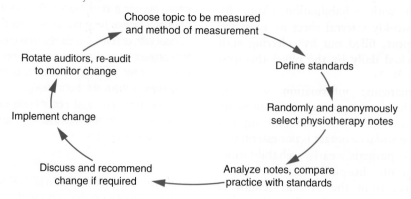

department is a useful first step. The topic chosen should have the potential for improvement and be responsive to physiotherapy, e.g.:

- percentage of problems resolved
- percentage of referrals or call-outs considered appropriate
- percentage of medical patients receiving discharge advice
- percentage of surgical patients discharged with pre-operative function.

An audit process can also be used as part of clinical education (Ivers *et al* 2012). If the full audit cycle (Fig 20.3) is not completed, the exercise is wasted.

Box 20.3 is an example of a biannual audit to monitor the efficacy of postoperative physiotherapy.

If it is felt that staff shortage is slowing patient discharges, this could be audited in association with the hospital discharge officer. Box 20.4 shows a method of collecting information for a delayed discharge audit.

We are the most available and abiding judges of our own work, e.g.:

- Am I allowing myself to get swamped with acute cardiorespiratory work and not tackling prevention or rehabilitation?
- Do I favour patients who are appreciative and co-operative rather than those who are demanding or depressed?
- Have I achieved the appropriate balance between patients' needs and my professional development?
- How do I handle my mistakes?

BOX 20.3

Postoperative audit

Standard	Patients will be able to climb one flight of stairs on their third postoperative day
Patients	Surgical patients admitted in March and September who were able to climb one flight of stairs pre-operatively
Method	Stairs assessment on third postoperative day
Audit meeting	Assess notes, identify cause of any shortfall, recommend change, agree who is to be next auditor and date of the next meeting to monitor change

BOX 20.4

In-patient delayed discharges

Patient	Ward
Date due for discharge:	
Cause(s) of delayed discharge	Social services/home circumstances ☐
	If yes, details:
	Staff shortage ☐
	If yes, which discipline:
	Other ☐
	If yes, details:
Date discharged:	

EDUCATION AND CONTINUING EDUCATION

Why is evidence ... so hard to transform into daily routines?

Flaatten (2012)

Needs of students and junior staff

It is the human qualities of supervisors that are often considered equal to, or more important than, clinical skills (Neville & French 1991), e.g.:

- enthusiasm, honesty and commitment
- respect for juniors and students so that they in turn respect their patients
- tolerance of a range of normality
- avoidance of labelling patients as difficult

- constructive relationships with medical and other staff
- willingness to say 'I don't know'
- ability to coax the nervous patient, soothe the fearful and encourage the weary.

Clinical placements play a major role in fostering motivation (Brindley 2013), and our finest clinicians should analyze their intuitive process so that they can pass on how they recognize subtle changes in a breathing pattern, sense a patient's motivation or adjust their treatment in response to barely-perceptible clues.

Junior staff and students also need:

- clarification of expectations
- assistance in setting feasible objectives and assessing whether these are met
- encouragement to work creatively and not become a clone of their senior
- regular feedback, case discussions and troubleshooting, while aiming at a balance of guidance and responsibility
- praise when due
- enjoyment in their work
- correction in a way that does not undermine confidence, especially in front of patients
- for junior staff and senior students, consultation on how closely they want to be supervised (Onuoha 1994)
- for staff after their first on calls, debriefing to encourage reflective practice
- for students, reinforcement of the curriculum emphasis on involvement of carers, expansion of community care and patient self-management (Roskell 2012)
- when possible, a simulated critical care experience, which can increase students' confidence and interest in the specialty (Ohtake *et al* 2013)
- encouragement to learn from patients, e.g. App. E, or structured feedback sessions with patients (Thomson & Hilton 2013)
- when available, a mentor who is not their manager or supervisor (Cole 2003)
- guided journal writing (Constantinou & Kuys 2013)
- time for reflection, using Fig 20.4 or social media (Rowe 2012)
- an information folder (App. A).

FIGURE 20.4 Reflective practice cycle

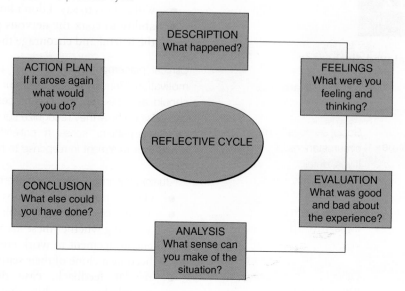

When asking a patient's permission for a student to be present, the student should be outside so that the patient feels free to refuse. Permission should also be sought for the student to read the medical notes (Wilkie 1997), and the patient advised, when appropriate, of the student's gender.

Patients often appreciate the extra time that students have to spend with them. As one supervisor said: 'it seems to me the patients really enjoy the interaction of having students around' (Davies *et al* 2011).

For qualified staff, a questionnaire is available to measure evidence-based practice (Bernhardsson & Larsson 2013). UK physiotherapists are granted 6 days a year minimum for education, on top of mandatory training (Dimond 2009 p.58).

> **PRACTICE TIP**
>
> Students can draw the lung and heart surface markings on a T-shirt as an aid to learning.

A team-based approach should be evident throughout pre- and postgraduate education (Weinstein *et al* 2013) and the teaching of communication skills has a positive effect on patient outcomes (Neumann *et al* 2012). Clinical practice on its own does not necessarily develop empathy (Thomson *et al* 1997), and this needs

to be facilitated rather than blunted by the casual insensitivities of the health system. For example, if there has been a ward round in which a patient's needs have been ignored, debriefing is required for the student afterwards. Supervisors should maintain awareness lest students feel obliged to conform to what may be 'normal' but is not acceptable. Box 20.5 is the experience of a student who would have benefitted from a debrief.

Competencies for on calls and weekends

The attributes required for competent practice have been itemized by Thomas *et al* (2008):

- practical assessment and treatment skills
- cognitive skills: theory, application of knowledge, interpretation of findings and reasoning
- attitude: empathy, professionalism and ethical awareness
- independent learning skills: learning methods, reflection, awareness of limitations
- critical thinking
- communication skills: verbal and written, including record keeping.

Staff numbers may allow weekend teams to contain a mix of experienced and inexperienced staff, but

BOX 20.5

A student's experience

The patient was looking beautiful. He'd been washed and his hair was combed. He looked a bit stony-faced, eyes gazing across the room. He's better today, I thought. I put my hands round his chest. 'Just take a nice deep breath' I said. I chatted away to him. I kept waiting for his next breath. 'You're looking well', I said. He still hadn't taken a breath. Unease grew. I finished a long sentence. My hands were glued to his chest. My eyes were glued to his eyes. Physios don't see dead patients do they? But I couldn't keep up the charade. Had I killed him? I backed away. I forgot everything except thinking 'I must leave the ward'. I found my supervisor and said 'I went to see Mr Jones but he was dead'. She said 'Oh fine'. I couldn't tell anyone about it for a year.

AI, 1990

evidence-based protocols have been used successfully by non-specialist physiotherapists working in the ICU (Hanekom *et al* 2013). A no-blame culture allows errors to be reported and reflected upon (Kiekkas 2011).

Clinical reasoning – learned or taught?

To prepare students for clinical practice, education should foster ethical wisdom and emotional curiosity.
Jensen & Greenfield (2012)

Clinical reasoning refers to the thinking and decision-making processes associated with clinical practice.

This can be learnt by examining different clinical reasoning models, exploring the differences in reasoning between novices and experts, and discussion with peers. For students, a case study may be discussed or role-played, followed by questions on clinical reasoning by educators and their peers.

Continuing education lays the foundation for lifelong self-evaluation. It also provides the opportunity for supervisors to show that compassion is fundamental for effective cardiorespiratory care, not is just an old-fashioned unscientific luxury.

When educators are humanistic in their training of students, the students become more humanistic in their care of patients.
Williams & Deci (1998)

CASE STUDY: Mr FF

What has happened to this 33 y.o. man from Abu Dhabi, who was admitted after eating a spicy Mexican meal?

History of present complaint
- Vomiting → back pain → collapse

Subjective

● Breathless

Phase one questions (Fig 20.5a)

1 Auscultation?
2 Percussion note?

Phase two questions

1 What might be developing?
2 Physiotherapy?
3 Outcome?

FIGURE 20.5a Mr FF on admission

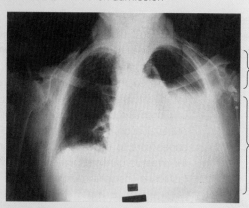

Blackness indicates air. Lack of lung markings indicates that the air is in the pleura, not the lung

Density of opacity, and lack of its location to a lobe, suggests pleural rather than lung pathology

CLINICAL REASONING

How helpful is this study which reported, in an uncontrolled trial, that people with an exacerbation of cystic fibrosis benefitted from *'rest, intravenous antibiotics, physical therapy, high-calorie diet and regular medical review'*.

Phys Ther (1994), 74, 583–93

RESPONSE TO CASE STUDY PHASE ONE

1 Auscultation?
- Breath sounds ↓ on the left

2 Percussion note?

- Hyperresonant L upper zone, stony dull L lower zone

What happened?
- Vomiting → ruptured oesophagus → empyema → development of gas-forming organism → pneumothorax

Management and progress
- Chest tube drained air and foul-smelling liquid from pleura.
- Fig 20.5b shows lung markings returned to L upper zone, indicating resolution of pneumothorax, but opacity is still present in L lower zone, suggesting continuing empyema, confirmed by stony dull percussion note.
- Blood gas deterioration → intubation, mechanical ventilation on volume control → increasing airway pressure (indicating ↓ lung compliance) → pressure control initiated.

FIGURE 20.5b

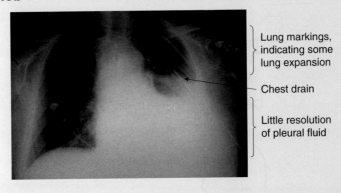

Lung markings, indicating some lung expansion

Chest drain

Little resolution of pleural fluid

RESPONSE TO CASE STUDY PHASE TWO

1 What might be developing?
- Acute respiratory distress syndrome, demonstrated by deteriorating blood gases, increasing airway pressure and initiation of pressure control ventilation.

2 Physiotherapy?
- Prone positioning, preventive respiratory care, musculoskeletal care.

3 Outcome?
- Patient improved (Fig 20.5c), recovered, decided to avoid spicy restaurants.

FIGURE 20.5c

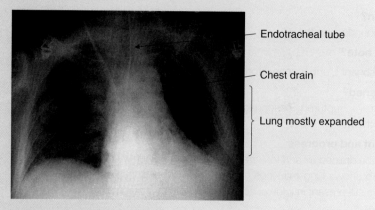

- Endotracheal tube
- Chest drain
- Lung mostly expanded

Response to Clinical Reasoning

This is all very nice but the plethora of interventions does not allow identification of which was helpful. Maybe it was the rest that was beneficial, maybe just natural recovery from an exacerbation.

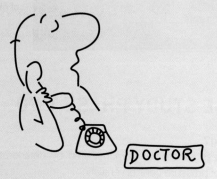

RECOMMENDED READING

Anon (2013) Understanding systematic reviews and meta-analyses. *Drugs Therap Bull*; **51**(10): 117–120

Bruton A, Garrod R, Thomas M (2011) Respiratory physiotherapy: towards a clearer definition of the terminology. *Physiother*; **97**: 345–9

Busari JO (2013) Clinical reasoning: reflecting on the decision-making process in respiratory medicine. *Breathe*; **10**: 413–417

Chang SM (2013) Should meta-analyses trump observational studies? *Am J Clin Nutr*; **97**: 237–8

Crowther DM (2013) A clinician's guide to systematic reviews. *Nutr Clin Pract*; **28**: 459–62

Edwards I, van Kessel G (2012) The development of moral judgment and organization of ethical knowledge in final year physical therapy students. *Phys Ther Rev*; **17**(3): 157–66

Fuller J (2013) Rhetoric and argumentation: how clinical practice guidelines think. *J Eval Clin Practice*; **19**(3): 433–41

Gasparyan AY, Kitas GD (2012) Best peer reviewers and the quality of peer review in biomedical journals. *Croat Med J*; **53**(4): 386–9.

Gunn H, Hunter H, Haas B (2012) Problem based learning in physiotherapy education: a practice perspective. *Physiother*; **98**(4): 330–5

Hess DR (2013) Science and evidence: separating fact from fiction. *Respir Care;* **58**(10): 1649–61

Nüesch E (2009) The effects of excluding patients from the analysis in randomized controlled trials. *BMJ*; **339**: 679–83

Rye KJ (2011) Critical thinking in respiratory therapy. *Respir Care*; **56**(3): 364–5

Stoller JK (2010) Implementing change in respiratory care. *Respir Care*; **55**(6): 749–57

Stratford PW, Riddle DL (2013) Assessing the amount of change in an outcome measure is not the same as assessing the importance of change. *Physiother Can*; **65**(3): 244–7

Swisher LL, van Kessel G (2012) Evaluating moral reasoning outcomes in physical therapy ethics education. *Phys Ther Rev*; **17**(3): 167–75

Glossary of abbreviations, definitions, symbols and values

If a definition is not here, see the index or Appendix H.
Values in [square brackets] are American.
Most values are approximate.

N = normal.
Δ = change, e.g. ΔV/ΔP = change in volume in response to change in pressure, i.e. compliance.
μ = micro-, prefix indicating 10^{-6}, i.e. 0.000001.
μm = micrometer or micron, i.e. one millionth of a metre, or 1×10^{-6} of a metre.
μmol = micromole, i.e. one millionth of a mole.
> = more than.
< = less than.
± = 'and/or' or 'with/without'.
~ = about.
Dot over symbol = value per unit time, e.g. $\dot{V}O_2$: oxygen consumption.
Line over symbol = mean value, e.g. $\overline{V}$: mixed venous.
Conversion of mmHg to kPa – multiply the value by 0.1333 (see also: App.G).

1RM one repetition maximum, i.e. the maximum load that can be moved once over full range of motion without compensatory movements.
A alveolar, e.g. P_AO_2.
a arterial, e.g. P_aO_2.
ABGs arterial blood gases.
ACBT active cycle of breathing techniques.
ACBT/AD active cycle of breathing techniques ± autogenic drainage.
ACE inhibitors angiotensin-converting enzyme inhibitor drugs.

ACPRC Association of Chartered Physiotherapists in Respiratory Care.
ACS acute coronary syndrome.
AD autogenic drainage.
ADL activities of daily living.
AF atrial fibrillation.
Air bronchogram visibility of airways on x-ray due to opacification of surrounding alveoli.
Airway (1) natural passageway for air to travel from atmosphere to alveoli, or (2) artificial device to hold open upper airway for relief of obstruction or to allow mechanical ventilation.
Airway closure closure of small airways, common in dependent lung regions at end-expiration.
Airway resistance see Resistance.
Albumin N: 40-60 g/l, [4.0-6.0 g/100ml].
ALI acute lung injury.
Alkalaemia alkalosis of blood.
Alveolar-arterial oxygen gradient see $P_AO_2-P_aO_2$.
Angioplasty invasive but non-surgical dilation of coronary artery stenosis, using catheter via femoral puncture, or laser.
Antioxidant substance which counteracts the effects of free radicals such as tobacco smoke.
AP anteroposterior.
Apnoea absence of breathing for >10 secs.
ARDS acute respiratory distress syndrome.
Arnold's nerve auricular branch of vagus nerve, responsible for the cough reflex in a small proportion of the population, whereby a cough can be facilitated by ear stimulation; also responsible for ear pain being an occasional early presentation of laryngeal cancer.

Ascites fluid in the abdominal cavity.

Aspiration (1) inhalation of unwanted substances (e.g. gastric acid or sea water) beyond the vocal cords, or (2) therapeutic removal of fluid or gas from a cavity such as the pleural space.

Atelectasis collapse of alveoli.

Atelectrauma damage to alveoli due to repetitive opening and collapse.

ATP adenosine triphosphate, a nucleotide which governs Cl^- secretion and Na^+ absorption, thereby regulating airway surface liquid.

Auscultation use of stethoscope to hear sounds from a body cavity.

Autoregulation ability of an organ to maintain constant blood flow despite changes in perfusion pressure.

BAL bronchoalveolar lavage: bronchoscopic washing out of bronchioles and alveoli with sterile saline for diagnosis.

Barotrauma air in the wrong place, e.g. pneumothorax or subcutaneous emphysema.

b.d. twice a day.

BiPAP bilevel positive airway pressure.

BIPAP biphasic positive airway pressure.

Blood pressure pressure exerted by the blood on the arteries. *see also:* mean arterial pressure.

Blood sugar 3.5–5.5 mmol/l before meals, rising after meals by a few mmol/l. ↑ in stress, ↑↑ in diabetes mellitus, ↓ in liver failure or starvation.

bpm breaths per minute or (heart) beats per minute.

Bradyarrythmia slow and abnormal heart beat.

Bradycardia resting HR <60/min in adults.

Bronchitis acute or chronic inflammation of mucous membranes of tracheobronchial tree.

Bronchopleural fistula communication between lung and pleura, caused by thoracic surgery, trauma or pulmonary disease.

Bronchospasm abnormal contraction of smooth bronchial muscle, causing narrowing of airway.

Bulla collection of air in lung tissue which is more than 1 cm in diameter, caused by alveolar destruction.

CABG coronary artery bypass graft.

Calcium N: 2.2–2.6 mmol/L.

C_aO_2 *see* oxygen content.

Cardiac output (CO or Q) blood ejected by left ventricle per minute, i.e. HR × stroke volume.
 – N: 4–8 l/min at rest, up to 25 l/min on exercise.

Catecholamine compound having sympathomimetic action, e.g. adrenaline.

cerebrospinal fluid (CSF) cerebrospinal fluid.

CCF congestive cardiac failure.

Central line catheter inserted into a large vein such as the internal jugular, subclavian or femoral for monitoring or the administration of thick fluids.

CF cystic fibrosis.

CHD coronary heart disease.

Cheyne-Stokes breathing episodes of rapid breathing, slow breathing and apnoea.

Chloride (Cl^-) chief anion in extracellular fluid,
 – ↓ levels in plasma: acidosis, some kidney problems, prolonged vomiting,
 – ↑ levels in sweat can be diagnostic of cystic fibrosis.

Closing volume closing capacity minus residual volume.
 – increases (becomes a greater proportion of FRC) with small airways disease, smoking, obesity and young or old age.
 – young person: 10% of VC.
 – age 65: 40% of VC.

Clotting studies (Broomhead & Mallett 2013)
 - ACT (activated clotting time). N: 100–140 secs. Monitors high-dose heparin therapy, e.g. during cardiopulmonary bypass.
 - APTT (activated partial thromboplastin time). Monitors low-dose heparin therapy. N: 30–40 secs.
 - Bleeding time. N: 3–9 mins.
 - FDPs (fibrinogen degradation products). N: <10 mg/ml.
 - Fibrinogen level. N: >150 mg/dl.
 - INR (international normalized ratio). Ratio of time blood normally takes to clot compared to increased time it takes to clot, e.g. for monitoring warfarin or detecting bleeding disorders. N: 1–3. Higher means increased clotting time and risk of bleeding, e.g. 2–4 for a patient on warfarin, 10 in a patient at severe risk of bleeding.
 - KPTT (kaolin partial thromboplastin time). N: <7 sec above control.
 - Platelet count. N: 140 000–400 000 mm^{-3}. Risk of bleeding with suction: <50 000 mm^{-3}. Spontaneous bleeding: <20 000 mm^{-3}.
 - PT (prothrombin time). N: 11–15 secs.
 - PTT (partial thromboplastin time). N: 12–30 secs.

CMV (1) controlled mandatory ventilation or conventional mechanical ventilation, or (2) cytomegalovirus.

CO (1) cardiac output, or (2) carbon monoxide.

CO_2 carbon dioxide.

Coagulation *see* clotting studies.

Cognition mental activities involved in acquiring and processing information.

Collateral channels airways between adjacent lung units which allow inspired gas to bypass normal airways if these are obstructed.

Consolidation replacement of alveolar air by substance of greater density, e.g. the inflammatory exudate of pneumonia.

COPD chronic obstructive pulmonary disease.

CPAP continuous positive airway pressure.

Creatinine electrolyte in plasma or urine, formed from muscle breakdown (end-product of normal muscle metabolism) and excreted by kidneys.
 – N in plasma: 50–100 μmol/l (0.6–1.2 mg/100ml).
 – ↑ in hypovolaemia or kidney failure, ↑↑ in septic shock.

Cryptogenic of unknown cause.

CT computed tomography.

CVP central venous pressure.
  N: 1–7 mmHg or 5–12 cmH$_2$O.
CXR chest x-ray.
Cytokine inflammatory product.
Decubitus side-lying.
  – right decubitus: lying on R side.
  – left decubitus: lying on L side.
Dependent underneath.
Derecruitment collapse of alveoli.
Desaturation ↓ oxygen saturation of haemoglobin in
  arterial blood.
Diastole ventricular relaxation.
DIC disseminated intravascular coagulation.
DNAR do not attempt resuscitation.
DO$_2$ see oxygen delivery.
DVT deep vein thrombosis.
Dysarthria difficulty speaking due to weak muscles.
Dysphagia difficulty swallowing.
Dyspnoea distressing breathlessness.
ECG electrocardiogram.
ECMO extracorporeal membrane oxygenation.
Elastance opposite of compliance.
EMLA eutectic mixture of local anaesthetics: cream for
  numbing skin before venipuncture.
Endotoxin toxin inside bacterial cell, released after
  destruction of bacterial cell wall.
Endurance capacity of muscle to sustain contraction.
Enteral via the gut.
Entonox analgesic gas mixture comprising 50% nitrous
  oxide and 50% oxygen, otherwise known as laughing gas.
Entrainment dilution of gas stream or aerosol with
  external gas such as room air.
Eosinophils inflammatory cells associated with
  hypersensitivity reaction.
  – ↑ in allergy e.g. extrinsic asthma.
Epiglottis cartilage which diverts food to oesophagus by
  closing over trachea.
ETCO$_2$ end-tidal CO$_2$.
  – N: 4–6%.
ETT endotracheal tube.
Extracorporeal outside the body.
Fatigue
  – central: reduced force generation due to events
    proximal to neuromuscular junction
  – peripheral: failure at or beyond neuromuscular
    junction.
FBC full blood count.
FET forced expiration technique.
FEV$_1$ forced expiratory volume in one second.
FG size of catheter or tube defined as the outside
  diameter in units of $1/3$ mm, e.g. 12 French Gauge
  catheter has outer diameter of 4 mm.
FiO$_2$ – fraction of inspired oxygen, expressed as
  decimal, e.g. F_iO_2 of 0.6 = 60% inspired oxygen, F_iO_2
  of 0.21 = room air.
Fluid overload 10% or greater increase in weight due to
  excess fluid.

FRC functional residual capacity.
FVC forced vital capacity.
Glottis vocal folds and space between them.
Glucose see blood sugar.
GOR gastroesophageal reflux.
H$^+$ hydrogen ion.
Haematocrit – concentration of red blood cells in
  blood.
  – N: 36–46% in women, 40–50% in men,
  – anaemia: <36%. polycythaemia: >55%.
Haemoglobin – respiratory pigment in red blood cells
  which combines reversibly with oxygen.
  – N: 11.5–15 g/100 ml in women, 14–17 g/100 ml in men.
  – ↓ in anaemia, ↑ in polycythaemia.
Haemoptysis coughing up blood ('frank haemoptysis' is
  coughing up pure blood).
Hb see haemoglobin.
HCO$_3^-$ bicarbonate ion concentration.
Hepatomegaly enlarged liver.
HF heart failure.
Hiccuping involuntary clonic spasm of intercostals and
  diaphragm followed by abrupt glottic closure, of
  unknown aetiology.
HME heat-moisture exchanger.
HR heart rate, N: 60–100 bpm.
HRCT high resolution computed tomography.
HVS hyperventilation syndrome.
Hypercapnia ↑ P_aCO_2.
Hyperdynamic status signalling onset of septic shock:
  galloping pulse, pyrexia, shaking chill, flushing of
  skin, high cardiac output, unstable BP.
Hyperkalaemia ↑ serum potassium.
Hypermetabolism ↑ energy expenditure by >10%.
Hypernatraemia ↑ serum sodium.
Hyperosmolar ↑ concentration of osmotically active
  ingredients.
Hyperoxia abnormally high oxygen tension in blood.
Hyperreactivity ↑ sensitivity to variety of stimuli
  – present in airways with asthma, sometimes
    present with COPD, bronchiectasis, CF, sarcoidosis,
    LVF.
Hyperventilation CO$_2$ removal in excess of CO$_2$
  production, causing P_aCO_2 <4.7 kPa (35 mmHg).
Hypervolaemia fluid overload.
Hypocapnia ↓ CO$_2$ in arterial blood.
Hypokalaemia ↓ potassium in blood.
Hyponatraemia ↓ sodium in blood.
Hypoventilation CO$_2$ production in excess of CO$_2$
  removal, leading to P_aCO_2 >6.0 kPa (45 mmHg).
Hypovolaemia ↓ blood volume due to e.g. haemorrhage
  or dehydration.
Hypoxaemia ↓ oxygen in arterial blood.
Hypoxia ↓ oxygen in tissues.
Hysteresis difference in compliance between inspiration
  and expiration, due to extra energy required during
  inspiration to recruit additional alveoli.
IABP intra-aortic balloon pump.

ICF framework International Classification of Functioning, Disability and Health (Ch. 2).

ICP intracranial pressure.

ICU intensive care unit.

I:E ratio *see* inspiratory:expiratory ratio.

Ileus gut obstruction, e.g. due to paralytic ileus, as indicated by lack of bowel sounds.

Infection presence of micro-organisms or their products in normally sterile tissue.

Infiltrate fluid, cells or other substance in tissue space, e.g. pulmonary interstitial infiltrate = fluid between capillary and alveolus, showing on x-ray as diffuse shadowing.

Inotropes drugs which ↑ force of cardiac contraction.

INR *see* clotting studies.

Inspiratory capacity volume inspired during maximum inspiration from resting end-expiratory position.

Inspiratory:expiratory (I:E) ratio duration of inspiration relative to expiration.

Insufflation blowing air into the lungs.

Intracranial hypertension ↑ intracranial pressure.

Intrapleural pressure pressure in pleural space.

Intrapulmonary pressure alveolar pressure.

Intrinsic PEEP trapped gas left in lungs at end-exhalation due to obstructed airways ± breathing through artificial airways.

IPPB intermittent positive pressure breathing.

IPPV intermittent positive pressure ventilation, i.e. mechanical ventilation.

IRV inspiratory reserve volume.

IS incentive spirometry.

Isotonic same osmotic pressure as body fluids, e.g. isotonic saline contains salt equal to that in body.

IV intravenous.

JVP jugular venous pressure.

kPa kilopascal (unit of pressure).

L left.

Lactate (in blood) serum lactate. N: <1 mmol/l, anaerobic metabolism: >2 mmol/l, poor prognosis: >3 mmol/l.

Laparoscopy minimal access incision through abdominal wall.

Laparotomy full surgical incision through abdominal wall.

LFT (1) lung function test, or (2) liver function test.

LTOT long term oxygen therapy.

LVF left ventricular failure.

Lymphadenopathy enlarged lymph nodes.

MAP *see* mean arterial pressure.

Maximal HR 220−age.

Maximum oxygen consumption maximal rate at which oxygen can be used by the body during maximal work, i.e. aerobic capacity, reflecting neural, cardiopulmonary and metabolic components of aerobic fitness and requiring $\dot{V}O_2$ to attain a plateau
  - ↑ with fitness, ↓ with advancing age but rate of decline slower in physically active people

  - N: 2 l/min or >25 ml/kg/min or 25 times resting level
  - COPD: typically 1 l/min
  - *see also* anaerobic threshold.

MDI metered dose inhaler.

Mean arterial pressure average pressure pushing blood through systemic circulation, i.e. cardiac output x peripheral vascular resistance
  - N: 80–100 mmHg
  - compromised circulation to vital organs: <60 mmHg
  - compromised circulation to injured brain: <80 mmHg.

MEF$_{50}$ maximum expiratory flow in mid-expiration.

MEP maximum expiratory pressure
  - N: 100 cmH$_2$O, inadequate cough: <40 cmH$_2$O.

mEq/l milliequivalents per litre of solution, e.g. of electrolyte concentration
  - also expressed as mmol/l.

mmHg millimetres of mercury (unit of pressure)

MH manual hyperinflation.

MI *see* myocardial infarction.

Micro one millionth.

Minute ventilation see below.

Minute volume or **minute ventilation ($\dot{V}_E$)** amount of gas expelled from lungs per minute, i.e. tidal volume × RR
  - N: 5–9 litres.

MIP maximum inspiratory pressure: assessment of respiratory muscle strength
  - N: minus 100–130 cmH$_2$O (men), minus 70–100 (women)
  - typical value for hypercapnic COPD: minus 55 (men), minus 40 (women)

Mixed venous blood blood in pulmonary artery.

MMEF maximum mid-expiratory flow.

mmHg millimetres of mercury.

MRI magnetic resonance imaging.

MRSA methicillin-resistant staphylococcus aureus.

Mucoactive affecting quality or quantity of mucus.

Mucokinetic accelerating mucus transport.

Mucolytic destroys mucin in mucus gel.

MV mechanical ventilation.

Myocardial infarction death of portion of heart muscle due to myocardial ischaemia.

Na *see* sodium.

Neuromuscular blockade chemical paralysis by neuromuscular blocking agents.

Neutropaenia ↓ neutrophils, i.e. <1.5 × 10^9, leaving patient vulnerable to infection.

Neutrophil white blood cell used for phagocytosis of bacteria but which in excess releases tissue-damaging enzymes as part of uncontrolled inflammation.

NICE National Institute for Care Excellence.

NICU neonatal intensive care unit.

NIV non-invasive ventilation.

NO nitric oxide.

Normovolaemia normal blood volume.

O_2 oxygen.

Oesophageal varices dilated veins in lower third of the oesophagus, at junction of portal and systemic venous systems, due to raised portal pressure.

Oliguria ↓ urine output, i.e. <20 ml/hr (normal 50–60 ml/hr).

Oncotic pressure osmotic pressure exerted by colloids.

Orthopnoea dyspnoea on lying flat.

Orthostatic hypotension/intolerance drop of >20 mmHg in systolic ± drop of >10 mmHg in diastolic BP on standing up.

Osmolality number of osmotically active particles per kg of solvent, and the most significant factor in the distribution of water between intracellular and extracellular fluid.

Osmolarity number of osmotically active particles per litre of solution.

-ostomy formation of artificial opening to skin surface.

-otomy incision.

OT occupational therapy/therapist.

Oxidative stress imbalance between generation and breakdown of oxygen free radicals (reactive oxygen species), accelerated under certain conditions including hyperoxia and hypoxia, which results in net gain of oxygen free radicals and potential for harm (Martin Grocott 2013).

Oxygen consumption amount of oxygen consumed by tissues each minute, i.e. CI × (C_aO_2–C_vO_2) × 10 ml/min/m^2,
 – N at rest: 150–300 ml/min/m^2 (if contributing values normal, i.e. CO 5 l/min, Hb 15 g/100ml, S_aO_2 97%, $S_{\bar{v}}O_2$ 75%),
 – critical illness: >600 ml/min.

Oxygen cost of breathing energy requirements of respiratory muscles and indirect measure of work of breathing,
 – N: one ml/l of ventilation.

Oxygen delivery (DO_2) volume of oxygen presented to tissues, i.e. CI × C_aO_2,
 – N: 600–1000 ml/min, i.e. ~25% of oxygen the tissues receive
 – may ↑ in hyperdynamic states.

Oxygen demand oxygen needed by cells for aerobic metabolism, estimated by $\dot{V}O_2$.

Oxygen extraction oxygen transferred from blood to tissues, i.e. C_aO_2 difference between arterial and mixed venous blood, equivalent to $\dot{V}O_2/DO_2$
 – N: 20–30%
 – 32% indicates ↑ oxygen demand or occasionally ↓ DO_2
 – <22% indicates damaged tissues unable to extract O_2, or hyperdynamic circulation e.g. early sepsis.

Oxygen extraction ratio ($\dot{V}O_2/DO_2$) ratio of oxygen consumption to oxygen delivery, indicating efficiency of tissues in extracting oxygen.
 – calculation: $C_aO_2 – C_{\bar{v}}O_2/C_aO_2$,
 – N: 25%
 – high oxygen extraction to meet excess metabolic needs: >35%
 – maximum for most tissues: 60–70%.

Oxygen transport transport of oxygen from lungs to mitochondria.

Oxygen uptake oxygen consumption.

P_{50} PO_2 at which 50% of haemoglobin is saturated with oxygen.
 – N: 27–28 mmHg.

PA postero-anterior.

Packed cell volume – equivalent to haematocrit
 – N: 0.36–0.46 (women), 0.40–0.50 (men)
 – ↑ in polycythaemia, ↓ in anaemia.

P_aCO_2 partial pressure of CO_2 in arterial blood
 – N: 4.7–6.0 kPa (35–45 mmHg).

Palliation alleviation of symptoms.

Panic attack rapid onset of fear accompanied by somatic symptoms.

P_aO_2 partial pressure of oxygen in arterial blood
 – N: 11–14 kPa (80–100 mmHg), declining by 0.55 kPa (4 mmHg) per 10 years.

P_aO_2/F_iO_2 ratio of P_aO_2 to inspired oxygen, more relevant than P_aO_2 alone, estimates shunt
 – N: 40 kPa (300 mmHg),
 – e.g. P_aO_2:F_iO_2 of 27 could mean P_aO_2 of 10.7 kPa at F_iO_2 of .40 or P_aO_2 of 16 kPa at F_iO_2 of .60.

P_AO_2-P_aO_2 alveolar-arterial oxygen gradient or A-a gradient: difference in oxygen tension across alveolar membrane, i.e. P_AO_2 minus P_aO_2
 – indicates efficiency of gas transfer, varies with F_iO_2
 – N on room air: 0.7–2.7 kPa (5-20 mmHg), reflecting normal anatomical shunt
 – ↑ on exercise, ↑ in the elderly, ↑ on supplemental oxygen, ↑ with diffusion impairment e.g. pulmonary oedema, fibrosis or ARDS.

PAP (1) peak airways pressure (peak inspiratory pressure) or (2) pulmonary artery pressure.

Parenchyma foamlike substance comprising gas exchanging part of lung, made up of alveoli, small airways, capillaries and supporting tissue.

Parenchymal lung disease disease affecting parenchyma, e.g. interstitial lung disease, pneumonia, TB, ARDS.

Parenteral other than through the gut, usually relates to intravenous feeding.

PAWP pulmonary artery wedge pressure
 – N: 5–15 mmHg
 – pulmonary congestion: 20 mmHg
 – pulmonary oedema: 25 mmHg.

P_{aw} mean airway pressure.

PC pressure contol ventilation.

PCA patient controlled analgesia.

PCV see packed cell volume.

PCWP pulmonary capillary wedge pressure (= PAWP).

PD postural drainage.

PE pulmonary embolus.

Peak cough flow N: 720 l/min.

PEEP positive end-expiratory pressure.

PEEPi intrinsic positive end-expiratory pressure.

PEFR peak expiratory flow rate.

PEG percutaneous endoscopic gastrostomy: surgical opening into stomach for enteral feeding.

PEP positive expiratory pressure.

Percussion (1) (therapeutic) clapping the chest wall to loosen airway secretions, or (2) (diagnostic) tapping chest wall to identify density of underlying tissue.

Percutaneous through the skin.

PF peak flow, i.e. peak expiratory flow rate.

pH measure of hydrogen ions in solution, i.e. inverse of log of hydrogen ion concentration
– N: 7.35–7.45.

Pharmacodynamics what a drug does to the body.

Pharmacokinetics what the body does to a drug.

PICU paediatric intensive care unit.

PIF peak inspiratory flow
– N: 40–50 l/min
– when breathless or with exercise: up to 200 l/min.

PIP peak inspiratory pressure.

Platelet count see clotting studies.

Plethoric florid complexion due to excess red blood cells.

Pleural pressure pressure in pleural space.

PN percussion note.

PND paroxysmal nocturnal dyspnoea.

PO_2 partial pressure or tension of oxygen.

Polycythaemia excess red blood cells due to late-stage lung disease, cyanotic congenital heart disease, high-altitude living or sleep apnoea.

Polypharmacy multiple medications ± more medications than clinically indicated.

Polysomnography recording of physiological parameters during sleep.

Postural hypotension ↓ BP of >5 mmHg on moving to upright position.

Potassium (K) electrolyte in plasma or urine
– N in plasma: 3.5–5.0 mmol/l.

P_{plat} plateau pressure on MV.

PR pulmonary rehabilitation.

p.r.n. 'as required', i.e. when the patient requests; usually relates to drug administration.

PSV pressure support ventilation.

$P_{tc}CO_2$ transcutaneous CO_2 tension.

$P_{tc}O_2$ transcutaneous oxygen tension.

PTSD post traumatic stress disorder.

Pulmonary artery pressure
– N: 10–20 mmHg (systolic 22, diastolic 10, mean 15)
– pulmonary hypertension: 25 mmHg.

Pulmonary vascular resistance
– N: 25–125 dyn.s.cm^{-5}.

Pulse pressure difference between systolic and diastolic pressures: indicates blood flow
– N: 40 mmHg
– ↑ with hypertension, ↓ with poor stroke volume
– dangerously low tissue perfusion: 20 mmHg.

Pulsus paradoxus weaker pulse on inspiration than expiration caused by expansion of pulmonary vascular bed on inspiration. i.e. excess negative pressure in chest
– occurs with severe acute asthma, hypovolaemic patient on MV, cardiac tamponade
– N: 10 mmHg, higher value indicating laboured breathing.

Purulent containing pus.

Q blood flow.

QoL quality of life.

Qs/Q_T shunt fraction.

R right.

Rapid shallow breathing index ratio of RR to V_T, e.g. patient with RR of 25/min and V_T of 250 ml/breath has rapid shallow breathing index of (25/0.25) = 100 breaths/min/l.
– used to judge if patients have the strength to wean from mechanical ventilation.

Recruitment opening up of alveoli.

REM rapid-eye-movement phase of sleep cycle.

Respiratory pump components that deliver oxygen to alveolar-capillary membrane and remove CO_2, i.e. respiratory centres, nerves, muscles, chest wall (thoracic cage + thoraco-abdominal interface).

Respiratory therapist (US) Respiratory physiotherapist (UK) combined with respiratory technician.

Resuscitation
– cardiopulmonary (CPR) – manual attempt to restart circulation and breathing
– fluid – replacement of intravascular fluids after dehydration, diarrhoea, vomiting, surgery, trauma or shock.

Reverse Trendelenberg positioning of the whole bed head up.

RFT respiratory function test.

RPE rate of perceived exertion.

RQ see respiratory quotient.

RV residual volume.

S_aO_2 saturation of haemoglobin with oxygen in arterial blood
– N: 95–98%.

Saturation oxygen saturation of haemoglobin in arterial blood.

Shunt proportion of blood passing through pulmonary vasculature without picking up oxygen
– N: 2% of CO.

SIMV synchronous intermittent mandatory ventilation.

Situs inversus transposition of organs in chest and abdomen to the opposite side, e.g. heart on right side.

SOB shortness of breath.

Sodium (Na) electrolyte in plasma or urine
   – N in plasma: 134–148 mmol/l [135–147 mEq/l].
Speech pathologist US term for speech language therapist.
S_pO_2 oxygen saturation by pulse oximetry, usually equivalent to S_aO_2.
Stokes Adams attack transient but pulseless loss of consciousness, often associated with complete heart block.
Stridor high-pitched sound produced by turbulent airflow through partially obstructed upper airway, heard on inspiration, expiration or both.
Stroke volume volume ejected from ventricle with each beat
   – dependent on preload, afterload and contractility, normally the same for each ventricle
   – N: 60–130 ml.
Subcutaneous emphysema collection of air under the skin.
Surgical emphysema subcutaneous emphysema.
$S_{\bar{v}}O_2$ *see* mixed venous oxygen saturation.
Syncope transient loss of consciousness, e.g. faint.
Systemic vascular resistance (MAP-CVP/ cardiac output) × 79.9
   – N: 800–1400 dyn.s.cm^{-5}
   – septic shock: <300.
Tamponade fluid in pericardium.
t.d.s. three times a day.
TENS transcutaneous electrical nerve stimulation.
Thoracentesis withdrawal of fluid from pleural cavity.
Thoracoscopy minimal access incision through chest wall.
Thoracotomy full incision through chest wall.
Tidal breathing breathing at tidal volume.
Tidal volume volume of air inhaled and exhaled at each normal sized breath
   – N: 7 ml/kg with spontaneous breathing, 7–10 ml/kg with MV, up to 12 ml/kg in acute respiratory failure.
T_I/T_{TOT} *see* tension time index.
TLC total lung capacity.
TLCO total lung transfer capacity for carbon monoxide.
Torr measurement of pressure (US) equivalent to mmHg.
Tracheal tube endotracheal or tracheostomy tube.
Transdiaphragmatic pressure diaphragmatic strength, measured by comparing oesophageal and gastric pressures using swallowed balloons. *See also* twitch diaphragmatic pressure.
Transpulmonary pressure as above.
Twitch diaphragmatic pressure measurement of diaphragmatic strength by bilateral phrenic nerve stimulation
   – N: 35 cmH$_2$O

   – weakness: typically 20 cmH$_2$O in patients with respiratory muscle weakness secondary to COPD
   – weak enough to require MV: 15 cmH$_2$O or less (Tobin *et al* 2010).
Upper respiratory tract nose (or mouth), pharynx and larynx.
Urea electrolyte in plasma or urine, formed from protein breakdown and excreted by kidneys
   – N in plasma: 2.5–10 mmol/l
   – dehydration: >8, hypovolaemia: >18, kidney injury: 55.
Urine output
   – normal: 1 ml/hr/kg, average 50–60 ml/hr
   – renal failure: <half normal.
V volume of gas.
v venous.
VAP ventilator-associated pneumonia.
Vascath vascular catheter, i.e. specialized central venous catheter used in dialysis.
Vasoactive drugs vasodilators and vasopressors.
Vasodilator drug which relaxes smooth muscle in blood vessels.
Vasopressor drug that constricts blood vessels.
VC (1) vital capacity, or (2) volume controlled ventilation.
V_D volume of dead space gas
   – N: for anatomical V_D: 2 ml/kg body weight.
V_D/V_T dead space in relation to tidal volume
   – N: 0.3, i.e. 30%, depending on body position
   – critical increase: 0.6.
Venous return blood returning to heart.
Venous admixture mixing of shunted venous blood with oxygenated blood, i.e. mixture of 'true' shunt which bypasses pulmonary capillary bed, and 'effective' shunt due to $\dot{V}_A/\dot{Q}$ mismatch
   – N: 5% of cardiac output.
VF ventricular fibrillation.
Vital capacity maximum volume of gas that can be exhaled after a full inspiration.
Volutrauma damage to alveoli due to overstretch.
V_T *see* tidal volume.
$\bar{v}$ mixed venous.
$\dot{v}$ volume of gas per unit time, i.e. flow.
$\dot{V}_A/\dot{Q}$ ratio of alveolar ventilation to perfusion,
   – N: 0.8 (4 l/min for alveolar ventilation, 5 l/min for perfusion).
$\dot{V}_E$ *see* minute volume.
$\dot{V}O_2$max *see* maximum oxygen consumption.
WCC *see* white blood cell count.
White blood cell count 4–10 10^9 cells/litre [4000–10 000/mm^{-3}]
   – bacterial infection: >10 000/mm^3
   – vulnerability to infection: <4000/mm^3.
WOB work of breathing (below).
Work of breathing N: 0.3–0.5 kg m/min or joules/l.

Credits page

All Figures, Tables, images and artwork *not* listed on this credit page are the authors' own work or the authors' own photos, and so do not require any credit lines, permissions acknowledgements or referencing citations.

The following Figures have all been reproduced with permission of the copyright holders, and the credit-lines are listed below:

Figure Number	Page number	Credit line
Fig. 1.2	6	Wanner A, Salathé M, O'Riordan G (1996) Mucociliary clearance in the airways. American Journal of Respiratory and Critical Care Medicine, 154, 1868–902
Fig. 1.14	26	Owens RL (2013) Supplemental oxygen needs during sleep. who benefits? Respiratory Care,Vol 58 (1), pp.32–47 (fig 1) 0020-1324
Fig. 2.28	60	© Michael Brauner/ISM/Science Photo Library
Fig. 5.1	146	Criner GJ (2000) Effects of long-term oxygen therapy on mortality and morbidity. Respiratory Care, 45(1), 105–18
Fig. 5.11	155	Van der Schans C (1996) Airway secretion management and oxygen therapy. In: Bach JR, Haas F. Pulmonary rehabilitation. Physical Medicine and Rehabilitation Clinics of North America, 7, 205–462
Fig. 5.14	163	Manning HL (2000) Dyspnea treatment. Respiratory Care, 45, 11, 1342–51
Fig. 5.18	169	Dolovich M, Newhouse M (1993) Aerosols: generation, methods of administration and therapeutic applications in asthma. In: Middleton EJ, Reed C, Adkinson N, *et al* ed. Allergy: principles and practice, 4th edn. St Louis: Mosby, 712–739.
Fig. 6.3a	182	© Shutterstock
Fig. 6.10	190	© Shutterstock
Fig. 9.1a	252	Hodgkin JE, Celli BR, Connors GLC (2009) Pulmonary Rehabilitation: Guidelines to Success. Elsevier (figs 21.4) p.338
Fig. 9.1b	252	Hodgkin JE, Celli BR, Connors GLC (2009) Pulmonary Rehabilitation: Guidelines to Success. Elsevier (fig. 10-2) p.132
Fig. 9.7	267	© Shutterstock
Fig. 10.1	281	© Cambridge News
Fig. 12.1	315	Menezes AR, Lavie CJ, Milani RV *et al* (2012) Cardiac rehabilitation and exercise therapy in the elderly: Should we invest in the aged? Journal of Geriatric Cardiology, 9(1), 68–75.
Fig. 13.4	336	Ringsberg MC, Åkerlind I (1999) Presence of hyperventilation in patients with asthma-like symptoms but negative asthma test responses. Journal of Allergy and Clinical Immunology, 103(4), 601–8
Fig. 13.6	341	Hagman C, Janson C, Emtner M *et al* (2011) Breathing retraining – A five-year follow-up of patients with dysfunctional breathing. Respiratory Medicine, 105, 1153e–115

Figure Number	Page number	Credit line
Fig. 14.2	349	Brockopp DY, Ryan P, Warden S (2003) Nurses' willingness to manage the pain of specific groups of patients. British Journal of Nursing, 12(7), 409–15
Fig. 15.4	361	Vogelsang NJ (1997) Patient, caregiver, and oncologist perceptions of cancer-related fatigue: results of a tripart assessment survey. Seminars in Hematology, 34(3), suppl.2, 4–12
Fig. 18.11	472	Hudak M, Bond-Domb A (1996) Postoperative head and neck cancer patients with artificial airways: the effect of saline lavage on tracheal mucus evacuation and oxygen saturation. ORL: Head and Neck Nursing website, 14, 1, 17–21
Fig. 18.13	483	Tobin MJ (2000) Weaning from mechanical ventilation: what have we learned? Respiratory Care, 45, 417–431
Fig. 19.6	499	Garradd J, Bullock M (1986) The effect of respiratory therapy on ICP in ventilated neurosurgical patients. Australian Journal of Physiotherapy, 32, 107–11
Fig. 19.12	516	Gattinoni L, Cairone P, Pelosi P, Goodman LR (2001) What has computed tomography taught us about the acute respiratory distress syndrome? American Journal of Respiratory and Critical Care Medicine. vol. 164 no. 9 1701–1711
Fig. 19.14	518	Albert RK (2000) Prone ventilation. Clinics in Chest Medicine, 21, 511–19
Fig. 20.1	530	Ntoumenopoulos G, Glickman Y (2012) Computerised lung sound monitoring to assess effectiveness of chest physiotherapy and secretion removal: a feasibility study. Physiotherapy, 98, 3, 250–255

The following Figures, Tables and Boxes have all been adapted and changed from the original sources but below are citation references to the research, for referencing purposes:

Item Number	Page number	Referencing citation
Fig. 1.1	5	Fully adapted from Fisher and Paykel
Fig 1.7	13	Fully adapted from West, J.B. (1995)
Fig. 2.8	47	Fully adapted from Wilkins, RL et al (2010)
Fig 2.15	53	Fully adapted from Hodgkinson DW et al (1993)
Fig. 2.27	60	Fully adapted from Hodgkinson DW et al (1993)
Fig. 2.29	62	Fully adapted from Jones PW (2001)
Fig. 2.32	65	Fully adapted from Anthonisen NR et al (1994)
Fig. 2.34	67	Fully adapted from materials available at Pneumacare Limited.
Fig. 3.3	76	Fully adapted from Cairo JM (2012)
Fig. 3.12	99	Fully adapted from Pezzulo AA et al (2012)
Fig 3.18	108	Fully adapted from BTS/ACPRC 2009, Tzeng 2000, and Mangera et al 2012
Fig. 3.25	119	Fully adapted from Martin SA, Pence BD, Woods JA (2009)
Table 3.1	83	Fully adapted from NICE 2012a
Table 3.5	109	Fully adapted from NICE 2006
Table 4.2	134	Fully adapted from New York Heart Association
Table 4.3	139	Fully adapted from Norgren et al 2007
Fig 5.3	147	Fully adapted from DoH (2010)
Fig. 5.6	150	Fully adapted from Fischer Paykell
Fig. 5.8	151	Fully adapted from Fischer Paykell
Fig. 5.9	152	Fully adapted from Haas F & Haas S (2000)
Fig. 5.12	155	Fully adapted from Haas F & Haas S (2000)
Fig. 5.17	168	Fully adapted from O'Callaghan C & Barry PW (1997)
Table 5.1	150	Fully adapted from Dodd et al 1998
Table 5.2	157	Fully adapted from assessment for Ambox (Young 2005, Duck & Barnett 2004)
Fig. 6.7	187	Fully adapted from Davis (1996)
Fig. 6.8	188	Fully adapted from Henleys
Fig. 6.9	189	Fully adapted from Henleys
Fig. 6.14	192	Fully adapted from Intersurgical
Fig. 6.15	194	Fully adapted from Banks et al (2010)

Item Number	Page number	Referencing citation
Box 6.1	178	Fully adapted from Hallenbeck (2008)
Box 6.2	179	Fully adapted from Bastow (2006)
Fig. 7.1	200	Fully adapted from Leboeuf, C (2000)
Fig. 7.4	206	Fully adapted from Taylor J. (2007)
Fig. 7.5	206	Fully adapted from Gooselink R (2004)
Fig. 7.7	212	Fully adapted from Medicaid
Fig. 7.10	216	Fully adapted from Philips Respironics UK
Fig. 8.1	224	Fully adapted from Rubin BK (2002)
Cartoon of humidification	224	Fully adapted from Ries *et al* (2010)
Fig. 8.2	225	Fully adapted from Morrison C (2000)
Fig. 8.3	227	Fully adapted from Intersurgical
Fig. 8.6	231	Marshall R & Holden WS (1963)
Fig. 8.7	232	Fully adapted from Paula Agostini
Fig. 8.8	235	Prasad SA & Hussey J (1995)
Fig. 8.9	235	Fully adapted from Fink JB (2002)
Fig. 8.11	235	Fully adapted from Henleys
Fig. 8.12	236	Fully adapted from Henleys
Fig. 8.14a	237	Fully adapted from VarioRaw
Fig. 8.14b	237	Fully adapted from PowerBreathe
Fig. 8.14c	237	Fully adapted from Henleys
Fig. 8.14d	238	Fully adapted from RC Cornet
Fig. 8.16	241	Fully adapted from Philips Respironics UK
Cartoon of cough control	241	Fully adapted from Milne A (1998)
Fig. 9.6	266	Fully adapted from Ries AL *et al* (1996)
Fig. 9.9	269	Fully adapted from Make (1994)
Fig. 10.2	281	Fully adapted from Long LG *et al* (1980)
Fig. 10.3	283	Fully adapted from SUPPORT (2010)
Fig. 10.4	283	Fully adapted from Fischer Paykell
Fig. 10.5	286	Fully adapted from Krechel SW, Bildner J (1995)
Fig. 10.6	287	Fully adapted from Wilkins RL *et al* (2010)
Fig. 10.11	290	Fully adapted from McIntosh N (1989)
Table 10.1	279	Fully adapted from Horrox (2002)
Table 10.2	285	Fully adapted from BMA 2010
Table 10.3	286	Fully adapted from APLS 2011
Fig. 11.1	301	Fully adapted from Wong–Baker Faces Foundation
Fig. 11.3	305	Fully adapted from Nikander K (1997)
Table 11.2	304	Fully adapted from APLS 2011
Table 11.3	306	Fully adapted from Schechter 2007
Box 11.1	304	Fully adapted from Gillespie 1989
Fig. 12.2	321	Fully adapted from Hamburg NM *et al* (2011)
Table 12.1	313	Fully adapted from McMurray *et al* 2012
Table 12.2	316	Fully adapted from NSF (2000)
Table 12.3	316	Fully adapted from RPE
Table 12.4	319	Adapted from ACPICR 2009)
Table 12.5	322	(Hamburg & Balady 2011)
Box 12.2	314	Adapted from ACPICR 2009 & Keteyian 2010
Box 12.3	317	BACPR 2012
Box 12.4	320	Adapted from ACSM (2010)
Fig. 13.2	330	Fully adapted from Gilbert C (1999)
Fig. 13.3	332	Fully adapted from Howell JBL (1997)

Item Number	Page number	Referencing citation
Fig. 13.5	336	Fully adapted from Rowbottom I and City Hospital, Edinburgh
Box 14.1	350	Adapted from Zimmermann (1998)
Fig. 15.1	356	Fully adapted from Pinnock H (2011)
Fig 15.2.	360	Fully adapted from Jensen G et al (2002)
Fig. 15.3	360	Fully adapted from Booth S (2008) modified
Fig. 16.3	371	Fully adapted from Reeder MK et al (1992)
Fig. 16.5	375	Fully adapted from Embling SA (1985)
Fig. 16.6	375	Fully adapted from Brennan TJ (2012)
Fig. 16.7	376	Fully adapted from Hall PA & Bowden MI (1996)
Fig. 16.11	383	Fully adapted from Bennetti F et al 1996
Fig. 16.15	389	Fully adapted from Adam SK & Osborne S (2005)
Fig. 17.1	411	Fully adapted from Stanchina M et al (2005)
Fig. 17.2	412	Fully adapted from Lindenmuth JE et al (1990)
Fig. 17.8	425	Fully adapted from Maunder RT et al (1984)
Fig. 17.14	429	Fully adapted from Lumb AB (2000)
Fig. 17.15	432	Fully adapted from Cohen C et al (1982)
Fig. 17.19	439	Fully adapted from Collier PS & Dohoo PJ (1980)
Cartoon of physiotherapist	454	Fully adapted from ACPRC Newsletter 11 (1987)
Fig. 18.2	457	Fully adapted from Branson RD (2007)
Fig. 18.4	460	Fully adapted from materials supplied by the University of Cleveland
Fig. 18.5	463	Fully adapted from Patman S et al (2000)
Fig. 18.7	465	Fully adapted from Nicholas Taylor
Fig. 18.8	468	Fully adapted from Branson RD (2009)
Fig. 18.9	469	Fully adapted from MacLean D et al 1989
Table 18.1	456	(Puntillo et al 2010)
Fig. 19.3	495	Fully adapted from Lu CW et al (2012)
Fig. 19.5	496	Fully adapted from Shalit MN & Umansky F (1977)
Box 20.2	531	(Suzanne Roberts, Whittington Hospital, London)

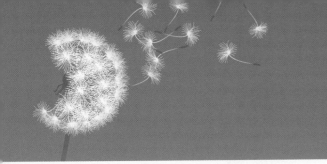

Index

oxygen cost of breathing 68–9
oxygen delivery 23
oxygen dissociation curve 17
    shift of curve 18
    steep portion 17–18
    upper flat portion 17
oxygen levels 68
oxygen therapy 145–6
    acute 152–3
    complications 146–8
    delivery devices 148–52
    head box 152
    heliox 157
    high flow (fixed performance) mask 148
    home oxygen 153–7
    hyberbaric 157
    low flow (variable performance) mask 148
    nasal cannula 149–51
    nasopharyngeal catheter 151
    neonatal 283
    oxygen chair 152
    reservoir systems 148–9
    T-piece 152
    transtracheal catheter 151–2
    tusk mask 149
oxygen transport 23
oxygen uptake 23
oxygenation 20

pacemaker 438–9
pacing 211–12
packed cell volume 77
paediatric intensive care unit (PICU) 300
    continuous positive airway pressure 302
    mechanical ventilation 302
    non-invasive ventilation 302
    pain management 300–1
    respiratory drugs 301–2
    tracheostomy 303
pain 40, 77, 96, 134
    assessment 375–6, 454
    in children 300–1
    in critical care 413
    in dying patients 363
    effects of 375
    in the elderly 348
    faces pain scale 301
    handling patients in pain 376
    management 374–8
    medication 376–8
    post-heart surgery 390
    post-surgery 371
    reduction in perception of 376
palliative care for children 307–8
palliative respiratory physiotherapy 355–6
    anxiety 362–3
    breathlessness 360–1
    communicating with dying people 358–9
    cough 361–2

    dehydration/thirst 362
    depression 362
    difficulty swallowing 362
    discomfort 363
    on dying well 364–5
    fatigue 361
    immobility 363
    insomnia 364
    management of symptoms 359–64
    nausea 363
    outcomes 365
    pain 363
    reactions of patients 356–7
    reactions of relatives 357
    reactions of staff 357–8
    secretions/death rattle 364
    stridor 362
    weakness 361
    where to die 358
pallor 44
palpation
    abdomen 46
    capillary refill time 48
    chest expansion 46–7
    hydration 48
    percussion note 47–8
    tactile vocal fremitus 48
    trachea 48
pancreatic damage 96
panic attacks 78, 339–40
paradoxical breathing 42–3
paralyzed people
    handling 459–60
    turning 460–1
parasuicide 508
parenchyma 40
Parkinson's disease 110
paroxysmal nocturnal dyspnoea 38–9, 134
partial-rebreathing bag 148–9
patient
    charts 34–6
    colour of 43–4
    follow up 475, 477
    history 38
    mobilization of 474–5, 476–7
    name 53
    notes 34
    preliminary checks 53
    state of 455–6
patient-controlled analgesia (PCA) 377
patients' rights
    consent 414–15
    end-of-life decisions 415
    moral rights 415
$PaCO_2$ 16
peak expiratory flow rate (peak flow) 61
peak flow 64
peer review 527
pelvic floor exercises 95